D1605146

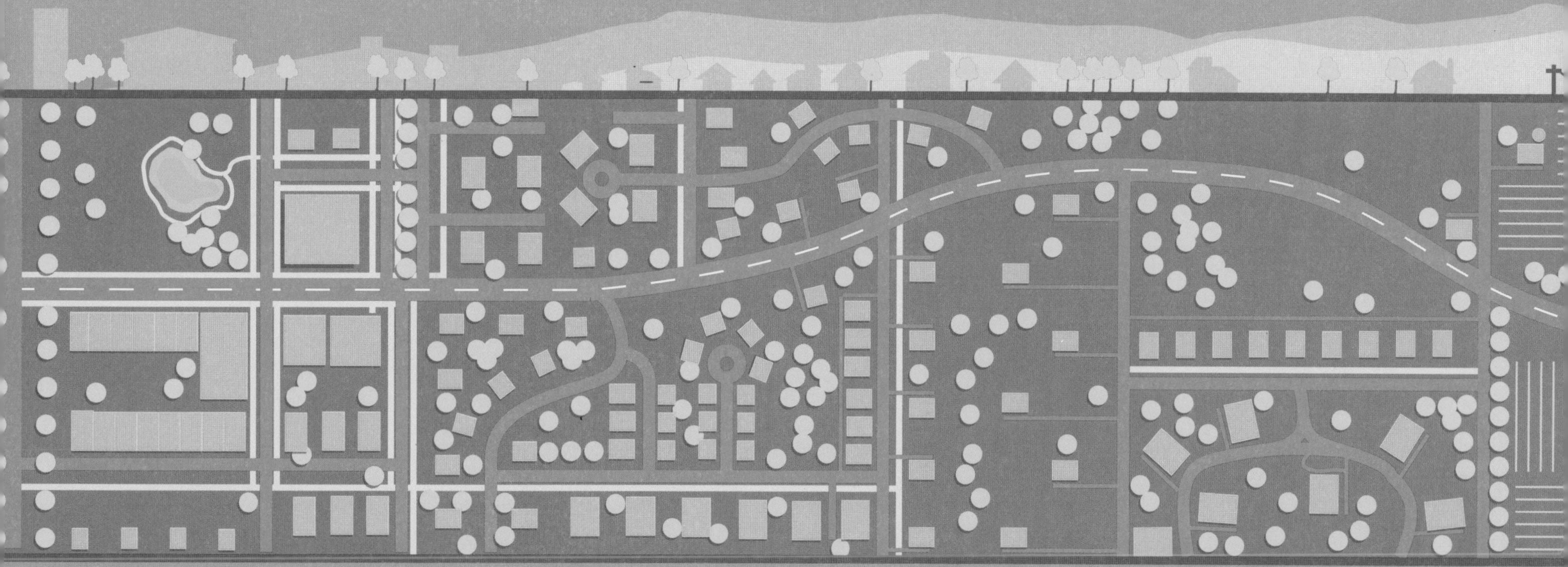

Shaping THE HEALTHY COMMUNITY

THE NASHVILLE PLAN

Shaping THE HEALTHY COMMUNITY

THE NASHVILLE PLAN

GARY GASTON • CHRISTINE KREYLING

with RON YEARWOOD • ERIC HOKE • JOE MAYES

NASHVILLE CIVIC DESIGN CENTER

NASHVILLE • VANDERBILT UNIVERSITY PRESS • 2016

Published by Vanderbilt University Press

First edition 2016
Printed in Canada

This book is printed on acid-free paper.

Design by Deborah Hightower Brewington,
Vanderbilt University Creative Services.

"Big City"

Words and Music by Merle Haggard and Dean Holloway

All references to "Metro" used in conjunction with
government departments refer to the Metropolitan
Government of Nashville & Davidson County.

All photographs unless otherwise noted are by Ron Yearwood,
Nashville Civic Design Center.

All photographs by Gary Layda were taken on behalf of
Metro Government.

Library of Congress Cataloging-in-Publication Data on file

LC control number 2015031362

LC classification number RA394.9G36 2015

Dewey class number 362.109768'55—dc23

ISBN 978-0-8265-2094-4 (cloth)
ISBN 978-0-8265-2095-1 (paperback)

To Betty Brown,
Ernest Campbell, and
Stephen McRedmond

The Nashville Civic Design Center would like to thank our generous partners for their support throughout this project:

Metro Public Health Department
Nashville Area Metropolitan Planning Organization
Tennessee Department of Transportation
Vanderbilt University

The Nashville Civic Design Center gratefully acknowledges those who have supported the process and the printing of *Shaping Healthy Community: The Nashville Plan:*

AARP Tennessee
AIA Middle Tennessee
cureHUNTER, inc.
Earl Swensson Associates
Greenways for Nashville
Gresham, Smith & Partners
Judy and Steve Turner
oneC1TY
Scott C. Chambers Fund
Southeast Venture
The Memorial Foundation
Urban Land Institute

We also wish to acknowledge the following sponsors:

Barge Waggoner Sumner & Cannon
Hastings Architecture Associates
Hawkins Partners, Inc.
H.G. Hill Realty Company
Lose & Associates
Tuck-Hinton Architects

Continuing support for the Nashville Civic Design Center is provided by the Metropolitan Government of Nashville and Davidson County, and the University of Tennessee College of Architecture and Design.

CONTENTS

FOREWORD

FOREWORD

Nashville is moving forward.

There are clear patterns that can be read in our city's success. Some aspects, such as a moderate climate and a central location, have always been part of Nashville's character. Then there are those we have made over time: a diversified economy, affordable living, business-friendly practices, an educated workforce, and a high quality of life. But quality of life—the well-being of individuals and society as a whole–is dependent on "quality of place," where the built environment, which we have the ability to shape, plays a tremendous role.

Covering over 530 square miles, Nashville's natural landscape is a diverse mixture of steep slopes, rolling hills, and plains, carved by a network of streams and rivers. We have worked to preserve large tracts of this landscape as open space for the recreation and contemplation of all Nashvillians. And the economic and cultural vibrancy of the city's built space extends from the urban core to the edges of Davidson County.

But the poor health rankings of our city, region, and state make it imperative that we consider how our built environment affects our citizens' quality of life. Once we understand this relationship, we must act accordingly. As we continue to grow, by a projected million new residents over the next quarter-century, it is critical that we form—and reform—our city to support and encourage active living. Then this generation and generations to come will be able to keep moving.

Establishing a healthier built environment for all Nashvillians—both current and future residents—is the focus of *Shaping the Healthy Community: The Nashville Plan*. Through historical, cultural, and structural analysis, this book explains how various factors in our existing and diverse built environments—downtown, traditional neighborhoods, suburbs, and rural areas—support, and sometimes undermine, active living for each of us. The book then prescribes how we can enhance the positives and mitigate the negatives to define a more health-sustaining "quality of place."

It is my vision that *Shaping the Healthy Community* will serve as guide, tool, and catalyst to conversations and creative actions that build toward a healthier Nashville so that we as a community, together, keep moving forward.

KARL DEAN
Mayor of Nashville
(2007–2015)

PREFACE

I remember a time when my father took his black doctor's bag around to make house calls. The city was smaller, the community was tighter—and maybe life was easier. But change is good and I would argue imperative. The secret is to design change so that it not only improves the economic and cultural growth of a community but also its health and well-being.

An individual's health is not primarily determined by healthcare, meaning the medicine one takes or visits to the doctor. Rather, 85 percent of health is governed by what we call "social determinants" such as education, socioeconomic status, personal habits, environment, and genetics.

We think of "environment" as social interactions with family and friends and daily habits, as well as the physical space in which we live, with its roads and buildings and green spaces—or lack thereof. This physical space is the "built environment," which, if well designed, can help promote health in every aspect of our lives by making healthier choices easier and more intuitive. Designing for health, however, requires the joint effort of individuals and communities, educators and local government, private business and industry.

This effort is sorely needed. Currently Tennessee holds the ignoble distinction of being one of the unhealthiest states in the union: 42nd of 50. And despite being the State's capital, Nashville/Davidson County ranks 13th out of Tennessee's 95 counties, according to the *2014 County Health Rankings* published by the Robert Wood Johnson Foundation. This study looked at various social determinants of health: access to care, obesity, smoking, and education rates as well as the physical environment, including such challenges to health as air pollution, drinking water violations, long commutes, severe housing problems, and driving alone to work. In physical environment Davidson County ranked last among the state's 95 counties.

The Nashville Civic Design Center has produced *Shaping the Healthy Community: The Nashville Plan* as a step in the direction of better health. The plan presented here focuses on how civic design and the built environment can change the face of our community. The book closely examines powerful health factors as they apply directly to our city and identifies specific areas for improvement in order to facilitate a conversation about how changes in our city can promote good health and well-being for all Nashvillians.

We are approaching a crisis point in American healthcare, and the answer will not be more doctors or hospitals or medicines. It will be creating healthier citizenry by changing the way we live at our core—creating a Culture of Health. And that starts at the local level.

Nashville is already a national leader in the healthcare industry, but I want nothing less than for us to be a national leader in *health.* As a physician and a policymaker, my mantra has become "make the healthy choice the easy choice." *Shaping the Healthy Community* is about just that.

SENATOR WILLIAM H. FRIST, MD

ACKNOWLEDGMENTS

ACKNOWLEDGMENTS

The Nashville Civic Design Center's (NCDC) work on the topic of health and the built environment has served as an ongoing and overarching focus of our organization during the past five years. NCDC's leadership on the topic of the built environment, its connection to public health, and its influence on quality of life in our region has been instrumental in shaping Nashville's approach to design interventions that can positively impact the health of our citizens.

NCDC's mission to elevate the quality of Nashville's built environment and promote public participation in the creation of a more beautiful and functional city for all is directly connected to this focus on health. Our practice spans a broad spectrum of collaborations: with government departments, elected officials, planners, designers, developers, neighborhood organizations, business leaders, and individual residents. We host community discussions, design workshops, lectures, design proposals, and case study research to help envision Nashville's future.

Work toward *Shaping the Healthy Community: The Nashville Plan* began in 2010 under the direction of then–design director Gary Gaston, with significant initial funding and support from the Nashville Public Health Department. Specifically, Dr. Bill Paul, director of the Metro Public Health Department, served as a pivotal partner during the duration of the project and contributed the "Scoping Nashville's Health" chapter to this book. Thank you, Dr. Paul, for your time, leadership, and patience.

Additional significant funding for *Shaping the Healthy Community* was provided by the University of Tennessee College of Architecture and Design, Vanderbilt University, the Nashville Area Metropolitan Planning Organization, the Tennessee Department of Transportation, Steve and Judy Turner, and the Memorial Foundation under the leadership of the late and much lamented J. D. Elliot.

The board would like to commend NCDC executive director Gary Gaston and author Christine Kreyling on their ability to coordinate and execute such a substantial and complicated undertaking.

Gary Gaston drafted the original grant for *Shaping the Healthy Community* in 2010 and served as project director and co-author; his work and dedication in seeing this through to completion has been unwavering. Writer and editor Christine Kreyling deserves our special appreciation for her patience, perseverance, and talent, which are unmatched. She has our deepest thanks for participating in this project; its success is uniquely owed to her involvement.

For a project that has transpired over such a lengthy duration, the board thanks the numerous and valuable individuals on the staff of the Nashville Civic Design Center who played a pivotal role in its production. First of all, a very special thanks and recognition to Ron Yearwood for his oversight and direction of the image production and editing for this publication. We also acknowledge Eric Hoke for his talents in creating dozens of the beautiful illustrations contained within these pages, and Joe Mayes for his assistance in research and with the final details to finish the book when it came to crunch time. Project manager Patricia Conway was responsible for getting the methodology and research process underway. NCDC research fellows Jill Robinson and Amy Eskind put in countless hours assembling content and verifying facts. Abby Wheeler exercised efficiency and accuracy in helping tie up many loose ends of the project and assisting with the project's rollout. The board would also like to thank the following interns who played a significant role in helping complete the book: Emma Grager, David Heyburn, Benjamin Jelsma, Nora Kern, Tyler McSwain, Kiera Mitchell, Wesley Rhodes, Kathleen Russell, Megan Scholl,

Sonica Sundri, Virginia Harr Webb, and Whitney Youngblood.

The Nashville Civic Design Center is grateful for the leadership and support of Mayor Karl Dean, who made improving the built environment and healthy living a major focus during his two terms in office. Merging public health onto the path of development and public investment has set this book, the Design Center, and the city of Nashville on a better journey.

As always, NCDC is extremely thankful for two of its longest partnerships: with the University of Tennessee College of Architecture and Design and with Vanderbilt University. From the inception of NCDC, the College of Architecture and Design, currently under the leadership of Dean Scott Poole, has contributed significant intellectual and financial support. Of particular note is NCDC's relationship with professor and former design director TK Davis. Each and every semester TK identifies projects in Nashville that enable his students to explore concepts, plans, and designs to advance urban design practice in the city; in every case his students lay the ground work for positive impact upon Nashville's neighborhoods.

Vanderbilt University Creative Services supplied the beautiful graphic design for this publication in the person of senior graphic designer Deborah Hightower Brewington. Vanderbilt University Press contributed its expertise for the book's publication under the leadership of director Michael Ames and supervision of Joell Smith-Borne.

Special recognition is due to Rick Bernhardt, executive director (retired) of the Metro Planning Department, and the entire staff of the Planning Department for its unwavering support of NCDC in general and this publication in particular; to Michael Skipper, executive director of the Nashville Area Metropolitan Planning Organization for critical financial support and strategic guidance; to Drew Mahan of Metro Archives and Beth Odle of the Nashville Public Library, who located historic photographs featured in this publication; and to NCDC board member and public relations guru Greg Bailey, for his guidance on the marketing initiatives related to the launch of *Shaping the Healthy Community*.

For a complete list of all partner groups, including government, professional consultants, academic institutions, and individuals, please refer to the "Documenting the Process" chapter of this book. The board also recognizes members of its Presidents' Council for supporting this publication: Tara Armistead, Greg Bailey, John Buntin, Scott Chambers, Mark Deutschmann, Hunter Gee, Kim Hawkins, Clay Haynes, Mike Kenner, Jeff Ockerman, Larry Papel, Ron Lustig, Clay Petrey, Craig Philip, David Powell, Jeff Rymer, Seab Tuck, and Manuel Zeitlin.

In closing, the board fully supports the choice of co-authors Gary Gaston and Christine Kreyling to dedicate *Shaping the Healthy Community* to the memory of three very important Nashvillians: Betty Brown, Ernest Campbell, and Stephen McRedmond. The influence and impact these individuals had upon Nashville's built environment, as well as their support of the mission of the Nashville Civic Design Center, was deeply felt. Their presence in Nashville was cherished and is greatly missed.

The Design Center acts every day to shape for the better the experience of living in, working in, and visiting Nashville. We believe you will find inspiration within this book to be a part of shaping the future of our city.

RYAN DOYLE
President, Board of Directors
Nashville Civic Design Center
2013–2015

PLANNING FOR HEALTH

"Cities are made, not born. A metropolis doesn't grow spontaneously like weeds in a lawn. A city is a willed artifact, embodying the evolving intent of the people who live in it as they react to specific conditions: geography and topography, climate and technology, demographics and economics, history and politics. This evolving intent may be read in three dimensions. A society projects its concept of the good life in the largest of its public works—its metropolitan form."[1]

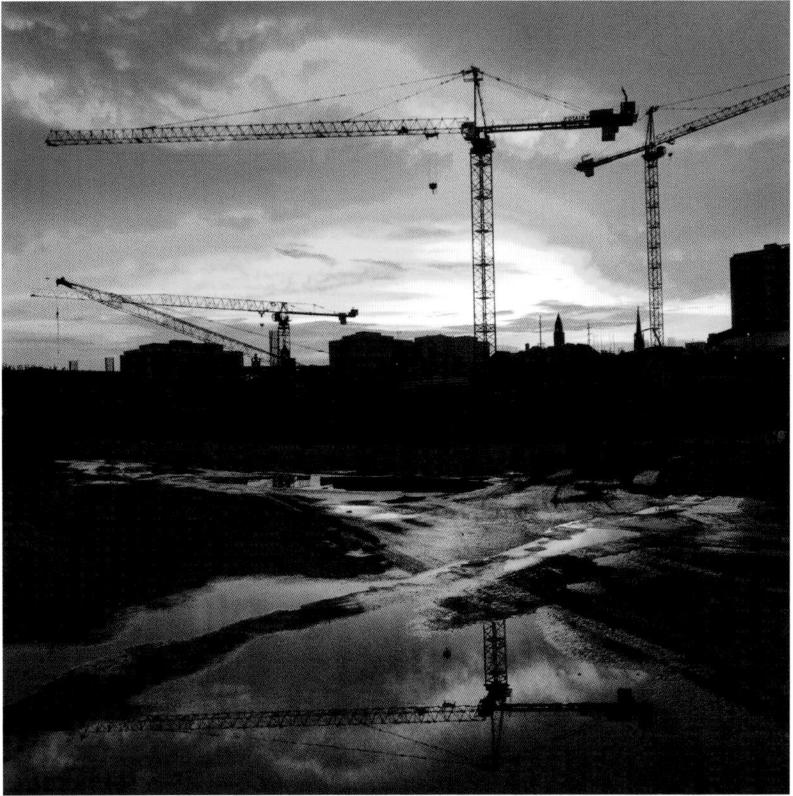

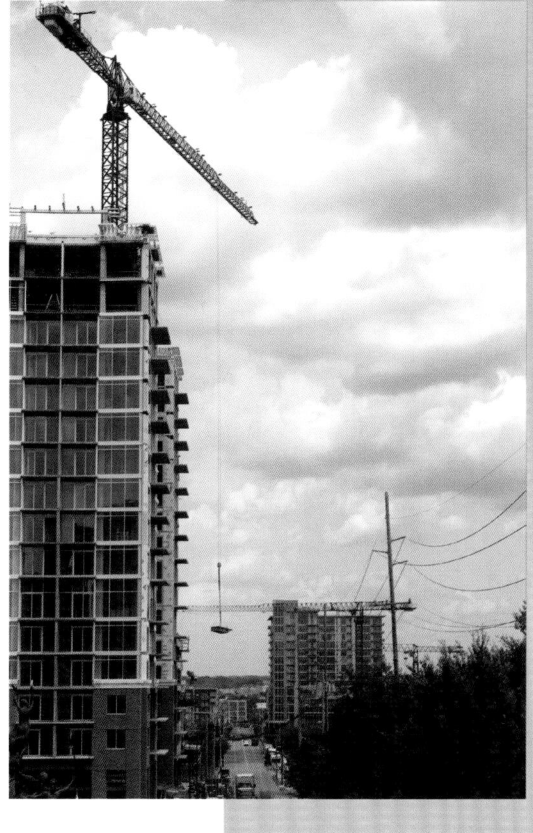

Nashville under construction. *(2010: Gary Layda; 2015)*

These are the opening sentences of *The Plan of Nashville,* produced by the Nashville Civic Design Center and published in 2005 by Vanderbilt University Press. As a general statement these words apply to all cities throughout history—to ancient Rome and Renaissance Florence, to 19th-century New York and 20th-century Los Angeles—and thus hold as true for Nashville today as they did in 2005. But in the intervening years since *The Plan* appeared, one aspect of society's conception of "the good life" has taken center stage: good health, as evinced in both the environmental health of the city as a whole as well as in the personal health of its citizens. This book is the latest record of the "evolving intent" of the citizens of Nashville: to make our city a healthier one.

The emergence of health as a focus for the study of metropolitan regions is a reaction to decidedly unhealthy conditions: the degradation of the environment—the habitat for people, animals, and plants alike—and the alarming rise of obesity and its related diseases in the United States are the most obvious. And perhaps that aging bulge in our population known as the baby-boom generation, increasingly sensitized to physical fragility, has ramped up anxiety about health. In any case, assessing the quality of life from the standpoint of individual and collective health, long the purview of public health officials, has become the new normal for the planning and design professions and for a city's political and private sector leadership.

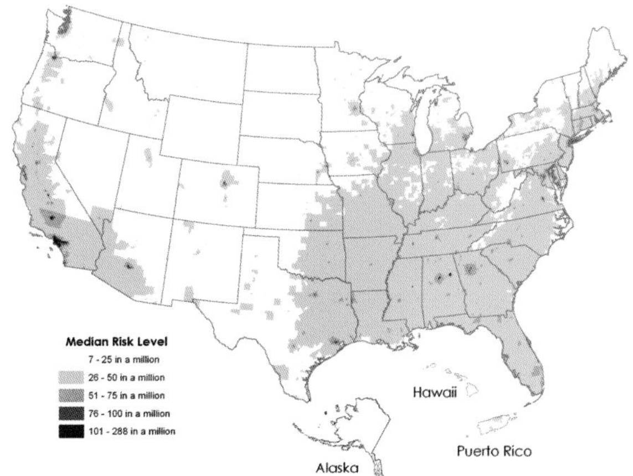

Map showing estimated cancer risk associated with toxic air pollutants. The darker the color, the greater the risk. Note: the Nashville metropolitan region is 51–75 cases in a million people, while the city has a higher risk at 76–100 in a million.[2] *(Map, 2005: US Environmental Protection Agency)*

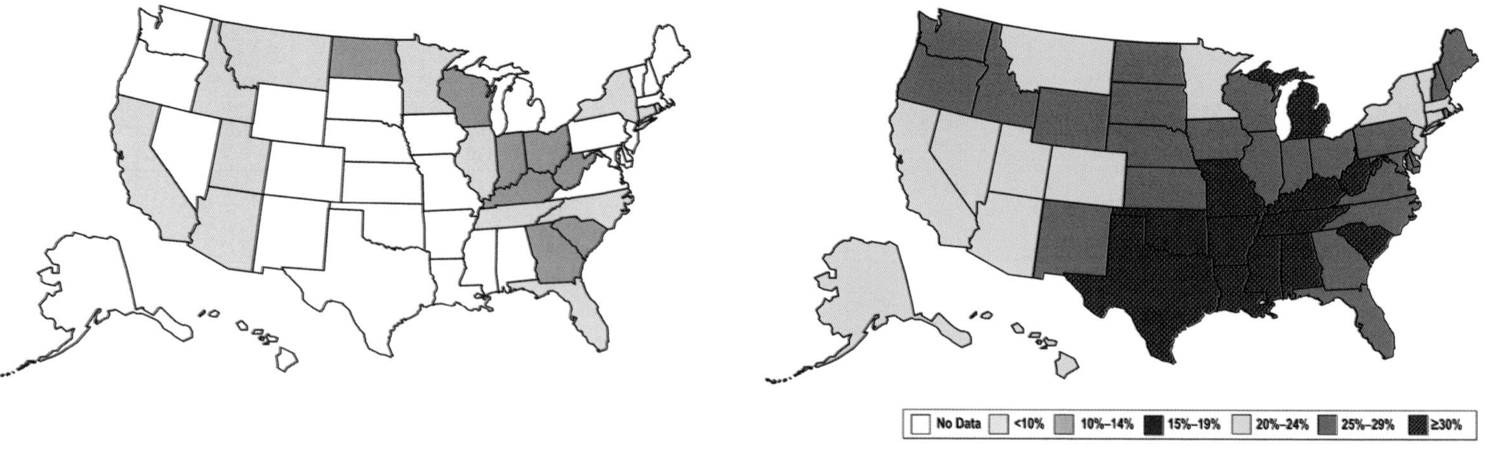

Obesity trends in the United States. Note that in 25 years Tennessee's rate has gone from 10–14 percent to 30 percent, the most dangerous category. *(Maps, 1985 and 2010: Centers for Disease Control and Prevention)*

FROM FRINGE TO MAINSTREAM

Two decades ago most Americans would have characterized as "beyond the fringe" anyone asserting that the car-centric and sprawling form of the American metropolis makes people sick. Public health professionals had already been warning about the tsunami of body fat engulfing our nation. As early as 1952 health researchers identified obesity as "America's No. 1 health problem" at the annual meeting of the American Public Health Association (APHA).[3] And they began to suggest links between our growing rates of obesity and our increasingly sedentary lifestyles.

It was not until the mid-1990s, however, that the relationship between urban form and environmental and individual health became a notable subject of research, according to a survey of scholarly articles published in the United States between 1950 and 2011.[4] For most of the second half of the 20th century, APHA focused on health-as-individual rather than health-as-contextual and on such issues as pasteurization, food safety, drug abuse, teen pregnancy, tobacco usage, and the HIV/AIDS epidemic.[5] During the 1960s the federal War on Poverty prompted attention to the links between low incomes and low health scores, but this research concentrated on housing rather than the more general urban form. It was only with the tremendous spike in obesity across the population and rising concerns about climate change that public health professionals and urban planners began to see the need for teamwork in reinventing preventive medicine.

There are many factors outside the scope of urban planning that impact individual health and morbidity: heredity, education, economic status, health behaviors, race and ethnicity, the American food industry, gun ownership, and so forth. Urban design alone, therefore, will not cure the nation's current health crisis. And a direct causal link between metropolitan form and health cannot be scientifically proven—at least at this point.

Nevertheless, "the way we move, or, more to the point, don't move has coincided with an alarming increase in disease," writes Robert Ivy, CEO of the American Institute of Architects (AIA). "Among our children, our nation's future, one third suffers from obesity. We need a diet, a design diet."[6]

Articles examining the links between automobile-dependent suburban form and physical inactivity first concentrated on diagnosis. In 2001, Richard Jackson and Chris Kochtitzky published *Creating a Healthy Environment: The Impact of the Built Environment on Public Health,*[7] a general guide to the topic. *Measuring the Health Effects of Sprawl: A National Analysis of Physical Activity, Obesity and Chronic Disease,* by Reid Ewing and Barbara McCann, appeared in 2003 and delivered "the first national study to show a clear association between the type of place people live [in] and their activity levels, weight, and health. The study . . . found that people living in counties marked by sprawling development are likely to walk less and weigh more than people who live in less sprawling counties."[8]

More recently the focus has been on treatment. Book-length studies such as *Urban Sprawl and Public Health* (2004),[9] *Understanding the Relationship Between Public Health and the Built Environment* (2006),[10] and *Making Healthy Places* (2011)[11] offer curative actions for the built environment. With the PBS documentary series *Designing Healthy Communities* (2012),[12] the subject of urban form and health entered the arena of popular discourse.

A more site-specific study appeared in 2013, when the American Institute of Architects partnered with the Massachusetts Institute of Technology's (MIT) Center for Advanced Urbanism to produce the *Health + Urbanism Report.*[13] This report explores eight metropolitan regions to establish a foundation for further research as part of a ten-year study "to analyze American cities and better understand links between health

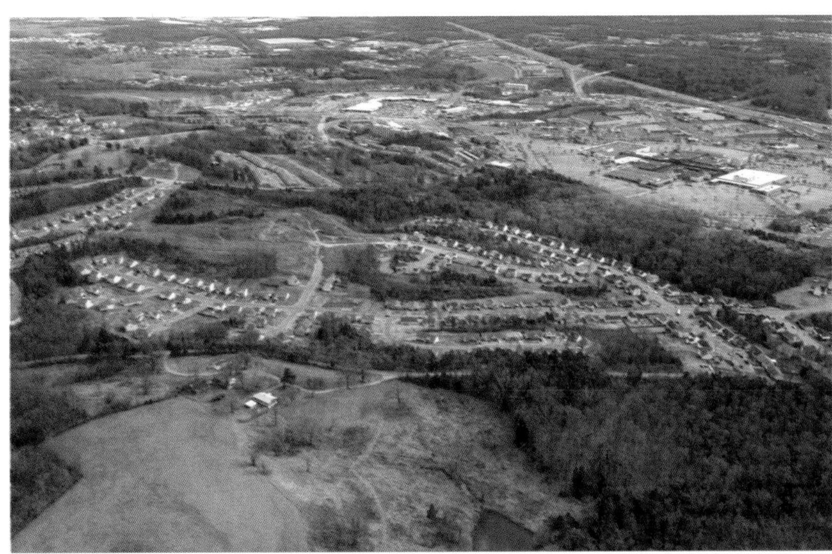

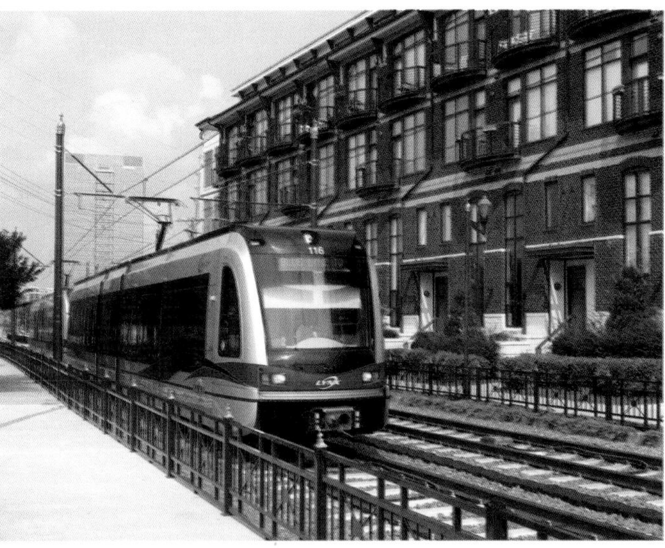

The nation's sprawling development patterns have coincided with the sprawl in American waistlines. *(2013: Gary Layda)*

Riders on the Lynx light rail transit in Charlotte, NC, experienced a drop in weight that researchers attribute to walking to and from transit stops. *(2011: Charlotte Area Transit System)*

factors and city form." The authors "detail key health outcomes and their relationships to various environmental, spatial, and population factors for each city."

The "Project Background" essay in the AIA/MIT report warns that much more research is necessary before the relationship between the physical design of cities and the physical health of people who live in them can be better understood. The authors question current thinking that automobile-dominant city form is the direct cause of many health problems, pointing out: "Despite the tremendous motorization of the American landscape from 1950 onward (three-fold increase per person), we have seen an increase in average US life expectancy of 7.4 years."[14] They also note: "A recent, well-executed longitudinal economics study found no evidence that suburban sprawl causes obesity. Instead, it determined that more obese people simply chose to live in suburbs."[15] Correlation is not necessarily causation.

Nevertheless, the correlations are adding up. For example, a study published in the *American Journal of Preventive Medicine* in 2010 examined the impact on riders of the Lynx light rail transit (LRT) in Charlotte, North Carolina. Researchers found that Lynx users, by walking to and from transit stops rather than climbing into their cars, experienced a 6.45-pound average weight loss and thus became 81 percent less likely than non-users to become obese over time.

"These findings suggest that daily LRT use provided assistance in weight control, independent of pre-existing differences in the built environment," the study states. "Importantly, LRT users and their comparison group were living in the same neighborhoods with similar commuting patterns, perceptions of neighborhood environments, and other potential confounders." Thus, "increasing the access to LRT transit for individuals to commute to work may help overcome some of the barriers to engaging in daily utilitarian exercise."[16]

No one questions that physical activity is an aid to better health. How to induce this activity is the question. For public health professionals attempting to prevent disease, there are two general approaches: trying to change the behavior of individuals one by one, or developing strategies to influence the habits of the population at large through changes in environment. In the case of obesity and its related diseases, intervention with individuals promises less overall success than environmental changes. Only a limited number of people will dedicate a block of time in their daily schedules to formal exercise: going to the gym, swimming laps, taking a walk, or biking in the park. But if walking or biking to a destination that an individual has to access in any case becomes socially acceptable and practical, this can have an impact on the individual and the larger population.

Unfortunately, the disciplines of public health and urban planning are still recovering from the divergent paths they took beginning in the 1950s. Research for the AIA/MIT report reveals "startling gaps of communication and knowledge between long-range planning initiatives, metropolitan area transportation planning efforts, and public/urban health problems."[17]

In addition, every city has its own topography, geography, and physical layout, as well as socioeconomic issues, precluding a one-size-fits-all approach. "When it comes to the design and form of cities," the findings on the eight cities suggest that "there are no silver bullets or universal solutions to urban health problems: each city has unique formal characteristics and fabrics that relate to spatially measurable urban health concerns."[18]

Hence the approach in this book, *Shaping the Healthy Community,* is to consider the formal characteristics and fabrics of Metro Nashville/Davidson County.

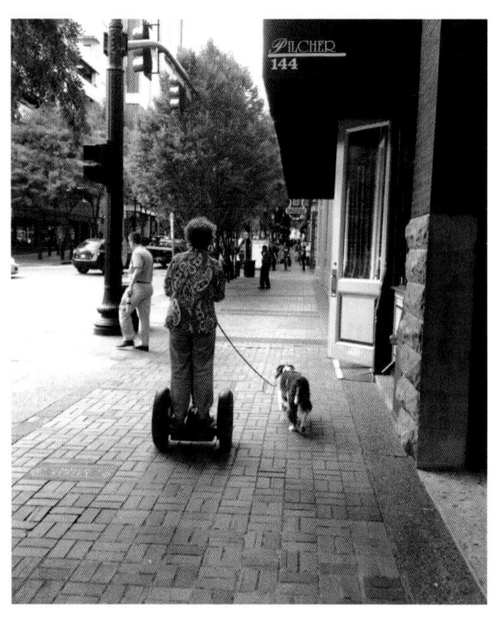

Dog "walking" on Nashville's Second Avenue. Americans' fondness for labor-saving devices has sharply reduced the amount of physical activity in our daily lives. *(2014)*

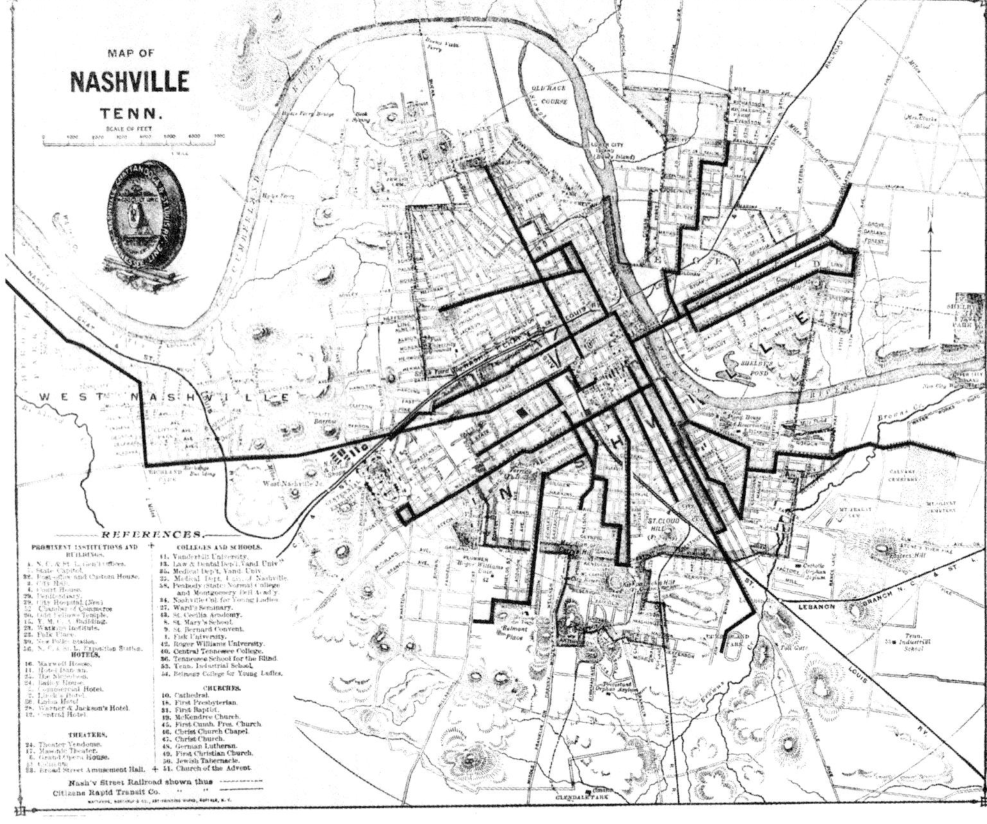

Historic streetcar lines. *(Map, 1897: Don Doyle,* Nashville in the New South, 1880–1920*)*

NOT EXERCISE BUT WORK

Before the invention and popularization of labor-saving devices, people's daily routines included frequent physical activity. And in the days before women entered the work force in significant numbers and the phenomenon of the stay-at-home dad appeared in our culture, the type of activity was largely segregated by gender. Men walked to the trolley or bus on their way to and from their jobs, climbed stairs to get to their offices. They cut their lawns with scythes, then push mowers. There were no snow or leaf blowers, just shovels and rakes.

Women hauled water for clothes washing,

The Couch Potato

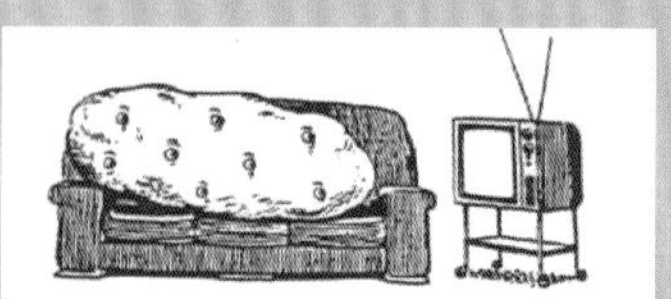

A "couch potato" or "sofa spud"; these terms evolved from "boob tuber." *(Drawing, 1970s: Robert Armstrong)*

The American predilection for inactivity entered the vernacular in the 1970s with the coining of the term "couch potato." The coiner, Tom Iacino, was part of a group of self-proclaimed "boob tubers" satirizing the exercise and healthy diet culture of Southern California. The "tubers" purported to sit on their sofas and watch TV—called the boob tube beginning in the mid-1960s—as a form of meditation. Since then, the couch potato has become the trademark for a variety of merchandise, entered the official lexicon of American English, and engendered protest campaigns by the Potato Anti-Defamation League and the British Potato Council, whose members argue that the expression maligns the image of the vegetable, which is actually low in fat and high in vitamin C.[19]

—CHRISTINE KREYLING

scrubbed garments by hand, then hung them to dry on a line outside. They beat carpets to dislodge dirt and debris, swept floors with brooms. They mashed and pureed foods by hand. Wood or coal was hauled for stoves and fireplaces.

Activities were also separated by race or ethnicity. Recent immigrants were relegated to the laboring class, a pattern that often holds true today. In the segregated South labor frequently fell to African Americans. Black women cleaned white people's houses, washed and ironed whites' clothes, cooked whites' food. Black men did the heavy lifting that whites didn't want to do.

Traditional neighborhood structure also played a role in inducing activity. Children walked to school, churchgoers to Sunday services, moviegoers to the local theater. The grocery, hardware store, and other shops supplying regular needs were within walking distance of homes.

A network of trolley lines coursed through the neighborhoods. People walked to the stop closest to their residences to access the merchandise and services downtown offered. When they disembarked, they walked again, to department stores and specialty shops, doctor and dentist, library and movie palaces.

All this activity was not considered "exercise" but "work." The devices that removed such activity from our lives—automobile, elevator, central heating, power lawn mower, automatic washers and dryers, vacuum cleaners, food processors—were universally welcomed. But the unintended consequences have been devastating to our physical and environmental health.

The internal combustion engines found in our automobiles, trucks, motorcycles, boats, and lawnmowers have severely eroded air quality. The runoff from our parking lots negatively impacts water quality. And when we stopped moving and infused large amounts of processed foods and sugary drinks into our diets, we got fat.

"Big City"

"I'm tired of this dirty old city.
Entirely too much work and never enough play.
And I'm tired of these dirty old sidewalks.
Think I'll walk off my steady job today.

Turn me loose, set me free, somewhere in the middle of Montana.
And gimme all I got comin' to me,
And keep your retirement and your so called social security.
Big City turn me loose and set me free."

—by Merle Haggard and Dean Holloway. Title track on the album *Big City* (Epic Records, 1981; released as a single in 1982). Copyright Sony/ATV Music Publishing LLC.

THE UNHEALTHY CITY

Americans as a society have traditionally had an ambiguous attitude toward cities. Take Thomas Jefferson. His ideal living condition was his big house in solitary splendor on his little mountain. Yet Jefferson was enamored of Paris during the years he spent there as ambassador to France (1785–1789). As he said about the city, "A walk about Paris will provide lessons in history, beauty, and in the point of Life."

But of course that was Europe, which had long ago tamed what was wild and free into managed landscapes. Our continent—what F. Scott Fitzgerald called "the fresh green breast of the New World"[20]—was colonized when the Romantic philosophy, which posits that a human being is at his or her best when closest to nature, shaped Western thought. The untrammeled nature found in such abundance here exemplified the state of freedom that has been a linchpin of our social thought ever since. American culture thus often views our cities as sites of personal constriction and a necessary evil—places to do business, not to call home.

For much of the nation's history, however, a dubious stance toward urban living was justified. That's because there was so much dying.

During the 19th century and into the 20th, life in urban centers was dangerous to one's health. The Industrial Revolution brought an influx of rural residents into urban areas where jobs were plentiful. A majority of the population lived in crowded, filthy, perilous conditions. There were no building codes to ensure safe and healthy dwellings. People were packed in like sardines—as many as 12 families per floor in New York City.[21] Sanitation systems and clean drinking water were largely nonexistent. Smoke from manufacturing plants polluted the air; industrial sites were often located near living quarters. Rubbish, including

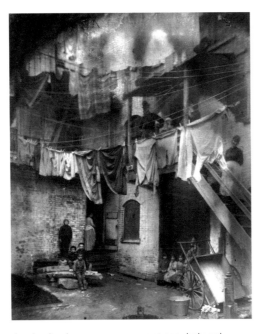

In *How the Other Half Lives,* photographer Jacob Riis documented the appalling living conditions of poor immigrants in the tenements of New York's Lower East Side in the latter decades of the 19th century. These circumstances were not unique to New York, however, but existed for the poor in many cities, including Nashville, before environmental interventions such as sanitation systems, building codes, and garbage collection. *(1890, Charles Scribner's Sons)*

dead animal carcasses, was not regularly collected. Food safety was not regulated.[23] Among the results were repeated epidemics of cholera, typhoid, yellow and scarlet fevers, diphtheria, and smallpox.

Until laboratory research by Louis Pasteur in the 1860s, and in the popular imagination for decades after, the "miasma" or "filth" theory of disease held sway. Miasma was thought to be a poisonous vapor filled with particles from decomposing matter. The bad air was identifiable by its foul smell.

"It is this odour which indicates the commencement of that condition known as crowd-poisoned atmosphere, and which, if allowed to increase, furnishes the specific germs which develop typhus, ship or jail fever," stated Dr. Edward H. Janes of the American Public Health Association in 1874.[24]

Because diseases were thought to be the product of environmental factors that poisoned the air within a locale, steps were taken to improve the environment. And because of the yoking of bad smells to bad health, those steps involved making the air smell less offensive to the human nose.

Doctors advocated for better personal hygiene and public sanitation. People were urged to wash their hands and bathe regularly, as well as keep clean households. Sanitary reformers pushed for city governments to build sewers and reservoirs, and develop a system for the regular collection of garbage and its incineration or burial. All these actions were medically helpful, even if the motivation was scientifically wide of the mark. What is significant for a larger consideration of the relationship between public health and urban planning is that these professions, new to the 19th century, joined together, often by means of public works, to treat the environment of the American metropolis.

The Civil War, paradoxically, occasioned improvements in public health. Frederick Law Olmsted began the linkage of landscape architecture, sanitation, and health during the war when he headed the United States Sanitary Commission, created to provide health-inducing conditions for sick and wounded soldiers.[25] After the founding of the American Public Health Association (1872), Olmsted became chair of its committee on "sanitary values and uses of shade trees, parks and forests."[26] He subscribed to the prevailing view that the density of urban populations, particularly of the poor, was at the root of the diseases afflicting cities. For Olmsted, open space and exposure to nature via parks and parkways, as well as the "buildings in a park" form of the

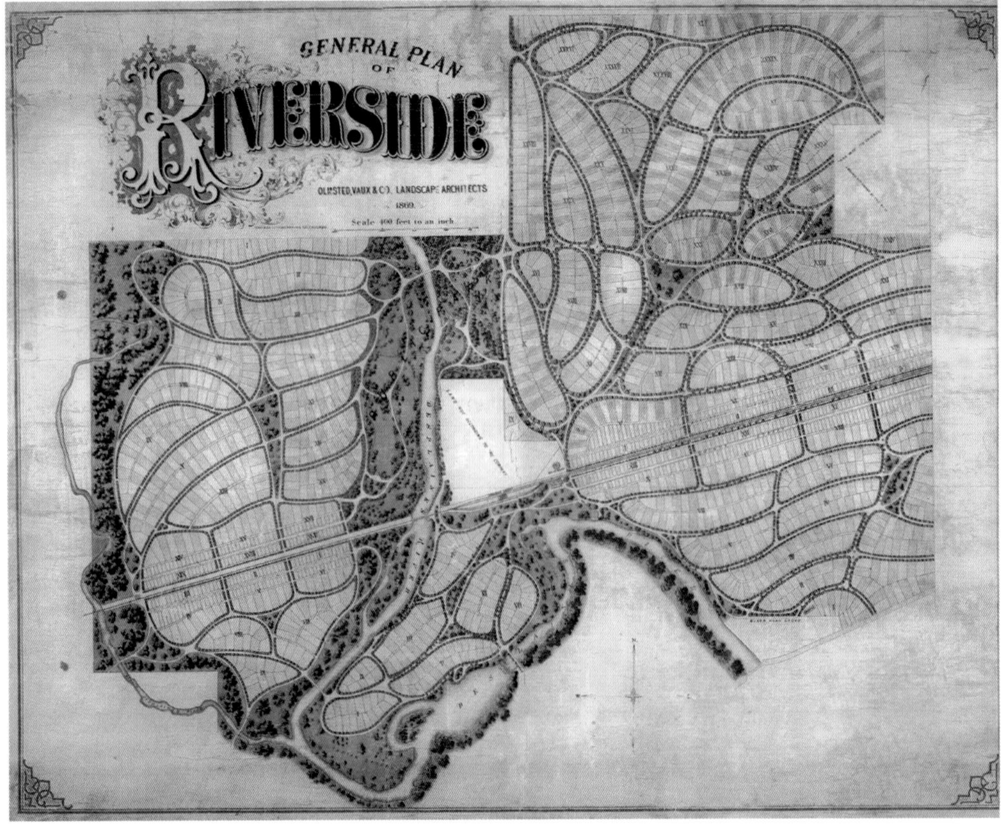

General plan of Riverside, Illinois, by Olmsted, Vaux & Co. Landscape Architects. Note the curvilinear, tree-lined streets interspersed with greenspace, and the more extensive parks along the banks of the Des Plaines River, features that influenced future plans of the upscale suburb.[22] *(Map, 1869: The Frederick Law Olmsted Society of Riverside)*

suburban neighborhood, were preventive medicines for physical as well as mental health.

The association of congestion with ill health was a major factor in leading Olmsted, with partner Calvert Vaux, to design the highly influential suburb of Riverside, Illinois, a 1,600-acre community west of Chicago.[27] Planning began in 1868. The first act of construction was a tree-lined parkway connecting Riverside to Chicago. Olmsted laid out lots with spacious yards along curvilinear streets—there are no right angles in nature—surrounding a village center. By 1900 Riverside had a Romanesque Revival village hall, a golf course, and clubhouse, thus establishing the defining elements of the archetypal suburb.

Density did exacerbate the spread of infectious diseases, but sprawling into the landscape was not the answer. That answer emerged only when medical scientists discovered that microorganisms were the cause—the "germ theory"—that air, water, insects, or bodily fluids were just the carriers, and that these epidemics could be controlled, and in the case of smallpox eradicated, through sanitation and immunization. Bad smells didn't make you sick.

Suburban living remained the American ideal, however, long after cities were able to control infectious diseases and install functioning sanitation systems and pure water supplies, which were largely in place by the 1930s. "In 1939, the American Association of Public Health [*sic*] published *Basic Principles of Healthful Housing* with a focus on pedestrian segregation from cars, the benefits of cul-de-sacs and introverted layouts of development, landscaping, and community design."[28]

By the post-WWII era, public health practice had focused on the biological causes of diseases rather than on environmental ones. City planners were preoccupied with securing federal funds for studies of transportation, housing, and other topics that would become the foundation for the urban renewal and interstate highway programs. The divergence between the two fields would remain until the end of the 20th century and the recognition of obesity as a medical, social, and economic problem.

UNHEALTHY NASHVILLE

Nashville experienced the same filthy conditions and epidemics common to other cities during the 1800s. Early settlers were relatively healthy because they dwelt on high ground, probably to avoid the frequent floods of the Cumberland River and its tributaries. As the population expanded into lower topographies, however, diseases appeared. Inadequate and improper sewage and rubbish disposal was the major culprit, according to medical historian John B. Thompson.[29]

Until almost the end of the 19th century,

"Water, water,
every where,
Nor any drop
to drink."

Samuel Taylor Coleridge, "The Rime of the Ancient Mariner" (1798)

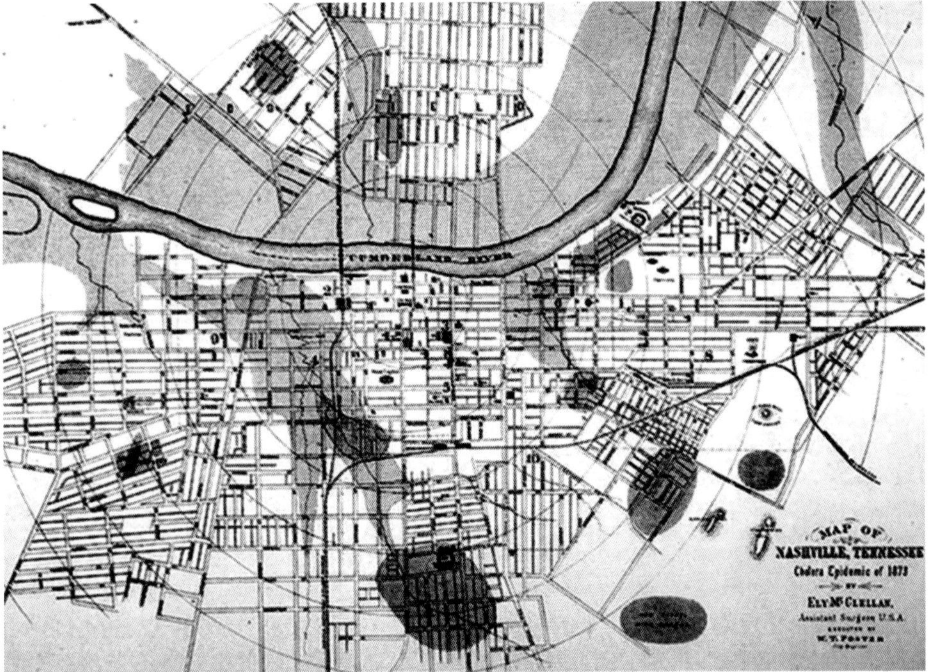

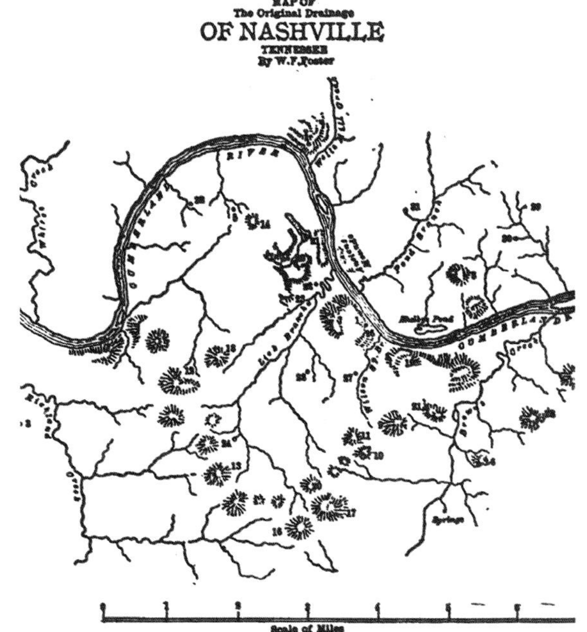

Left: Map of Nashville's cholera epidemic of 1873. The disease was concentrated in low-lying areas where contaminated water often overflowed the banks of streams and the Cumberland River, saturating the water table that wells tapped for drinking water. *(Engraving, 1873: US National Library of Medicine)*

Right: Map of the original drainage of Nashville by W. F. Foster, as published in *Early History of Nashville* by Lizzie P. Elliott. The filigree of waterways, coupled with the limestone shelf lying close to the earth's surface, delivered contamination to areas of low-lying terrain. *(Map, 1911: Board of Education, Nashville; rep. Kessinger Publishing)*

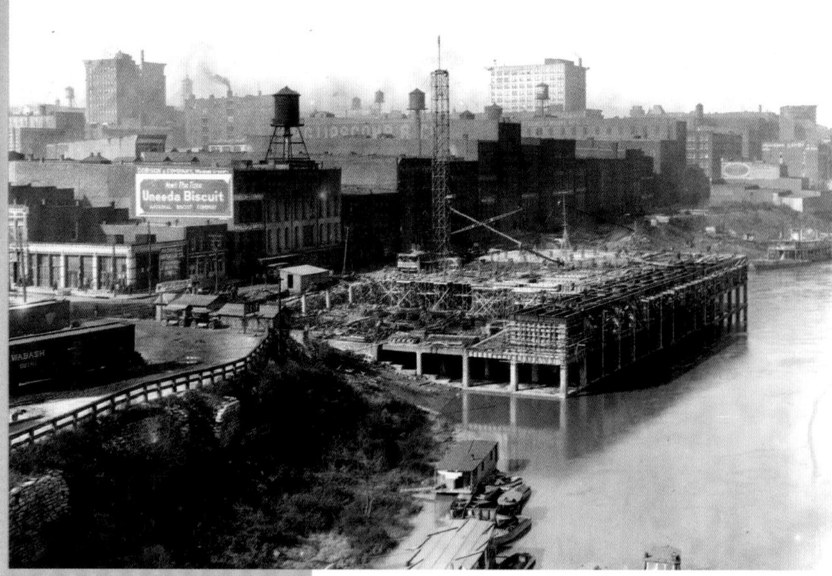

Nashville's air quality during the era of soft coal usage was visibly poor. This photograph of the working riverfront, with the Nashville River & Rail (later Ozburn-Hessey) Terminal under construction on the riverbank, illustrates how the bad air pervaded downtown. *(1922: Metro Nashville Archives)*

Thompson writes, "garbage was left lying in the streets, human excrement flowed along the surface, especially on rainy days, and the water from wells and springs was exceedingly dangerous to drink." Hogs rooted in the muddy streets and alleys, the only regular agents of garbage "collection." "Milk filled with sediment was sold daily from carts in the streets."[30]

The town's first case of smallpox was recorded in 1817, of cholera in 1833. Cholera epidemics occurred in 1849, 1850, 1866, and 1873; in the latter outbreak more than a thousand people died. Although the epidemics were more dramatic, "the continuous toll from typhoid fever and dysentery was much greater until the advent of modern antibiotic therapy," Thompson adds.[31]

The poor in general, and African Americans in particular, were especially victimized by unhealthy living conditions. In 1890 the death rate for whites was 13 per 1,000 people; for blacks it was 25 per 1,000.

While the unsanitary conditions were typical of urban areas in general, their lethal effects were "compounded by Nashville's location on a limestone shelf situated very close to the surface, so that very little water falls on Nashville that does not make its way into the surrounding streams and eventually into the Cumberland River"[32]—both sources of drinking water.

Even after construction of a city reservoir on the river bluffs south of town (now Rolling Mill Hill) and a pumping station on the lower bluff, the contamination persisted because there was no filtration system. The water for the reservoir was pumped from the Cumberland River, but Brown's Creek, a major conduit of the "polluting effluent," emptied into the river *above* the intake.[33] In addition, the reservoir water was primarily used for cooking, cleaning streets, and extinguishing fires, according to historian Don Doyle. The majority of families relied on wells for drinking water, but used outdoor privies, which contaminated the thin soil and the water table in the limestone beneath.[34]

In 1877 Dr. John Berrien Lindsley, the city's public health official, reported that Nashville had the highest death rate in the nation and the fifth highest in the world. Even when water and sewer lines were laid throughout the central city in the 1880s, few families could afford the hookup, much less the plumbing and "water closets." According to Doyle, "By 1898 the city's population of over 80,000 could count no more than 682 toilets, 212 bathtubs, and 52 urinals."[35]

Then there was the air quality—or lack thereof. Soft coal used to heat buildings and power locomotives blackened the air and left a patina of soot on everything from drying laundry to the lining of lungs. Under these circumstances, the flight to the suburbs was a logical move.

The 1873 epidemic stimulated the creation of a permanent board of health that joined forces with city government to construct a new water supply system.[36] A new reservoir on Kirkpatrick Hill—now called the 8th Avenue Reservoir—was finished in 1889; a new sewage system was completed in 1895. In response to the discovery of harmful bacteria, Nashville began chemical treatment of its water supply in 1908.

The ultimate triumph over infectious diseases in Nashville was, as in other cities, the result of collaboration between public health professionals and the city's planning and public works departments. Today it is chronic, rather than infectious, diseases that plague Nashville, many of them associated with the obesity that is a fact of life for an increasing number of Americans—and Nashvillians. And it is apparent that, to help control these diseases, once again the fields of public health and planning must join together.

DESIGN AND HEALTH

"Whether combatting obesity through the development of more pedestrian-friendly cities and neighborhoods that encourage active, healthy lifestyles, or preventing the onset of noncommunicable diseases such as asthma by ensuring access to cleaner air and outdoor environments, the relationship between the physical design of cities and the health of the people who live, work, and play there must be better understood," writes Robert Ivy of the American Institute of Architects. "Good design cannot be an afterthought. We need to ensure that holistic thinking about the relationships of our buildings, infrastructures, streetscapes, and public landscapes is investigated and understood at the very beginning of the development process. Future generations will hold us accountable for what we have done to ensure their health. We owe it to them and to ourselves to work for their gratitude."[37]

Shaping the Healthy Community represents a coming together of public health and planning disciplines to investigate the relationships of Nashville's buildings, infrastructures, streetscapes, and

Nashville, Water, and a Healthy City

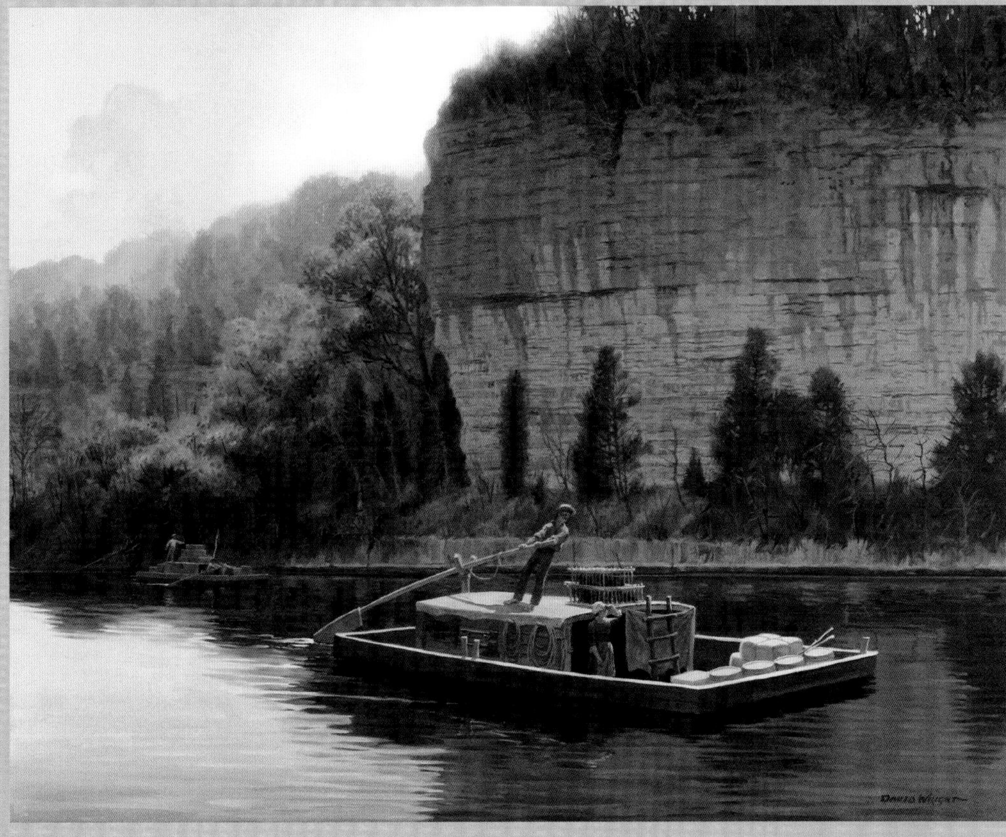

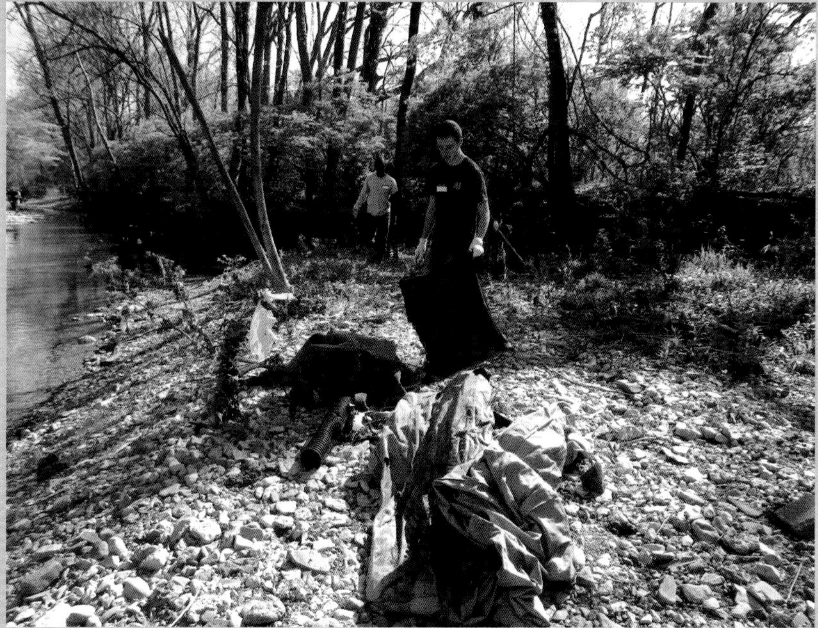

Nashville's river life during the 19th century is depicted in "Drifting Downriver: Flatboats on the Cumberland." *(Painting, 2013: Courtesy of David Wright, davidwrightart.com)*

A less idyllic scene: volunteer garbage pickup on the banks of Mill Creek. *(2015: Paul Davis, Cumberland River Compact)*

There are many determinants for shaping a healthy city, but none is more vital than the stewardship of its waters. While our future well-being certainly depends on the quality of all our natural resources, the health of our water is critical.

Prior to the arrival of mostly European settlers, the Cumberland River and its tributaries supported herds of buffalo, elk, bear, and deer. The region's early inhabitants shared these abundant hunting grounds long before Nashville's founders arrived by land in the winter of 1779 and by river in the spring of 1780.

From the beginning, the waters of the Cumberland have served as our lifeline, moving our commodities to market, watering our crops, nourishing our families, and allowing us to teach our children the joys of fishing, swimming, and exploration. The same rivers and streams have supported abundant and diverse communities of fish, mussels, crayfish, and other aquatic life.

Through the first half of the 20th century, as in other cities across America, Nashville took for granted the services of its waterways, routing untreated industrial and sanitary waste directly to rivers and streams. As the population grew, the city's waters could not assimilate the volume of waste and maintain healthy conditions. The wastewater system was unsustainable.

In 1958 the Central Wastewater Treatment Plant just north of downtown began operation. Additional treatment plants opened in 1961 and 1975.[38] But in so-called "combined sewer" systems such as Nashville's, which collect sewage and stormwater runoff in a single-pipe network, heavy rainfall can cause overflows. The excess stormwater and sewage is then released untreated into an adjacent body of water. The result is serious water pollution.

Beginning in 1990 Metro Water Services undertook an aggressive program to reduce the volume, frequency, and duration of sewer and collection system overflows to the Cumberland River. By 2002, 33 miles of the Cumberland had been restored to meet federal and state water quality standards. Between 1990 and 2007, combined sewer overflows were reduced in frequency by 59 percent, in volume by 72 percent, and in duration by 83 percent. An additional 90 miles of Nashville's streams have also been removed from the list of impaired waters through a concentrated effort to identify and eliminate their sources of pollution.

These improvements were a great beginning, but much more remains to be done in order to restore and

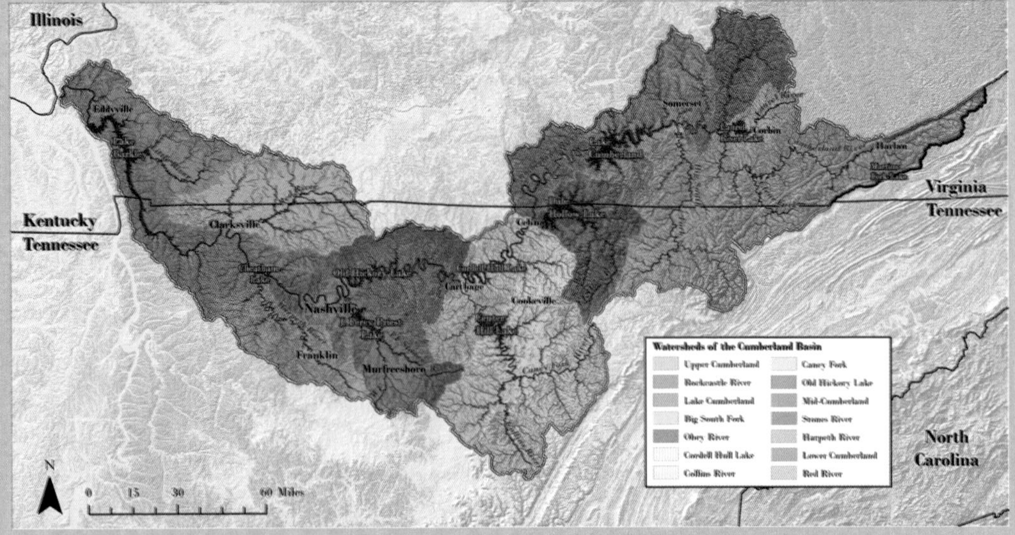

Watersheds of the Cumberland River Basin. *(Map, 2014: Cumberland River Compact)*

protect Nashville's rivers and streams. Within Metro Nashville are all or a portion of twelve sub-watersheds to the Cumberland River. Among these are Whites Creek, Browns Creek, Marrowbone Creek, Sycamore Creek, Mansker Creek, Stones River, and Mill Creek. More than 300 miles of these rivers and streams currently do not meet Tennessee's criteria for their designated uses: drinking water, recreation, habitat for aquatic life, agriculture, industry, or navigation. In summary, they fall short of our expectations for healthy waters.

Today Metro Water Services—together with local engineering and design professionals and volunteers—are making a determined effort to replace the city's obsolete water infrastructure and to manage rainfall in innovative ways that can help restore poor quality streams and preserve the healthy ones. Among the examples of their collective work:

- The Clean Water Nashville Overflow Abatement Program represents an estimated $1 billion to $1.5 billion community investment in rehabilitation of the city's aging infrastructure and in improving water quality in the Cumberland River and its tributaries throughout Davidson County.
- Metro Nashville's "Low Impact Development Manual" offers developers a design path that attempts to mimic the land's natural hydrology. This is accomplished through the conservation of natural features combined with stormwater management strategies designed to infiltrate, store, and reuse, or return to the atmosphere the rain water that falls on a site. The city offers incentives to projects that use the manual.
- Nashville's *Green Infrastructure Master Plan* provides guidance for managing stormwater to prevent it from overwhelming the sewer system. Examples include green roofs, urban trees, rain gardens, and permeable paving. This approach reduces the need for more capital-intensive alternatives while enhancing neighborhood amenities.
- The Riverfront Park restoration is transforming the city's relationship with the Cumberland River by creating new recreational and cultural opportunities along downtown's east and west riverbanks. Phase three will expand riverfront amenities and provide easy downtown access for canoes, kayaks, and paddle boards.
- The "Unified Flood Preparedness Plan" was completed by Metro Water Services in January 2013 in response to the catastrophic floods of May 2010. The plan aligns flood protection, control, and mitigation strategies to 22 "damage centers" throughout the county.

These examples suggest the magnitude and complexity of water issues that must be successfully addressed in the years ahead. Priorities include providing safe drinking water, appropriately managing waste water and stormwater runoff, minimizing flood risks, providing safe and abundant opportunities for recreation and education in our rivers and streams, and restoring and protecting in-stream habitats for fish and other aquatic life. Each of these is a substantial task; collectively they will require unparalleled vision, public support, political will, and capital commitment.

In order to meet our future challenges, the following eight actions are recommended:

- Implement restoration plans that recognize and reduce the pressure that a growing economy places on stream ecosystems.
- Protect and preserve those rivers and streams that are currently healthy.
- Further expand the use of green infrastructure, naturally capturing water so we do not have to collect and treat it.
- Increase citizen engagement and stewardship for our water through education, conservation, clean-up activities, and citizen-driven restoration projects across our county.
- Remain vigilant to prevent compromising Nashville's excellent water resource managers and the policies they work to implement.
- Continue to increase access to, and opportunities for, recreational enjoyment of our rivers and streams.

Great cities have great rivers. The Cumberland River flows through our city for more than 50 miles. It is the river that brought us, that has sustained us for more than 230 years, and that will help define our future.

—PAUL SLOAN, board chair, Cumberland River Compact, and former deputy commissioner, Tennessee Department of Environment and Conservation

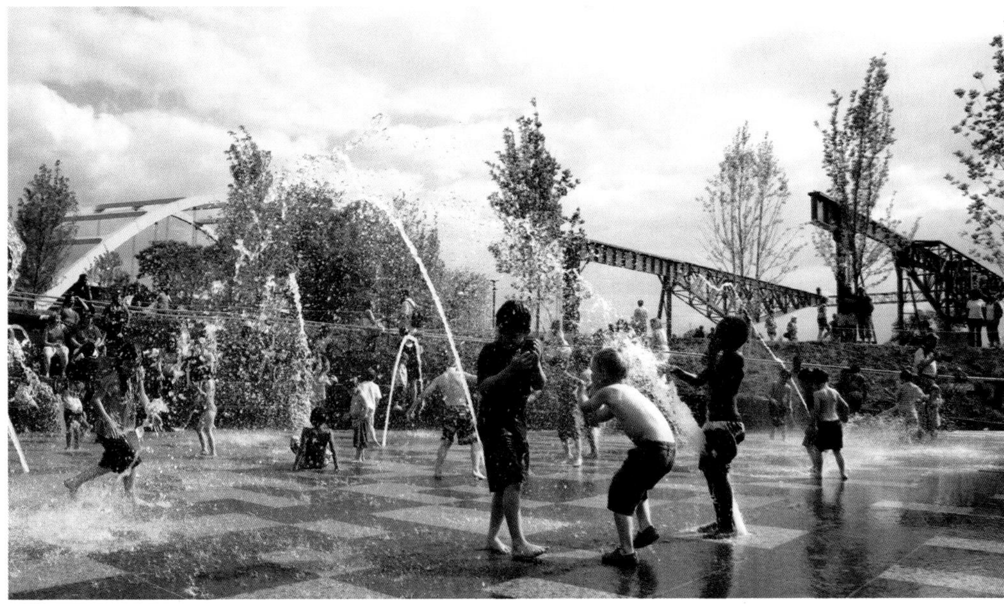

Cumberland Park on the East Bank; this play park was designed to be an activity center for children as part of the redevelopment of Nashville's downtown riverfront. *(2013: Hawkins Partners, Inc.)*

public landscapes in order to apply "holistic thinking" to the public and private development processes. This book sets forth specific strategies for overcoming some of the barriers to health currently structured into Nashville's built environment. Given that there are particular nuances to each development site and situation, however, *Shaping* is also a general call to assess the health impacts of proposed projects as an essential and routine part of each design process, using the assessment of traffic impacts as model and precedent. This book provides a framework for integrating health impact assessments (HIA) into the shaping and reshaping of our city.

The terrain most in need of reshaping is that of the post-World War II suburb. More Nashvillians—over 400,000—live in areas characterized by suburban patterns of development than in any other development pattern, such as urban or the downtown core. Suburban development also consumes more land—38 percent—than other development patterns within Davidson County. The reformation of suburbia into a more health-promoting environment can have the most significant impact on our land mass and our population as a whole. But these areas cannot be demolished and rebuilt wholesale.

BEWARE UNINTENDED CONSEQUENCES

Among the many lessons to be learned from the great suburbanization era is that the comprehensive application of a planning formula can and will produce unintended consequences. The general formula for the period from 1950 to 2000 was low density, segregated land uses and a transportation infrastructure dedicated to the personal vehicle and characterized by an overdependence on wide arterials and limited access highways. Among the associated unintended consequences: vehicular congestion, vast amounts of carbon emissions, and a sharp decrease in the average American's level of daily physical activity.

In reaction, density, mixed-use, and multimodal transportation options have become the triple-mantra of planners today. Many developers have embraced this approach, in part because density enables them to get maximum utility—and profit—from their land purchases.

There is no question that denser development can reduce sprawl and conserve open space. It is also true that a mixture of land uses, with daily needs located within walking distance of residences, can induce more physical activity than will drive-and-park development. And access to a variety of transportation modes can reduce fossil fuel consumption and curb carbon emissions, as well as enable people to walk to transit, bike to work, and so forth. Yet this formula, if applied without attention to context, will undoubtedly produce unintended consequences as well. It is incumbent upon us to try to anticipate those consequences as we plan how we are to live in the 21st century.

Let's begin by considering the qualities of suburban living that were so attractive to the people who moved outward in the second half of the 20th century. Yes, one of the motives was racial and socioeconomic homogeneity. But there were more positive yearnings at work.

For people used to living so close to their neighbors that conversations were inadvertently shared, a suburban home on a larger lot promised privacy. Rather than an ambiance of street noise, the suburbs offered quiet. The surrounding greenspace provided trees and a big yard in which kids could play and Fido could romp, without encountering dangerous traffic. There was also room for the patio and grill, perennial border, vegetable garden, and maybe even a swimming pool. This was the middle-class American lifestyle that evolved from an object of desire into a cultural expectation.

Today desires have shifted, in part because of the unintended consequences that accompanied the ranch house on the big lot. But it is only fair to acknowledge that urban living—touted as the obvious choice for millennials, seniors, and every hipster between these age brackets—will

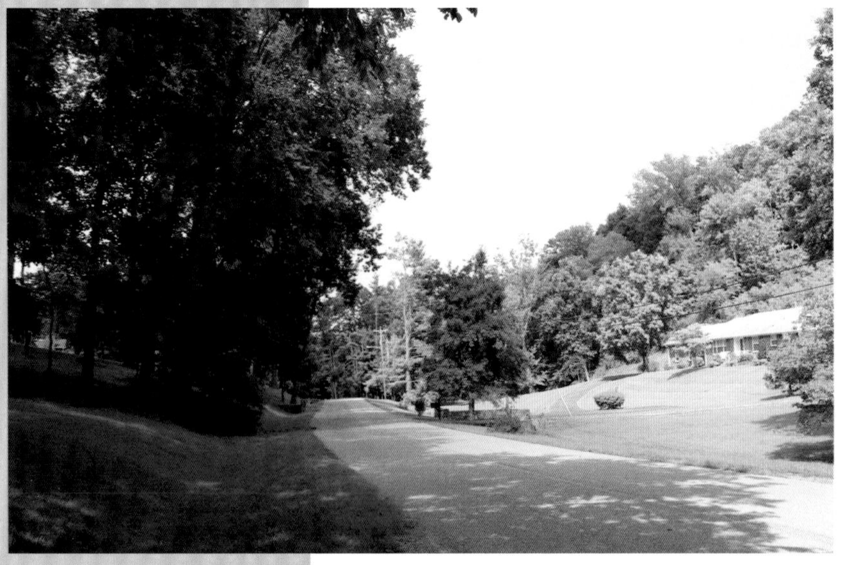

The suburban idyll, here pictured on Jocelyn Hollow Road in West Meade, became a cultural expectation in America after World War II. *(2015)*

be less private than suburban living. In addition, a mixture of land uses is frequently noisier, especially for those who live near drinking, dining, and entertainment venues. And public, or at least private-but-shared, greenspace must be provided as a replacement for the lawns and patios. Urban design can mitigate the negative effects of increased density and mixed land uses, but only if planners and designers recognize that some effects are in fact negative and plan and design accordingly.

It is also important to recognize that a change to the built environment "meant to address one health concern may simultaneously worsen another health concern. For example, creating more pedestrian access by building sidewalks and crosswalks in a neighborhood may increase levels of physical activity in an attempt to address health issues of obesity and diabetes. However, if these sidewalks are located close to high levels of automobile traffic or highways, the exposure to air pollution and the risk of asthma and other respiratory diseases actually increases."[39]

The same is true for housing. Los Angeles planners have prioritized infill in the form of transit-oriented development (TOD) along its light rail lines, which were constructed to improve air quality by offering an alternative to the personal vehicle. These transit lines, however, lie in the same corridors as freeways and major arterials, which are highly congested and therefore have highly polluted air. The city is now struggling to mitigate the air quality impacts on the residents of the infill housing.[40] This is an example to keep in mind as we consider dense residential infill on our arterials.

"On more general environmental terms," warn urban designers Jocelyn Drummond and Alan Berger, "there is a huge contradiction in advocating for only higher density living conditions across the country, while promoting better urban health. A deep body of scientific research shows that increases in density inevitably lead to major declines in biodiversity. Stream quality is damaged roughly in step with increasing density/impervious cover. Up to a threshold, more density simply means more environmental damage for water quality/biodiversity.[41] If environmental concerns are to be taken as part of the solution to the urban health conundrum, then advocating for higher density must be carefully situated and measured."[42]

Shaping the Healthy Community is situated in Metro Nashville/Davidson County. Within this boundary, this book analyzes the various development patterns present here and now. Case studies of specific Nashville neighborhoods further demonstrate the importance of context in devising tactics for the reformation of our built environment.

Nashville is the place we have made for ourselves. The strategies taken to make it a healthier place we must make for ourselves as well.

It's all in the details. Both of these multifamily developments on East Nashville's Woodland Street are within walking distance of public transit and the shops, restaurants, and bars of Five Points, as well as having easy access to the green spaces of Shelby Park and Bottoms. But their designers responded to the challenges of similar urban sites with different degrees of success.

The East End Lofts are set above the sidewalk, protecting the privacy and access to daylight of first-floor residents. At 715 Woodland, the first floor units are at street grade; residents therefore must keep windows covered, blocking natural light, or risk subjecting themselves to the curious gaze of passersby. *(2015)*

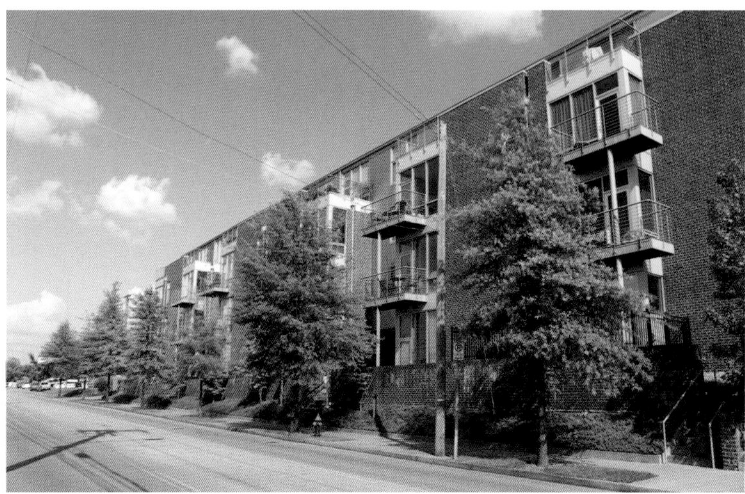

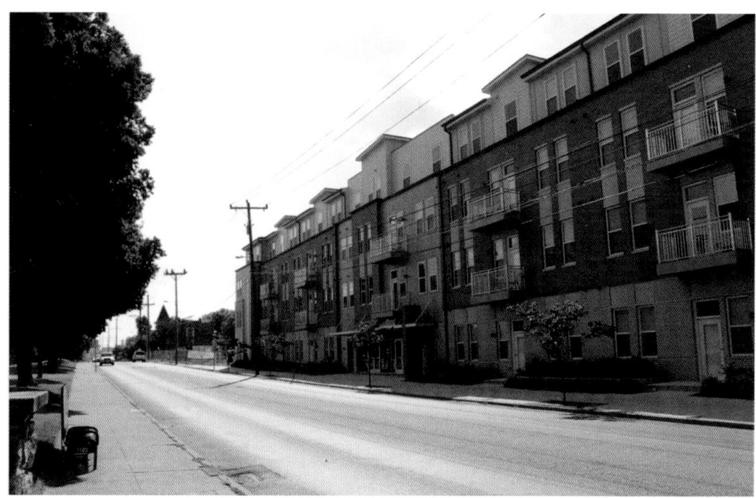

Girding the Grid

On May 1, 2010, exactly one month after Mayor Karl Dean created the Office of Environment and Sustainability, rain began falling in Nashville. By the time the rain stopped, Nashville was in the throes of the worst flood in its history—a "thousand-year flood" as many called it, attempting to give some perspective to its rare magnitude. Ten people died in Davidson County alone, and 31 percent of the State of Tennessee was declared a federal disaster area.

The stated mission of Metro's Office of Environment and Sustainability is to lead projects and initiatives in three areas: reducing greenhouse gas emissions and energy use, improving alternative transportation alongside "smart growth planning strategies," and conserving open space and natural resources "for the health and environmental benefit of Nashville residents and visitors." These goals project a progressive vision for a 21st-century American city looking to grow responsibly and have the potential to ease the negative impacts of climate change by reducing water and electricity usage, and by more effectively managing large volumes of stormwater.

Flood mitigation is the driving force behind the West Riverfront Park in downtown. The $100 million project proposes a 2,100-foot-long flood wall as well as a stormwater pumping station. Metro has already spent $127 million to purchase and demolish 267 flood-prone homes and reinforce the Metro Center levee.

Experts agree, for the most part, that no single weather event can be linked directly to the rising global temperatures associated with climate change, and the Nashville flood of 2010 is no exception. As Eric Pooley, now senior vice president for strategy and communications at the Environmental Defense Fund, told the *Nashville Scene* two months after the deluge, however: "In a warmer world, that kind of thing will happen more often. So if you liked the Nashville flood, you're going to love living in a warmer world."[43]

Love it or not, a warmer world is all but certain: 10 of the hottest years on record in the United States have fallen within the last 15 years. With policy action at the federal level stalled indefinitely and no serious state-level climate change efforts in place for Tennessee, the only choice for cities like Nashville is to deal with adaptation—coping as much as possible by building and retrofitting an urban environment that is less carbon-intensive and better able to withstand climate change effects.

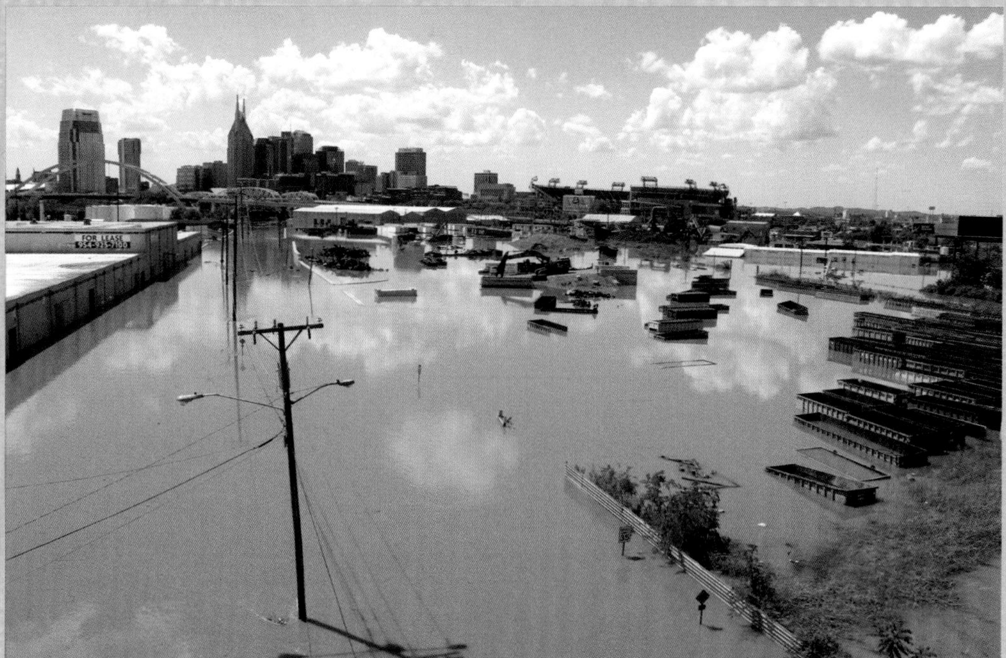

Development in floodplains + too many impervious surfaces + too much rain + too much stormwater runoff = Nashville's May 2010 flood. The city got a wake-up call on the potential impacts of climate change. *(2010: Kaldari, Wikimedia Commons)*

Nashville does not have a climate change action plan, per se, on file with the EPA. (Chattanooga is the only Tennessee city that does.) Nevertheless, Nashville has developed the *Green Infrastructure Master Plan,* which addresses sustainability issues in some key areas. They include "green infrastructure," rainwater harvesting, green roofs, urban trees, stormwater control, and low-impact development—plus a range of ideas for funding and incentivizing such measures. "The goal of [Green Infrastructure]," according to the city's Master Plan, "is to design a built environment that remains a functioning part of an ecosystem rather than existing apart from it." Insofar as this is possible, the plan at least provides for a conscientious approach to development.

In October 2010 Mayor Dean formalized the Complete Streets program by way of executive order to ensure that, going forward, public roads are designed to accommodate more than just cars. The first new street constructed under the directive is the 28th to 31st Avenue Connector, which includes dedicated space for pedestrians, cyclists, and a new mass-transit route, as well as LED lighting, a rain garden in the median (designed to both collect water for irrigation and also divert stormwater away from the road), and bioswales (gardens that work as drainage filters). The city has actively encouraged bike usage through its public programs, including the free Green Cycle program and the rental-via-kiosk B-cycle system.

Another measure intended to reduce the climate impact of the city is Nashville: *Naturally,* the open space plan adopted in April 2011, which calls for "the acquisition and preservation of 22,000 acres of undeveloped land in Nashville over the next 25 years" and the

The green roof of the Music City Center is currently the largest in the southeast at 175,000 square feet, just over four acres. *(Jamie Meredith – TMG Studio, 2015)*

"transition [of] 110 acres (20 percent) of the suitable impervious surfaces in downtown to pervious surfaces or natural plantings in the next 10 years." So far, land acquired under the plan includes Stones River Farm (600 acres), Ravenwood Country Club (180 acres), Cornelia Fort Airpark (130 acres), and Southeast Park (600 acres).

The largest and most visible evidence of the city's low-impact development ambitions is the massive new Music City Center (MCC), erected with environmental sustainability in mind. A Metro ordinance stipulates that renovation or construction of public buildings larger than 5,000 square feet or more costly than $2 million must be designed to LEED silver certification standards. To that end, the structure includes a few notably eco-conscious features, among them a 360,000-gallon collection tank designed to store rainwater that will in turn be used for irrigation and to flush the building's hundreds of toilets. The top of the center includes a 175,000-square-foot green roof "designed to mimic the rolling hills of Tennessee," as the center's official website declares, along with a 200-kilowatt solar array to help power HVAC and some escalators. The newly extended Korean Veterans Boulevard, which borders the MCC to the south, is another "complete street" project.

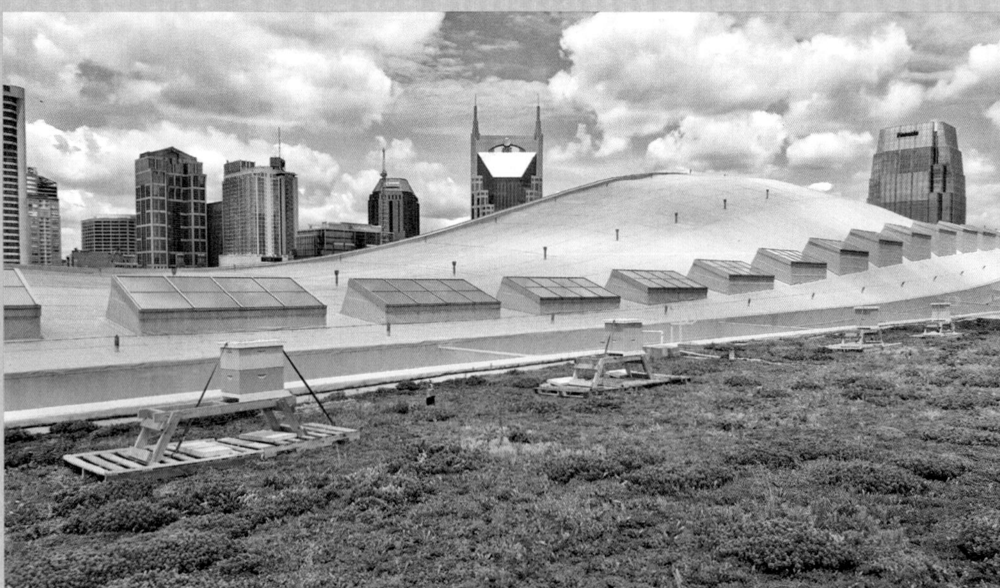

Beyond the convention center's shadow, the city offers a green roof credit for private properties equal to $10 multiplied by the square footage of green roof installed. (The rebate is applied to the monthly sewer charge.) Green roofs can help reduce the heat island effect in cities—caused by the predominance of asphalt and other hard surfaces—and one can see how an array of such roofs, distributed throughout the urban core, might be helpful to some degree. Nashville Energy Works, a partnership between Metro, TVA. and Nashville Electric Service, provides up to $700 in rebates to homeowners who undergo an energy evaluation and are able to achieve at least 15 percent in projected energy savings.

Other large Nashville-area enterprises have also taken steps to reduce their carbon footprint. In early 2013, the Bonnaroo Music and Arts Festival announced the installation of 196 solar panels on its Manchester, Tennessee, property, capable of generating 61,000 kilowatts per year, or about 20 percent of the event's power needs. Vanderbilt University's Board of Trust voted in April 2013 to convert the school's coal-fired power plant to natural gas—a $29 million project that was completed in 2015. In a press release, Vanderbilt vice chancellor Jerry Fife said the conversion, which he described as "consistent with the university's increasing commitment to sustainability efforts across campus," would have another tangible benefit: it would "eliminate the daily traffic of large trucks transporting coal to the plant."

Some adaptive measures will require vision at the state level. For instance, permeable pavement can help reduce ponding during a downpour, but Tennessee Department of Transportation (TDOT) regulations currently do not allow these surfaces on major roads. (A few test patches have been installed throughout the state, and Deaderick Street in downtown Nashville was retrofitted with permeable pavement for its renovation.) Stress on the power grid due to increased energy demands will be a concern. The Tennessee Valley Authority, which is responsible for generating the power that Nashville Electric Service distributes throughout the city, issued a Climate Change Adaptation Plan in 2012 that strikes all the right notes. In short, this is an important concern and raises many separate issues we must work to address, but it offers few specific action recommendations.

Lack of a cohesive statewide adaptation strategy may become problematic soon, especially concerning water resources in fast-growing pockets of the state like Middle Tennessee. It remains to be seen whether city-level measures alone will suffice in the face of rising temperatures and their attendant hazards. Meanwhile, transit will become a more pressing need if the population continues to grow. Nashville has at least instituted an intelligent approach toward sustainability and adaptation.

—STEVE HARUCH, contributing editor, *Nashville Scene*

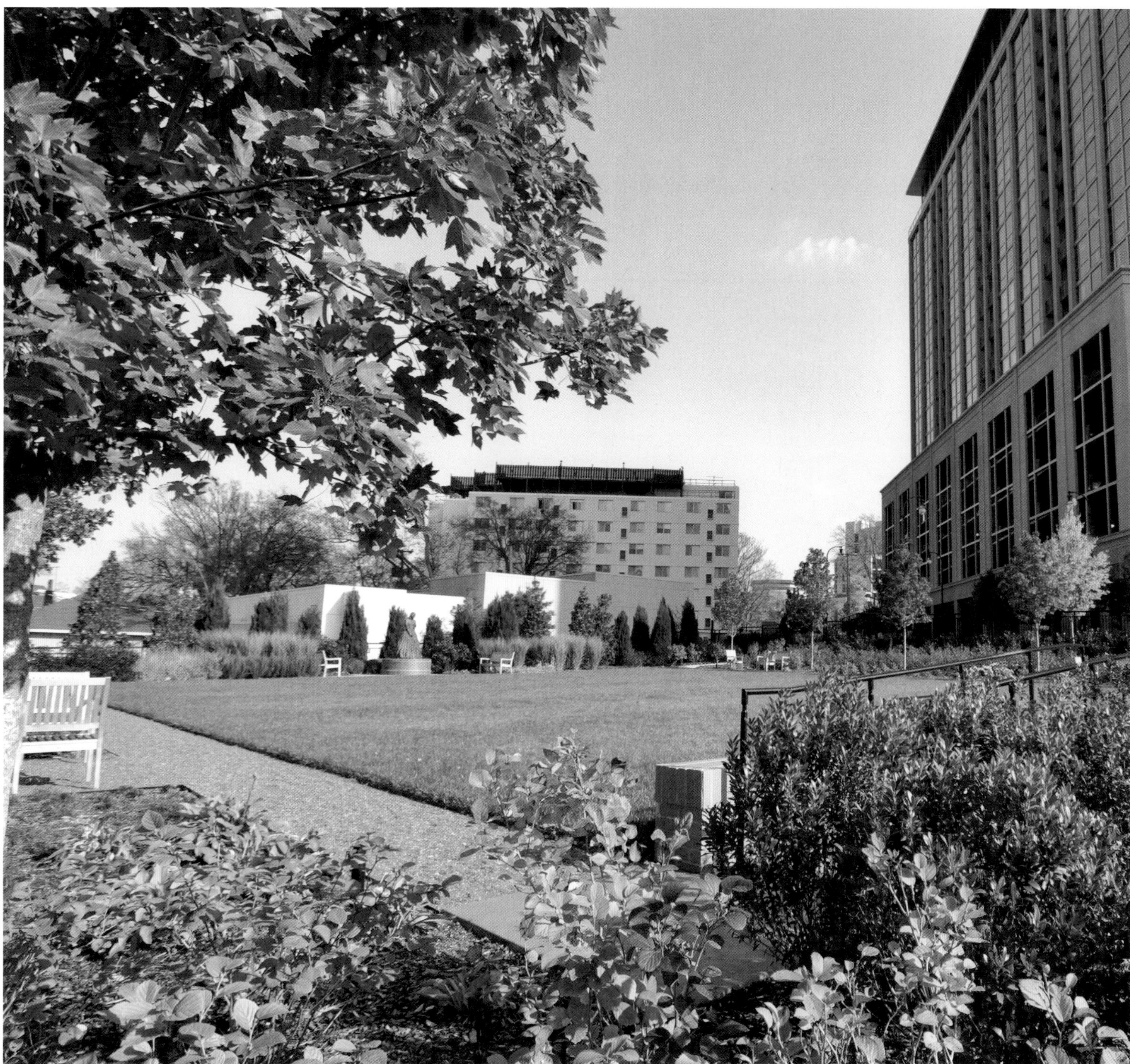

Adelicia Park is a private park protected under a conservation easement through partnership with The Land Trust for Tennessee. *(2007: Laura Brown)*

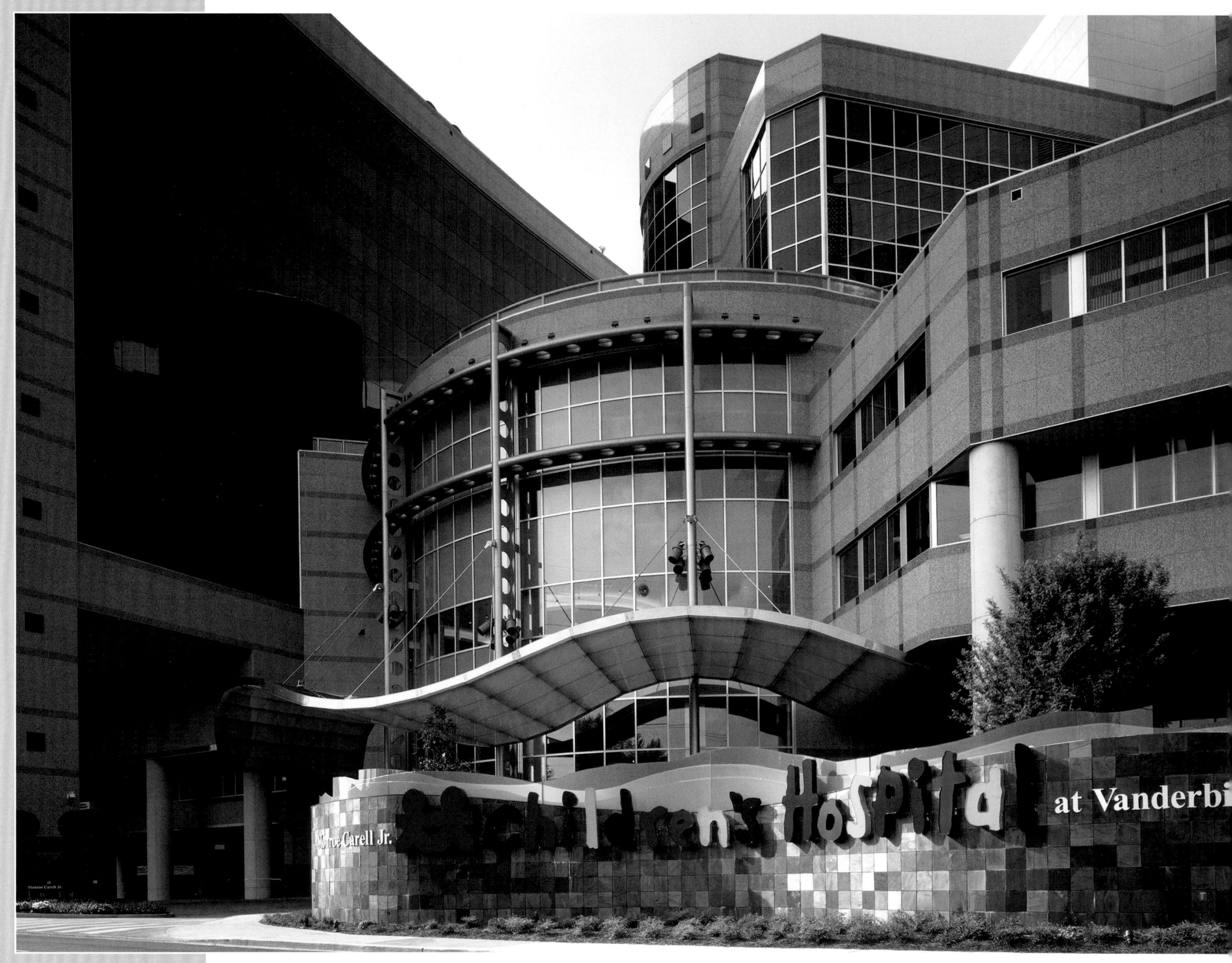
Monroe Carell Jr.
Children's Hospital
at Vanderbi

Bill Paul, MD, MPH
Director, Metro Public Health Department

Nashville is an epicenter of medical research, innovation, and entrepreneurship, all while boasting some of the best hospitals in the country. Does that make Nashville the healthiest city? No. As vital as it is, medical care focuses primarily on people who are already sick. If we want to live long and healthy lives, we need to pay attention to living well and avoiding sickness in the first place. Just as there is more to cars than auto repair, there is more to health than medical care.

In the United States, we spend about $8,000 per person per year on medical care: more than any other country. Yet our "vital signs" for premature mortality and infant mortality are below average for the developed world. According to the Organization for Economic Cooperation and Development (OECD), life expectancy at birth in the US ranks 26th of 34 OECD member nations. Our infant mortality rate ranks a dismal 31st.[1]

This disconnect between money spent on health care and actual health outcomes is *not* explained simply by the fact that so many Americans are uninsured. Medical care has less influence on our health and well-being than many people think. In 2005 about 45,000 Americans died because of lack of insurance.[2] Of those, hundreds were probably Tennesseans and dozens were Nashvillians who died because they had no coverage. About the same number of people die each year from motor vehicle accidents. These are significant numbers, but they pale in comparison to other categories of preventable death. For example, tobacco kills around 435,000 Americans per year, and unhealthy diets join with lack of physical activity to kill approximately 400,000 Americans per year.

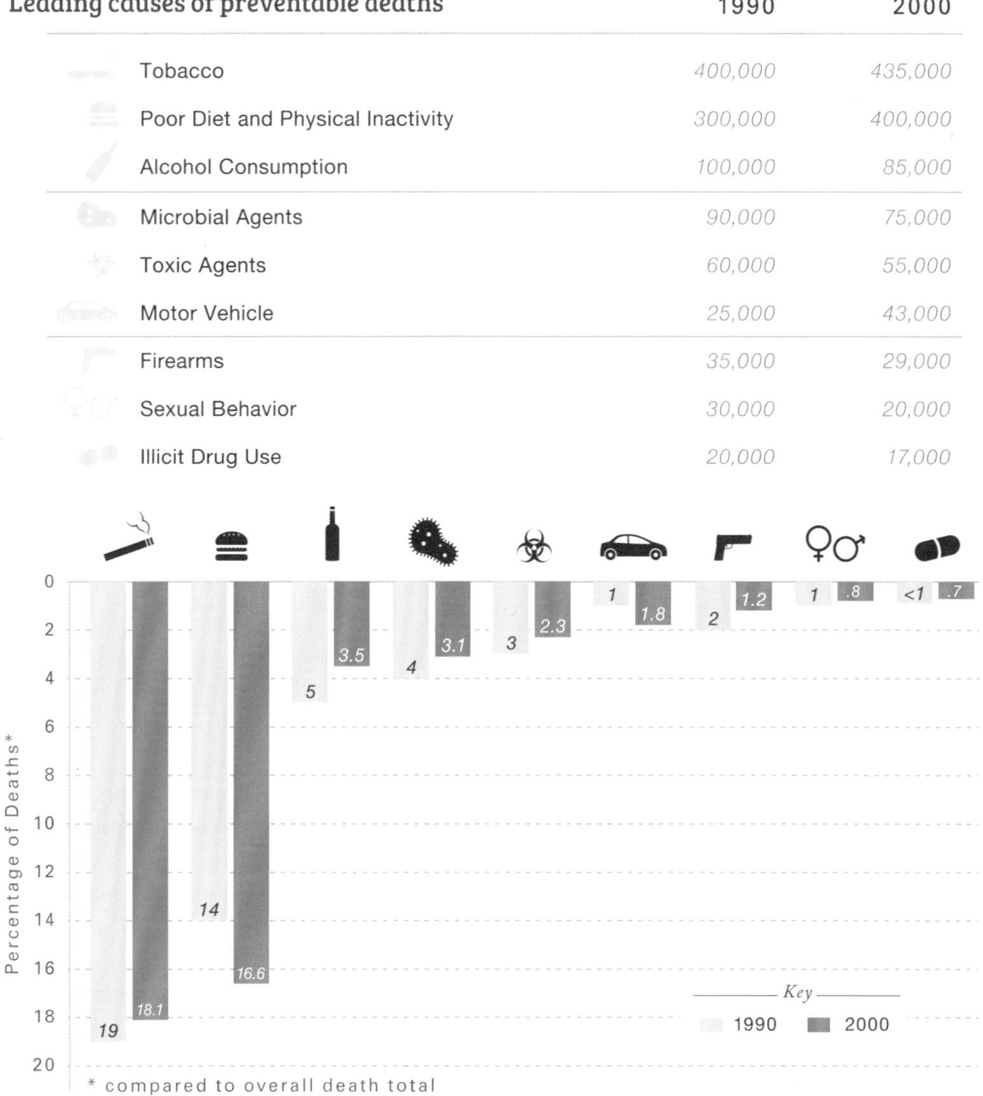

Leading causes of preventable deaths	1990	2000
Tobacco	400,000	435,000
Poor Diet and Physical Inactivity	300,000	400,000
Alcohol Consumption	100,000	85,000
Microbial Agents	90,000	75,000
Toxic Agents	60,000	55,000
Motor Vehicle	25,000	43,000
Firearms	35,000	29,000
Sexual Behavior	30,000	20,000
Illicit Drug Use	20,000	17,000

Opposite page: The Monroe Carell Jr. Children's Hospital at Vanderbilt University Medical Center is one of numerous state-of-the art hospitals in a city known for its health care infrastructure. *(2013: Scott McDonald © Hedrich Blessing/Courtesy of ESa.)*

The nation's leading causes of preventable deaths. *(2012: Janey Nachampasak, NCDC)*

HEALTH

Contributors to premature death in the United States. *(2012: Janey Nachampasak, NCDC)*

The NashvilleNext community meetings, part of the Metro Planning Department's process for developing a new general plan for the city, have given people the chance to contribute ideas for making Nashville a healthier city. *(2013: Metro Planning Department)*

Proportional contribution to premature death

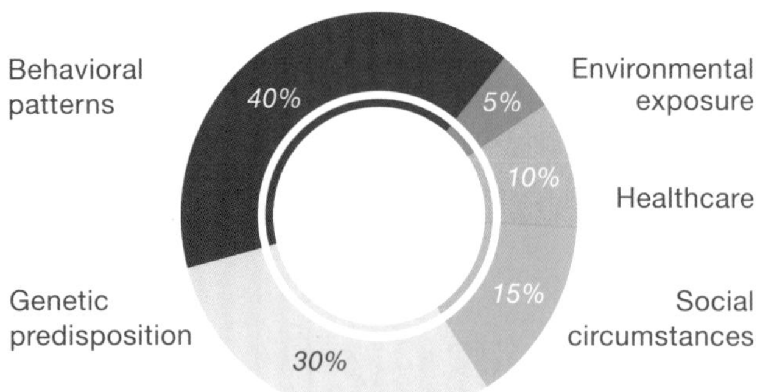

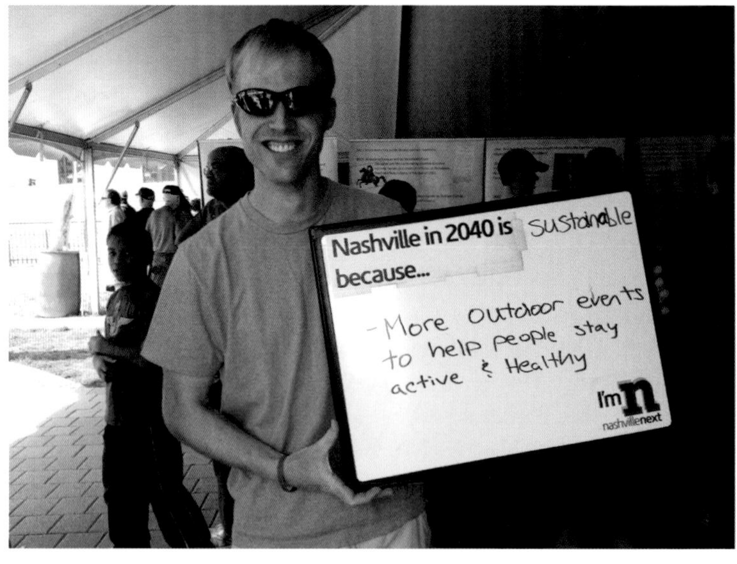

Nashville in 2040 is sustainable because...
- More outdoor events to help people stay active & Healthy
I'm n
nashvillenext

"Health is a state of complete physical, mental, and social well-being and not merely the absence of disease or infirmity."

Preamble to the Constitution of the World Health Organization as adopted by the International Health Conference, New York, 19–22 June 1946; signed on 22 July 1946 by the representatives of 61 States (Official Records of the World Health Organization, no. 2, p. 100) and entered into force on 7 April 1948.

We must consider health broadly. Even when we do focus on disease and infirmity, we must remember that nonmedical factors play a major role. Our risk of becoming ill and dying early is shaped by five major factors: genetics, social conditions, health behaviors, environmental exposures, and medical care. Of these five, medical care can prevent about 10–15 percent of early deaths. If we stopped using tobacco, adopted healthier diets, got regular physical activity, wore seatbelts, and moderated our alcohol intake, however, we could prevent 40 percent.[3]

Beyond behaviors and habits, social conditions shape our health in many ways throughout our lives. Each of us is exposed to different places, life events, stresses, and supports that shape our health and well-being. These include our parents' health before we are born, their skills at parenting, whether our basic needs for shelter and food are met, our education, the strength and habits of our social networks, and even the amount of control we have over our lives.[4] The choices and behaviors that cause 40 percent of our early mortality are influenced by a lifetime of experiences as well. Media and marketing, social norms, laws and regulations, convenience, accessibility, and affordability can all make us more or less likely to eat an apple a day or a burger and fries, to drink skim milk or sugary soda, to walk two miles daily or stay glued to our chair and computer screen.

The physical form of our cities shapes our behavior. It influences whether we drive, bike, or walk to work, whether healthy food is available close to home, and whether there are safe places to play, to enjoy nature, to interact with neighbors. So the cities we build can have a more profound impact on our health and well-being than the hospitals we build. Cities that intentionally support health and healthy behaviors by policy and by design will enjoy a healthier population than those that do not.

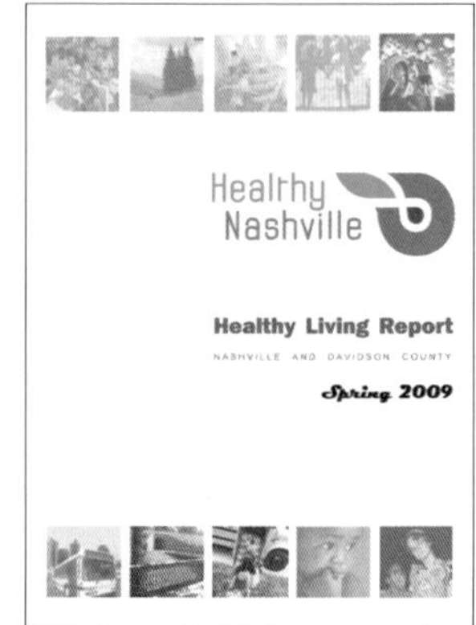

The Healthy Nashville Leadership Council's status update on the health of the community. *(2009: Metro Public Health Department)*

NASHVILLE'S HEALTH EXAM

Since health is defined broadly and influenced by many factors, sizing up the health of a city goes beyond looking at disease statistics. The Healthy Nashville Leadership Council (HNLC) periodically undertakes a community health assessment—a process akin to a comprehensive medical exam, in which the whole community is the patient.

A doctor listens to the patient's symptoms and history, asks questions about habits, family, living and working conditions. Then she examines the patient and may order specific studies like x-rays and laboratory tests. Different organ systems are checked, a diagnosis is made, and a prescription is given.

Like a comprehensive exam at the doctor's office, a community health assessment is thorough. The health council examines the community by listening to leaders and ordinary people, asking questions, and at times ordering special studies. We can also look into key "systems" in our community that have an impact on our health and quality of life, such as education, transportation, food, housing, and health care.

When the Healthy Nashville Leadership Council assessed Nashville's health in 2003, the key health priorities identified for Nashville at that time were obesity, tobacco use, and racial and ethnic disparities in chronic diseases. The health council conducted partial reassessments in 2006 and in 2009, prioritizing similar issues. In 2009 the group made recommendations for promoting healthy eating, active living, and prevention of unhealthy weight gain with a Healthy Living Report.[5]

During 2013, the Healthy Nashville Leadership Council (HNLC) completed a community health assessment for Nashville, the first phase of Mobilizing for Action through Planning and Partnerships (MAPP). Using this nationally recognized process for community-based, data-driven strategic planning, the HNLC will help Nashville address community health issues during the next five years.

NASHVILLE'S VITAL SIGNS

One way to size up our community's health is to pay attention to what's killing us. The number and causes of deaths are important "vital signs." Untimely or premature deaths can provide particular insights that help inform plans to improve community health.

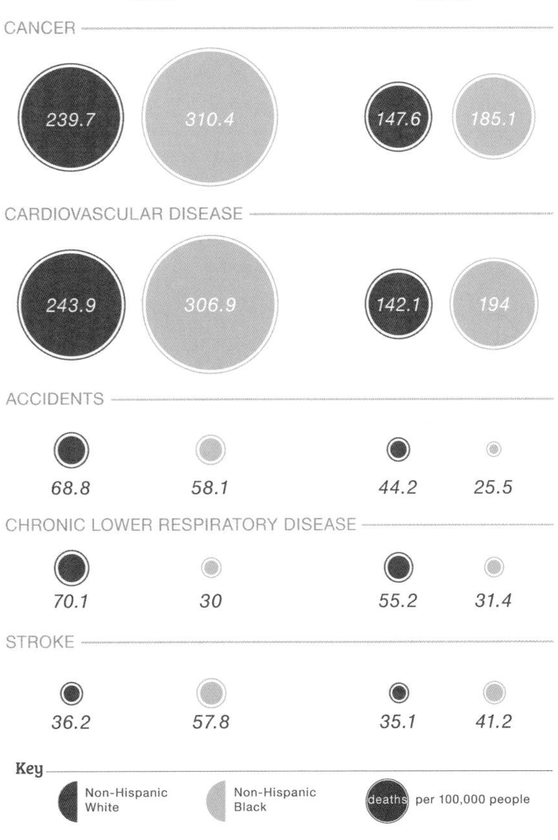

"A healthy Nashville has a culture of well-being, where all people have the opportunity and support to thrive and prosper."

Nashville MAPP 2013 vision statement.

This chart of leading causes of death in Nashville shows the disparity by gender and race. *(2012: Janey Nachampasak, NCDC)*

Leading causes of death and years of life lost to them in Nashville. *(2012: Janey Nachampasak, NCDC)*

Leading causes of death ranked by frequency with corresponding age-adjusted mortality rate, and years of potential life lost (YPLL) for Davidson County, TN, 2011

DISEASE/CONDITION	NUMBER	RATE*	YPLL
Cancer	1,115	190.8	9,941.5
Cardiovascular Disease	1,088	187.6	7,385
Accidents	302	49.1	6,864
Chronic Lower Respiratory Disease	301	54.2	1,665
Stroke	213	38.2	1,175
Diabetes	154	26.2	1,622.5
Alzheimer's	149	27.5	70.5
Suicide	74	11.4	2,064
Nephritis, Nephrotic Syndrome & Nephrosis	72	12.5	581.5
Chronic Liver Disease and Cirrhosis	68	10.7	1205.5
Pneumonia and Influenza	68	12	377.5
Homicide	50	7.3	2,017.5

**Rate = Deaths per 100,000 people*

Source: 2011 Mortality Data, Metro Public Health Department

Epidemiologists with the Metro Public Health Department analyzed the 4,826 deaths that occurred among Davidson County residents in 2011[6] and reported that cardiovascular disease and cancer were by far the most common causes of death, followed by accidents, chronic lung diseases, and stroke. Non-Hispanic blacks had higher rates of death for the major causes of death, with the exception of chronic lung disease and accidents.

To describe premature mortality in Nashville, the team analyzed years of potential life lost, using 75 years of life—the average longevity in Tennessee—as a benchmark. A count of years of potential life lost (YPLL) for a particular disease or cause represents the sum of the years that lives were cut short, that is, the differences between each person's age at death and age 75. For example, someone dying of cancer at age 65 would contribute 10 years of potential life lost to the total for cancer, while a victim of homicide at age 20 would contribute 55 to the total for homicide.

The biggest contributors to early death in Nashville are chronic diseases. Heart disease and cancer are top causes of death, as well as top contributors to years of potential life lost, for Davidson County. Nashville does not stand out here: these are nationally the top killers.

Improving our health behaviors can prevent cardiovascular disease, cancer, stroke, and respiratory disease—all among the leading causes of death. We could have a major impact on these chronic diseases and on medical costs, disability, and early deaths if we could reduce tobacco use and make healthy food and regular physical activity the rule rather than the exception.

Injuries (accidents, suicides, and homicides combined) caused 426 deaths, accounting for over 10,000 years of potential life lost, more than heart disease or cancer. Accidents (including sleep-related deaths of infants, motor vehicle accidents, and accidental drug overdoses) were the third leading cause of death and contributor to years of life lost. Violent deaths (suicide and homicide together) tend to affect younger people and account for the fourth leading cause of years lost. Injury-related deaths—whether accidental or intentional—are deaths that are preventable, not inevitable.

TRACKING RISKY BEHAVIOR

Since smoking, poor diet, and lack of physical activity are major contributors to the top diseases that cause us to die prematurely, public health officials track these behaviors in the population. In order to do so, they use the Behavioral Risk Factor Surveillance System, a state-by-state telephone survey designed and coordinated by the US Centers for Disease Control (CDC). In Tennessee, these data are collected annually, and since 2005, the state designed the survey so that estimates are available for Davidson County.

There are reasons to be cautious when looking at data of this type. First, the number of interviews done is small enough that Nashville can have some random ups and downs from year to year in its results. Second, like residents of other cities, many Nashvillians have eliminated their landline telephones. Until 2011, only landlines were included, but the survey methods changed in 2011 to include interviews of people who only have a cell phone. The change of methods has resulted in year-to-year comparisons that are not meaningful, so 2011 and 2012 results are not presented here.

Smoking is the leading cause of preventable death in the United States. Smoking rates fell nationally as clean indoor air laws, increased taxes, and other measures made more places smoke-free. Smoking is becoming more of an exception

Current Smokers

Tennessee
Davidson

Body Mass Index (BMI) Chart for Adults

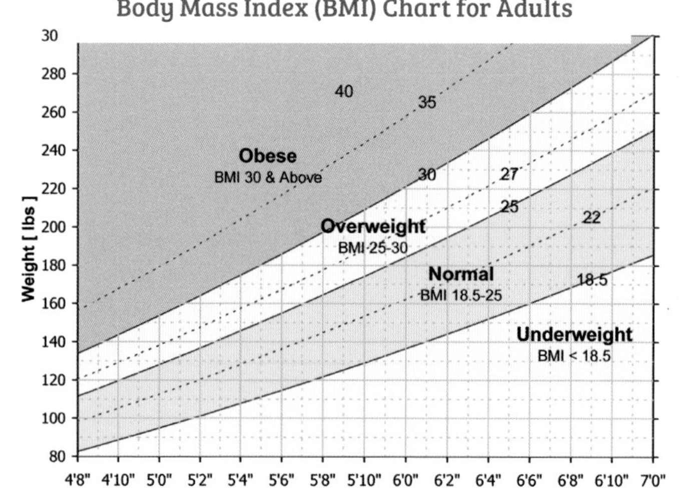

Diabetes

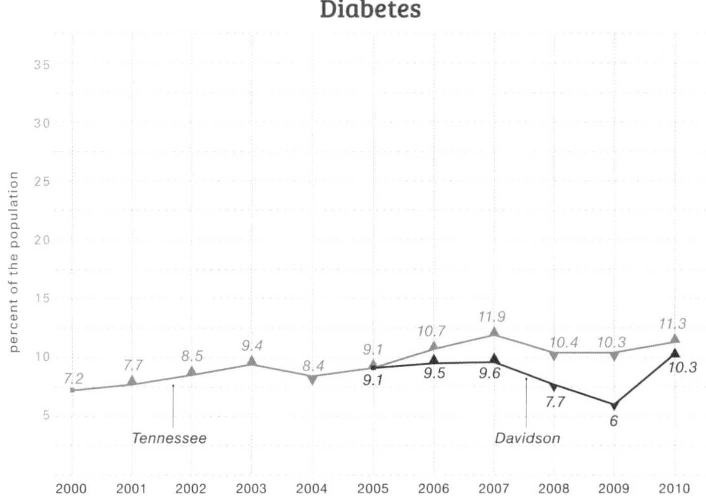

Overweight or Obese

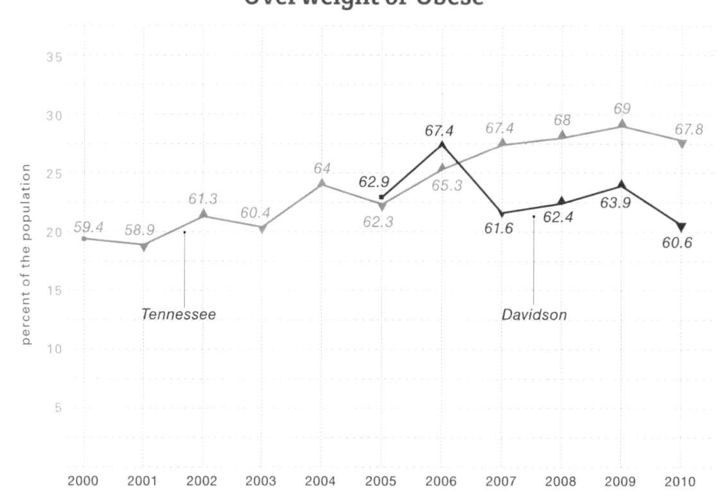

Clockwise from top left: Declining rates of smoking show the impact public policies can have on unhealthy behavior. *(2012: Janey Nachampasak, NCDC)*

For adults, overweight and obesity ranges are determined by using weight and height to calculate a number called the body mass index. BMI is used because, for most people, it correlates with their amount of body fat. An adult who has a BMI between 25 and 29.9 is considered overweight. An adult who has a BMI of 30 or higher is considered obese.[8] *(BMI Chart created by Vertex42.com. Used with permission. www.vertex42.com/ExcelTemplates/bmi-chart.html)*

Charting the weight gain in Nashville and Tennessee. *(2012: Janey Nachampasak, NCDC)*

Diabetes in Nashville and Tennessee. *(2012: Janey Nachampasak, NCDC)*

than a rule. One out of every five or six adults is still a smoker in Tennessee and in Nashville, but both showed declining rates in recent years. This is the expected result of the cigarette tax and clean indoor air law that were implemented in 2008. These findings help demonstrate that healthier places and policies can impact behavior in a beneficial way.

Obesity is connected to a host of diseases, including diabetes, cardiovascular disease, some cancers, and arthritis. Rates of obesity are an indicator of poor diet and lack of physical activity in a population. In national, state, and municipal populations,[7] obesity has been climbing steadily and dramatically in the last five decades to the point where two-thirds of adults in Davidson County are overweight or obese. Recent data suggest a decline in obesity in Davidson County and a leveling off for the state overall. This could be a promising sign that Tennesseans are eating healthier food and getting more physical activity, but after so many years of increasing obesity, we shall want to see improvement in several measures of the epidemic over several years to be confident the tide has turned.

Along with obesity, diabetes among adults has also been rising in Tennessee, again with some possible leveling off seen in the years from 2008 to 2010. In Davidson County, the numbers appear to have swung erratically the last two years.

The ten census tracts with the highest premature mortalities average a 41 percent poverty rate, 17 percent unemployment rate, and a 16 percent vacancy housing rate. Conversely, the ten census tracts with the lowest premature mortalities average a 9 percent poverty rate, 4 percent unemployment rate, and a 9 percent vacancy housing rate. *(Map, 2013: Jill Robinson, NCDC)*

Careful measurement in future years will determine whether there is a real trend.

There are signs that the rising tide of overweight and obesity in children is starting to turn around. The CDC reported that many states are showing declines in obesity among preschool-aged children participating in federal programs during the years 2008 to 2011. Unfortunately, Tennessee was one of three states with obesity rates that actually worsened over those years.[9] However, among school-aged children there is some better news in Tennessee. Schoolchildren in Davidson County and twelve other counties in the state have charted declines in rates of obesity and overweight between the 2007/08 and 2012/13 school years. In Metro Nashville Public Schools during the same period, the percent of overweight and obese schoolchildren declined from 39.9 percent to 36.1 percent.[10]

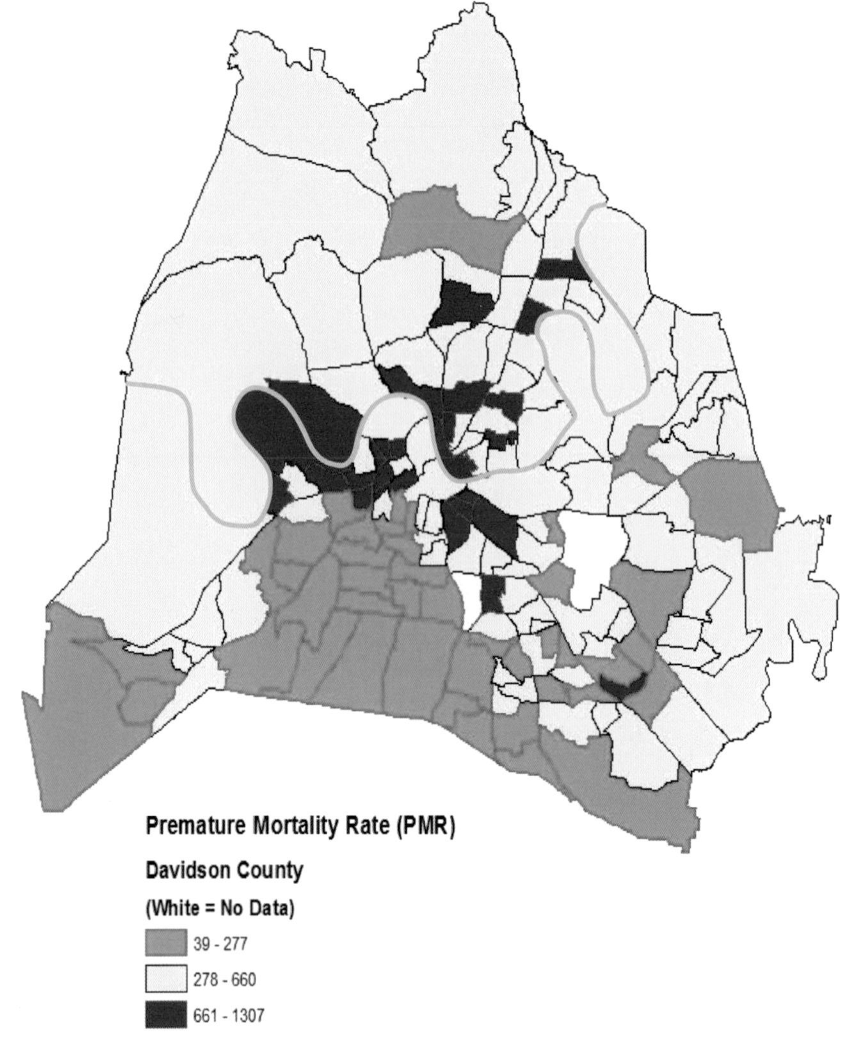

HEALTH AND PLACE

One of the most powerful predictors of an individual's health is the address where he or she lives. Within Davidson County, for example, risk of chronic disease varies widely by census tract. One countywide survey showed that in some census tracts most adults were neither overweight nor obese, while in other tracts the majority were obese. In some census tracts less than 15 percent of residents had hypertension, while in others 49 percent or nearly half did.[11]

Neighborhoods are typically separated by socioeconomic status, and areas with high levels of poverty experience poorer health and higher mortality. One study in Boston found that the likelihood of early death was 39 percent higher in census tracts with at least 20 percent of people living in poverty than in census tracts with less than five percent living in poverty.[12]

In Nashville, premature mortality varies widely by neighborhood, with the highest mortality occurring in areas with a high percentage of people living in poverty. The healthiest 25 percent of Nashville's census tracts have premature mortality rates at or below 277 deaths per 100,000 people, while the sickest quartile have rates that are all above 660, reflecting roughly twice the risk of early death.

Economics obviously shapes individuals' health and well-being. Money buys access to healthy food and safe, stable housing. Neighborhood environments can also influence health in positive or negative ways. For example, neighborhoods that have more abundant opportunities for physical activity and access to healthy food can support better health for their residents.

People can benefit by living in healthier places even if they are poor. A Chicago study found that residents of public housing who were randomly assigned to move to low-poverty areas developed less obesity and diabetes than those who moved to high-poverty areas.[13] Another study identified neighborhood effects on mental health.[14] Boys from poor families who moved from high-poverty public housing to lower poverty neighborhoods experienced less anxiety, depression, and dependence problems than those who stayed in public housing.

In addition, racial segregation can be unhealthy. Neighborhoods in American cities tend to be racially segregated. Many high-poverty neighborhoods have predominantly African American residents. But the differences in social environment

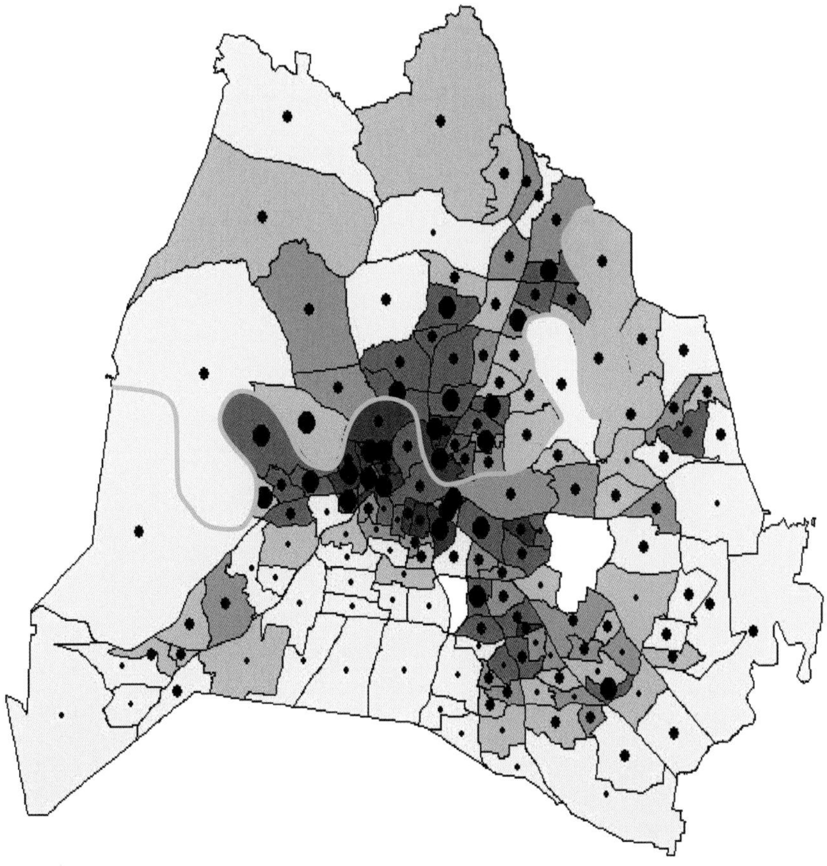

Percentage Below Poverty

Davidson County

(White = No Data)

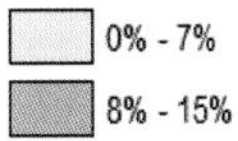

0% - 7%

8% - 15%

16% - 23%

24% - 41%

42% - 84%

Premature Mortality Rate (PMR)

Davidson County

39 - 277

278 - 660

661 - 1307

The ten census tracts with the highest premature mortalities average a 41 percent poverty rate, 17 percent unemployment rate, and a 16 percent vacancy housing rate. Conversely, the ten census tracts with the lowest premature mortalities average a 9 percent poverty rate, 4 percent unemployment rate, and a 9 percent vacancy housing rate.
(Map, 2013: Jill Robinson, NCDC)

How Davidson County Stacks Up

The United States ranks poorly compared to other developed nations when it comes to life expectancy. But how do the number of years people in Davidson County are expected to live compare with other places in Tennessee and the world?

The table below offers a global context for Davidson County and two other Tennessee counties: Shelby County, a poor urban county that includes Memphis, and Williamson County, a wealthy neighbor to Davidson. In 2009, Davidson County looked like Mexico or the Czech Republic when it came to life expectancy calculations. Shelby County looked more like Libya or Malaysia, and Williamson County looked most similar to Canada.

—JILL ROBINSON
NCDC research fellow

	Life Expectancy	*1989*	*1999*	*2009*
State	Davidson, TN	69.9	71.5	73.7
	Shelby, TN	68.6	70	72.1
	Williamson, TN	73.5	76.2	78.6
Global	Bolivia	56.6	60.6	63.5
	Bosnia & Herzegovina	63.9	71.2	72.5
	Canada	74	76.3	78.3
	Chile	70.2	73.4	75.6
	China	66.4	69.5	71.6
	Czech Republic	68.2	71.4	73.4
	Ecuador	66	70.2	72.2
	Italy	73.3	76	78.2
	Libya	65.3	69.7	71.8
	Macedonia	69.1	70.6	71.8
	Malaysia	67.9	69.9	72.1
	Mexico	67.5	71.7	73.8
	Oman	67.6	71.7	74.3
	Russia	62.9	59	60.7
	Slovenia	68.7	71.6	74.7
	Somalia	43.4	46.2	48.2
	South Korea	66.7	71.6	76
	Sudan	50.7	54.2	57
	Syria	66	70.2	72.3
	Tunisia	66.3	70.4	71.9
	United States	71.6	74.1	76.2

Source: Institute for Health Measures and Evaluation (University of Washington, 2009). Life expectancy by county and sex (US) with country comparison (Global), 1989, 1999, 2009. Retrieved August 6, 2013 from *www.healthmetricsandevaluation.org/tools/data-visualization/life-expectancy-county-and-sex-us-country-comparison-global-1989-1999-2009#/data-methods*

(2013: Janey Nachampasak, NCDC)

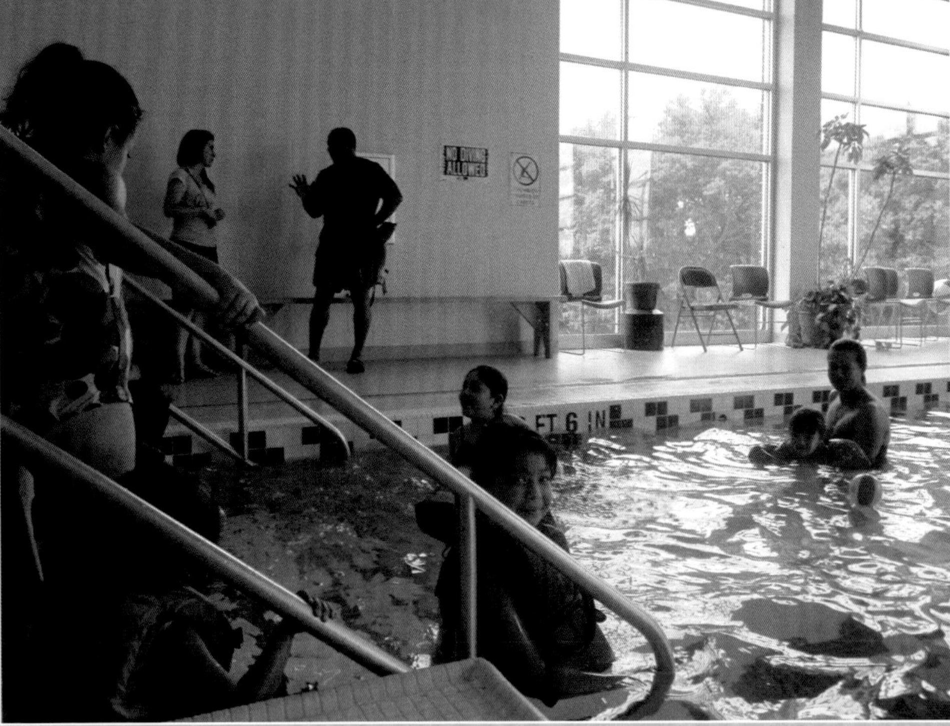
Family swim program at Coleman Park Community Center involves both parents and young children in active swim play time with an instructor. *(2013: GROW program)*

Childhood Obesity

Almost one in four children in Tennessee is either overweight or obese; a quarter to almost half of these children will stay that way as adults. In the clinic, I see infants drinking soda out of their bottles, and three-year-olds who weigh more than 100 pounds with enlarged livers and the inability to sleep lying down. Much of the debate about obesity focuses on individual behavior: too many calories in and too few out. While this contributes to the problem of obesity, it neglects the context in which individuals live.

Context often determines whether families have access to green spaces to run and play, whether these spaces are free from crime, well lit, and distant from traffic that could threaten the safety of a running child. Knowing the importance of context, our city government has increased the amount of green space in Nashville and doubled the number of available, affordable community recreation centers.

Given that one in three children born in the year 2000 is at risk of developing Type 2 diabetes, and that healthy behaviors happen within one's family and community, the Monroe Carell Jr Children's Hospital at Vanderbilt and Metro Parks and Recreation embarked on a unique partnership in 2008. The resulting Nashville Collaborative develops and tests community-based programs aimed at reducing childhood obesity in Davidson County.

We found we could amplify health just by better utilizing the resources we have. We could sustain use of the community recreation centers for routine health for both children and their parents, and shift early childhood growth patterns toward normal. The key was to teach families how to use the centers. One year later, these families were still engaging in weekly physical activity at the recreational centers. This is how you can tip the balance from disease to health.

The Nashville Collaborative also identified and addressed the barriers to utilizing the centers more fully. We learned that most people walk to their neighborhood community recreation centers. For these families, common barriers for going outside include crime rates, lighting, street safety, speed limits, and a finding that surprised us: stray dogs. In fact, families tell us that stray dogs are one of the main reasons they don't send their children outside to play. Many of these families choose to let their children stay inside and watch media, seeing this as the safer choice. Identifying the issue of stray dogs and then examining how our city can implement and enforce existing policies is an example of a potential pivot point for changing how families utilize their community resources to reinforce and sustain healthy habits.

—SHARI BARKIN

professor of pediatrics; William K. Warren Foundation chair; division director, General Pediatrics; director, Pediatric Obesity Research, DRTC; Vanderbilt University School of Medicine

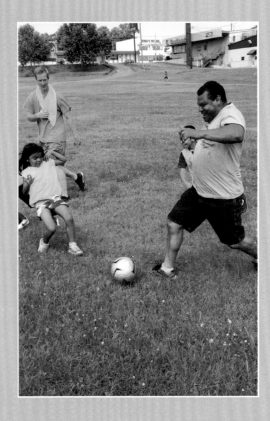
Parents and children being active together in our green spaces. *(2013: GROW program)*

based on race, while important, do not explain all of the differences in health. A Baltimore study found that typical racial disparities in hypertension, diabetes, and obesity in women were lessened or eliminated in a low-income neighborhood where blacks and whites live together under similar socioeconomic conditions.[15]

THE AIR WE BREATHE

Clean, healthy air prevents asthma episodes, doctor and hospital visits, lost work and school days, and even deaths. While smoking and exposure to secondhand tobacco smoke are important, the quality of Nashville's air is a critical environmental health issue.

The Environmental Protection Agency (EPA) develops National Ambient Air Quality Standards based on known and measurable health hazards from carbon monoxide, sulfur dioxide, nitrogen dioxide, particles, and ozone. Nashville's success in achieving clean air is measured by the number of days in the year that the air here meets these National Standards. In recent years, Nashville has met the goal. In 2014, EPA ozone standards were met 100 percent of the days of the year. According to Metro, the highest 2012–2014 three-year average at the ozone monitoring sites was 70

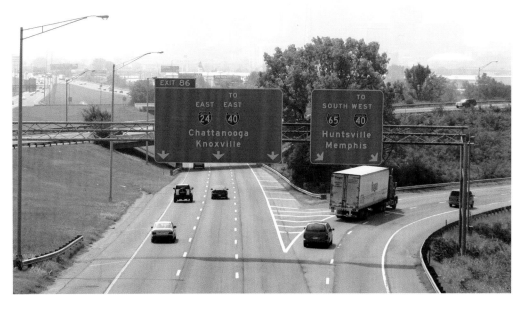

The white smog shrouding Nashville is caused primarily by pollutants exhaled by the internal combustion engines found in our automobiles, trucks, motorcycles, lawnmowers, and boats. Drivers log over 21 million miles in and through Davidson County each day, and Nashville's daily average of nearly 35 vehicle miles driven per person is much higher than the national average.[16] *(2011: Gary Layda; infographic, 2013: Janey Nachampasak, Eric Hoke, NCDC)*

DAVIDSON COUNTY

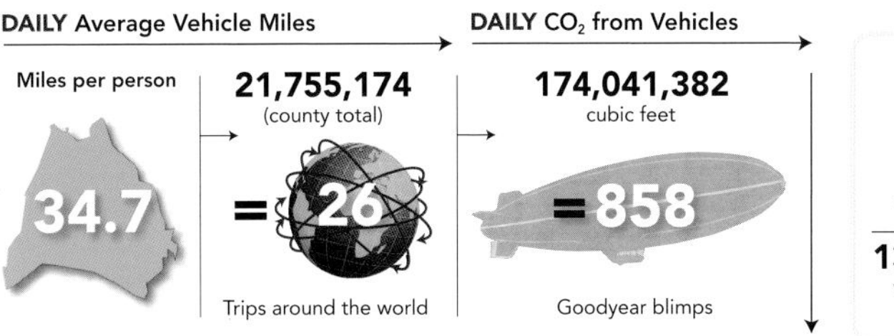

60% daily trips =/< 5 miles — 13,053,104 vehicle miles

If 1/2 of these were [walking, biking, transit] — 6,526,552 vehicle miles

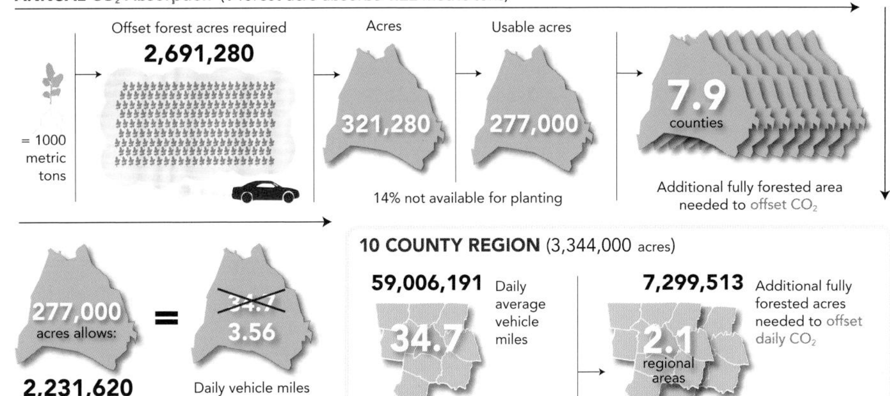

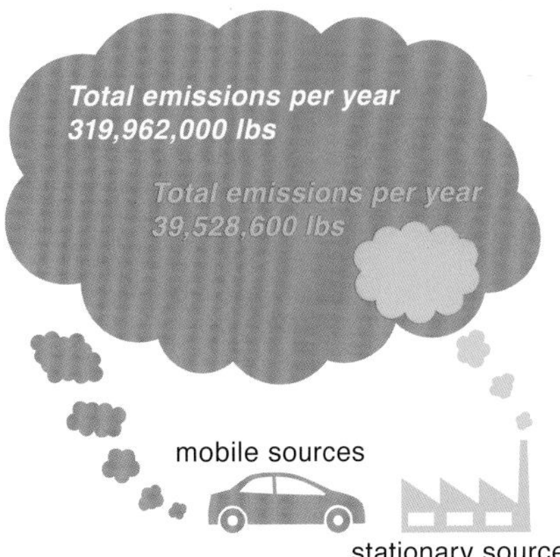

Left: In Davidson County, mobile sources emit 89 percent of the five pollutants reported by the Metro Public Health Department, while stationary sources emit only eleven percent. *(Infographic, 2013: Janey Nachampasak, Eric Hoke, NCDC)*

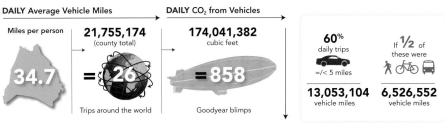

Source: 2010 Annual Report, *Metro Public Health Department*

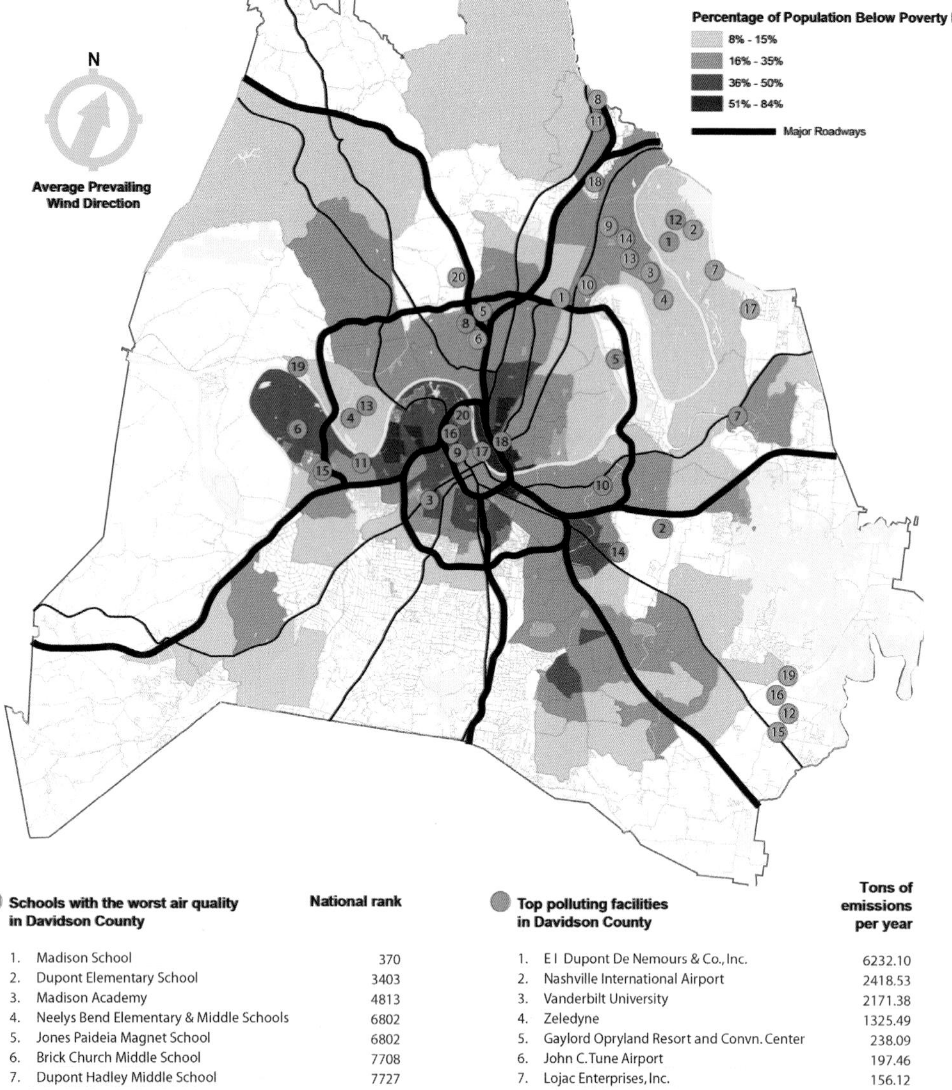

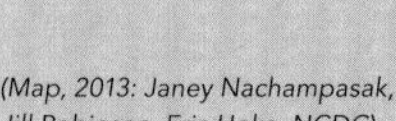
(Map, 2013: Janey Nachampasak, Jill Robinson, Eric Hoke, NCDC)

Schools with the worst air quality in Davidson County	National rank
1. Madison School	370
2. Dupont Elementary School	3403
3. Madison Academy	4813
4. Neelys Bend Elementary & Middle Schools	6802
5. Jones Paideia Magnet School	6802
6. Brick Church Middle School	7708
7. Dupont Hadley Middle School	7727
8. Metro Christian Academy	8320
9. Amqui Elementary School	9096
10. St. Joseph School	10150
11. Goodlettsville Middle School	10150
12. Antioch High School	10613
13. Madison Nazarene Christian Academy	11898
14. Stratton Elementary School	12034
15. Mt. View Elementary School	12414
16. John F. Kennedy Middle School	12664
17. Andrew Jackson Elementary School	12953
18. Gateway Elementary School	13161
19. Thomas A. Edison Elementary School	13376
20. Goodlettsville Elementary School	13431

Source: *content.usatoday.com/news/nation/environment/smokestack/index*

Top polluting facilities in Davidson County	Tons of emissions per year
1. E I Dupont De Nemours & Co., Inc.	6232.10
2. Nashville International Airport	2418.53
3. Vanderbilt University	2171.38
4. Zeledyne	1325.49
5. Gaylord Opryland Resort and Convn. Center	238.09
6. John C. Tune Airport	197.46
7. Lojac Enterprises, Inc.	156.12
8. Worldcolor Nashville	110.94
9. United States Tobacco Mfg., LP	107.14
10. Gibson Guitar Co.—Electric Division	99.76
11. Innophos, Inc.	91.69
12. Fiberweb, Inc.	74.05
13. M M Nashville Energy, LLC	73.20
14. Vought Aircraft Industries, Inc.	71.54
15. The Mulch Company	70.15
16. Werthan Packaging, Inc.	69.80
17. Marathon Petroleum Company, LLC	69.50
18. Magellan Terminals Holdings, LP	69.31
19. Haileys Harbor, Inc.	68.32
20. Metro Central WWTP	68.28

Source: *www.epa.gov/ttn/chief/net/2008inventory.html*

parts per billion, which is below the 2008 eight-hour ozone standard of 75 parts per billion. This current 2008 eight-hour ozone standard is scheduled to be lowered in 2015. If the new eight-hour ozone standard is exceeded, the Metro Public Health Department will work with the Tennessee Air Pollution Control Division and the EPA to develop a plan for bringing the area back into alignment with the existing standard as expeditiously as possible.

One barrier to meeting EPA standards is the weather. Specifically, episodes of extreme heat and drought adversely affect air quality. Put simply, ozone is created by a chemical reaction facilitated by high temperatures and low humidity. Most of our ozone problem results from a mix of motor vehicle exhaust and summer weather. If our summers get hotter, our air quality will suffer. To meet any new, more stringent standard, we shall have to continue to enforce controls on motor vehicles and other sources of pollution. Replacing older, "dirtier" vehicles with newer, cleaner vehicles will help. But to really achieve cleaner and healthier air, we will need to find additional transportation strategies that reduce the burden of vehicle exhaust in our region.

THE TENNESSEE CONTEXT

Although Davidson County ranks high in comparison to the rest of Tennessee, Tennessee is not the healthiest state in the United States. *America's Health Rankings* is a widely publicized index that ranks health measures state by state. The 2014 *America's Health Rankings* put Tennessee in 45th place overall. Strengths mentioned in that ranking system included ready availability of primary care physicians and high immunization coverage. Challenges included a high violent crime rate, high prevalence of sedentary lifestyle (rank 49 of 50), and high infant mortality (rank 41 of 50).[17]

COMPARING NATIONAL PEERS

People are often interested in knowing how Nashville compares to similarly sized cities in the South as well as in other regions of the country. Although unscientific, this type of comparison can provide some ideas and insights about differences among cities in factors that influence premature mortality, health habits, and well-being.

One pattern that is evident in these county comparisons—true also of different areas within a county— is that communities with more college graduates and less poverty experience less premature death. Affluence and education correlate with better health behaviors, fewer preventable hospitalizations, and fewer premature deaths.

Within Tennessee, Williamson County is the healthiest. Only seven percent of its children live in poverty and a high percentage of its population attended college. Looking beyond state lines, Portland, Oregon; Austin, Texas; and Charlotte and Raleigh-Durham, North Carolina, have lower premature death rates, lower smoking rates, lower obesity rates, and less physical inactivity than other cities on the list. They also have a higher percentage of college graduates than the less healthy cities.

There are some surprises. Raleigh–Durham, one of the historic strongholds of tobacco production, currently has one of the lowest rates of smoking and is closest to the national benchmark among comparison cities. This metropolitan area also meets or is close to national benchmarks in the other measures. Raleigh–Durham has a comparatively low child poverty rate, although not extremely low as in Williamson County. Denver, Colorado, and Portland, Oregon, have rates of childhood poverty comparable to Nashville's, yet have lower overall mortality rates, better health behaviors, and fewer preventable hospitalizations.

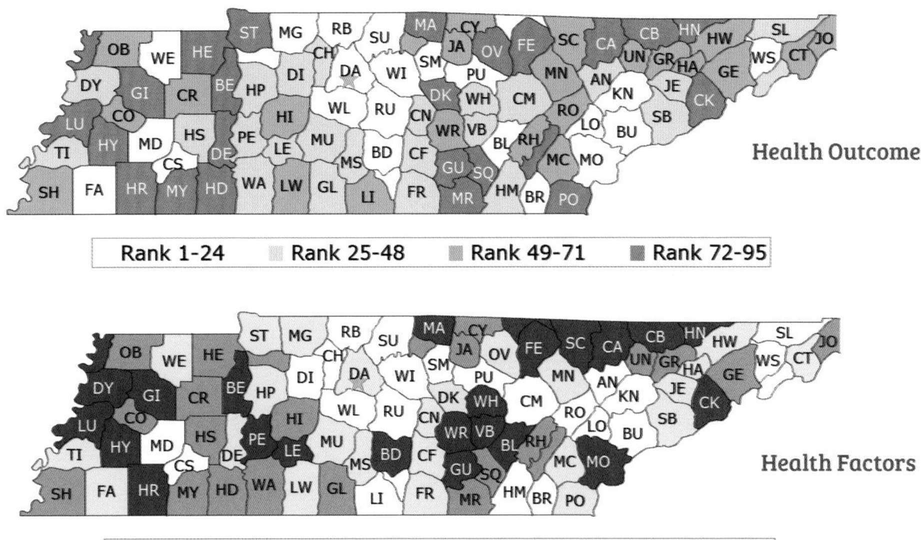

The *County Health Rankings* is an annual report that summarizes key health-related measures for counties across the United States and presents county rankings within each state.[20] The 2013 County Health Outcomes (measures of disease and premature death) list Davidson County as 13th healthiest among Tennessee's 95 counties overall. Areas of relative strength were health behaviors (ranked 6th) and clinical care (ranked 16th). Premature death in Davidson County was ranked 19th. The Health Factors map (measures of things that influence disease and death such as behaviors, clinical care, social and economic factors, and the built environment) reveals a more challenging set of factors for which Davidson County ranked 67th, including the third highest rate of violent crime in the state. The healthiest county in Tennessee is Williamson County, which is also the wealthiest. *(Maps, 2013: University of Wisconsin Population Health Institute)*

DIAGNOSES

To sum up this overview of health measures for Nashville, there are some key areas where our city could make progress toward better health and longer lives.

First, the rising tide of obesity is the epidemic challenge of our generation. National statistics suggest that this epidemic is a new phenomenon in the last 50 years. The rising rates of diabetes, whose complications include loss of eyesight, loss of limbs, kidney failure, as well as cardiovascular disease, are part of the same epidemic. Recent projections suggest that by 2030, 63 percent of adults in Tennessee will be obese (at least 30 pounds overweight) and that a 5 percent reduction in average body mass index could save $13.8 billion in cumulative obesity-related medical costs over 20 years.[18] Some studies have predicted declines in life expectancy in the United States because of this epidemic.[19]

Second, tobacco still kills, but lower smoking rates in Nashville and across the country are an example of real behavioral change that is saving lives. Some of the key strategies that made smoking less common, such as smoking bans in public places and tobacco taxes, demonstrated that healthier behaviors can be encouraged through policies that create healthier places.

Third, although the numbers of deaths are smaller than for chronic diseases, injuries—including accidents and violent death from homicide and suicide—are significant contributors to early mortality. Public safety and community prevention strategies are needed. Safety is a high priority for Nashville and is both a matter of personal and community responsibility.

Fourth, good health is not distributed fairly and equitably across communities. At a local level, where you live affects how well and how long you live. The unhealthy impacts of obesity, tobacco, and injury risks are important to address everywhere, but especially in places where people live in environments with fewer choices and opportunities for healthy living.

This comparison with peer cities uses the *County Health Rankings* for selected health indicators. Larger counties from Tennessee are included, along with a list of urban counties that are similar in size to Nashville/Davidson.
(2013: Janey Nachampasak, NCDC)

COUNTY City State	Population	Premature Deaths	Preventable Hospital Stays	Motor Vehicle Crash Death Rates (per 100,000)	Commute Alone	Adult Smoking	Adult Obesity	Physical Inactivity	Some College	Children in Poverty	Violent Crime Rate (per 100,000)
MECKLENBURG Charlotte NC	913,639	6,351	49	11	77%	16%	26%	20%	71%	21%	679
TRAVIS Austin TX	1,026,158	5,559	57	12	73%	17%	25%	18%	70%	25%	434
DENVER Denver CO	610,345	7,661	44	13	69%	20%	18%	16%	67%	31%	569
JEFFERSON Louisville KY	721,594	8,405	70	13	81%	24%	34%	29%	66%	24%	607
WAKE Raleigh-Durham NC	897,214	5,212	51	11	80%	15%	26%	18%	77%	15%	301
MULTNOMAH Portland OR	726,855	6,649	43	8	63%	17%	24%	16%	71%	25%	526
FAYETTE Lexington KY	296,545	7,043	54	12	80%	18%	31%	24%	73%	24%	636
MARION Indianapolis IN	890,879	9,229	74	12	82%	26%	30%	26%	58%	31%	1,146
TULSA Tulsa OK	601,961	9,162	63	15	81%	24%	29%	29%	62%	23%	846
JEFFERSON Birmingham AL	665,027	11,049	54	19	84%	22%	32%	29%	64%	28%	727
JACKSON Kansas City MO	705,708	8,979	61	14	82%	23%	33%	26%	62%	24%	828
DUVAL Jacksonville FL	857,040	9,643	79	17	81%	21%	28%	26%	61%	24%	836
DAVIDSON Nashville	635,710	8,664	68	16	81%	20%	30%	27%	64%	31%	1,202
KNOX Knoxville	435,725	7,981	59	16	85%	20%	31%	28%	69%	17%	582
SHELBY Memphis	920,232	10,334	65	19	82%	19%	34%	29%	60%	29%	1,377
WILLIAMSON	176,838	3,914	58	10	80%	14%	24%	19%	81%	7%	137
RUTHERFORD	257,048	6,919	92	15	85%	20%	30%	27%	63%	18%	447
STATE OF TN		9,093	86	22		24%	32%	30%	55%	26%	667
NATIONAL BENCHMARK		**5,466**	**49**	**12**		**14%**	**25%**	**21%**	**68%**	**13%**	**66**

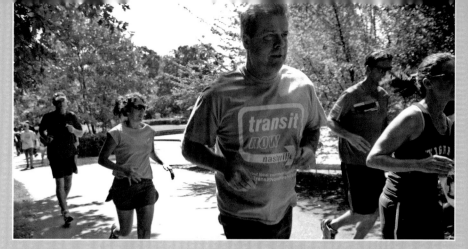

The NashVitality Movement

In 2010, Nashville was awarded a two-year, $7.5 million Communities Putting Prevention to Work (CPPW) grant from the Centers for Disease Control and Prevention to accelerate the city's progress in promoting healthy eating, active living, and obesity prevention. The Metro Public Health Department worked with the office of Mayor Karl Dean, various Metro departments, and community partners to create a collaboratively developed Community Action Plan for healthy change in Nashville.

Nashville's approach for CPPW was to develop and support a variety of visible projects that make healthy choices easier for as many people in Nashville as possible. All those invested in the Community Action Plan worked with schools, employers, youth serving organizations, and places of worship to create policies and shape the environment so that healthy choices were more prominent, more visible, and more likely to be the default choices.

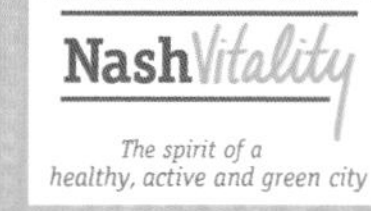

The efforts are tied together in an overarching brand and campaign, NashVitality. More than 20 projects set in motion and boosted changes to make healthy choices easier.

Here are a few accomplishments of the Nashville community that reflect the spirit of NashVitality:

- School gardens gained momentum, with 46 gardens active and a school garden policy developed to support ongoing efforts.

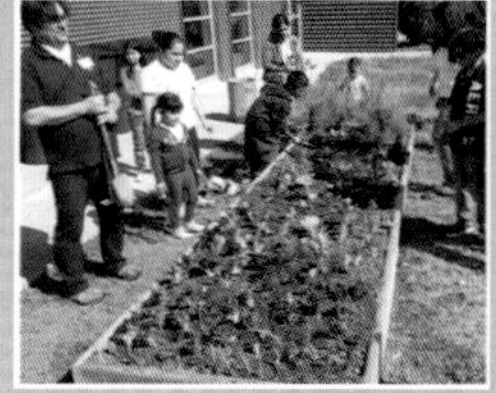

- At last count, over 80 community gardens were up and running. The University of Tennessee's agricultural extension office hired a person to provide technical assistance for community gardens.
- Several organizations that serve youth outside of school implemented healthier policies. Metro Parks and Recreation, Martha O'Brien Center, Rocketown, and others took a stand for limiting junk food served and promoting physical activity in after school settings affecting thousands of children and youth.
- The Metro Health Department composed a challenge and a guide to help communities of faith institute healthy policies. Several faith communities ranging from 100 to 10,000 members established covenants to make their places of worship nonsmoking and to promote physical activity and healthy food.

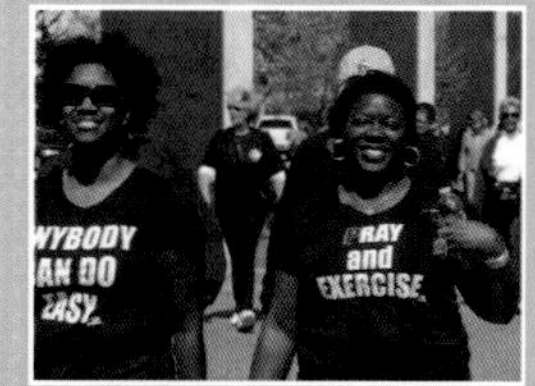

- Healthy food became easier to find in some of Nashville's food desert neighborhoods. Four corner markets began carrying and promoting fresh produce, whole grain bread, and low fat dairy products.

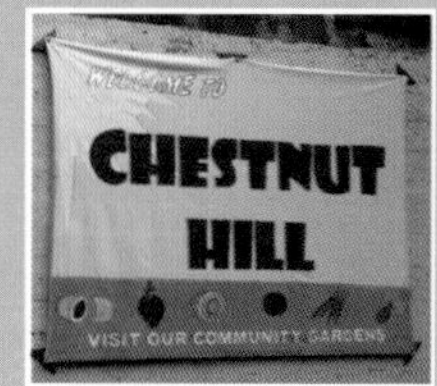

- Four out of Nashville's five birthing hospitals committed to policies that create a more supportive environment for new mothers to choose to breastfeed. Local businesses and employers, as well as Metro government departments, took steps to accommodate breastfeeding.
- The Metro Health Department staff developed a toolkit to help employers promote healthy worksites. This "Prescription for a Healthy Workplace" is part of Mayor Dean's workplace challenge, which promotes sustainability and voluntarism, as well as healthy policies and practices at work. Metro departments and over 100 area businesses have taken up the challenge so far, many adopting policies supporting physical activity, active commuting, healthier food in the workplace, smoke-free worksites, and support for nursing moms.

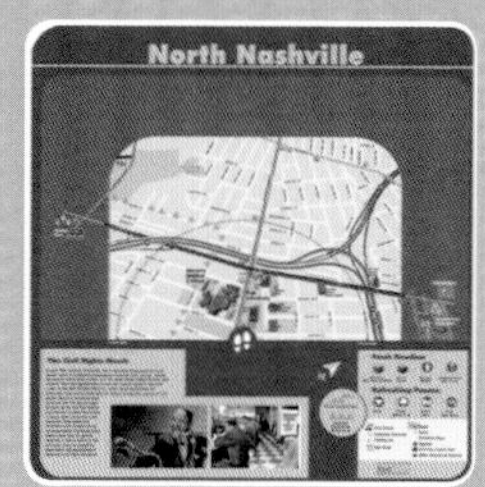

- Nashville's bike share program received major upgrades, including Nashville Green Bikes, which are free recreational bikes deployed mainly for use on greenways, and Nashville B-cycle, which offers commuter-oriented bikes deployed at transit stations, universities, and other key sites in the downtown and urban areas.

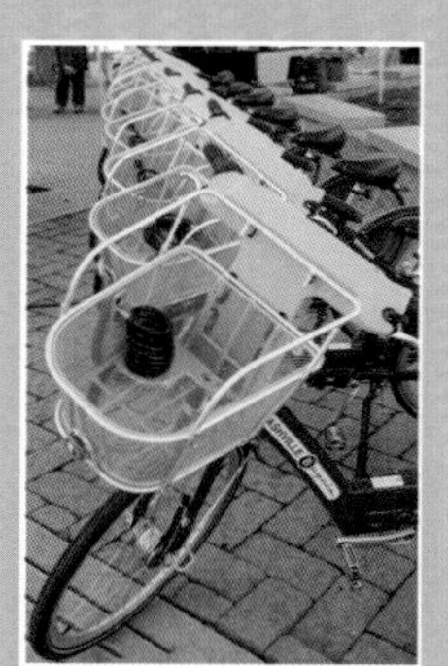

- To promote safer conditions for physical activity in neighborhoods plagued by loose animals, Metro Public Health helped bring partners together so that the Nashville Humane Association could more effectively make no-charge spay and neuter services available in high-need areas of the city where animals running at large cause a public safety problem.

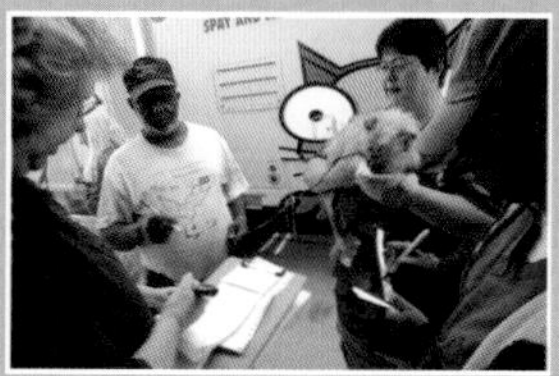

Mayor Karl Dean heading the pack at the Mayor's 5K Challenge. Dean personally led other high-profile, high-impact initiatives, such as the Walk 100 Miles Challenge. He also made significant commitments to making Nashville's infrastructure healthier, including acquisition of open space for permanent preservation, budget commitments to sidewalks and greenways, and a complete streets policy to make public rights-of-way more supportive of pedestrians, cyclists, and transit. *(2011: Gary Layda)*

NashVitality logo. *(2010: Metro Public Health Department)*

Community gardens help teach students about growing fresh foods. *(2013: GROW program)*

Walk for health by a faith-based organization. *(2012: Metro Public Health Department)*

Gateway signage for the Chestnut Hill neighborhood expresses the collective pride in the community's gardens. *(2013)*

The CPPW team developed signs and maps that highlight healthy places in Nashville and safe ways to walk and bike to destinations. *(Signage, 2013: Nashville Public Works)*

B-cycle Station at the Downtown Public Square. *(2012: Gary Layda)*

Mobile spay and neuter clinics. *(2011: Metro Public Health Department)*

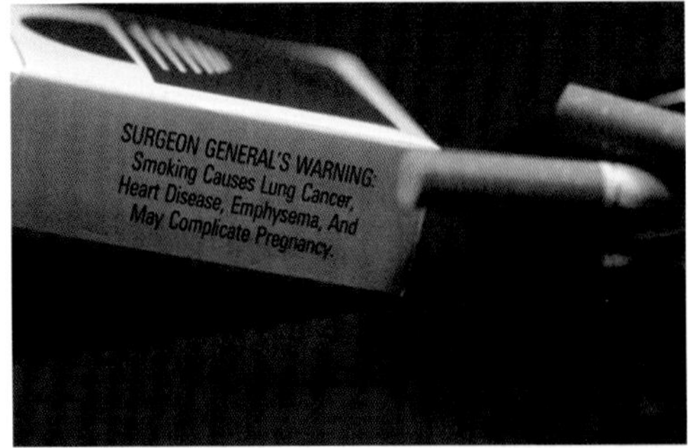

The US Surgeon General's warning about the ill effects of smoking now appears on every pack. *(n.d.: Centers for Disease Control and Prevention)*

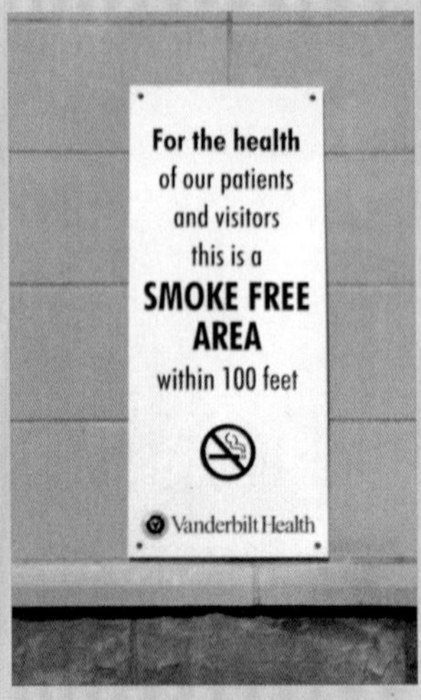

Vanderbilt University Medical Center prevents smoking within 100 feet of hospital and clinic entrances. *(2013)*

PRESCRIPTION: WHAT WORKS?

Improving our health will take both personal responsibility and community action. We routinely make choices as a community to address problems that individuals cannot or should not have to solve individually. We create schools, support police and fire departments, and build roads with signs and guardrails, all in an effort to improve our public safety. Rather than educating every person to boil every drop of water he or she drinks, we invest in clean potable water for everyone.

Individual medical care is expensive and is not a sure path toward better health. Some people argue that individual education and personal responsibility are the only strategies we need. These strategies are important, but they have not turned the tide.

A lesson from tobacco is that unhealthy behaviors can become less common, but it takes more than individual responsibility and education. After all, educational efforts to reduce smoking had little effect. It was policy and environmental changes that helped actually reduce the percentage of people who smoke.

Tobacco taxes, laws that reduce nonsmoker's exposure to smoke, hard-hitting marketing that shows the dangers of smoking, and policies that limit access to tobacco contributed to a decline in smoking; many lives have been saved as a result. A large component of what worked for limiting tobacco was a focus on creating healthier places. Public places and workplaces are now smoke-free, and the number of places that allow smoking continues to shrink. The State of Tennessee provides printable signs for businesses to post informing patrons about the laws regarding smoking indoors.

Public health officials have been talking about exercise and healthy food for generations, but it is clear that the battle against obesity's health toll has not been won with talk and education alone. For obesity prevention, change will not be simple. We cannot recommend that anyone quit eating. The roots of the obesity epidemic are intertwined with agriculture policy that subsidizes production of fattening foods, food marketing and availability, the design of our communities, and our ingrained habits. There will not be one single magic bullet; no one intervention is likely to turn the situation around in a few short years.

Even though this is a complex issue, we can and must take action. There are several resources that point communities toward doing "what works" for prevention of obesity and chronic disease.[21] The common denominator in many of the reports and recommendations is that healthy living needs to be built into everyday life. If opportunities to be healthy are ubiquitous, woven into the fabric of the city, and supported by a rich network of social support and encouragement, our health will improve. The automatic or default choices need to be healthy choices. Our health will continue to decline and our medical costs will continue to skyrocket if staying healthy is an uphill slog on a narrow path. Currently, individuals are surrounded by unhealthy choices and sternly admonished to seek out the inconvenient, unaffordable choices that require heroic willpower.

How do we weave healthy choices into the fabric of the city? By intentionally and systematically making decisions that favor safety, routine physical activity, and access to healthy food. Whenever we have an opportunity to shape our neighborhoods, streets, schools, workplaces, and places of worship, we must change policies, systems, and the environment to create healthier conditions everywhere.

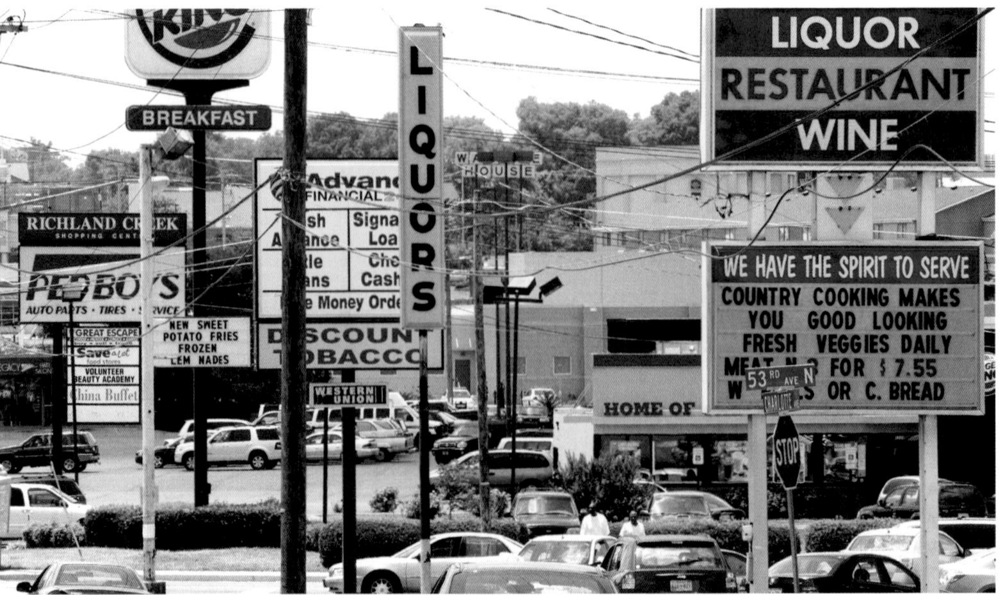

Built environments that create a negative atmosphere for health—little or no walkability, unhealthy food and beverage choices—are a way of life on Davidson County's commercial corridors. *(2012: Gary Layda)*

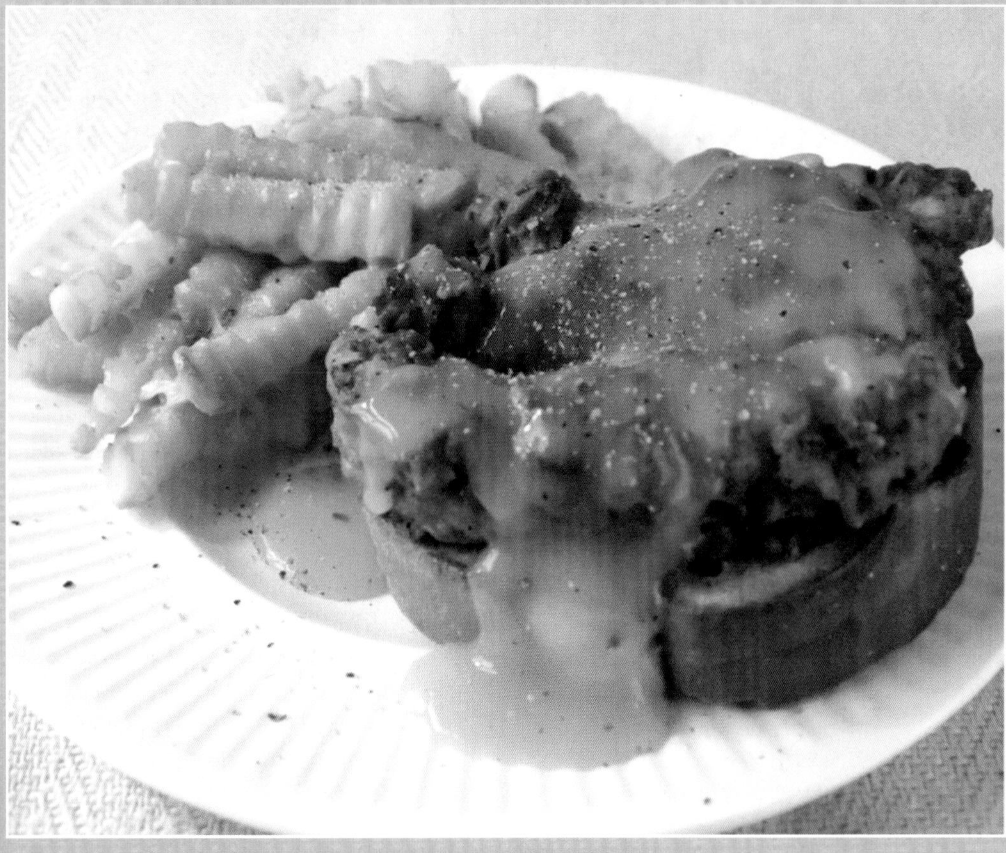

The all-American, all-fried meal.
(2015: Teresa Blackburn)

Smothered in Cheese and Swimming in Gravy

In June of 2013, the American Medical Association formally classified obesity as a disease. Critics of the new policy warned that abruptly declaring one-third of Americans—the estimated number of our citizens with a body mass index of 30 or higher—"ill" or "sick" would lead to a reliance on drugs or surgery for treatment, rather than lifestyle changes. In "Why Labeling Obesity as a Disease is a Big Mistake,"[22] however, Geoffrey Kabat suggests that what needs treating is "what has been called the 'obesogenic' society."

I encountered this society at its most ponderous during a cross-country road trip. Let me explain that my husband and I were traveling with our three dogs and one cat, which condemned us to nights in the only kind of motels that tolerate menageries: cheap. Nearby dining options were equally economical. We foreswore the usual assortment of fast food franchises, reasoning that we had a fighting chance to garner a salad with dressing on the side and a fish that was poached or grilled in places that serve food on plates rather than encased in Styrofoam.

In the so-called "heartland," however, we usually searched in vain for items that were un-fried, uncheesed, or meatless. Here's a sampling from the menu of a Nebraska eatery that touts its "homestyle cookin'."

- "Thick cut all-beef bologna fried and served on a toasted brioche bun [*sic*]," with two slices of American cheese, breaded and deep-fried pickles, and a separate plate of "fresh fried tater chips."
- "Farmboy Omelet" (three eggs) is "stuffed" with "spicy sausage, diced potatoes and melted American cheese" then "drowned" in sausage gravy and topped with shredded cheese.
- "Big Texas Burger: Two tasty patties stacked high with onion rings and American cheese, all served between two grilled cheese Texas toast sandwiches."

Mac and cheese comes embedded with chunks of bacon and chicken. The BLT sports "an incredible eight strips of bacon," with chicken an optional add-on. Fries are "smothered" with chili and cheese, the "loaded" baked potato "heaped" with cheese and bacon. Even the "Pot Roast Hash" is served "covered in cheddar."

And then there's "The Big Max," whose promo is set off in a special box. "Think climbing Mount Everest is a challenge? Well, try this one on for size. Two pounds of ground beef on a large homemade bun topped with choice toppers. Four pounds total!!! Are you tough enough to try? If you can polish this baby off in less than an hour, we'll give you a free shirt and hang your picture on the wall."

No mention is made of the fact that you'd have to scale Everest to work off Max's calories.

Kabat writes: "We tend to over-estimate and idealize what the individual can do by resisting the prevailing current." When that current is one of melted cheese and sausage gravy, the swimmers in it are going to find themselves stuffed, smothered, and drowned.

—CHRISTINE KREYLING

This article originally appeared in *Nfocus Magazine,* August 2013.

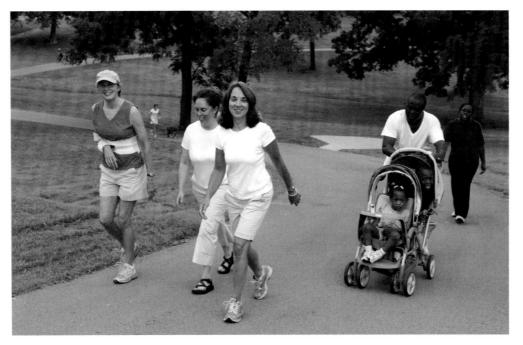

A Mayor's Walk and Bike Ride on the Stones River Greenway. Built environments that provide opportunities for physical activity and social interaction can play a role in creating positive health outcomes. *(2010: Gary Layda)*

FITNESS VERSUS FATNESS: UNDERSTANDING AND PREVENTING OBESITY

Most people think of obesity as a personal issue. When the topic comes up, the conversation turns toward lifestyle choices and weight loss. Personal responsibility for health behaviors is important, but it is hard to fathom how our current situation—where a majority of Americans are overweight or obese—could have resulted from a surge in personal irresponsibility affecting almost every corner of our society.

Gaining weight is easy

Obesity rates started climbing in the US in the 1970s.[23] There have been many changes in our culture and environment that have made it easy to consume excess calories, get less physical activity, and gain unhealthy pounds.[24] The rise of automobile dependence altered the design of our lives and our communities so that we hardly ever need to walk. Additionally, long hours watching television, fewer meals cooked at home, the rise of fast food, increasing portion sizes, proliferation of sweetened beverages, the convenience of drive-through restaurants, labor-saving household devices such as clothes dryers and even electric window and door openers, are some of the many cultural and environmental changes that contribute to a rise in obesity rates. All of these factors create the "obesogenic environment," an environment that promotes weight gain and deters weight loss. We do not have to point to massive character flaws linked to unhealthy weight gain. It seems as though everywhere we turn there is an opportunity to get fatter. According to a recent review in *The Lancet,*[25] people are reacting normally to an "obesogenic environment."

Losing weight is difficult

There are many weight loss strategies out there—usually a combination of eating fewer calories and burning more by being physically active. But as almost anyone who has shed pounds can attest, people who intentionally lose weight are seriously challenged to keep from regaining it. The reasons, which defy conventional thinking that only focuses on willpower, have just recently begun to emerge.

Dietary researchers such as Dr. David Ludwig of Boston Children's Hospital have conducted studies that seem to counter the simple wisdom of "a calorie is a calorie." Diets high in carbohydrates, especially refined carbohydrates and

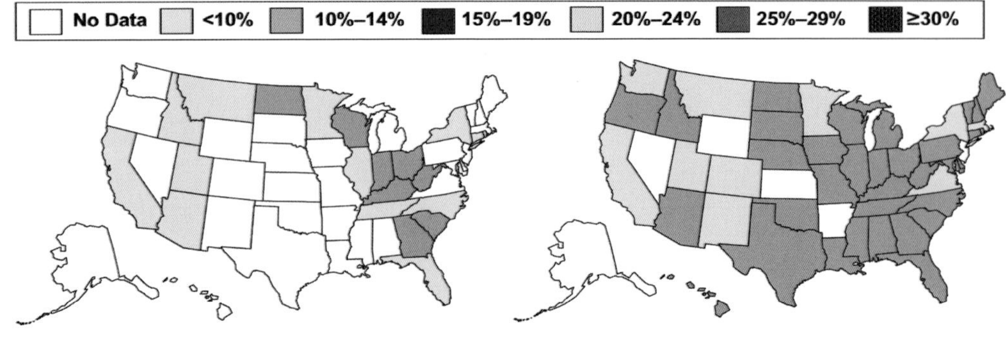

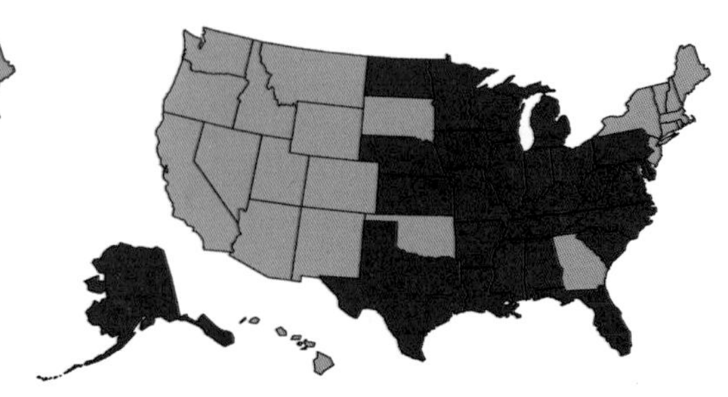

Obesity trends among US adults between 1985 and 2010. Note: each map represents five years of change. *(Maps, 2010: Centers for Disease Control and Prevention)*

sugars, exacerbate hunger and reduce metabolism—exactly what you don't want to happen if you are trying to keep weight off.[26]

There is also the observation that the human body seems to adapt to weight loss by fighting to regain the poundage, as if the body were starving. "Researchers have known for decades that the body undergoes various metabolic and hormonal changes while it's losing weight," writes Tara Parker-Pope in a 2011 article in the *New York Times*.[27] These changes inhibit the body's expenditure of energy, while at the same time increasing appetite—just like the body on the high carb diet. An Australian study discovered that these changes persisted for a year following weight loss, even after people began to regain the weight they lost.[28] These findings suggest, according to the Australian research team, "The high rate of relapse among obese people who have lost weight has a strong physiological basis and is not simply the result of the voluntary resumption of old habits."

Rena Wing, a professor of psychiatry and human behavior at Brown University's Alpert Medical School and co-founder of the National Weight Control Registry, admits that these physiological changes probably do occur. But for Wing, the larger problem is environmental. "We live in an environment with food cues all the time," Wing says. "We've taught ourselves over the years that one of the ways to reward ourselves is with food. It's hard to change the environment and the behavior."[29]

So for weight loss to be successful, a person must avoid foods that exacerbate hunger and overcome a strong biological push to regain lost weight, while navigating a food environment that is flooded with cues to eat.

Preventing excess weight gain

Because weight loss is difficult, prevention of unhealthy weight gain is important for everyone, not just those with an identified weight or health problem. Setting the course for a lifetime of healthy weight should begin in infancy and early childhood. Studies point to breastfed babies being at lower risk for obesity, while bottle-fed infants who begin solid food before four months of age have a six-fold risk of being obese at age three.[30]

Prevention for infants and children depends not on their knowledge or responsibility, but on the choices that adults in their lives offer them. Children need to be offered healthy food and routine physical activity, rather than a diet of high-calorie junk food and unlimited screen time.

Fitness trumps fatness

Once the pounds are on, it is difficult for most people to slim down to a "normal" weight, but even modest weight loss can have health benefits. Long-term studies show that a sustained moderate weight loss of just 10 percent improves control of blood sugar and high blood pressure, and can improve cholesterol levels and heart function.[31]

There is evidence that improved cardio respiratory fitness—one result of regular physical activity—can reduce many of the health hazards of obesity, even without weight loss. The Aerobic Center Longitudinal Study followed over 80,000 people over a period of 35 years. In one analysis of this study, mortality was measured in fit versus unfit men in three weight categories. The risk of death was lower for obese, fit men than for lean men who were not fit. It was better to be "fat and fit" than "unfat and unfit." Further, those who were "fat and fit" experienced rates of early death similar to the rates for normal-weight people.[32] This finding supports the notion that, even if a person does not lose weight, many of the health hazards of obesity can be erased by routine physical activity.

Gaining weight is easy. Losing weight is difficult. As communities aim to address the obesity epidemic, focusing solely on helping obese individuals lose weight will fall short. Our strategies should prevent unhealthy weight gain in the first place, and also improve fitness and health for those who are now overweight and obese, whether they achieve weight loss or not. Successful solutions will not focus on obesity, but on creating healthier food environments and opportunities for everyone to be physically active as part of their everyday routine, no matter their age or how they are shaped.

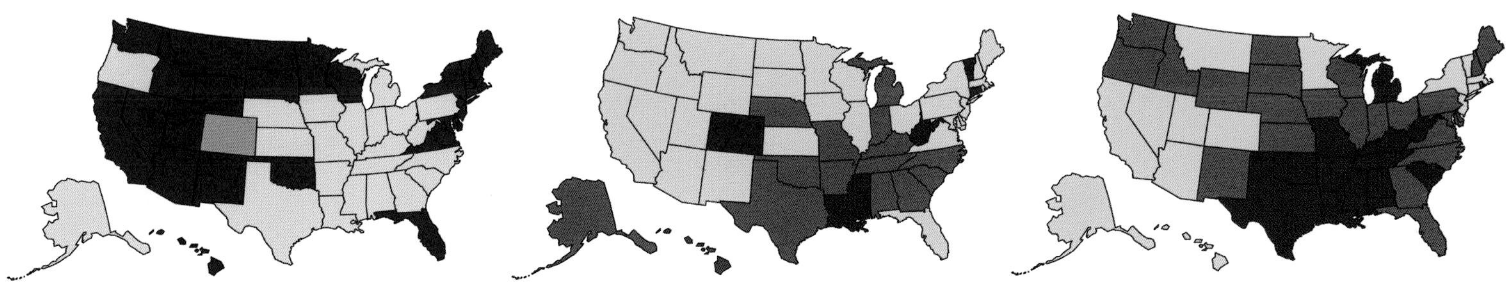

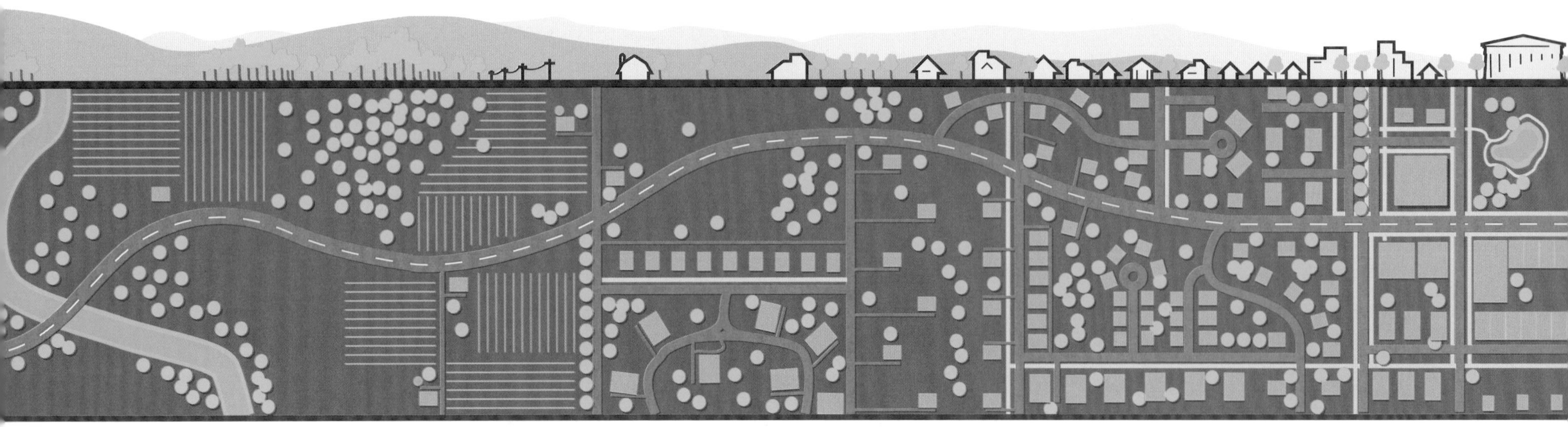

Shaping THE HEALTHY COMMUNITY

THE NASHVILLE PLAN

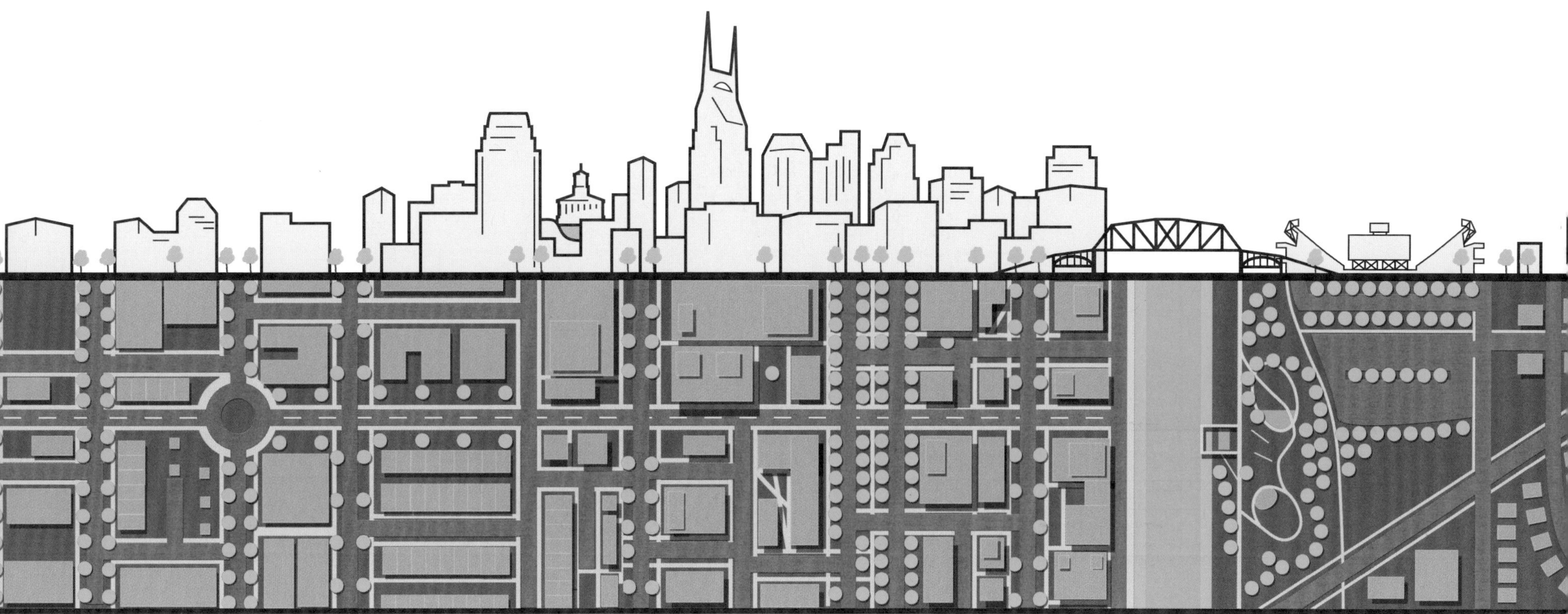

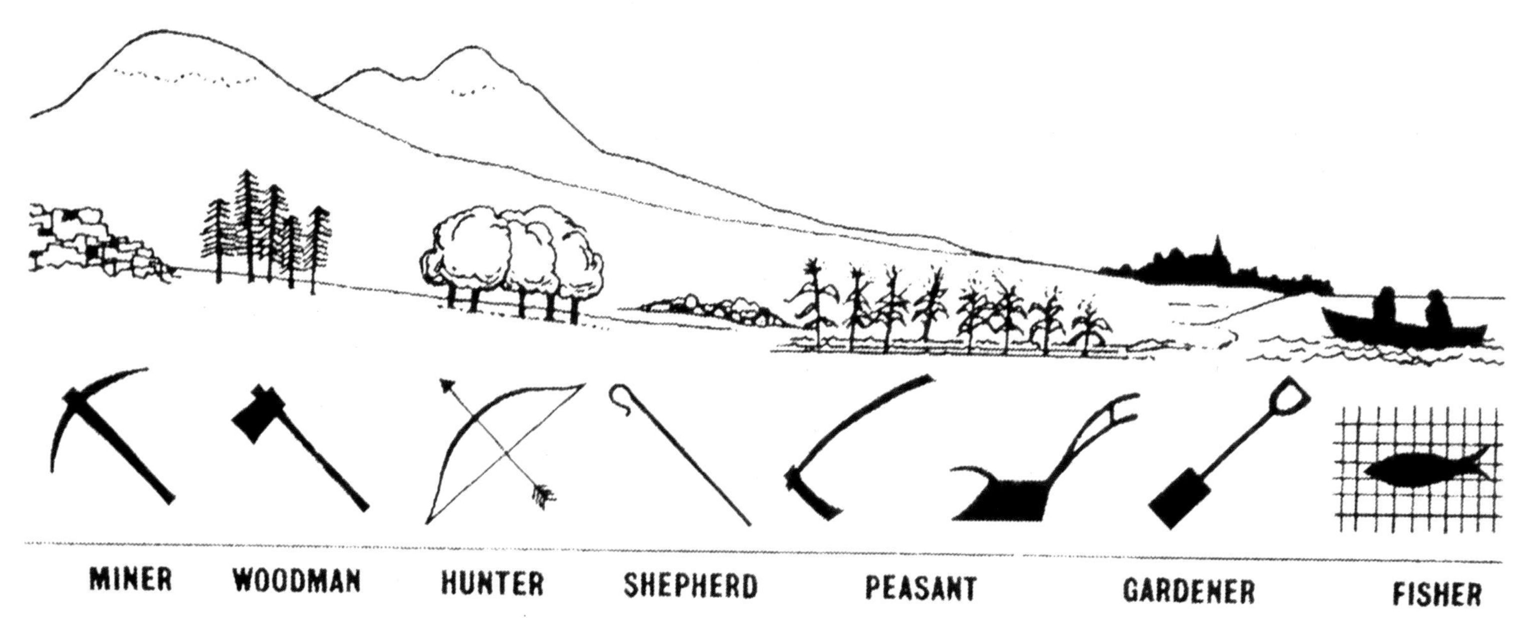
MINER
WOODMAN
HUNTER
SHEPHERD
PEASANT
GARDENER
FISHER

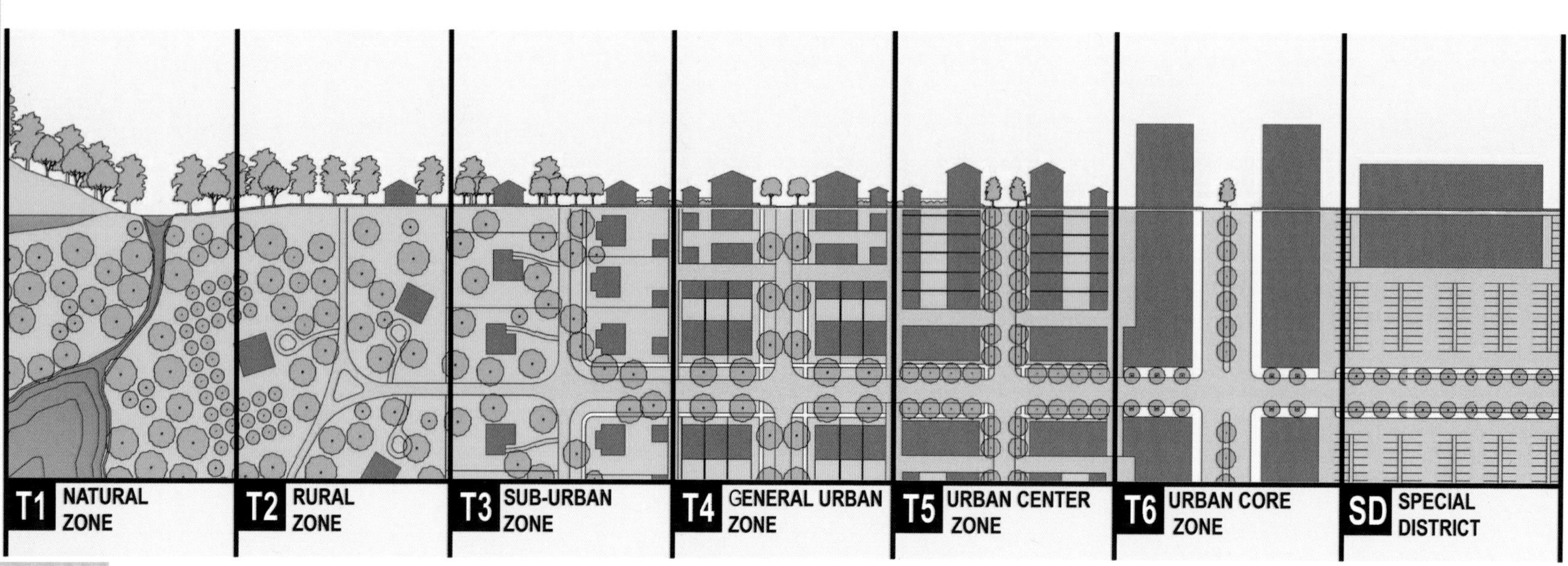
T1 NATURAL ZONE
T2 RURAL ZONE
T3 SUB-URBAN ZONE
T4 GENERAL URBAN ZONE
T5 URBAN CENTER ZONE
T6 URBAN CORE ZONE
SD SPECIAL DISTRICT

THE TRANSECT

The verb "transect" means to cut or divide crossways or transversely, as in slicing through the rings of a tree. In the natural sciences the noun is used to refer to a selected strip of land that exhibits a range of habitats in order to measure and monitor the distribution of plant or animal populations within a given area.

But human beings also have habitats in which they thrive or decline. In the 19th century, industrialization dramatically altered human living conditions. The Scottish biologist and sociologist Patrick Geddes (1854–1932) was one of the first to link this new habitat with negative social outcomes: poverty, disease, and crime.[1]

Geddes believed, along with the influential English art and social critic John Ruskin, that just as the evolution of animals and plants is influenced by habitat, so also human social behavior is related to the spatial form in which it occurs. By the same kind of careful observation scientists devote to the natural world, therefore, social scientists could determine the intimate and causal connections between the social development of the individual and the cultural and physical environment.

Geddes thought it was possible to improve social outcomes by changing the spatial form in which people lived. His illustration of the relationship between human settlement and natural context, called the "Valley Section," was the precursor of the application of the concept of the transect to urban planning.

Fast forward to the late 1990s, when New Urbanists Andres Duany and Elizabeth Plater-Zyberk (firm: DPZ) developed a categorization system that organizes the elements of the human environment on a scale from the natural and least developed to the densest urban spaces. They called this system the "Transect."[2]

Duany and Plater-Zyberk were responding to the then-prevalent method of categorization by land use and density. They thought that the *form* of development impacted how people functioned within it and that separated-use zoning systems encouraged a car-dependent culture and land-consuming sprawl.

Duany and Plater-Zyberk studied walkable American development patterns—the traditional neighborhood or small town established before the automobile became the dominant mode of personal transportation. They found that transects within towns and city neighborhoods revealed areas that were less urban and more urban in character. This urbanism could be analyzed as natural transects are analyzed.

From their analysis DPZ produced an alternative model for a zoning code. The seven transect zones provide the basis for neighborhood structure, which requires walkable streets, a mixture of land uses, transportation options, and housing diversity. The T-zones vary by the ratio and level of intensity of their natural, built, and social components. Because the zones are based on the physical form of the built and natural environment, this transect-based code is called a form-based code. The model code, the SmartCode, was released by DPZ in 2003.[3]

The transect forms the basic armature of *Shaping the Healthy Community: The Nashville Plan*. This is in part because the transect recognizes distinct forms of settlement patterns. And inducing healthier behavior requires tailoring strategies to the specifics of each context in order for them to be effective. What applies to downtown would not work in a rural setting.

In addition, Metro Nashville's Planning Department uses the transect system as the basic planning tool in its new General Plan, *NashvilleNext*, as well as in its *Community Character Manual*, to guide new development. Thus the strategies proposed here can be easily adapted to planning efforts, in particular to assess the health impacts of specific development proposals.

Because of their farm-to-market ancestry, Nashville's pikes are radial in character and often exhibit the spectrum of transect zones from rural to downtown core. (Charlotte Pike is probably the best example of this phenomenon.) These pikes are a focus of this book because they present the greatest opportunity for reshaping the built environment of Nashville with more transit-oriented development.

Top: Geddes' Valley Section from ridgeline to shoreline. It is the first transect to show natural conditions with their associated human presence, presented only in terms of exploitation—a 19th-century conception. *(Diagram, 2008: Duany Plater-Zyberk & Company)*

Bottom: Natural–urban core transect illustration with elements drawn in section above and plan below. *(Diagram, 2008: Duany Plater-Zyberk & Company)*

1 2 3 4 5 6 7

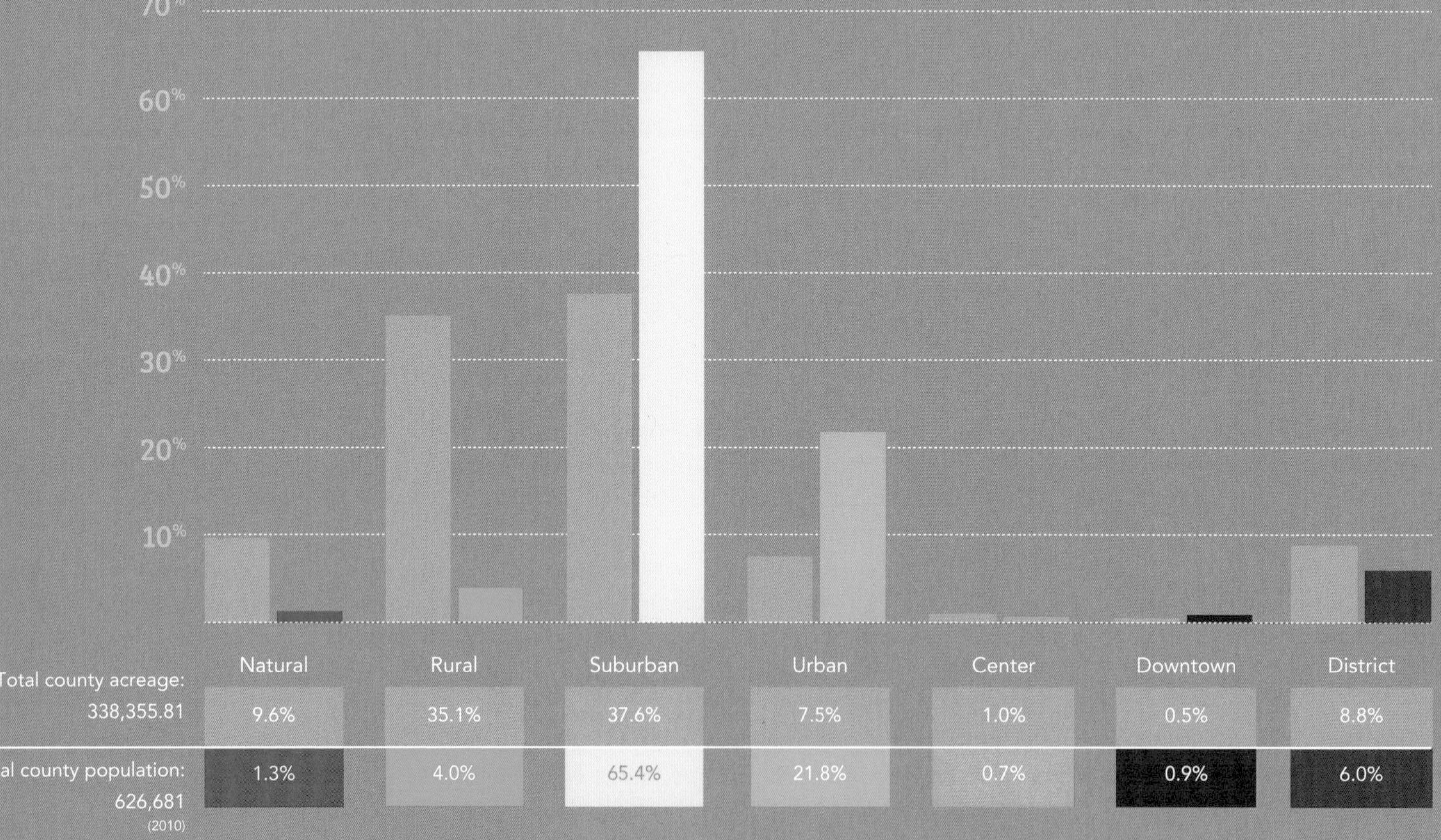

	Natural	Rural	Suburban	Urban	Center	Downtown	District
Total county acreage: 338,355.81	9.6%	35.1%	37.6%	7.5%	1.0%	0.5%	8.8%
Total county population: 626,681 (2010)	1.3%	4.0%	65.4%	21.8%	0.7%	0.9%	6.0%

These statistics show the population and size of each transect zone. That the suburban zone has the highest population of any zone and occupies the most land indicates that this development pattern is the dominant one in Nashville. This fact represents the most significant challenge in reshaping Nashville's built environment to be a more health-enabling one.

(Table, 2013: Metro Planning Department)

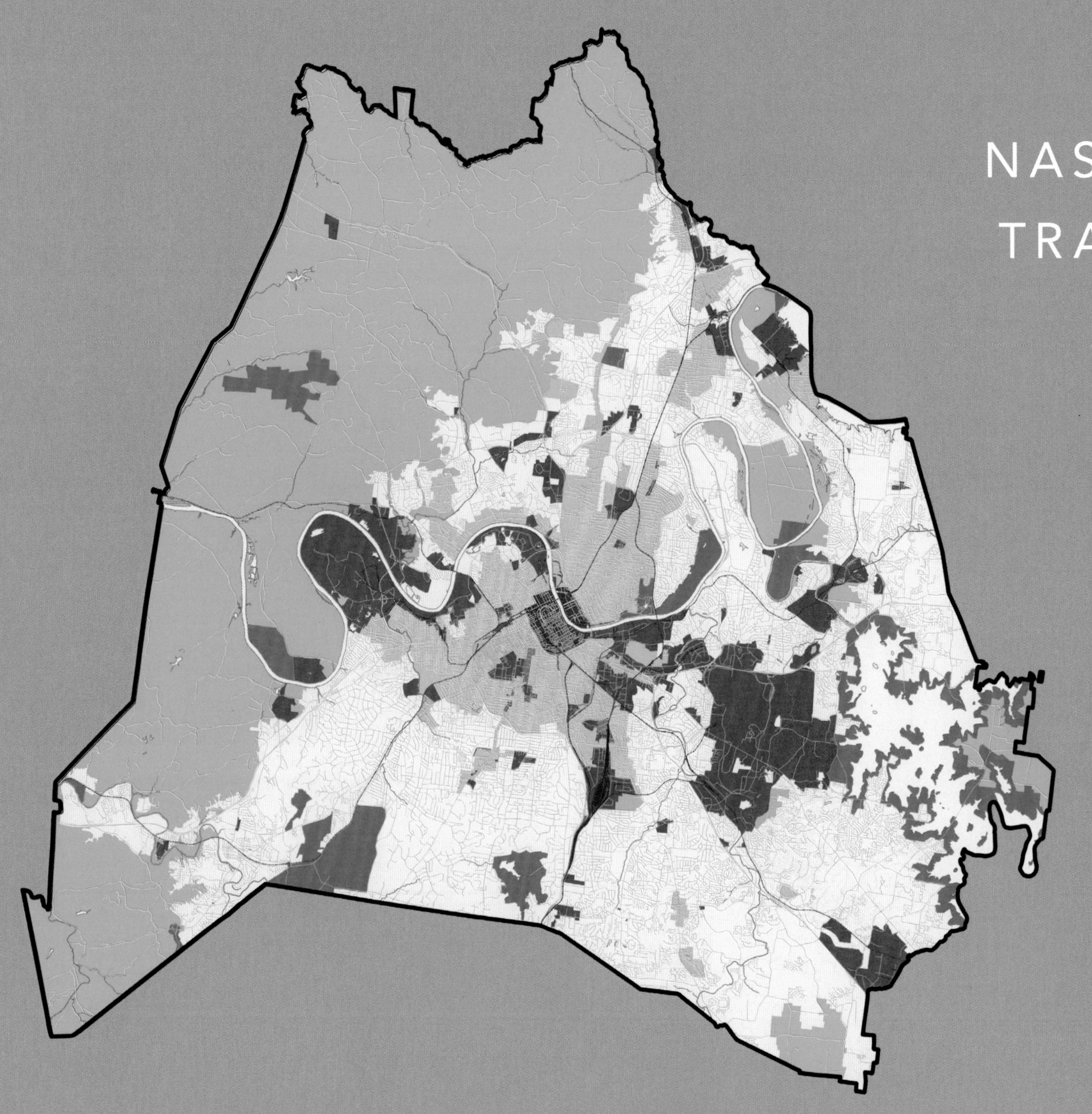

THE NASHVILLE TRANSECT

Davidson County with transect zones highlighted. Note: descriptions and historical evolutions of individual zones within the transect are contained in the subsequent chapters devoted to each zone. (Map, 2014: Metro Planning Department)

THE FACTORS

The Nashville Civic Design Center staff conducted a review of national and international research literature and determined six aspects of the built environment within all zones of the transect that impact health. These are called "factors."

These factors are used zone by zone to analyze and evaluate quality-of-health issues in Nashville. Each factor plays a part in shaping daily life. By continually improving their positive impact, we can make our city healthier for all our residents.

NEIGHBORHOOD DESIGN AND DEVELOPMENT

TRANSPORTATION

WALKABILITY AND PEDESTRIAN SAFETY

FOOD RESOURCES

HOUSING

OPEN SPACE AND PARKS

NEIGHBORHOOD DESIGN AND DEVELOPMENT

Neighborhoods look and function differently in rural, suburban, and urban areas. But each neighborhood, while different in form, contains the same factors or ingredients.

How these factors are exhibited—their relative strength or weakness—reflects design and development choices made in response to history, culture, economics, and politics. Thus suburban communities, designed to be auto-centric, typically lack the multimodal transportation connectivity present in urban neighborhoods. And the low population density of traditional rural communities determines the relative absence of proximity to goods and services when compared with suburban and urban neighborhoods.

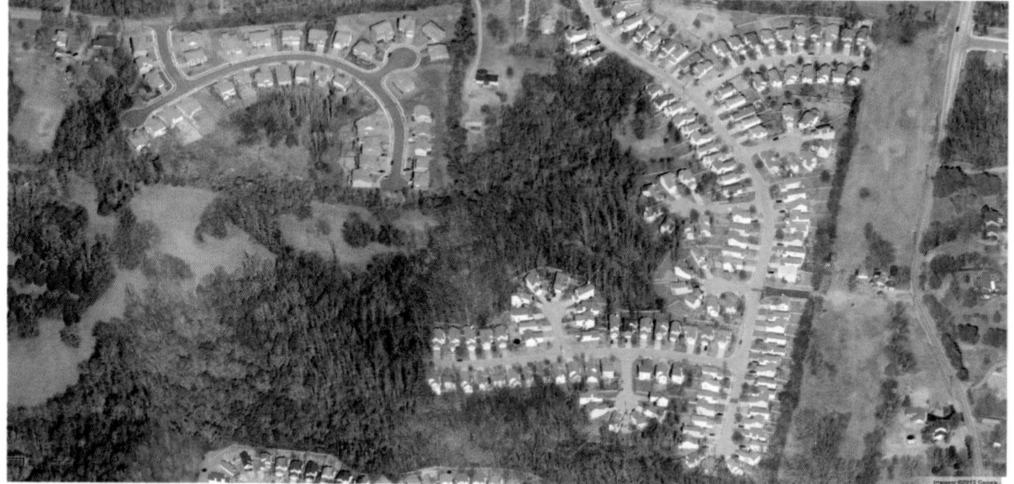

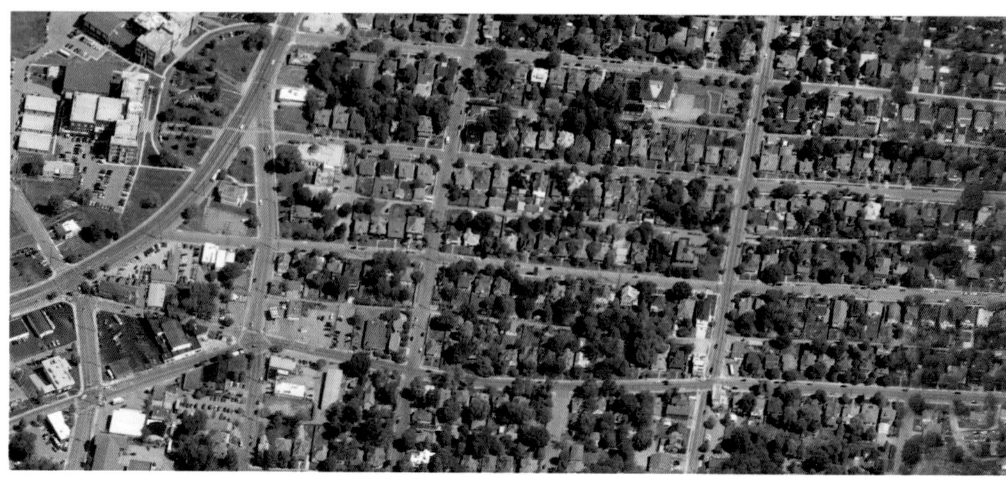

Aerials illustrating the forms of suburban (Hermitage) and urban (East Nashville) transect zones in Nashville. *(2013: © Google)*

Urban Design and Daily Life: Learning from Madison, Wisconsin

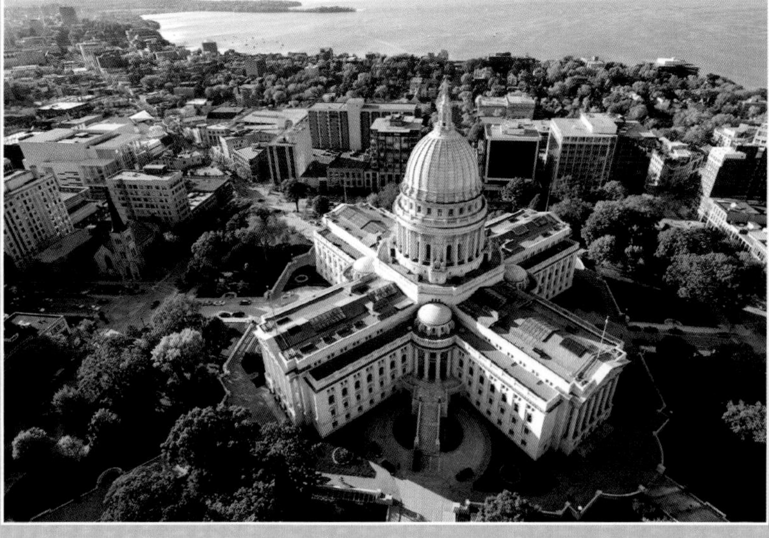

Aerial view of the Wisconsin State Capitol in downtown Madison, looking northwest. In the background, left to right: the University of Wisconsin-Madison campus, Picnic Point, and Lake Mendota. *(2011: Jeff Miller; © Board of Regents of the University of Wisconsin System)*

View of the Memorial Union from Lake Mendota. *(2014: Gary Gaston, NCDC)*

During the seven years I lived in Nashville (2002–2009), I enjoyed many of the things that are now garnering Nashville the reputation it deserves as a fun and interesting place to visit and live. My time in Nashville included graduate studies at Vanderbilt University's Peabody College in community research and action. I also worked on urban design, planning, and community development with the Nashville Civic Design Center and the Metropolitan Development and Housing Agency.

In the summer of 2009, I moved to Madison to teach and do research at the University of Wisconsin–Madison. I was eager to experience and understand Madison, a city with a strong reputation among urbanists, academics, and social activists. Upon arrival I was immediately struck by the contrasts in the built environments of Madison and Nashville and the ways these differences influence people's daily lives.

First, some background on Madison: Centered on a one-mile-wide and four-mile-long isthmus between two lakes, Madison is the state capital and home to the University of Wisconsin (1849). A city of approximately 240,000 residents within city limits containing less than one-fifth the land area of Nashville-Davidson County, Madison is the seat of Dane County, home to about 510,000 residents spread across more than twice the land area of Davidson County.

As these numbers suggest, Madison has a fairly densely populated downtown and, although the area does have suburban sprawl similar to most US cities, the degree of sprawl is not nearly as extensive as Nashville's. Unlike many small and mid-sized cities, the center of downtown Madison is the hub of most types of activity, and property values reflect this. Living in the heart of the city is more expensive than living in most of the surrounding suburbs.

The basic plan of Madison was established in the 1830s, prior to its selection as the state capital. Its design by civic booster James Doty, who had no professional training in architecture or urban planning, was influenced by Baroque principles.[4]

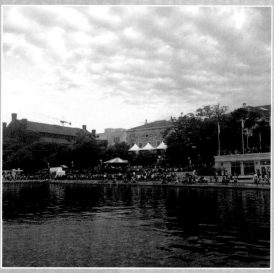

For instance, the city has streets emanating from the State Capitol in cardinal directions that intersect diagonally with the primary street grid, creating numerous Capitol vistas—similar to L'Enfant's plan for Washington, DC. Also like Washington, buildings in downtown are not permitted to be taller than the base of the Capitol's dome to preserve the building's visual dominance. Instead of the corporate towers, often with logos, that dominate most US cityscapes and emphasize the importance of enterprise and wealth, Madison's skyline is a reminder of democratic ideals.

The first professional designer to study the city was John Nolen, who graduated from the newly established Harvard School of Landscape Architecture after instruction by Frederick Law Olmsted Jr. In 1911 Nolen devised his plan for the future growth and development of Madison as both the capital of the state and the home of its university. This plan exerted particular influence on the city's park system.[5] Madison's faithfulness to these early plans has served the city well.

When I host visitors to Madison for a summer weekend I can offer them a wide array of activities. Our day might begin with a bike ride to the Capitol Square, the geographic and civic centerpiece of the city that serves as the site of the Saturday farmers' market, where nearly 200 independent vendors sell local produce and other foods. From there we can walk down State Street, a one-mile stretch of shops, restaurants, bars, and sidewalk cafes that connects the Capitol and the University campus and is off-limits to private automobiles. The primary campus destination is the Memorial Union, which sits on the shore of Lake Mendota and boasts a large public terrace occupied during the summer by people picnicking or taking in free music performances or movie showings. There is also access to the lake for swimming, canoeing, windsurfing, sailing, and paddle boarding.

In sharp contrast with Nashville, no limited-access highways come through or near the city center. Large surface parking lots are also a rarity in downtown Madison. Thus the numerous neighborhood festivals, public beaches, nature preserves, museums, and the free public zoo and botanical garden are all not only accessible by foot, but also enjoyable to walk to because they are

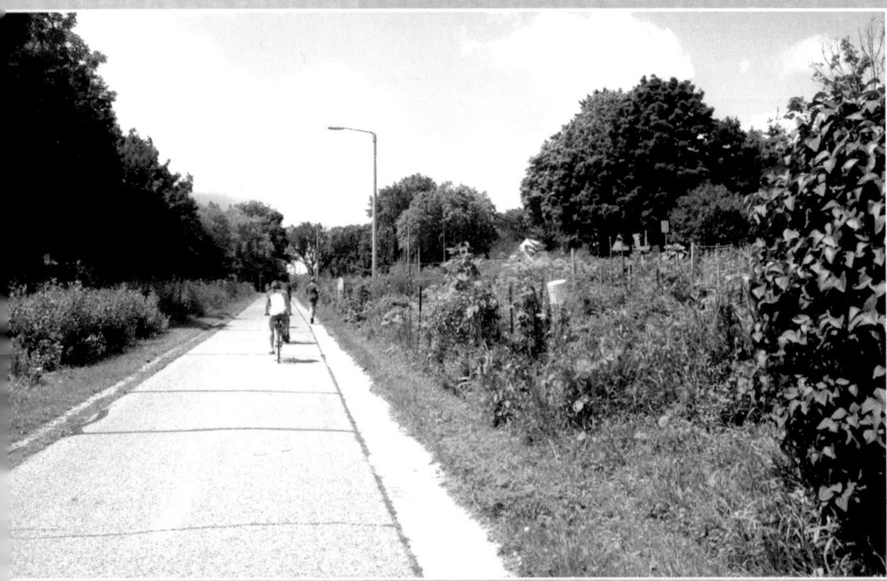

Two-way bike path through a community garden. *(2014: Gary Gaston)*

connected by contiguous urban fabric.

Madison has more parks and playgrounds per capita than any other US city and also tops the list for community garden plots per capita.[6] It also has some of the best urban bicycling infrastructure in the country,[7] including more than 200 miles of dedicated bike paths. These paths are heavily used throughout the summer for recreation as well as commuting, and are maintained in the winter for year-round bike commuters. The city's pedestrian infrastructure is also extensive and generally well maintained. Despite winter weather that can be extreme, many Madisonians remain active. Cross-country skiers and ice skaters take advantage of infrastructure that is designed and maintained for those seasonal uses. Ice fishing, ice boating, and kite boarding across the frozen lakes provide further evidence of the extent to which physical activity is wired into at least some parts of the culture in the city.

Although Madison is continuing with attempts to enhance the livability of its built environment—for example, redeveloping formerly industrial properties running through the center of the isthmus and improving the water quality of its lakes—it already provides a good example of a mid-sized city that has implemented many of the urban design principles contained in this book and *The Plan of Nashville* before it. To explore the intersection of health and the built environment, then, we should ask: How does Madison compare with Nashville on indicators of health?

It's clear that on average, residents of Dane County, WI, are healthier than residents of Davidson County, TN, with lower rates of physical inactivity (18 percent Dane; 27 percent Davidson), adult obesity (25 percent Dane; 30 percent Davidson), smoking (14 percent Dane; 17 percent Davidson), and fewer daily long commutes made driving alone (22 percent Dane; 30 percent Davidson). A higher percentage of Dane county residents have access to recreational opportunities than do Davidson residents. These environmental and behavioral factors are associated with divergent health outcomes between the two counties. For example, Davidson's rates of diabetes and infant mortality are both nearly 50 percent higher than Dane's.[8]

A look at population characteristics, however, reveals that there are many other differences that may help account for divergences in health outcomes. Dane County's rate of child poverty (14 percent) is less than half of Davidson's rate (29 percent); median household income is higher in Dane ($61,790) than in Davidson ($46,676); and while whites make up about 60 percent of Davidson's population, they account for close to 85 percent of Dane's.

Despite Dane County's relatively small nonwhite population, however, it has some of the most extreme black-white disparities in education, employment, income, criminal justice, and health in the country. In 2011 the unemployment rate in Dane County was 4.8 percent for whites and 25.2 percent for blacks; the rate of child poverty was 5 percent for whites and a staggering 75 percent for blacks.[9] Through a variety of pathways, these socioeconomic inequities manifest as health disparities between races.[10]

Living in poverty in Dane County typically means living in suburban neighborhoods that are relatively disconnected from civic institutions, services, and the amenities and numerous recreational opportunities described above. Four times as many black women receive insufficient prenatal care as compared to the proportion for white women, and black teens living in Dane County are more than four times as likely to be arrested than their white peers. The disparity in arrests across races is even greater for adults.[11] These inequities compound (through the mechanisms that Dr. Bill Paul's chapter in this book describes) to create disparities in life expectancy. In Dane County's case, however, these disparities are even more highly correlated with race than they are in Davidson County.

Civic leaders and designers in Madison have invested considerable resources and creative energy to shape an urban environment capable of promoting well-being. The cityscape is a draw for new residents and visitors, and provides real benefits to many of the city's residents. Madison's inequities related to race, however, bring into focus the fact that even the best urban designs cannot meaningfully counteract the ill effects of poverty and racism, at least not by themselves.

Many in Madison are realizing that for the benefits of a healthy city to be widely shared, people must have real power to shape the environments and systems that impact their daily lives. As in many other places in the United States, public health and urban planning practitioners are studying community organizing and working with grassroots initiatives to understand how empowerment can relate to place-making and the relationships between place and well-being.

Thus there are two lessons that Nashville can learn from Madison. First, shaping the built environment so that it promotes walking, biking, and recreation can provide real community benefits, including improved health among residents. Second, considerations of power and equity must be central to these transformations, both in process and in outcomes, for their benefits to be widely shared. Both of these lessons will be critical for Nashville as it shapes a healthier city.

— BRIAN D. CHRISTENS, associate professor of human ecology, University of Wisconsin–Madison

TRANSPORTATION

Most Davidson County residents rely on cars for transportation. More active transportation forms, however, such as walking, biking, or catching a ride on public transit, aid in healthy living. Reducing auto dependency alleviates air pollution, increases physical activity, reduces stress, and increases mobility for those whose age or finances limit their ability to drive. Residents in urban areas need increased opportunities to walk or cycle between home and work, shopping, and school. Those in a more suburban context require better linkages between pedestrian/cycling routes and transit. Rural residents may carpool/vanpool.

Pedestrian, cyclist, and driver safety has impacted road design and led to the installation of traffic calming devices. Transit-oriented development (TOD), created through new construction or the adaptation of existing neighborhoods, is a method of planning that clusters development around existing or planned transit services, as well as cycling or walking pathways.

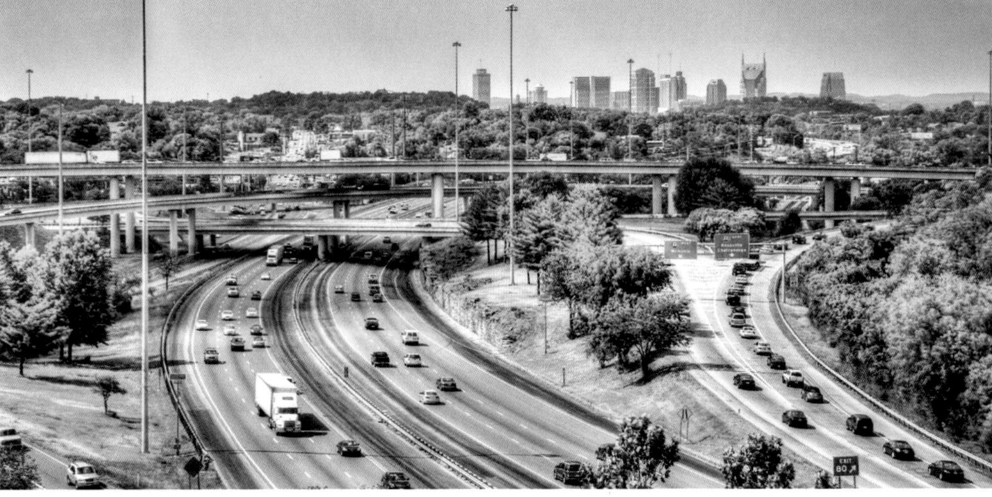

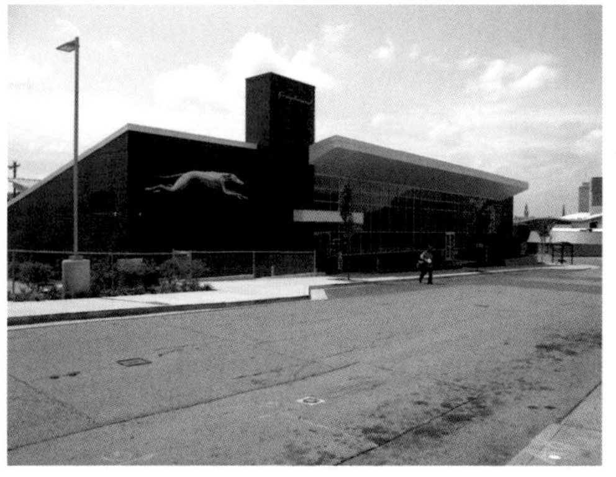

Nashville has the basic personal and commercial modes of transportation found in cities. The challenge for the built environment is to make it easier to use the ones that increase activity in daily life. *(2012–2015: NCDC; top left: 2012: Bruce Can, ElevatedLens.com)*

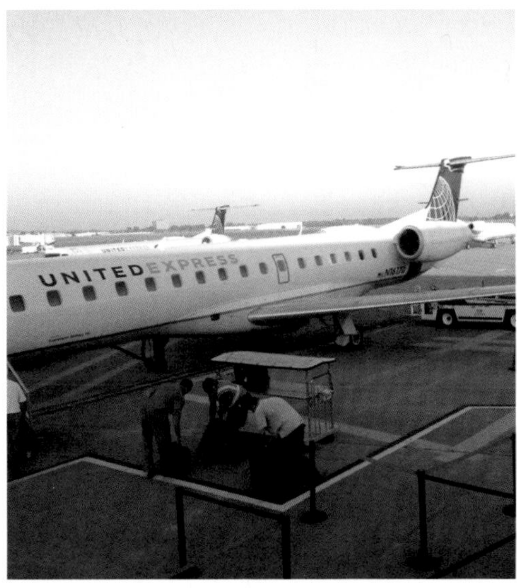

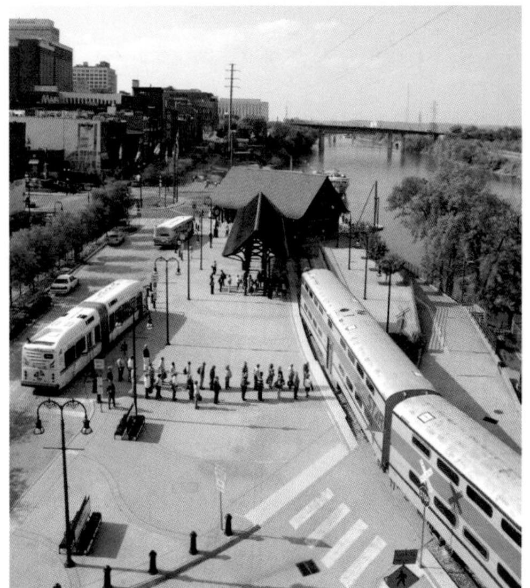

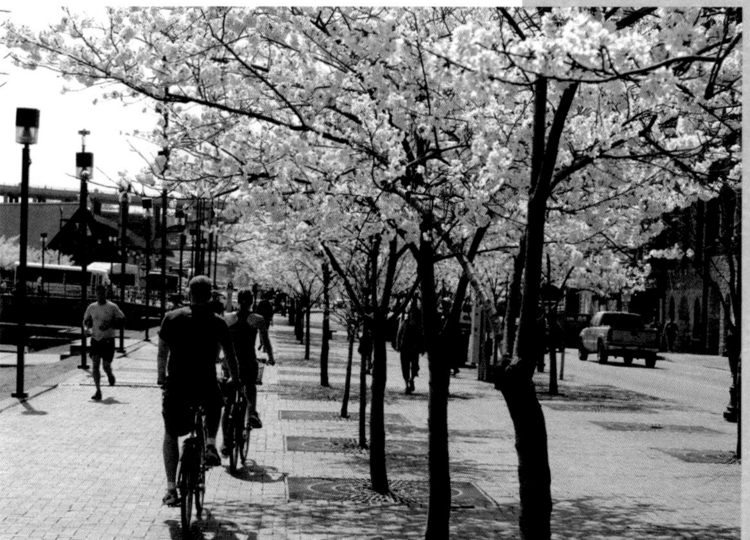

The Complete Street: Theory and Practice

The concept of complete streets to enable safe access for all users of all ages and abilities is an excellent goal. Benefits include safety, economic development, and health. From a safety perspective, studies show a dramatic reduction in accidents and severity of injury with the implementation of complete streets.[12] Economic development studies show that public investment within the right-of-way enhances the overall streetscape, improving property values and lease rates, and creating stronger neighborhoods.[13] Health is also improved: when citizens are offered safe and comfortable environments for walking and cycling, they are more likely to adopt daily habits using these modes of travel. And the environmental health of cities benefits from fewer car emissions and the added street trees and planting zones.

From typical street to complete street. A new half-mile segment of roadway constructed to complete street principles opened in Nashville's Gulch neighborhood in June 2015. *(2013: Hawkins Partners, Inc.; 2015)*

The realization of this goal, however, takes more than civic willpower.

Accommodating pedestrian, cyclist, automobile, and mass transit traffic all within the same right-of-way on every street may be desirable—and even achievable—in a greenfield situation. When open land is under development planners can allocate sufficient space for each mode of travel. The difficulty comes with retrofitting our existing cities, where street rights-of-way take up about one-third of our land area in urban areas and have carved out their dimensions through the years.

One hundred years ago, when the personal vehicle was not yet omnipresent, street rights-of-way were designed to balance the needs of vehicles, streetcars, and pedestrians. Many streets were also shaded with canopy trees, making the pedestrian environment attractive and comfortable.

In the second half of the 20th century, however, street design tilted out of balance. The car took over the street. Dimensions were determined by the goal of maximizing car capacity for mobility, ease of access, and turning movements.

Personal car storage also figures into rights-of-way in the form of on-street parking. These cars buffer the pedestrian from moving vehicles, providing more safety, and add to the city's coffers through parking meters. But privately owned parked cars occupy space that could be used for bike lanes, wider sidewalks, and street trees that benefit all.

In the last decade, planning for the bicycle and related bike infrastructure has been increasing, as has transit use. This rise of transportation alternatives to the passenger car coincides with statistics showing fewer and fewer American youth and young adults getting drivers' licenses, once thought an undeniable rite of passage.

Given the jockeying among all of the different users and their needs within the limited space, providing for all of them all of the time creates understandable conflicts within the developed city. Our existing urban rights-of-way are limited in width. Widening can cause unwelcome consequences, such as carving away valuable developable land or affecting historic or contextually important structures that are built to the edge of the right-of-way.

Many cities have developed creative ways of balancing all of these users within complete streets programs. Strategies include:

- "Road diets," in which, for example, a four-lane roadway is reconfigured to two vehicular travel lanes with a turn lane, giving back 10 to 12 feet for one of the other transportation modes. Vehicle lanes can also be reduced in width, from the once standard 12 feet wide—the width of an interstate lane—to as narrow as 10 feet. Width reduction has the added benefit of constricting vehicular speed, which increases pedestrian and cyclist safety and comfort level.
- Dedicated transit lanes enhance the speed and efficiency of this mode to make it more competitive with personal vehicles.
- "Bike boulevards" provide bicycle priority with a low-speed lane parallel to the dominant street or arterial. Protected bike lanes or cycle tracks, which are designed with physical buffers like landscaping or bollards between moving vehicles and cyclists, can be created by removing car lanes in road diet programs.
- The elimination of on-street parking on one or both sides of the street creates space for alternative transportation users. This strategy is sometimes difficult because of the income lost due to parking meter removal.

Ultimately, a complete streets approach is not necessarily about providing for every use in every street, but about the consideration of every use within the overall transportation network.

—KIM HAWKINS, Hawkins Partners Landscape Architects

WALKABILITY AND PEDESTRIAN SAFETY

Walking is a key component in an active lifestyle. The ability to walk easily and safely within a community is critical to achieving the recommended daily physical activity of 30 minutes for adults and 60 minutes for children.

A mixture of land uses—such as retail, schools, office, and other commercial destinations—within walking distance of residential areas enables pedestrian activity. Streets laid out in a fine-grained network make walking routes more direct and efficient, thus more inviting.

The built environment can encourage walking with wide, well-maintained sidewalks, crosswalks, minimal curb cuts, and traffic calming in pedestrian areas. Enhancements such as shade trees and street greenery improve the experience. Good, human-scaled lighting, animal control, and community engagement through watch organizations or neighbors sitting out on their front porches increase feelings of safety and security.

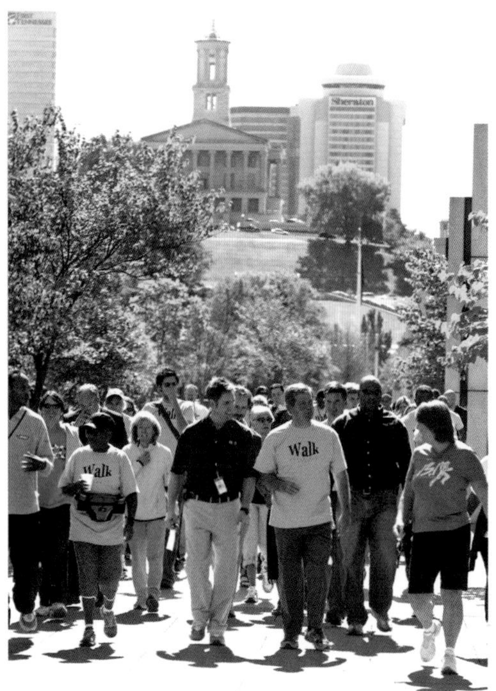

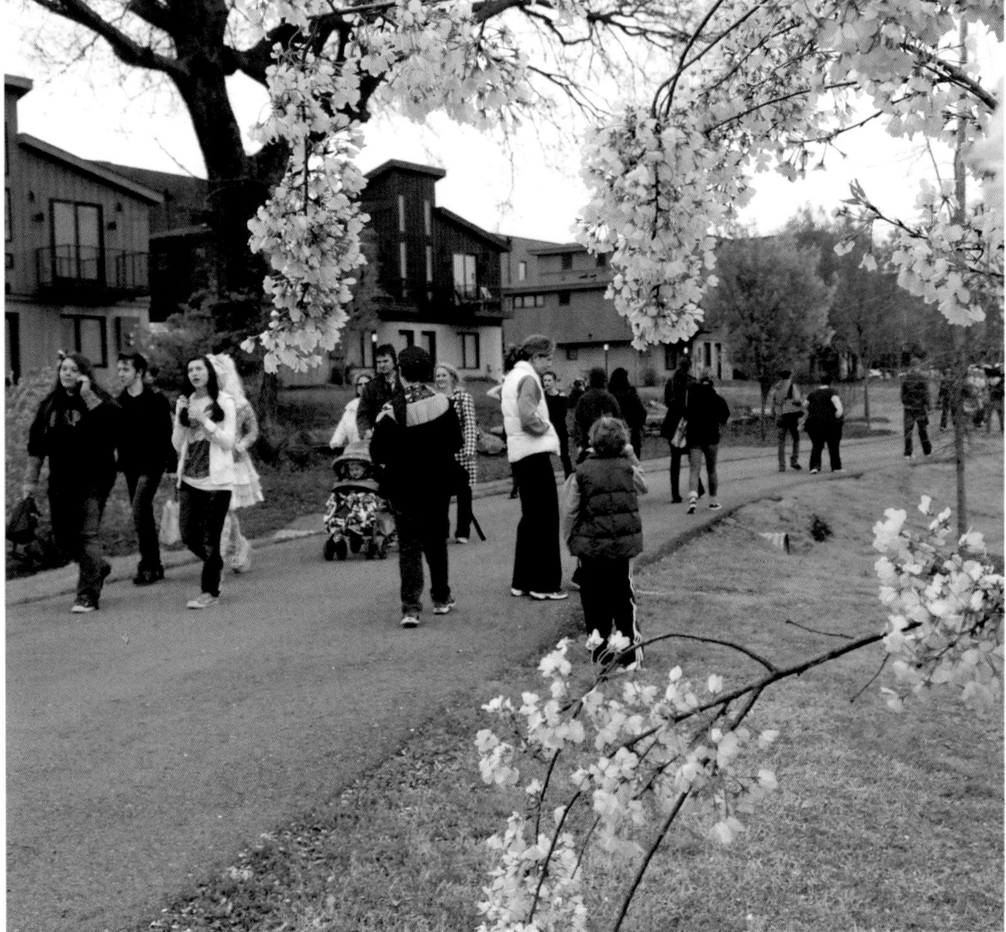

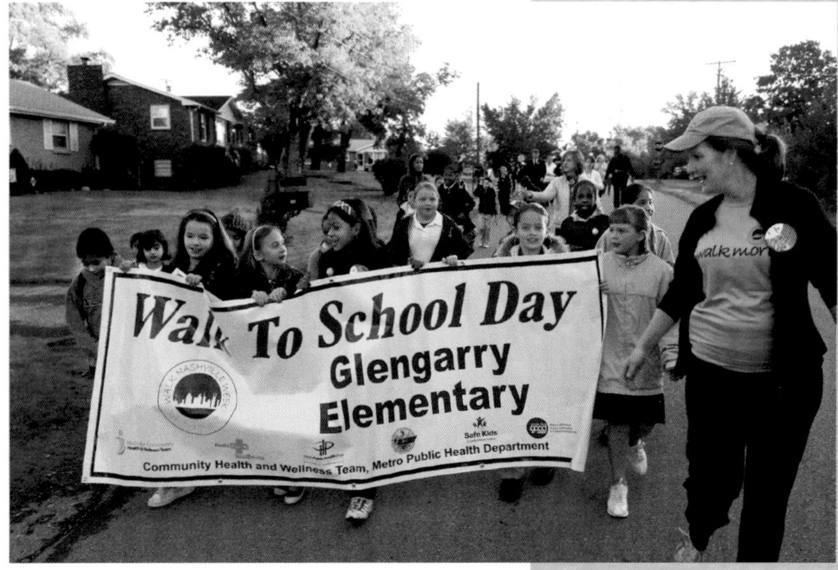

Nashville has walkable neighborhoods. For many Nashvillians, however, walking is a staged special event and not part of daily life. *(2009–2013: Gary Layda)*

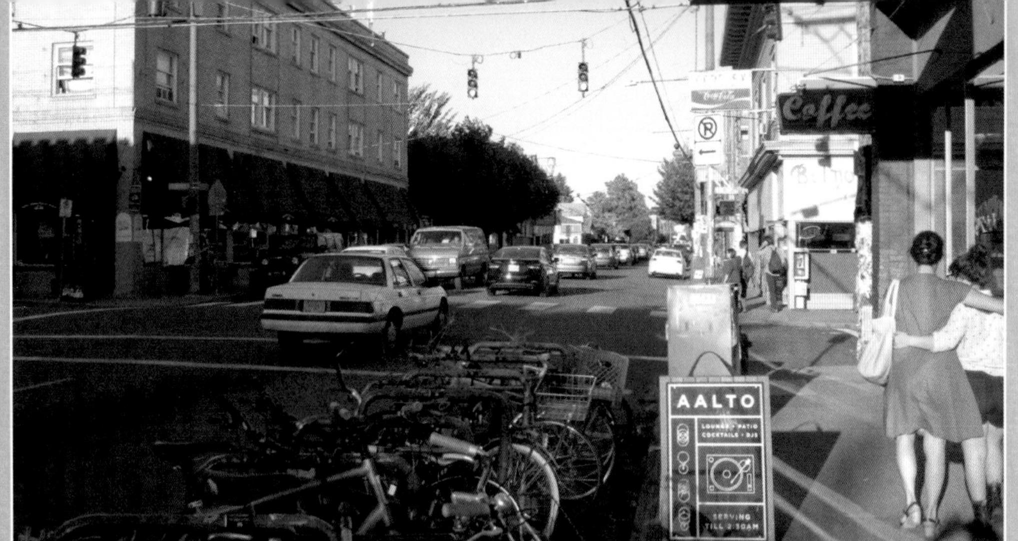

Belmont Street in the Sunnyside Neighborhood of Portland, Oregon. *(2015: Wing Grabowski)*

The 20-Minute Neighborhood

Good ideas are often a lot easier to talk about than to actually understand. That is certainly the case when discussing such ideas as "walkable communities," "active lifestyles," or "healthy neighborhoods." In considering the relationships between the environments in which we live and healthful living, wouldn't it be great if we could visualize what a neighborhood or community would be like if the ingredients of active and healthy living actually came together? Not only could we have a common vision of such an environment, we could look around Nashville and Middle Tennessee to see if there are places that are approaching this vision—or could approach such a vision with some combination of interests, resources, and creative thinking.

The idea of "20-Minute Neighborhoods" might be just such a conceptual tool. In 2012 the city of Portland, OR, updated its long-range development scenario with what is now called "The Portland Plan." Core goals included a range of desires for sustainable living: active and healthy lifestyles, energy conservation, improved community connections, and equity. The "20-Minute Neighborhood" concept became a tool to help inform decisions about growth, development, and livability as Portland entered the 21st century. Simply put, a 20-minute neighborhood is a place with "convenient, safe, and pedestrian-oriented access to the places people need to go to and the services people use nearly every day: transit, shopping, quality food, school, parks and social activities . . . all that are near or adjacent to housing."[14]

In short, the Portland folks took the concept of a "walkable environment" and described it as a place where people "go and get to" in about 20 minutes. The 20-minute time-frame actually came from planning literature that evolved in the 1920s as cars began to replace walking and transit in most American cities. While fast walkers can obviously go farther, it was generally accepted then, as now, that 20 minutes of walking equates to about a quarter of a mile. The concept is elegant in its simplicity: Is it possible to meet most of the needs of daily living within 20 minutes of where one lives?

In Nashville, as in Portland, the movement toward car-dependency quickly replaced any thought of maintaining such neighborhoods, especially as suburban growth exploded at the end of the Second World War. Cheap fuel, good roads, available land, and growing family incomes for the most part accelerated car-dependent development. Only those who did not share in the economic growth of the times remained dependent on public transportation.

The idea of 20-minute neighborhoods helps us now regain a vision of a future that we know has growing value as the price of transportation increases, our need to become and stay physically fit becomes more obvious, and we understand more than ever the delicate balance of life in our fragile environment.

What are the core ingredients of a 20-minute neighborhood? The Portland folks borrowed heavily on "walkable environment" research and came up with the following elements:

- Building scales that are comfortable, that is, not too intimidating for pedestrians
- Mixed-use and dense development near neighborhood services and transit
- Distinct and identifiable centers and public spaces
- A variety of connected transportation options together with lower speed streets laid out in a grid or some pattern featuring frequent connectivity
- Accessible design of housing and services

For many these characteristics describe those familiar older neighborhoods that were developed before the car was king. One thinks of East Nashville, for example. For others, these characteristics represent attributes of "new urban" design. Several new developments across Middle Tennessee ascribe to at least some of these attributes.

The power of the 20-minute neighborhood idea, however, does not only lie in finding such neighborhoods in perfect harmony with the concept. The power lies in how we think about growth and development across Nashville and Middle Tennessee, using the core concepts of a 20-minute neighborhood as we anticipate our future over the next 25 years or so.

If we apply the idea of a 20-minute neighborhood to any proposed development or public investment, we inherently are asking questions about three attributes of any development proposal:

- Distance: How easy is it to travel by foot, bike, or transit?
- Destinations: Are businesses (including food) and public facilities nearby?
- Density: Are there sufficient numbers of residents, employees, and income to support these businesses and public facilities?

By just asking these questions we can take the idea of the 20-minute neighborhood and apply it to a specific project or proposal. Although the opportunity to create a new 20-minute neighborhood from scratch will obviously be rare, the walkable qualities of any proposed development or project will surface as these questions are asked and answered. Therein is the power of the 20-minute neighborhood idea: it helps us understand, and therefore support, projects that promote walking, access to important services, access to transit, and a more affordable and satisfying living environment—an environment that makes healthy living a part of each day, not dependent on trips to the gym.

To begin a change in thinking to reflect the 20-minute neighborhood idea, Portland launched a fascinating analysis that mapped distance, destination, and density variables across the city. As one would expect, some areas actually approached the 20-minute neighborhood threshold. Others did not. The conversation that has followed this analysis has focused on where such neighborhoods are appropriate and where other models are better. That is a productive discussion that has engaged many citizens who previously were not involved in linking development questions with daily living.

There just may be something in the 20-minute neighborhood idea for Nashville and Middle Tennessee. If healthy living is our goal, any tool that helps us evaluate the impacts of public and private investments on our health could be of great value. The 20-minute neighborhood tool not only helps us talk about healthy living, it helps us evaluate investments in healthy living.

ED COLE, former director, Environment and Planning, Tennessee Department of Transportation; former director, Transit Alliance of Middle Tennessee

FOOD RESOURCES

Food is essential for life. And the quality of the food consumed can have a significant impact on the consumer's health.

Ideally, grocery stores featuring fresh foods would be located in close proximity to residential areas and reachable by sidewalks, bike paths, and public transit. But in so-called "food desert" communities, the available foods are heavily processed products high in fast sugars and fats, a chronic problem for residents without access to an automobile.

Alternative methods to supply healthy foods include mobile markets, community supported agriculture (CSA) programs, farmers' markets, and farm stands. Community gardens and community kitchens also increase the local availability of fresh foods and foster community identity as well as entrepreneurship.

Public schools have become a source of education and outreach. Lunchroom menus are evolving in a healthier direction, and "backpack" programs include an increasingly diverse array of foods for youth to bring home.

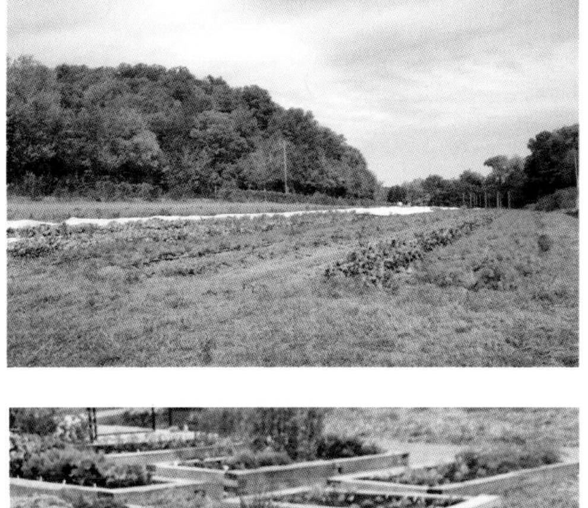

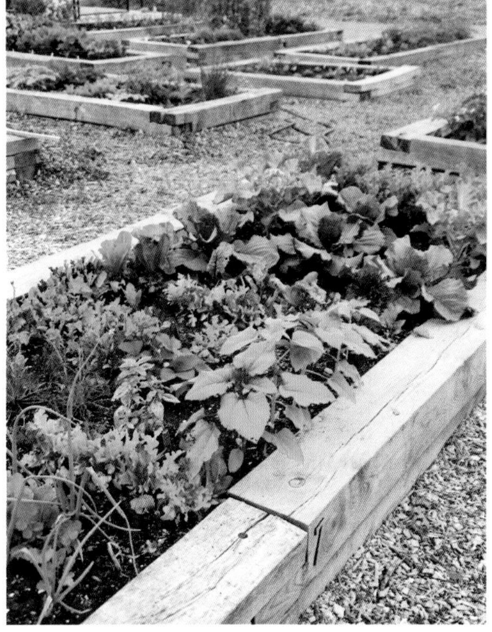

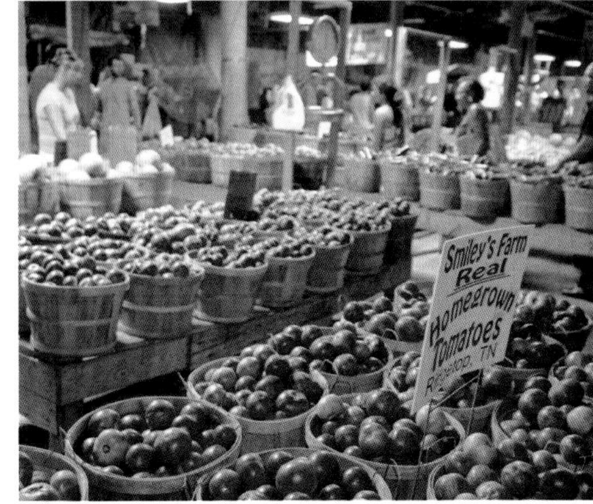

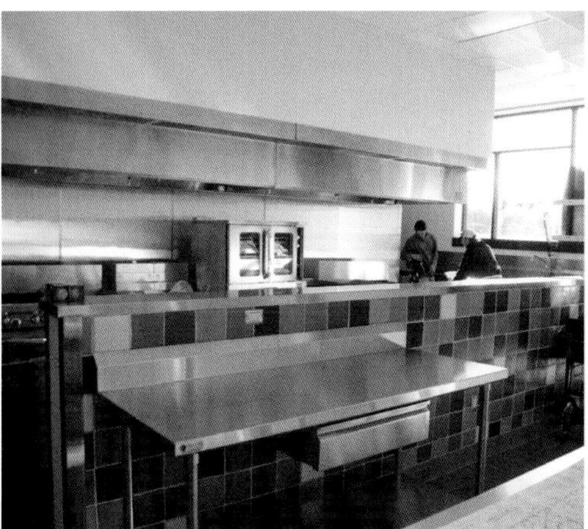

Healthy food resources in Nashville. Clockwise from top: farm in Bells Bend; raised garden bed in urban yard; farm stand; commercial incubator kitchen for local food entrepreneurs at Casa Azafrán; Farmers' Market. *(2011–2013: NCDC; 2009: Gary Layda)*

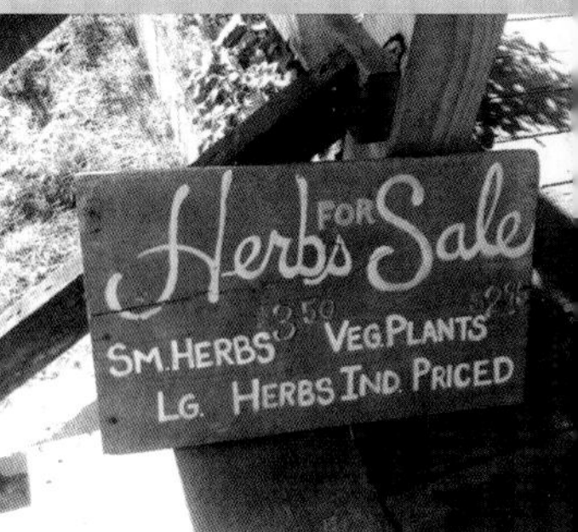

Eating Our Way to a Healthy City

Have you ever wondered where your food comes from? I sometimes ask at Portland national chain food markets: "Can I buy something grown in Oregon?" I usually get a blank stare because there is so little from Oregon in these markets.

Nashville, like Portland, is sitting in the midst of one of the world's most food-abundant places. Why is it so difficult to buy food grown in Nashville? The answer is that we import most of the food we eat.

This problem is not an isolated one. A study of the Cleveland region estimated only 1 percent of the food consumed in the region was grown there. In Portland we import an estimated 90 to 95 percent of the food we purchase from outside the Portland region. Research sponsored by the *USDA Sustainable Agriculture Research and Education Program*[15] found that the total food and food-related products purchased outside the Portland region is about $4.7 billion a year.[16] If we can substitute 10 to 20 percent of the food currently imported from outside the region with food produced regionally, we can increase regional wealth by between $470 million and $940 million annually.

Not only can we make money, we can save money by moving the food dollar to locally produced, nutrient-dense, healthy foods. The YMCA of Central Tennessee estimates that by 2013 Tennessee will be spending $2.81 billion a year on the health care costs associated with obesity. Now we are talking real money!

Strategies to get people walking, visiting parks and open spaces, and living in housing that is near employment and in walkable neighborhoods are all important for the 21st century healthy city.

We are what we eat and what we eat influences our economic prosperity. Nashville can take realistic steps to rebuild the local food economy and help the private market offer healthy food choices. Nashville, like other regions that have created regional food strategies,[17] can eat its way to human and economic health.

Based on our experience in Portland and our review of multiple regional plans I recommend the following strategies:

1. **Define the food economy.** The food economic cluster includes production (growing), processing, distribution, and consumption industries. Taken together, this is a significant economic engine. In the Portland region, the food cluster includes 16,150 firms, 155,903 employees, and a 2008 payroll of $2.97 billion.
2. **Focus on productive capacity.** Determine by careful research the extent to which the Nashville region can feed itself on locally sourced fresh fruits, vegetables, dairy, and meat products. Locate the best soils and microclimates for crop production suitable to the region. Support innovative technologies, such as aquaponics, that can re-occupy old warehouses as closed-loop food factories.
3. **Increase the demand for local foods.** Several related strategies and tools provide places to start:
   - Expand farmers' markets so there is one in every city, town, and large neighborhood.
   - Increase the supply of local food in regional markets and corner stores.
   - Encourage schools, hospitals, and other large institutions to purchase more local food.
   - Increase participation in community supported agriculture (CSAs).
   - Encourage the use of locally grown products in local restaurants and catering businesses.
   - Regionalize purchasing strategies for major market chains and fast food establishments to make it more efficient for these venues to buy local food products.
   - Support innovations such as developing smartphone applications to help inform interested shoppers of food origins.
4. **Increase the supply of local foods.** Our research indicates that regions need new strategies to support their local food economies. These strategies include:
   - Make it easier to grow food in cities.
   - Support community design for food, including permanent homes for farmers' markets and community gardens.
   - Implement transferable development-rights-type programs focused on protecting agricultural lands in the urban-rural fringe. This enables increased development in areas served by infrastructure, meanwhile protecting prime agricultural lands.
5. **Increase farm profitability.**
   - Support producer cooperatives or other organizations to help farmers brand, process, market, and distribute their products.
   - Provide information on good farm business practices.
   - Create and support networks designed to find and facilitate the next generation of farmers.
   - Provide information on traditional bank and innovative sources of capital for farmers.
   - Enable farm- and food-related businesses in rural areas to generate farm income by means such as food tourism and business incubation centers.
6. **Increase our human and social capital to support the food economy.** To maximize the potential of the food economy all public policy channels—schools, health care institutions, social services agencies, and civic leaders—need to work together to advance the entire food system.

—ROBERT WISE, associate principal, Public Policy and Strategic Planning, Cogan Owens Greene

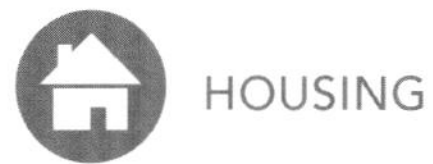

HOUSING

Nashvillians can and do live in a wide variety of dwellings and densities: single-family homes, attached-wall townhomes, duplexes and larger apartment blocks, lofts and garage flats, condos they own, and apartments they rent.

Within a neighborhood a diversity of housing types and prices offers a range of options for an array of family modes for the entire cycle of life, allowing residents to age in place while maintaining social and community ties. This can have a significant and positive impact on mental as well as physical health.

Health issues for individual units include the number of people living in a household and the proximity to highways and other air quality and environmental hazards. The environmental quality of the materials used during construction—many currently contain carcinogens—and the state of a home's repair can affect human health, particularly through interior air quality, and lead paint and asbestos remain issues of concern in older homes.

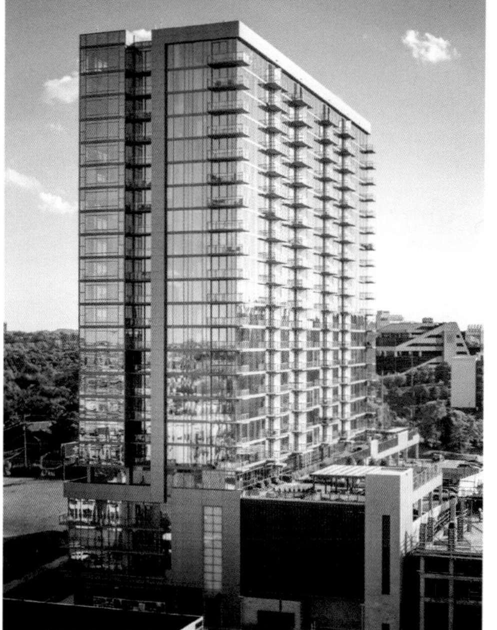

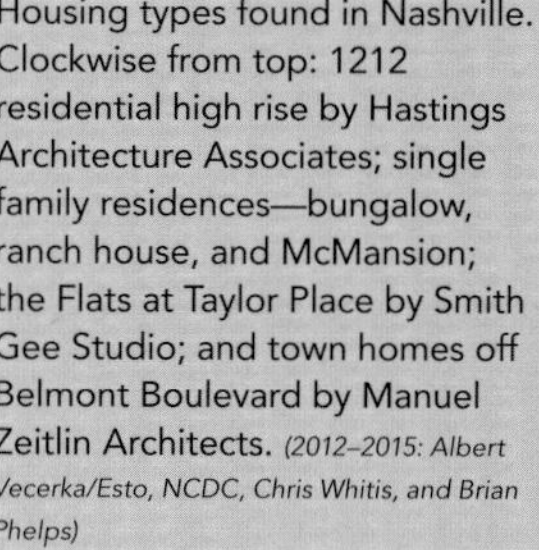

Housing types found in Nashville. Clockwise from top: 1212 residential high rise by Hastings Architecture Associates; single family residences—bungalow, ranch house, and McMansion; the Flats at Taylor Place by Smith Gee Studio; and town homes off Belmont Boulevard by Manuel Zeitlin Architects. *(2012–2015: Albert Vecerka/Esto, NCDC, Chris Whitis, and Brian Phelps)*

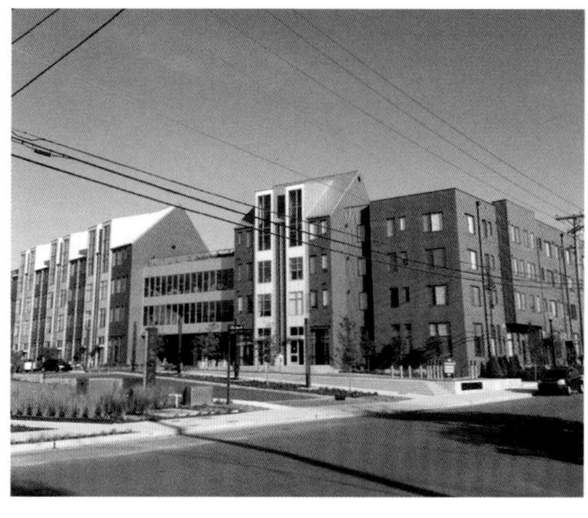

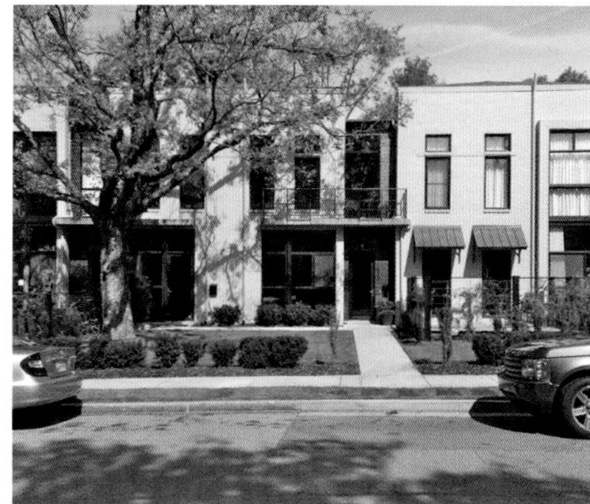

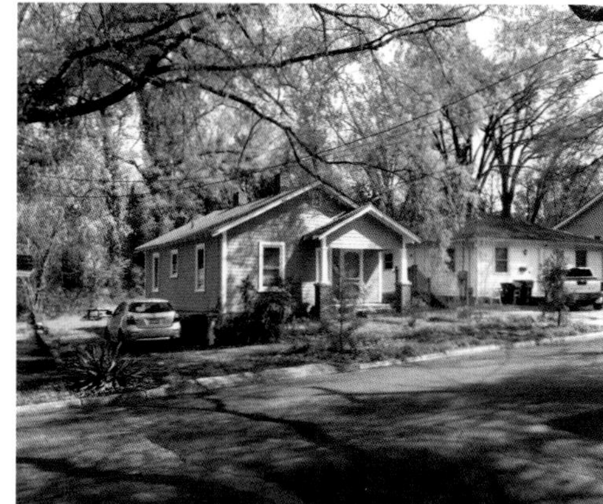

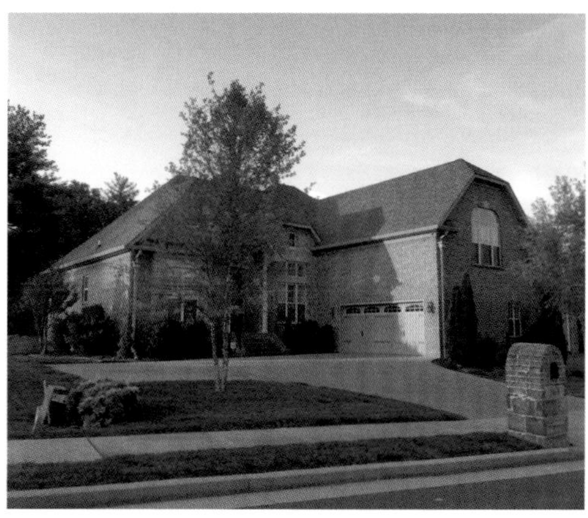

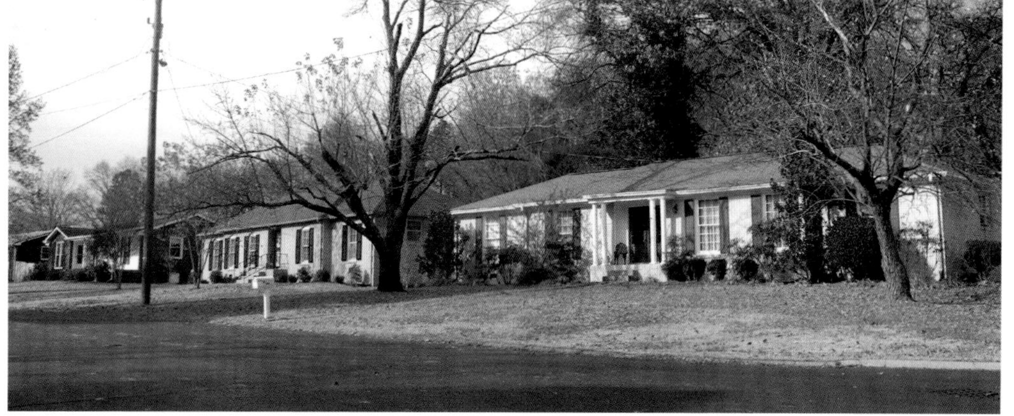

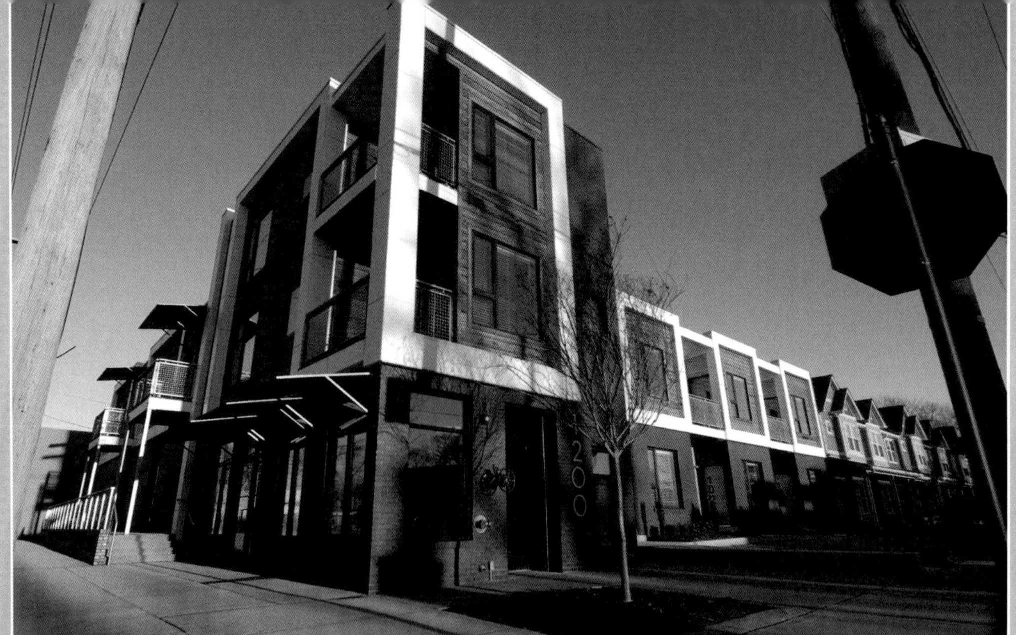

3rd and Chestnut Apartments in the Chestnut Hill neighborhood provides 10 affordable units and 1,500 square feet of commercial space. *(2015: Urban Housing Solutions)*

Housing for All

A household is considered cost-burdened if the occupants must spend more than 30 percent of their income on housing. In Davidson County, statistics from the federal Department of Housing and Urban Development show that 100,000 households are cost-burdened, which is roughly 40 percent of the city's population.[18]

"When people must allot more than 30 percent of their income to housing, they often skimp on preventive health and quality foods," says Loretta Owens, former executive director of the nonprofit The Housing Fund.[19] Therein lies a major link between housing and health.

Severely cost-burdened heads of households aged 50 and over spend 43 percent less on food and 59 percent less on health care compared with otherwise similar households living in housing they can afford.[20] For the younger set not having access to stable housing—which results in frequent moves and even homelessness—has been found to hamper a child's success in school. These problems can persist even after children are in stable housing, according to new research conducted at Vanderbilt University.[21]

Subsidized housing alleviates the cost burden by making up the difference between 30 percent of household income and the cost of rent, effectively holding the cost for the resident to 30 percent of income. There are not enough subsidies for all who need them, however. Thus, as noted above, nearly 100,000 households are under extreme financial pressure.[22]

The average rent in Nashville is increasing at a pace among the fastest in the nation, according to Moody's Analytics. Apartment rents are up 18 percent since 2009, while median household income in Nashville has grown by only 5 percent. More than half of renters in Nashville are considered cost-burdened.[23]

In order for Nashville to respond to this unfortunate reality, the city must place greater focus on policies to expand housing accessibility. Strategies to create more affordable housing in Nashville include those described below.

Provide a consistent revenue source for the Barnes Housing Trust Fund. The construction of affordable units requires subsidies because rents do not cover building costs. In 2013, the Metro Council created the Bill Barnes Housing Trust Fund (named in honor of Reverend Bill Barnes, who advocated for such a fund for more than 50 years). The Barnes Fund sponsors the development of housing for households that earn less than 80 percent of the US Department of Housing and Urban Development determined median household income—currently $49,335.[24]

Initial funding for the Barnes Fund was $3 million; the city pledged an additional $500,000 for 2014. But the contribution is largely symbolic when compared to other peer cities, according to a report by researchers at Vanderbilt University. Consider the commitments made by other second and third tier cities: the affordable housing fund for Austin, TX—$65 million; Charlotte, NC—$86 million; Minneapolis, MN—$73 million; Seattle, WA—$145 million.[25] The Barnes Fund clearly needs a dedicated, recurring revenue source.

During much of the 20th century the federal government funded low-income housing, but that source has waned. To fill the gap, Tennessee created a state housing trust fund in 2006 and has awarded approximately $15 million in competitive grants to Davidson County projects, including Room In the Inn transitional housing and Oasis Center residential housing for troubled teens. In 2012 projects in our city received $2.3 million from the state trust fund for building or rehabilitating 49 housing units, including two units of transitional housing for women who are victims of domestic violence and their families. A small portion of the funds went to rent subsidies for 32 households. These are worthy projects, but their impact is dwarfed by the numbers. According to Vanderbilt professor James Fraser, Nashville will need to construct 113,000 new affordable housing units, averaging to 3,800 per year, just to meet the expected growth for the region. With the increasing need for housing citywide, rising prices due to low supply could create even more cost-burdened households.[26]

Preserve the existing supply of lower cost housing. Due to the current rage for housing in Nashville's older neighborhoods, infill developers are demolishing smaller homes and replacing them with substantially larger structures to maximize their profits. This phenomenon has the effect of decreasing affordability.

A number of these neighborhoods, or portions of them, lie within preservation zoning overlay districts. But the demolitions continue, in part because the houses being bulldozed are from the 1950s and 1960s. This vintage does not have protection because they were not classified as "contributing" to the architectural character of the neighborhood when the buildings in a district were surveyed before the installation of the overlay. Houses from these periods might now qualify for contributing status under the federal 50-year standard if the districts were resurveyed by the staff of the Metro Historical Commission.

For neighborhoods without preservation zoning protection, housing rehabilitation zones can provide incentives for developers and property owners to rehab, rather than demolish and build new.

Adopt policies that encourage mixed-income neighborhoods. What is called "inclusionary zoning" requires a portion of new housing developments to be set aside for affordable housing. Many local advocates propose that families earning less than 60 percent of the county's median income should qualify. In return, developers can receive density bonuses, zoning variances, or expedited permits, thus reducing construction costs. This program can be voluntary or mandatory and may offer developers the option of paying into the housing trust fund, rather than actually building the affordable units, or the choice of building affordable units off-site.

This strategy uses market activity to increase the city's supply of affordable housing and disperses affordable units throughout the county, fostering mixed-income communities. Research has found that mixed-income schools are associated with higher academic performance and that families that moved from high-poverty to low-poverty neighborhoods experienced educational improvements, as well as mental and physical health improvements.[27]

Increase shared-equity housing. In 2010 the nonprofit organization The Housing Fund, Inc. received a stimulus-funded grant from the larger Neighborhood Stabilization Program (NSP) to start a shared-equity program, Our House. An income-eligible buyer in the program purchases a home with a 1 percent down payment and Our House provides an additional 25 percent. If the homeowner subsequently decides to sell, the owner must sell to an income-eligible buyer. If the house has increased in value, Our House and the homeowner split appreciation proceeds. The 25 percent Our House investment remains in the home, keeping it affordable.

There are currently 33 homes in the program, with plans for at least 100 by 2017. Though small, this program offers buyers homes in decent neighborhoods with lower mortgage payments.[28]

Combine affordable housing projects with transit-oriented development (TOD). Households in auto-dependent neighborhoods spend about 25 percent of their budgets on transportation. For those in walkable neighborhoods with convenient transit options, the transportation expense is 9 percent.[29] Housing is more affordable if a household's transportation expenses are reduced. Planning new affordable housing near transit corridors is a logical way to accomplish this. The Denver TOD Fund, for example, allocates monies for preserving and creating 1,000 affordable homes along transit corridors.[30]

Increase home energy efficiency support, which can provide substantial cost savings to low-income households. In January of 2013, Nashville was one of five cities selected by Bloomberg Philanthropies and Living Cities' to create Financial Empowerment Centers.[31] With the $2 million grant, Nashville provided no-cost energy efficiency and stormwater mitigation work to more than 150 low-income homeowners, many in Chestnut Hill. Over 980 volunteers completed home energy improvements, which included such upgrades as insulation, weather stripping for doors and windows, and low-flow showerheads.[32] The weatherization program extended the affordability and livability of aging housing stock, much of which dates to the 1930s.

In 2013, the Nashville Energy Works program offered 100 homeowners in North Nashville no-cost evaluations and upgrades as part of the Go Green North Nashville campaign—a partnership between the Mayor's Office, Tennessee State University, Hands On Nashville, and Village Real Estate Services. Additionally, Nashville Electric Service and the Tennessee Valley Authority are providing 50 home energy audits to qualifying North Nashville homeowners.[33]

To minimize land costs in housing development, increase the supply of accessory dwelling units and cottage-style courtyard housing. An accessory dwelling unit, also known as a "granny flat," is a self-contained second living unit that occupies the same lot as the main residence. For the homeowner ADUs offer an independent housing option for the owner's grown children starting out, elderly parents downsizing, or unrelated families looking to establish themselves—and a revenue stream to offset construction costs.[34]

Cottage-style developments typically feature small homes—rarely more than 2,000 square feet and often vertical in form to conserve land costs—with front porches, traditional materials and styles, grouped around a common green space.[35] In Nashville, examples include Germantown Court in North Nashville and Fatherland Court on the Eastside.

Expand existing home repair assistance programs. Home rehabilitation programs have the ability to improve the livelihood of occupants by extending the livability of their homes.

—REVEREND BILL BARNES,
WITH AMY ESKIND AND KION SAWNEY, NCDC

"Concentrated poverty is the enemy of good schools, the enemy of safety, the enemy of health, the enemy of employment. Affordable housing should be dispersed throughout the city."

—Reverend Bill Barnes

OPEN SPACE AND PARKS

Public open spaces in Nashville range from the visibly structured to natural settings. *(2010–2015: Gary Layda; NCDC)*

Today most Americans view access to public open space as a basic right of citizenship. Such space provides important opportunities for improving public health.

For children and adults, outdoor recreation aids in physical fitness. Simply being outdoors decreases stress and enhances focus. A variety of public open spaces—parks, greenways, waterways (so-called "blueways")—offer occasions for active as well as passive uses: organized sports, hiking, cycling, horseback riding, walking, wading, birding, boating, picnicking, playing fetch in a dog park, climbing a jungle gym, exploring nature, strolling by a stream, and sitting on a bench. All foster the physical and mental health of a community.

Our public green spaces also contribute significantly to the city's tree canopy, which has a positive impact on the environment. Trees improve air quality and mitigate respiratory illness, help cleanse storm water, and reduce the urban heat island effect.

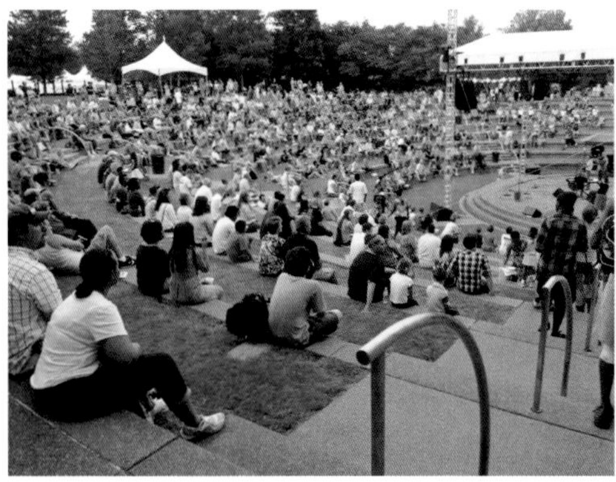

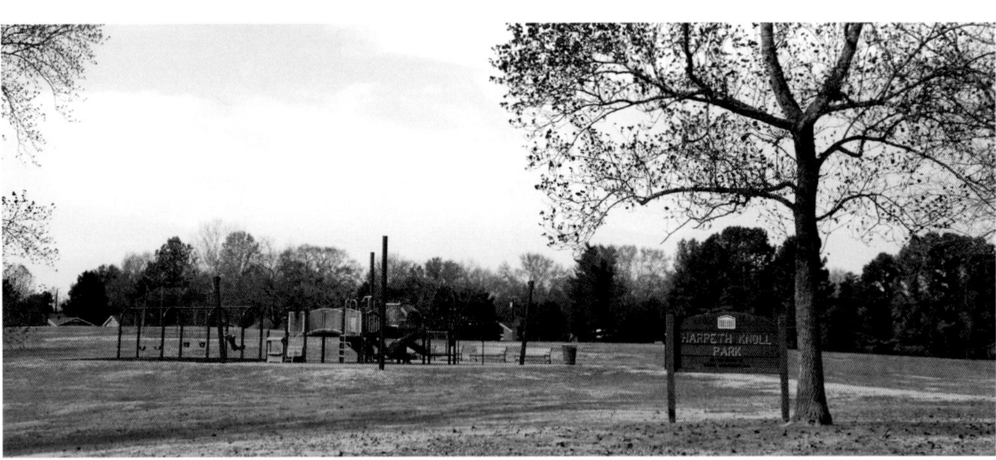

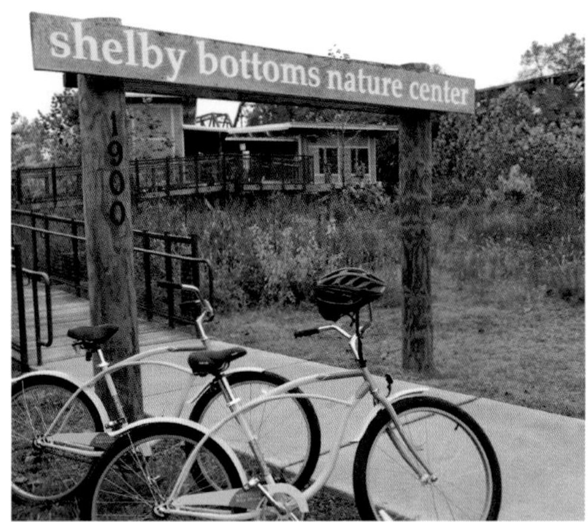

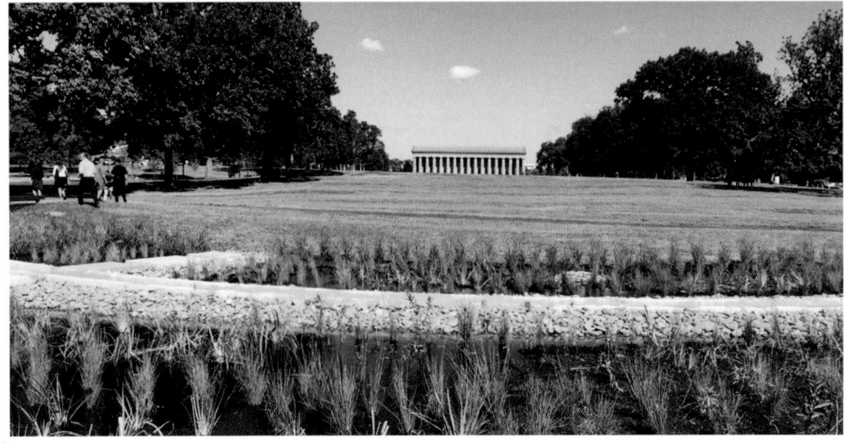

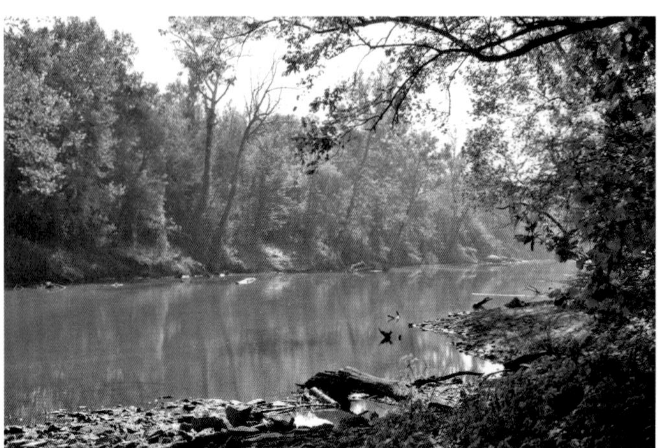

The Stewardship of the Land: Nashville's Parks and Greenways

We think of Nashville's public parks and greenways as our greenest civic spaces. This may be true in terms of color, but not in terms of the other "green": environmental sustainability.

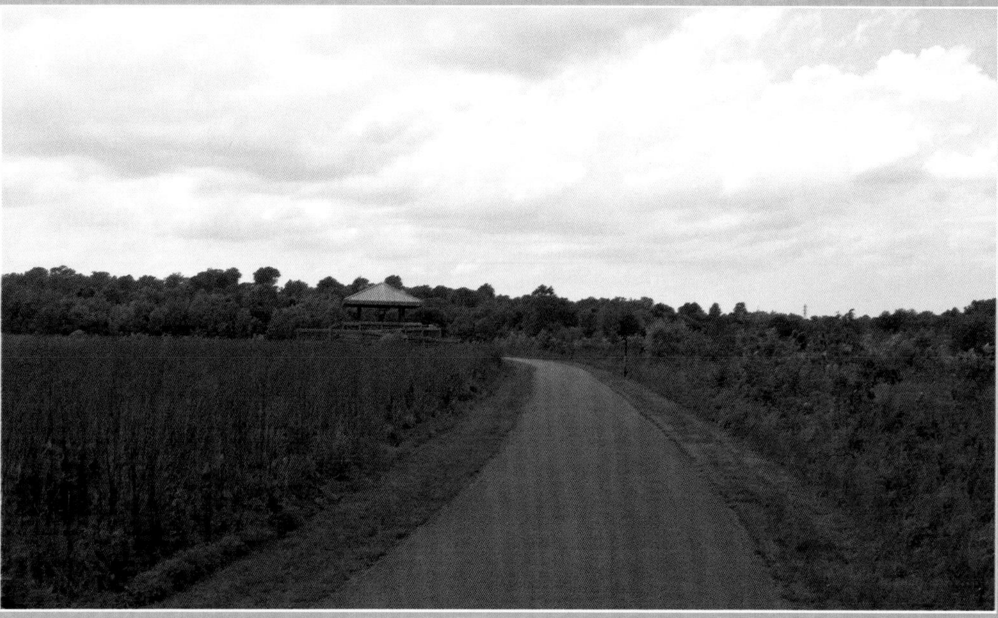

Shelby Bottoms greenway with observation deck in background. This is the one area in the Bottoms where the Parks Department, with the assistance of the Friends of Shelby Park and Bottoms, is maintaining a large open meadow. *(2015)*

The Living Landscape

Ecosystems are dynamic. Changes within an ecosystem are called succession, "the stepwise, gradual, generally plant-dominated, replacement of one set of plant and animal species (natural community) by another set until establishment of a 'climax community'" that will stand until disrupted. "Each plant community is a distinct living-space for an animal community thriving within. As plant communities change, so do the animal communities."[36]

Existing conditions in an ecosystem can be disrupted dramatically by "disturbances." Examples of natural disturbances include wildfires, tornados, insect and disease epidemics, ice storms, floods, and droughts. Human disturbances range from forest clearing for agriculture to timber harvesting, wildfire suppression, application of fertilizers and pesticides, introduction of non-native species, irrigation, and global warming.

An example of long-standing human disturbance in many parks and greenways is the highly unnatural state of watersheds. Streams that feed into the Cumberland River and its tributaries have been channeled into masonry culverts. In floodplain landscapes formerly used for agricultural purposes, water is concentrated into steep-sided drainage ditches that enhance the speed of the flow into the Cumberland River. This kind of engineering deprives native plants and wildlife of hydration and aquatic habitat.

Clear patterns of plant succession can be observed in the recent history of various segments of Nashville's greenways system. Floodplain landscapes, where land was formerly farmed, evolved into open meadows that are now rapidly being occupied by shrubs and trees. This pattern is also occurring in areas of our parks that were once mowed as lawns and have more recently been left to grow.

Unfortunately, the occupiers are dominated by non-native and invasive species like bush honeysuckle, privet, Bradford pear, and others. These invaders create a hostile environment for native plants and animals. Exotic bush honeysuckle, for example, replaces native forest, shrubs, and herbaceous plants by its invasive nature and early leaf-out. Recent studies suggest that the bush also releases toxins that prevent other plant species from growing in the vicinity.[37]

The park and greenway environment has changed for human users as well. Scenic vistas have been lost and the Cumberland River is becoming ever more invisible, even from paths within a stone's throw of the riverbank. Pedestrians, especially those on the unpaved trails, can become disoriented because they can't see through the thicket.

Mow or No

Metro's Parks and Recreation Department staff are trying to see through the metaphorical thicket of chronic underfunding for daily operations. During the past three mayoral administrations, the Department has added significantly to its landmass. Under Mayor Karl Dean alone 3,000 new acres have been acquired as part of the fulfillment of the open space plan Nashville: *Naturally* (2011). This is the good news.

The bad news is that during these same administrations, the Parks' maintenance budget has been routinely cut, adding up over the years to total reductions of approximately 32 percent. According to Parks director Tommy Lynch, between 2008 and 2015 "we lost $3 million in our operating budget and 29 people. In terms of full-time-equivalents, we're down from 673 to 563 people, and more than one-third of those were in maintenance." There is more territory to cover and fewer staff to manage it.

By necessity, Parks administrators have turned to a land management strategy of "mow or no." Acreage that is used passively—as opposed to ball fields, golf courses, and so on—is either mowed as lawn on an approximately monthly basis or left to grow untrammeled. The result in the untrammeled areas is the advance of exotic invasives and the decline of native plant and animal habitat.

The Parks Department is currently developing a natural resources management policy for acreage that possesses "scenic, ecological, geological, or recreational value that provides significant habitat for native plants and animals, provides land and open space for passive recreational opportunities and is worthy of restoration, protection and preservation." Once the policy is in place, selected parklands will be designated as "natural areas." Then land management plans will be developed for specific properties.

The fact that so many potential natural areas require restoration rather than preservation, and the underfunding of Parks' budget, however, place severe restrictions on implementation of any future plans.

More than Money

A better-funded Parks Department, however, will not by itself necessarily lead to better land stewardship. This will require a comprehensive analysis of current versus best practices in terms of environmental sustainability.

For example, open spaces not designated as natural areas and not used for active recreation could become meadows cut twice a year rather than lawns mowed once a month, reducing labor and increasing natural habitat. Goat and sheep herds could be used for grazing, thus decreasing fuel and labor costs—four-footed herbivores don't get benefits and pensions—and reducing vehicle emissions. Controlled burning of parklands not immediately adjacent to development is a technique increasingly recommended to restore natural cycles to the land.

Additionally, Nashville's parks and greenways lack a comprehensive recycling and composting program. Containers for recycling—forget composting—are available only within Parks Department buildings and outdoors at the relatively small Cumberland Park on the East Bank. Plastic bottles, aluminum cans, paper plates, banana peels, and orange rinds of joggers, walkers, and picnickers all go to the landfill. Parks staff say this is the cheapest method of waste management because so many park users do not sort before they toss. A broad-based education program, perhaps coordinated with Metro schools, would make Nashvillians better recyclers.

Good Stewardship

Nashville's parks and greenways can provide many different kinds of experiences. In addition to recreation, these include the contemplation and understanding of natural resources. Viewsheds through meadows and forests to the Highland Rim and the Cumberland River and its tributaries, as well as riparian areas, hills, ridges, floodplains, and floodways, enable us to apprehend Middle Tennessee's major defining landscape features. The observation of wildlife—mammals, aquatic species, birds and insects, and distinct varieties of vegetation—allows us to appreciate the intricate relationships in these ecosystems.

The Parks Department has begun taking steps to renaturalize some watersheds within its territories. Implementation of the Centennial Park master plan brings the historic Cockrill Spring, which had been buried and drained to a sewer, back to the surface. A portion of its stream will be filtered through a wetland garden before being used for irrigation and pumped into Lake Watauga to improve its water quality.

A $2 million restoration of the stream corridor through the Shelby Park Golf Course is a project of the Tennessee Stream Mitigation Program, a subsidiary of the nonprofit Tennessee Wildlife Resources Foundation, in partnership with Metro Parks. The water corridor, which has flowed downhill in concrete channels, will become a naturally flowing stream again, feeding Lake Sevier.

These are good steps, but they are baby steps. Lands in the public trust require thoughtful, planned stewardship, a task which is much more encompassing than mowing and weed-eating.[38]

—CHRISTINE KREYLING

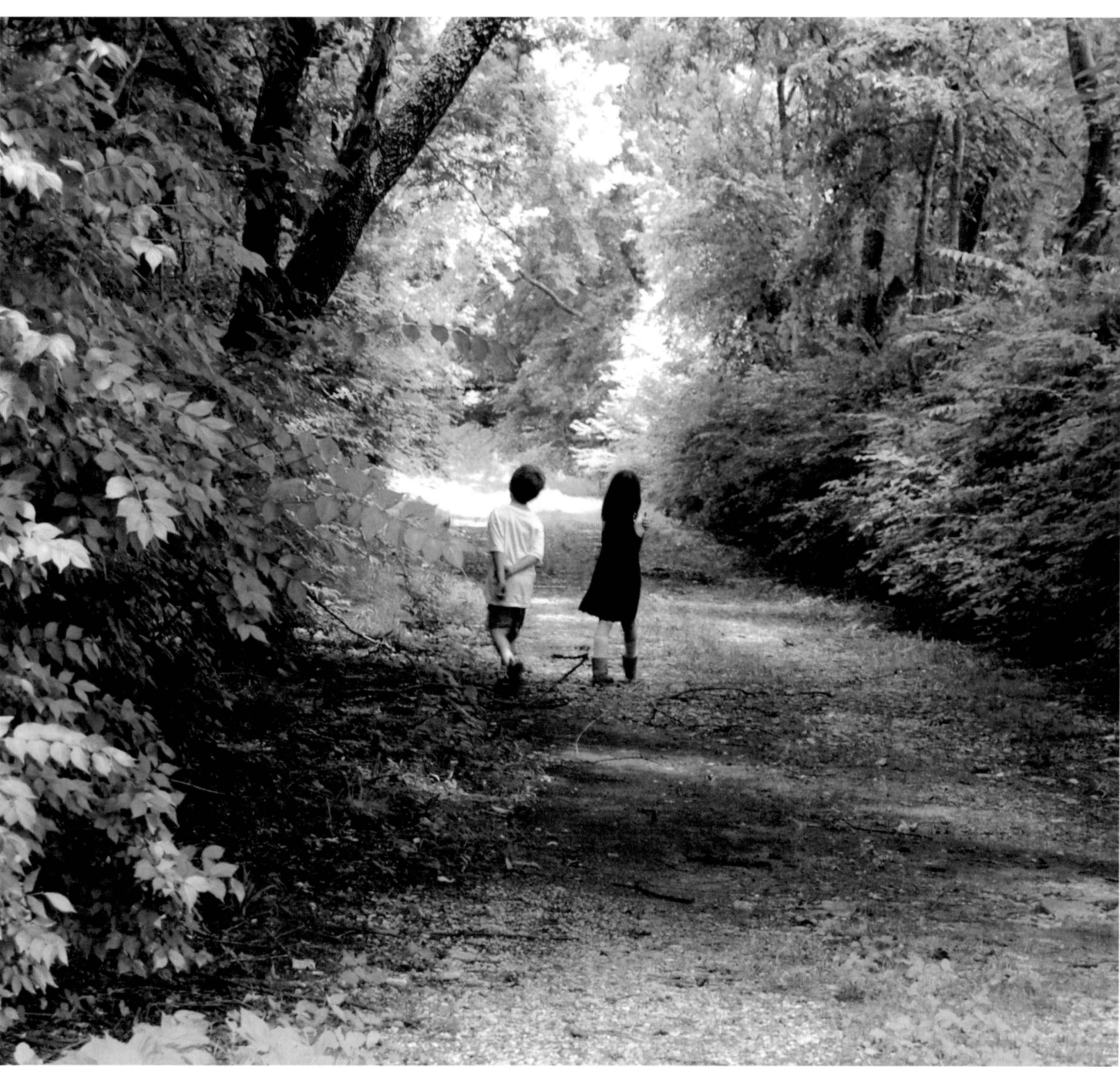

Glen Leven Farm. *(2012: Land Trust for Tennessee)*

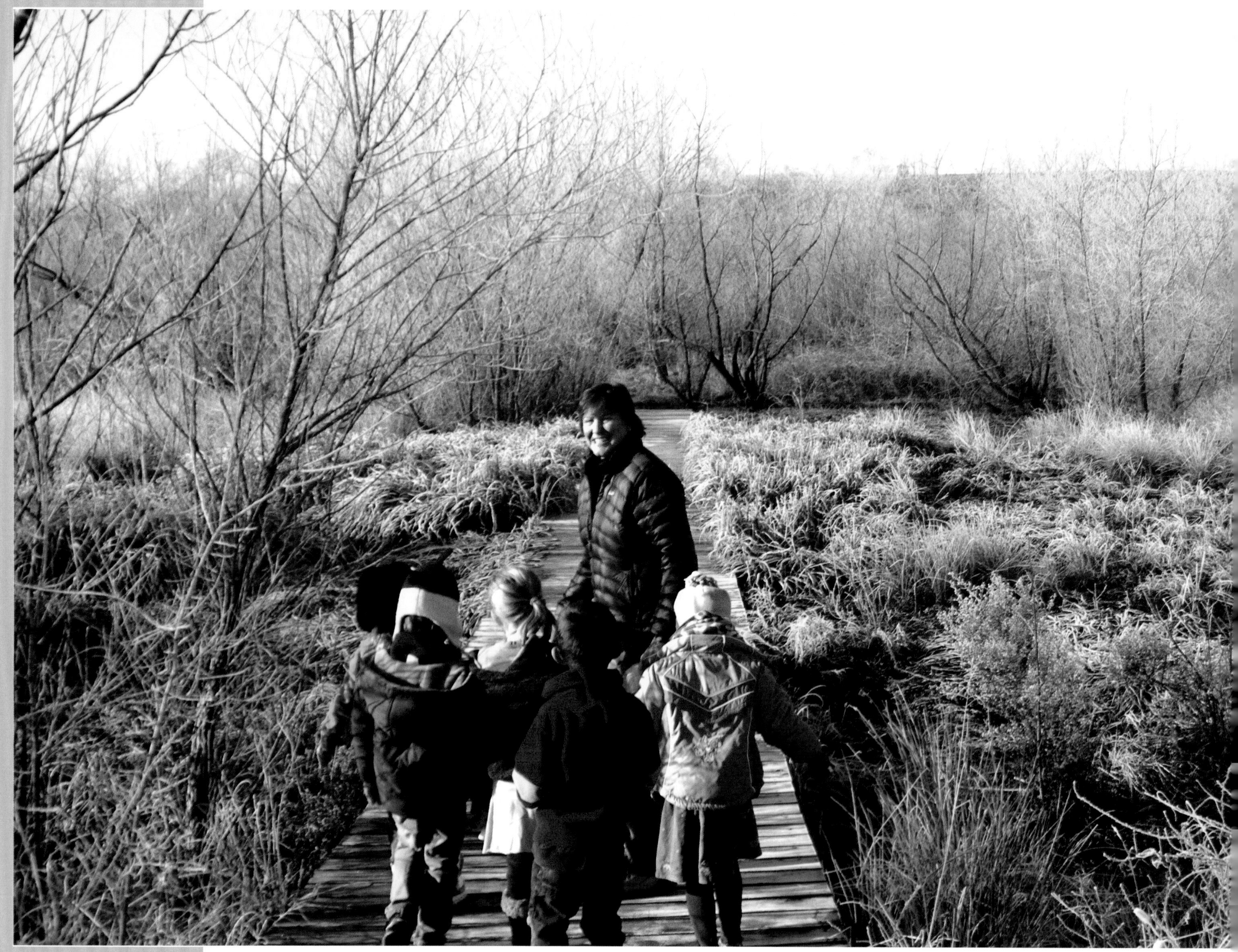

CYNTHIA LEE

During my working years I was a sixth grade math teacher. I tried to connect what I taught with the outside world.

One day I learned that the bluebirds were in trouble, so I asked myself, "How can I incorporate this in the sixth grade math classroom?" We constructed bluebird boxes, placed them on a farm, then monitored growth and made graphs.

In a few years we created a new position at school to create more opportunities for students to connect what they were studying in the classroom with the natural world. I took on the job as Director of Outdoor Education and Lower School Naturalist. I was then able to find many opportunities for our students in every grade.

We began a program at the University School of Nashville to raise trout in the classroom. First graders learned about water organisms and watched the trout evolve from eggs. While learning to write and spell, the students were excited to find the right word to describe what was going on with the trout.

Sometimes our kids struggle in the classroom to stay seated in their chairs. But when they walk outside, they light up. They start thinking in different ways. It's like this is their natural place.

When I read Richard Louv's *Last Child in the Woods,* the book synthesized a lot of what I'd learned as a teacher. There are things that a child cannot learn within the walls of a school. We have to have outdoor places that we can easily take our kids to. That's why our public parks are so important. I took my students on a walk across the Shelby Pedestrian Bridge [now Seigenthaler Bridge] and we discussed how the founding Nashvillians traveled down the river to get here and start the city.

One of my favorite places for kids was and still is the garden at Warner Parks. The children would sit among the vegetables and draw. We'd talk about organic growing, about compost. The garden motivated us to plant box gardens at school. When do you see kindergarteners want to eat a radish? When they grow it themselves.

When I taught I started an outdoor program for children to go bicycling, mountain biking, and hiking. But there are challenges to outdoor activity. The way the streets are designed and the fact that car drivers are not aware of bikes make it unsafe. Being able to ride your bike to work, to play areas, to school would be a wonderful change for us. The city is building new bikeways; they should include a bike park with an obstacle course, which I've seen out west. It's great exercise: A kid can ride over a bridge, up and down, and over a berm. Of course, the adults have to be willing to let them fall.

I've been taking 10th graders on a four-day camping trip for 13 years, and every year it gets harder. That's because of phones—students today are more and more connected to their phones. They communicate, text, play games, surf the web, listen to music, and in general turn to their phone to alleviate boredom. It's difficult to pull the students away from their electronic devices and truly appreciate the nature around them.

But kids do rise up to challenges. For them, white water rafting or trying to find their way up a rock cliff or along an obscure path are natural challenges that are fun to solve.

Research shows that time spent in the natural world, even as little as 15 to 20 minutes a day, lessens the symptoms of depression, and even more so with a two- or three-day trip. For kids with attention deficit disorder, being outside helps them become more focused. They go back to class and their teacher would say to me, "Wow! They really do well outside. I haven't observed them like this in the classroom." The child is more self-confident because he/she has been successful and had fun—it carries over.

Young adults today have not had many outdoor experiences, so they need a guide or a group to take them. The first time I offered a canoe trip on the Duck River to a young women's group, I wasn't sure how many people would sign up. We had 44 on a Saturday morning. We swam in the river rapids and looked into caves. At least 10 of those women have gone back and done it again. Two of them bought canoes. All they needed was to be shown how.

Until you experience being on a river, the problem of polluted stormwater runoff is too abstract. But once you see how beautiful the river is, how many plants and animals live there, it changes the way you think. And if we learn to love these places we'll do a better job of taking care of them.

Metro Parks' nature centers have amazing programs. You go on a guided bird walk and all of a sudden you know the names of some birds and can distinguish their calls. You become interested and might even go birding by yourself. Our community is hungry for experiences of nature. Why else would 250 people sign up for the Mayor's geology walk?

1

STRATEGIES

Use greenways to link open spaces around the county with each other and with commercial and residential development.

Utilize contextual architecture, native plantings and unobtrusive lighting for civic buildings to minimize environmental impacts.

Limit the amount of parking and vehicular traffic in natural areas by restricting car storage to the perimeter of parks.

Provide public transit access whenever possible, and make natural areas more accessible to walkers and cyclists from surrounding communities.

Create walking and hiking paths segregated from vehicular circulation.

Make maps of trails in public open space easily accessible.

Use selected areas of parks that were formerly farmland and meadowland as demonstrations of agricultural practice for educational purposes and to preserve local food resources.

Identify and preserve existing open space in Davidson County as an environmental and educational resource for citizens and visitors.

Conserve and/or restore a diversity of habitats for native plants and animals.

THE NATURAL TRANSECT ZONE

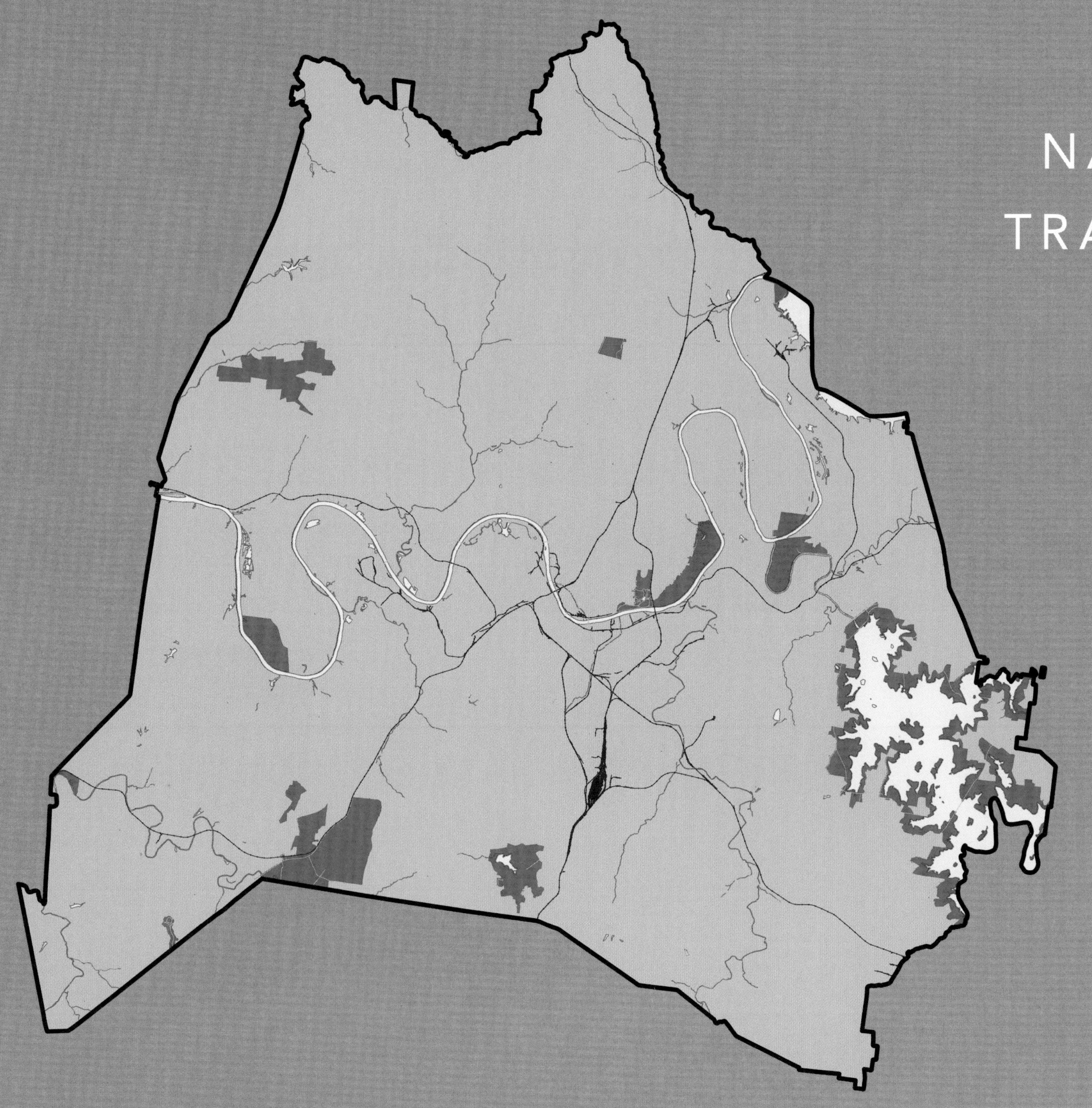

Davidson County, highlighting all areas in the natural transect zone. Examples include state and Metro parks such as Warner Parks, Radnor Lake State Natural Area, Beaman Park, Bells Bend, Shelby Bottoms, Cedar Hill Park, Peeler Park, Stones River Bend Park, and Hidden Lakes State Park. Note that highly urbanized parks, such as Centennial and Riverfront Parks, are not considered natural areas because they have been largely transformed from their original natural setting. (Map, 2014: Metro Planning Department)

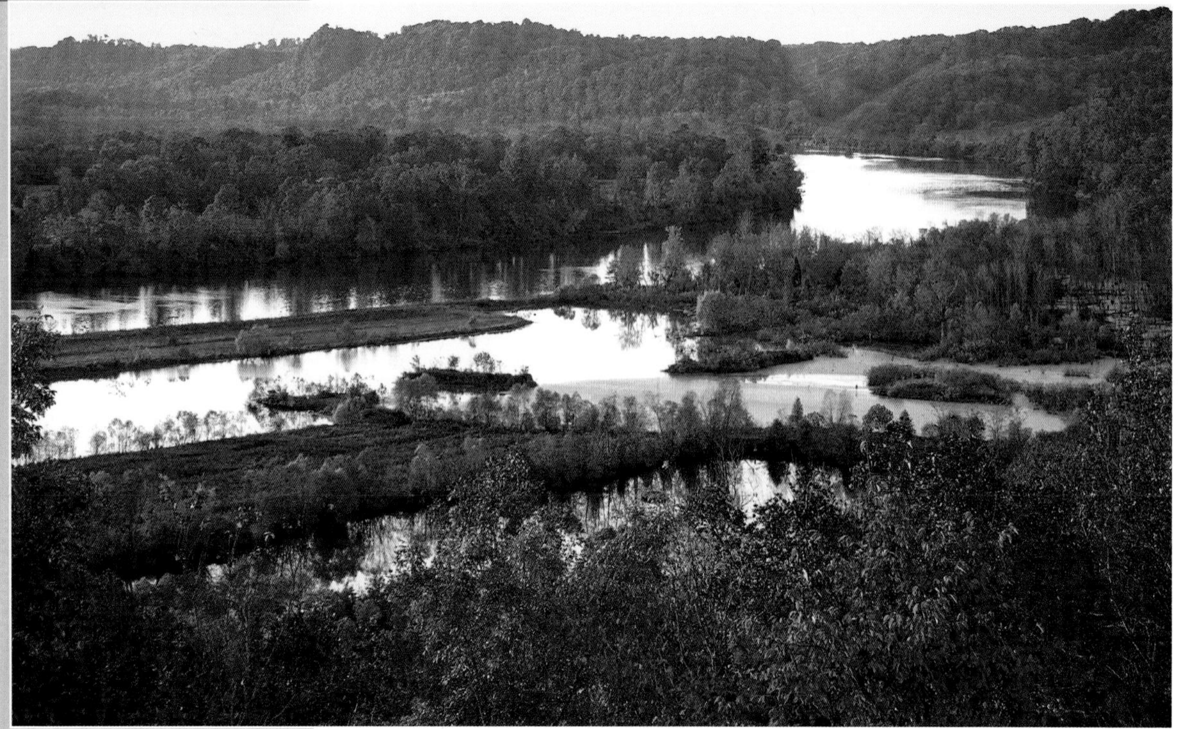

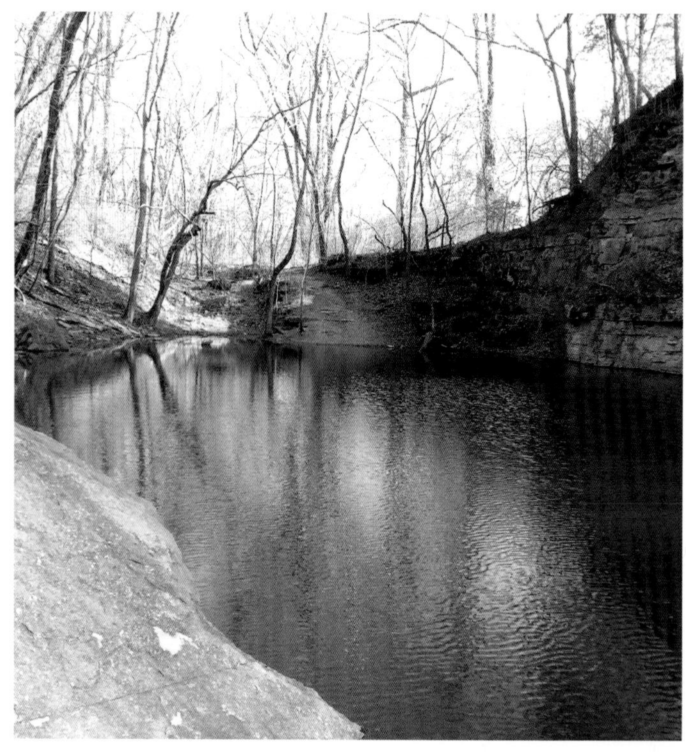

The riparian corridor of the Cumberland River, part of Davidson County's natural transect zone. The corridor serves many valuable functions: filters sediment from runoff before it enters the water, protects banks from erosion, serves as potential storage area for floodwaters, provides food and habitat for wildlife, and preserves open space. *(2013: Gary Layda)*

Hidden Lakes State Park. Located in southwest Davidson County, the park features many hiking trails as well as views of the Middle Tennessee Veterans Cemetery. *(2014: Joe Mayes, NCDC)*

Elementary school children on a field trip in Edwin Warner Park learn about the park's natural inhabitants. *(2012)*

THE NATURAL WORLD

Nashville's open spaces are the lungs through which the city breathes. This is metaphor, of course. But Nature as metaphor for health and freedom has had a powerful impact on the American mind.

The founding mind of Thomas Jefferson, to take one example, preferred "the woods, the wilds, and the independence of Monticello" to what he saw as the superior "wealth" but greater "misery" of the city.[1] And for that irascible Yankee, Henry David Thoreau, the human condition was dependent on the natural world. "Our village life would stagnate if it were not for the unexplored forests and meadows which surround it," he wrote in *Walden*. "We need the tonic of wildness. . . . We can never have enough of nature."[2]

An equally influential thread in our culture, however, is what the *New York Times* recently described as "that American will to leave one's mark on God's exquisite canvas, even if it means inexorably changing it."[3]

The pace of "inexorable change" in Nashville has quickened in recent years. Which makes the need to preserve our open spaces all the more compelling.

Our civic identity as a place, not only of man-made monuments, but also of forests and meadows, hills and plains, depends upon it.

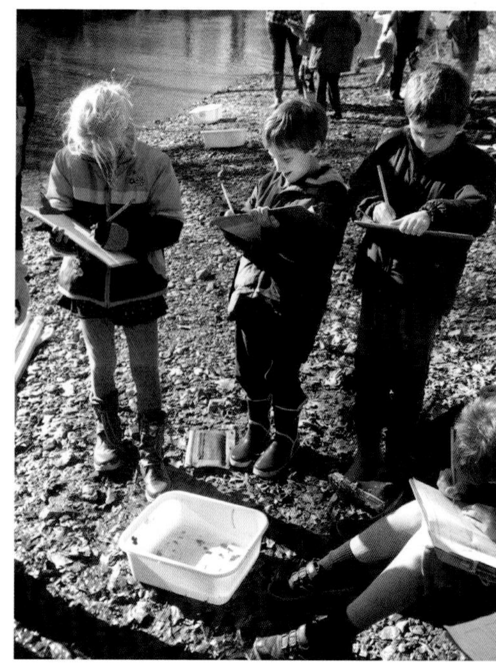

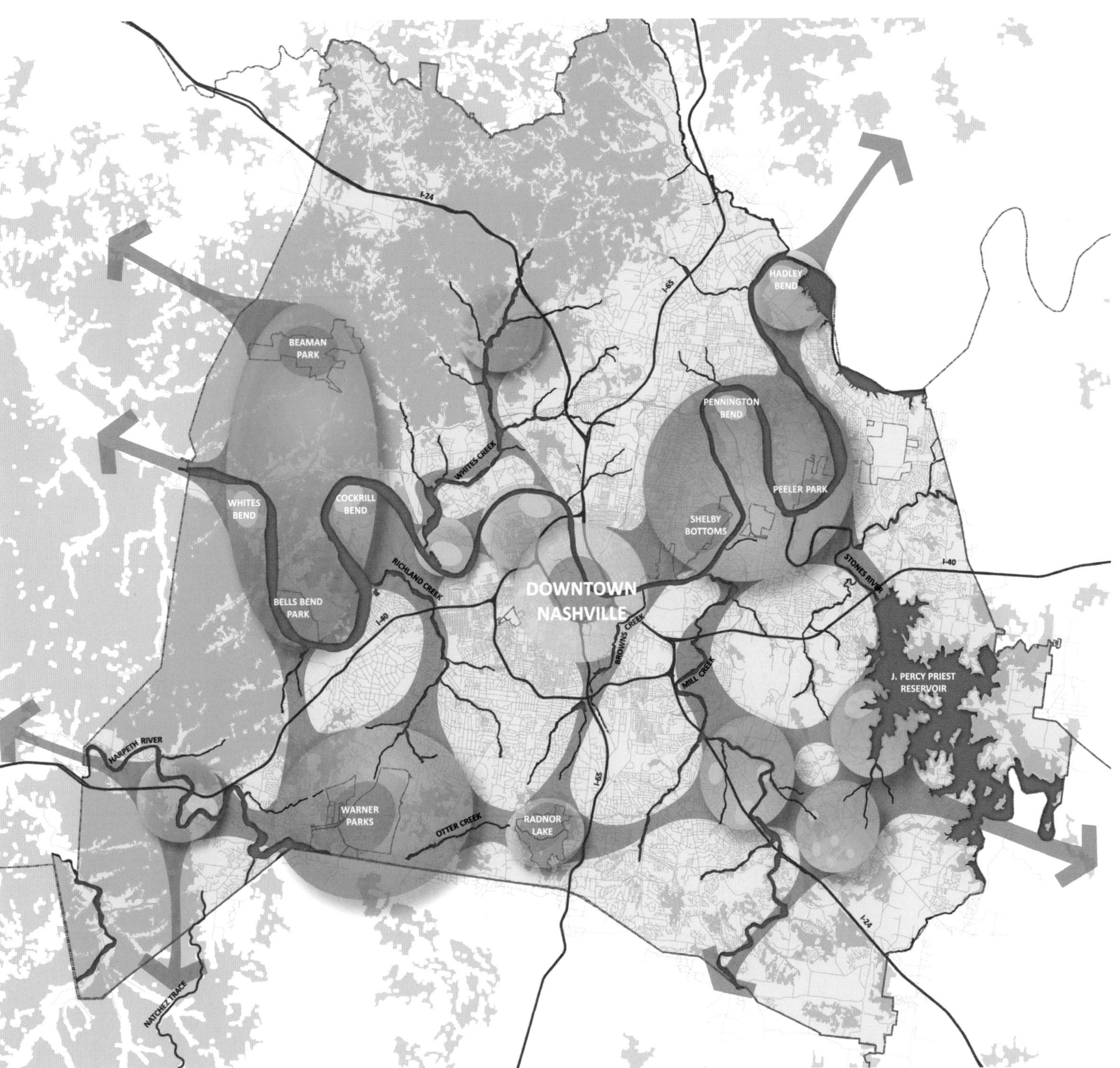

Open space vision as defined by Nashville: *Naturally*, the first conservation plan for Davidson County.[4] The plan calls for protecting each of the nine bends of the Cumberland River, as well as creating large protected spaces in each corner of Davidson County around a central "heart of green" in the downtown core. *(Plan, 2011: Hawkins Partners, Inc.)*

NATURAL ZONE BASICS

For planning purposes, natural transect zones exhibit the following characteristics:[5]

- **Large expanses of land, often publicly controlled, and undisturbed by development**
- **Land uses limited to open space and parks**
- **Public open spaces serving as refuges, where people can enjoy the scenery and participate in low impact, informal recreation**
- **Found adjacent to urban, suburban, and rural transect zones**
- **Privately owned land permanently protected by conservation easements or other preservation tools that remains in a natural and undeveloped state. Often in these cases, steep slopes, waterways, location within a scenic view shed, or agricultural significance make the land undesirable for conventional development**
- **Few buildings; existing structures usually designed to avoid eroding the natural environment and generally associated with civic and public benefit uses (e.g., nature centers or community centers)**
- **Narrow internal roads without sidewalks that follow the topographical contours and other natural features**

The natural transect zone compromises 32,500 acres, or roughly 9.6 percent of the total land area of Davidson County. Of that total, 17,990 acres is land and 14,510 is water.[6]

SHAPING HEALTH IN THE NATURAL TRANSECT ZONE

STRATEGY: *Use greenways to link open spaces with each other and with commercial and residential development.*

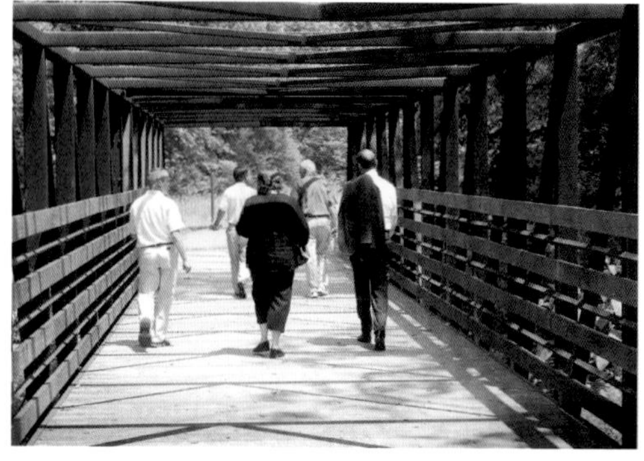

Pedestrian bridge crossing the Stones River links greenway segments and decreases commute time for greenway users. *(2009: Gary Layda)*

STRATEGY: *Within natural areas, civic buildings should avoid visual prominence and be sited to minimize environmental impacts.*

STRATEGY: *Use native plants in informal groupings where landscaping is added at entrances and buildings.*

"The quality of life in Nashville is intrinsically bound to its history and beauty. Rolling hills, striking river bluff views, and serene forests are essential to the character of our city."

—Karl F. Dean, Mayor 2004–2015
Nashville: *Naturally* (2011)

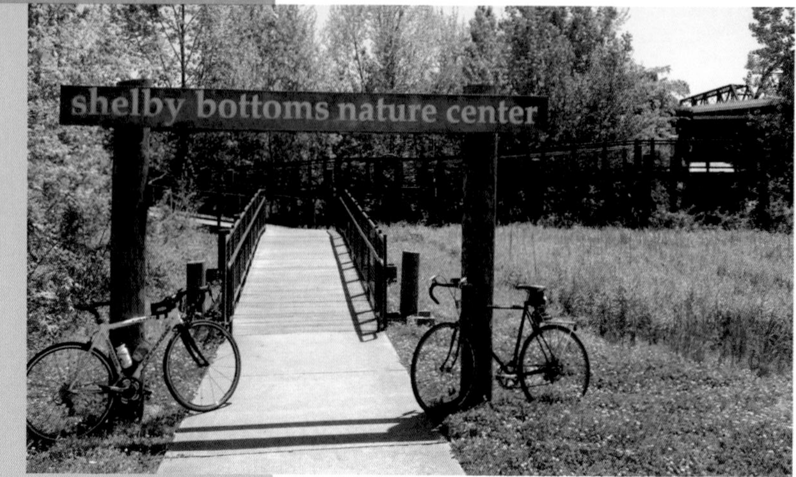

The Shelby Bottoms Nature Center responds to the landscape with its use of natural materials and its elevation on piers due to its floodplain location. Signage complements the park's natural vegetation. *(2014)*

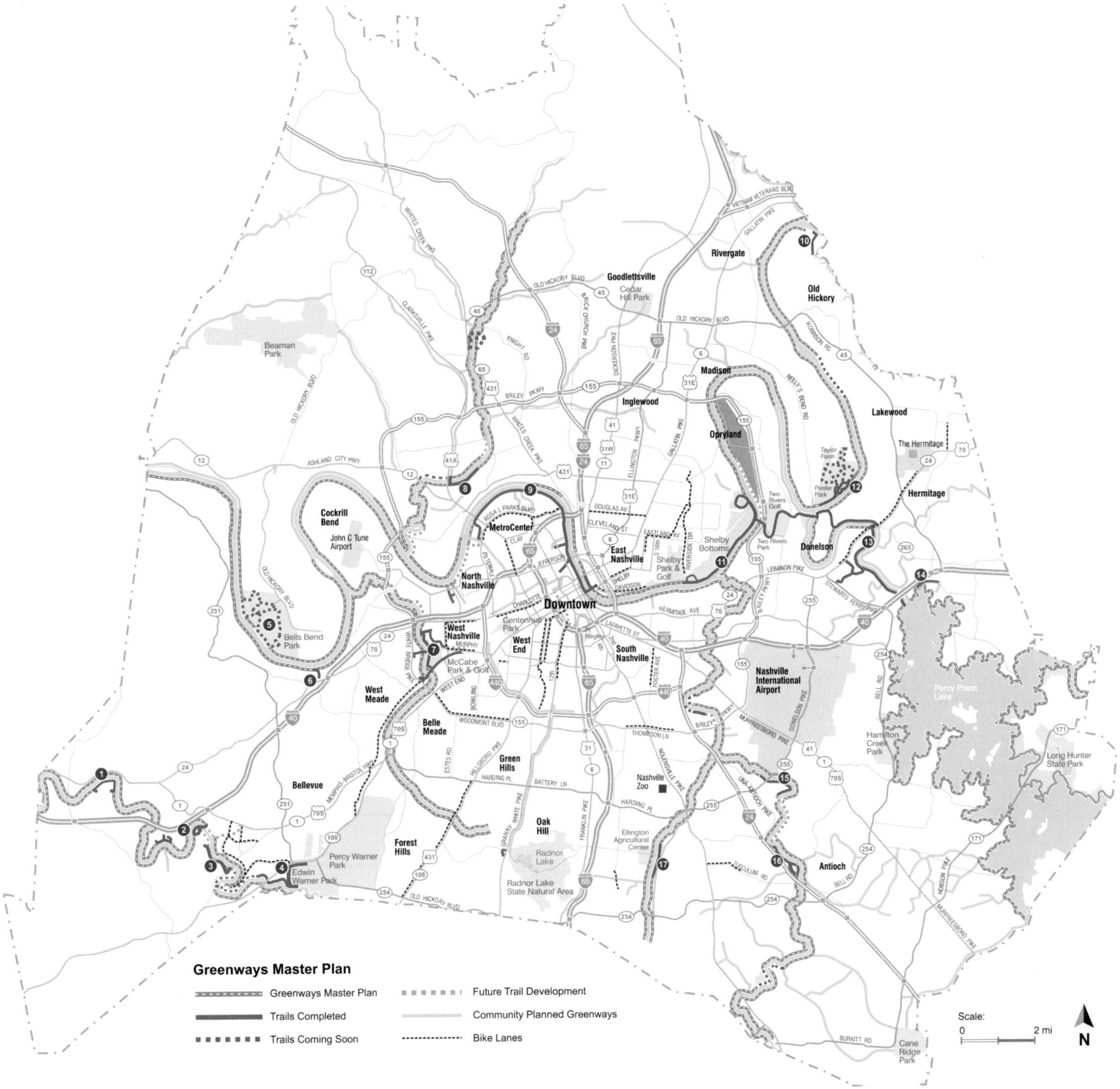

Greenways Master Plan

Greenways Master Plan
Trails Completed
Trails Coming Soon
Future Trail Development
Community Planned Greenways
Bike Lanes

Scale: 0 2 mi

N

Greenways Master Plan, showing existing and planned greenways throughout Davidson County. The Metro Nashville Parks and Recreation Department is about 90 percent of the way toward the goal of having a greenway trail within two miles of every neighborhood/community in the county. The longest continuous path is the 27-mile stretch from Percy Priest Dam to the Tennessee State University campus.[7] *(Map, 2013: Metro Parks Department)*

STRATEGY: *Lighting should be provided selectively and limited to safety purposes near community buildings and campgrounds to avoid nocturnal wildlife disturbance.*

STRATEGY: *Minimize noise, especially amplified noise, to avoid wildlife disturbance.*

STRATEGY: *Limit the amount of parking and car traffic in natural areas by restricting car storage, whenever possible, to the perimeter of parks.*

Car emissions in natural areas degrade air quality for park users and wildlife. Promoting alternative forms of transportation, as well as perimeter parking will help decrease the presence of cars. Keeping natural areas free of toxins and trash preserves water and air quality.[8]

Parking placement should avoid environmentally sensitive features and be arranged in small groupings rather than aggregated on large flat areas. Pervious paving and other low impact designs reduce stormwater runoff.[9] Parking areas should be designed to avoid environmentally sensitive features and to blend with existing land contours and vegetation.[10]

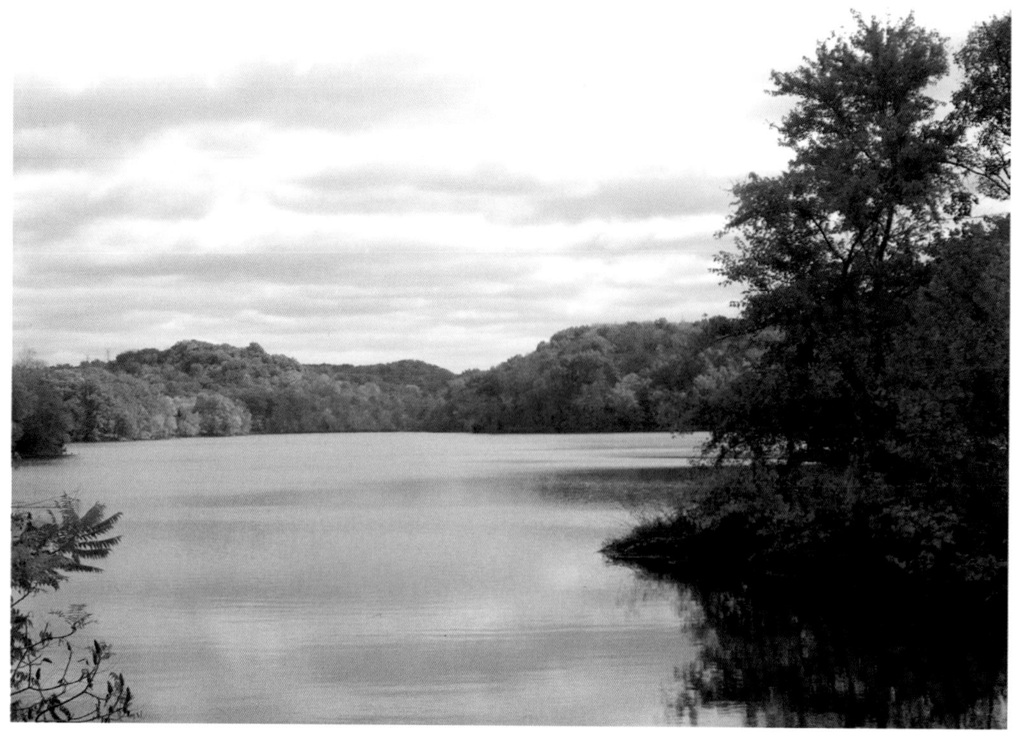

Radnor Lake State Natural Area has limited artificial lighting; the park closes at dark, and neither dogs nor runners are permitted on the pathways that surround the lake. *(2013)*

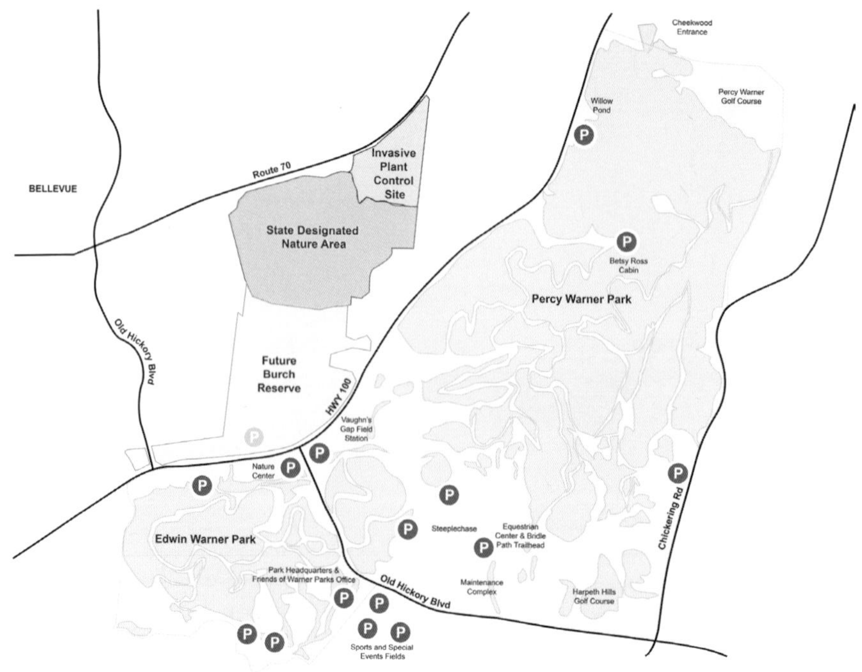

Parking locations in Percy and Edwin Warner Parks. Note how much of the available car storage lies at the perimeter, with that inside the natural area located adjacent to specific attractions. *(Diagram, 2015: Eric Hoke, NCDC)*

Historically, the ends of the streetcar lines reached various parks, including Warner Parks. This map shows the different routes that provided park access based on a 1928 streetcar map. The red routes represent the streetcars and the blue routes represent the bus lines added in 1926. *(Diagram, 2015: Eric Hoke, Joe Mayes, NCDC)*

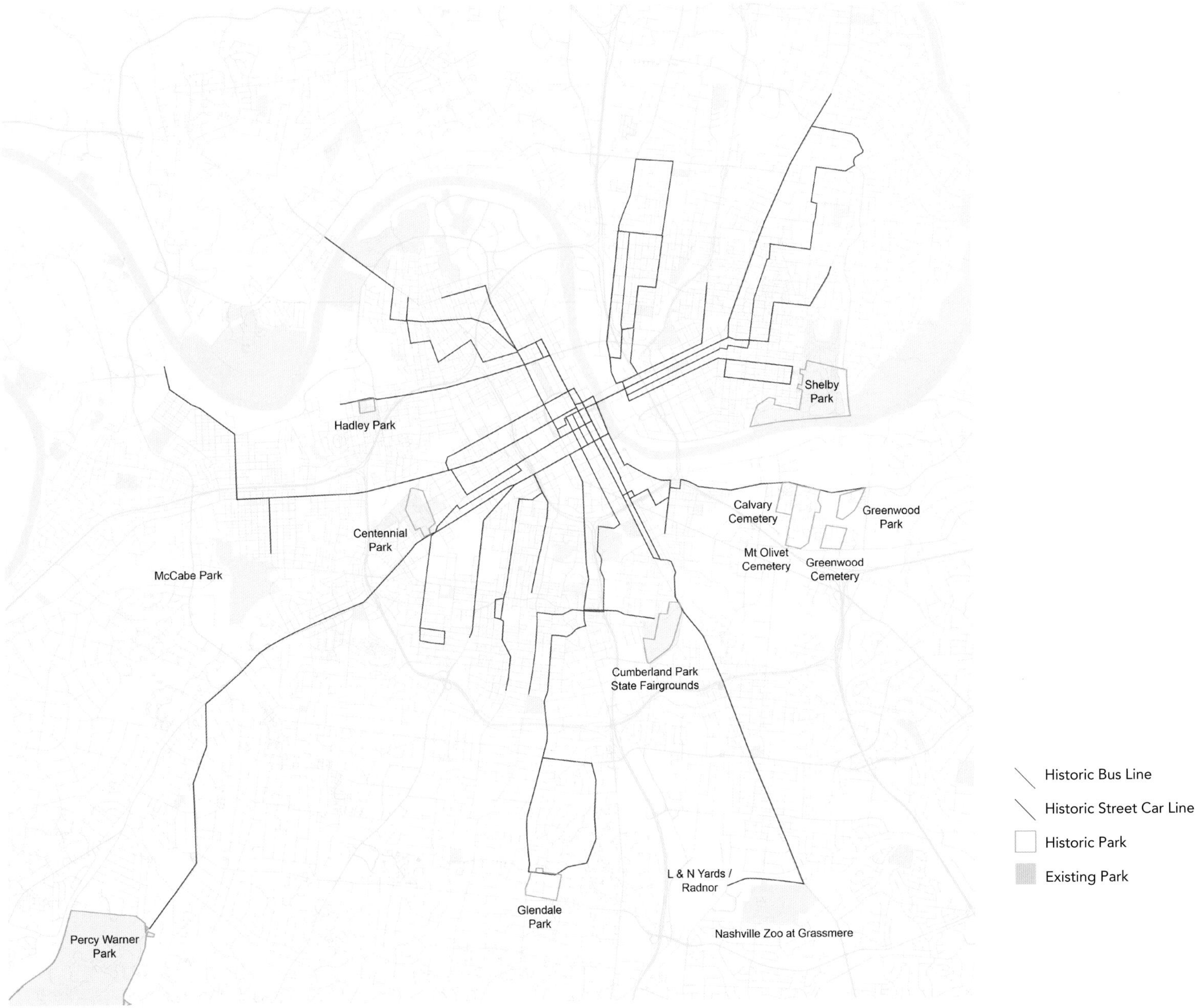

Shelby Park
Hadley Park
Calvary Cemetery
Greenwood Park
Centennial Park
Mt Olivet Cemetery
Greenwood Cemetery
McCabe Park
Cumberland Park State Fairgrounds
L & N Yards / Radnor
Glendale Park
Nashville Zoo at Grassmere
Percy Warner Park

Historic Bus Line
Historic Street Car Line
Historic Park
Existing Park

STRATEGY: *Provide public transit access to natural areas.*

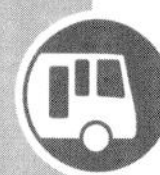

Golden Gate Park, located in San Francisco, and Nashville's Shelby Park and Bottoms both lie in urban areas. Note that one half of Shelby borders the Cumberland River, providing an opportunity to increase access points via the proposed blueway (page 243 in Downtown chapter). *(Rendering, 2015: Eric Hoke, NCDC)*

Main entrance into Shelby Park from Davidson Street. This entrance is not prioritized for pedestrians or cyclists, but rather for cars. While the recently redesigned Davidson Street includes the city's longest stretch of protected two-way bicycle lanes, bicycle lanes and sidewalks terminate prior to entering the park, where users of these travel modes must merge with car traffic. This entrance should be redesigned to accommodate automobiles, pedestrians, and cyclists alike. *(2014: ©Google; Visualization, 2015: Eric Hoke, NCDC)*

STRATEGY: *Make natural areas more accessible to walkers and cyclists from surrounding communities.*

STRATEGY: *Provide bicycle parking adjacent to community buildings and near natural attractions inaccessible by bikes.*

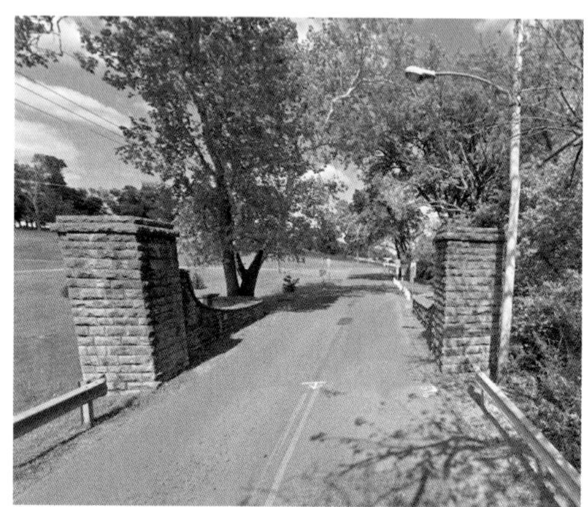

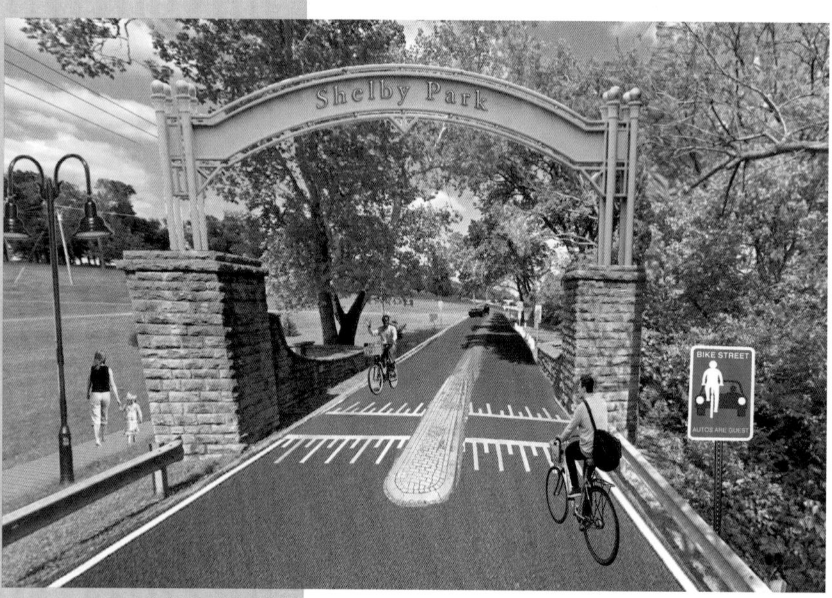

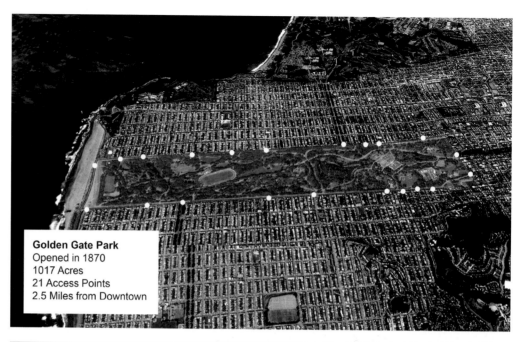

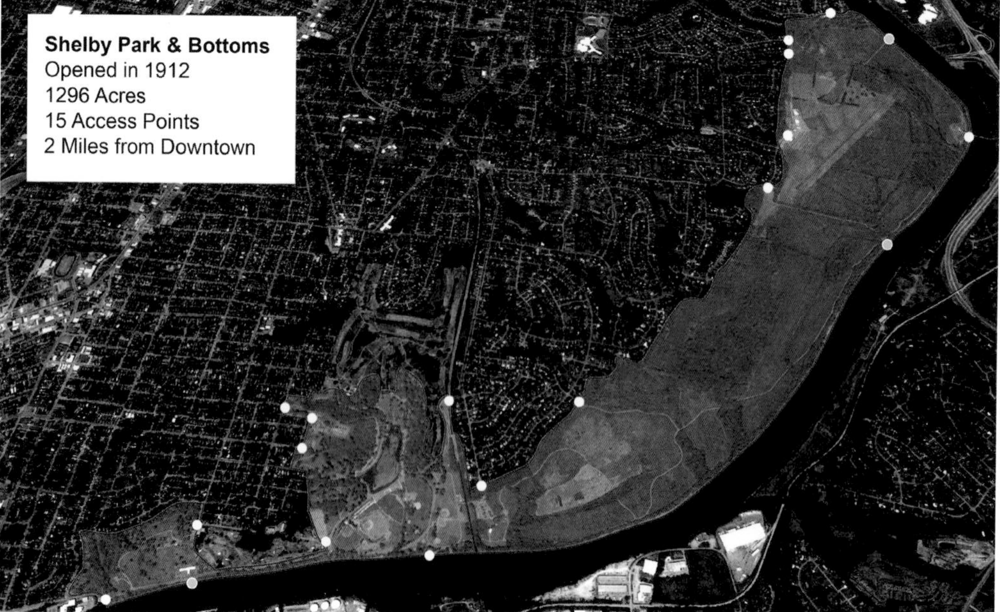

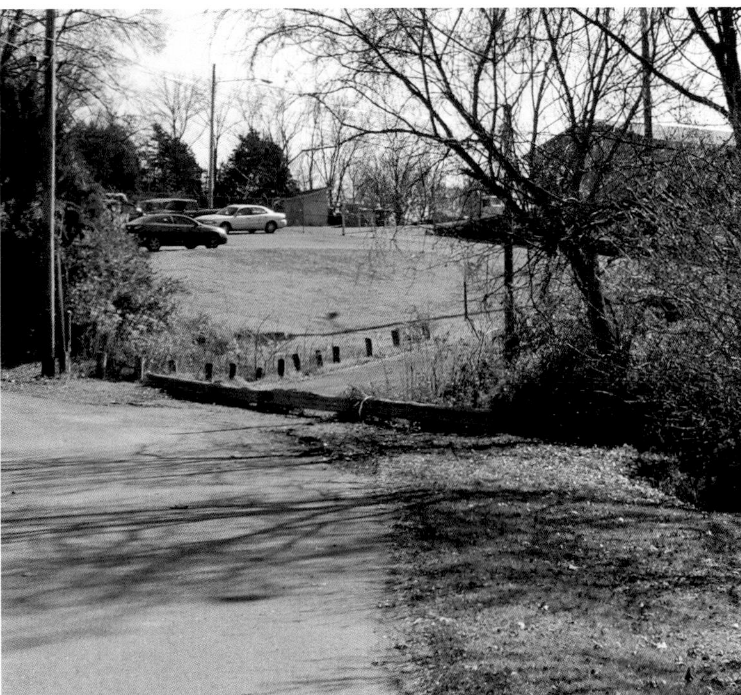

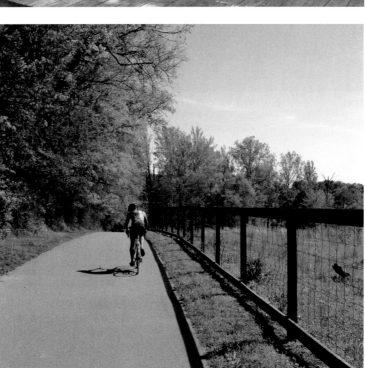

Metal barrier at entrance to Cedar Hill Park for blocking car access is also a barrier, if unintended, for cyclists and pedestrians. *(2015: Joe Mayes, NCDC)*

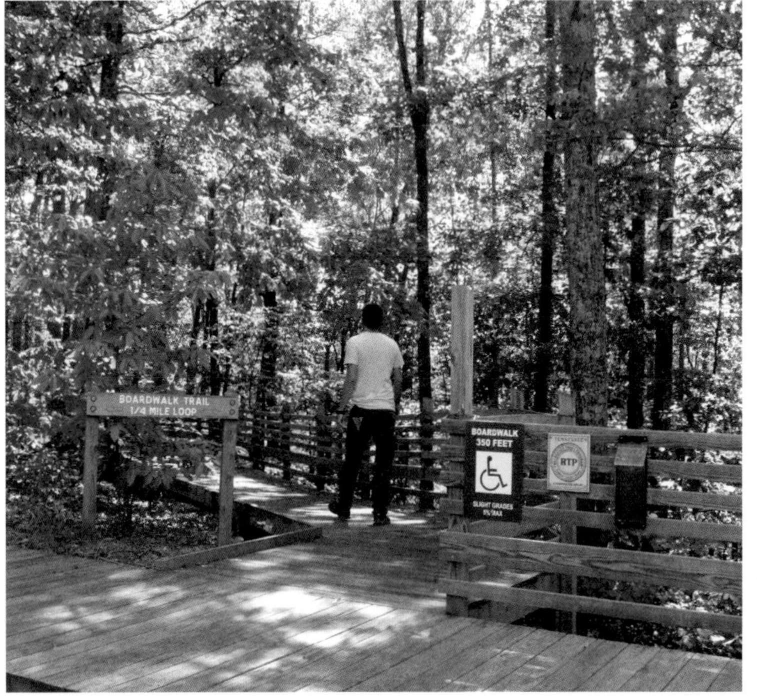

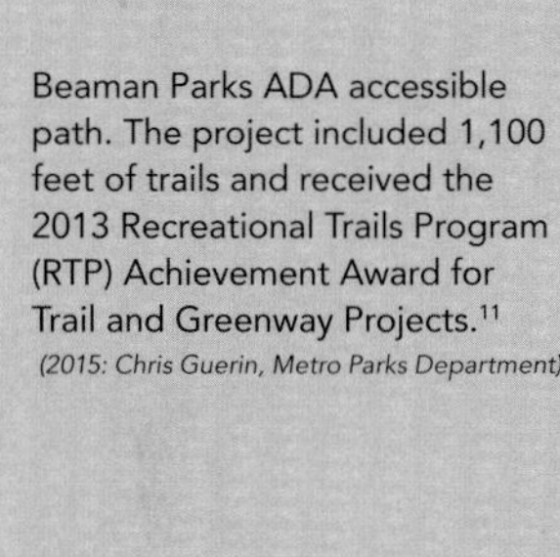

Beaman Parks ADA accessible path. The project included 1,100 feet of trails and received the 2013 Recreational Trails Program (RTP) Achievement Award for Trail and Greenway Projects.[11] *(2015: Chris Guerin, Metro Parks Department)*

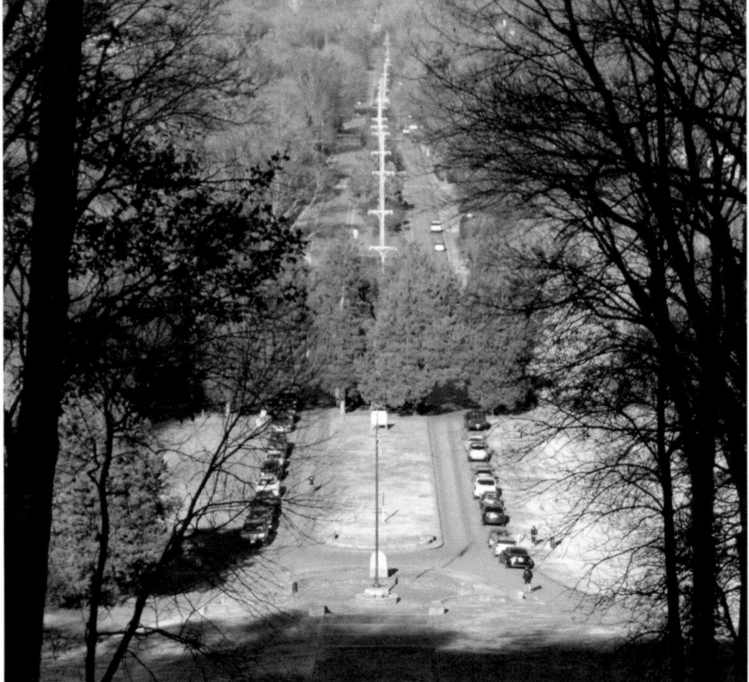

Entrance to Percy Warner Park that is walkable and bikeable. Photo from Lea's Summit shows where the old streetcar path was located in the middle of Belle Meade Boulevard. *(2015: Joe Mayes, NCDC)*

Music City Bikeway passing through Stones River Bend Park. Those willing and able to commute via bike can do so without competing with cars for space on the road. *(2014)*

View of 600-acre Stones River Bend Park, acquired in 2012 by Metro. This large tract of farmland could provide land for organic farming and grazing, thus promoting local food production.[12] *(2012: Gary Layda)*

STRATEGY: *Use selected areas of parks that were formerly farmland and meadowland as demonstrations of agricultural practice for educational purposes and to preserve local food resources.*

STRATEGY: *Create walking and hiking paths segregated from vehicular circulation. Make maps of trails in public open spaces easily accessible.*

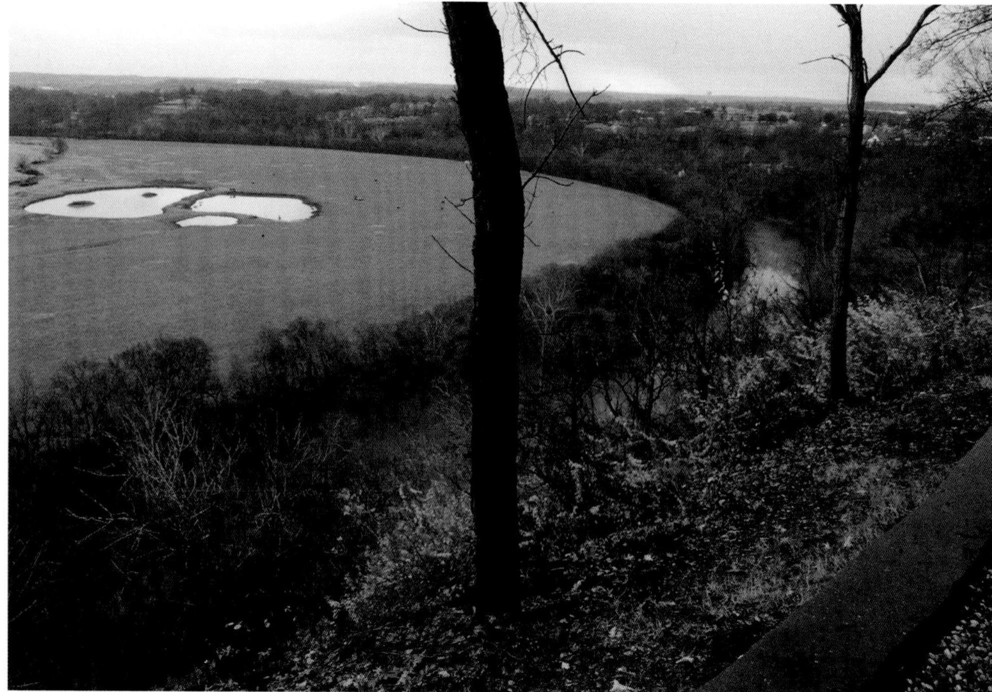

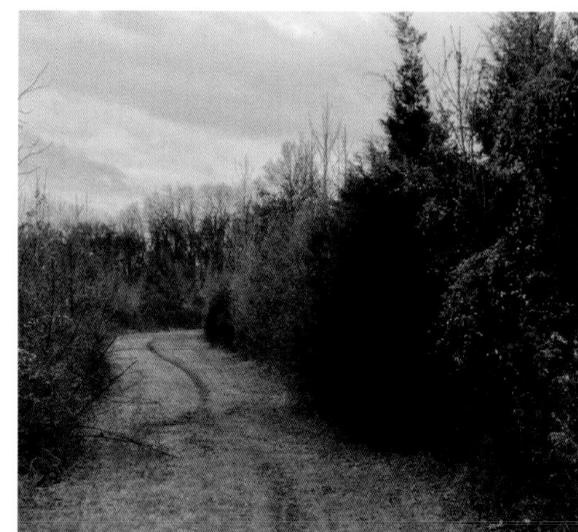

Hiking trail in Shelby Bottoms. *(2013)*

Road in Warner Parks offers tree coverage and low speed limit to promote the safety of pedestrians using the hiking trails that frequently cross the road. *(2009: Gary Layda)*

Map at trailhead in Edwin Warner Park shows trail lengths and connectivity. *(2015: Joe Mayes, NCDC)*

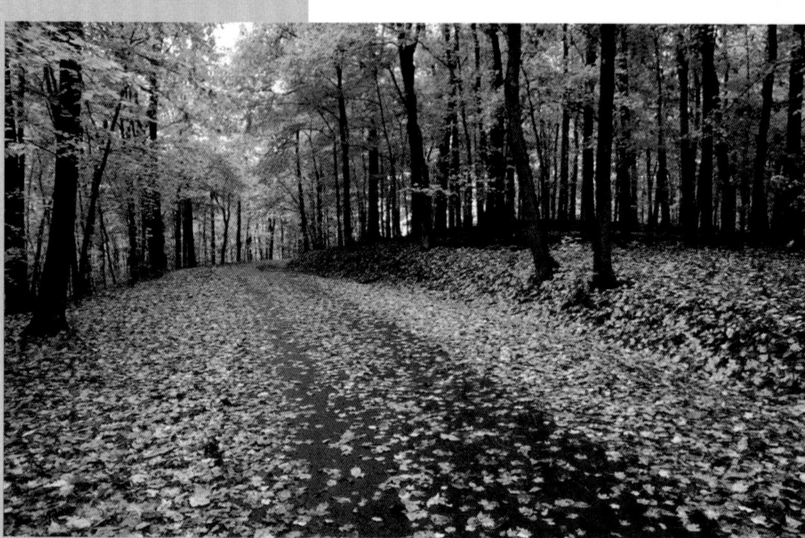

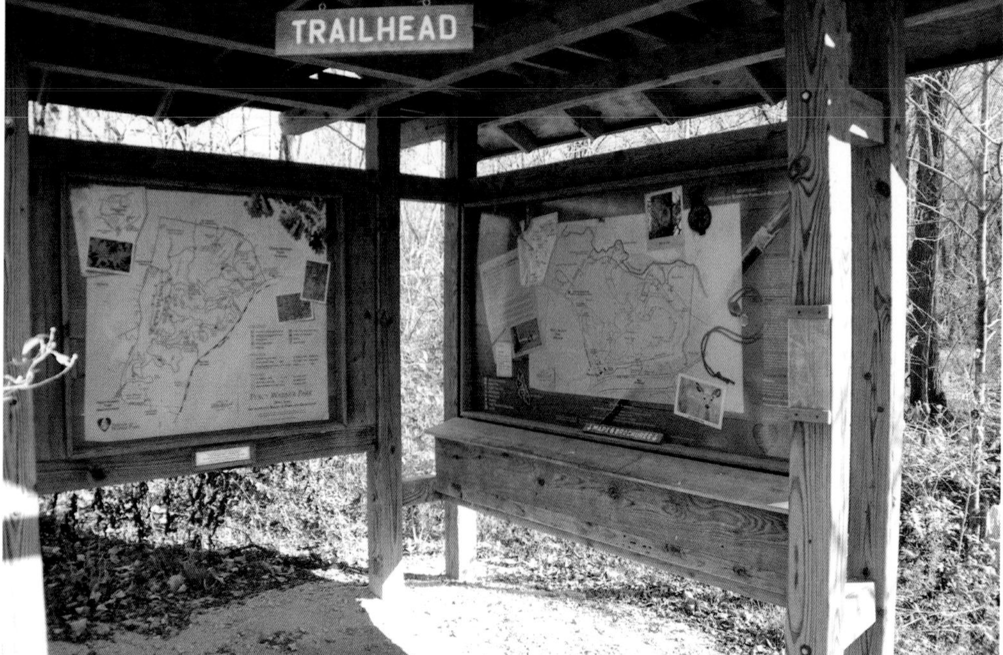

Every Child Outdoors

"Nature-deficit disorder" is a term coined by Richard Louv, who writes about the connections between family, nature, and community. In his 2005 bestseller, *Last Child in the Woods,* Louv brought to national attention sobering data showing that kids are plugged into electronic media and have lost their connection to the natural world.

By 2010, Louv's Children and Nature Network found that children were spending an average of 7.5 hours per day in front of electronic screens, compared with 30 minutes a day of unstructured time outdoors. This disparity has led not only to poor physical fitness among our youth but also to long-term mental and spiritual health problems. The dramatic decrease in time spent outdoors has raised significant behavioral and health issues, including childhood obesity, attention deficit disorder, and depression. Emerging research reveals that, in addition to reducing the risks associated with not spending time outdoors, the positive effects of spending time in nature may have significantly greater impacts on a child's physical, cognitive, and social development than imagined. This research and information has sparked a worldwide movement to introduce more kids to the wonders of nature through various planned and spontaneous activities.

In response to these statistics, Warner Parks Nature Center has been a leader in the Tennessee Every Child Outdoors Coalition, promoting opportunities and experiences that connect children, as well as parents and teachers, with the outdoors. The installation of Nature-Play, a kid-friendly interactive area in the park, the integration of unstructured time during field trips, and facilitated exploration programs are just some of the ways in which we hope to reconnect today's youth with their intrinsic wonder for the natural world.

—VERA VOLLBRECHT
director, Warner Parks Nature Center

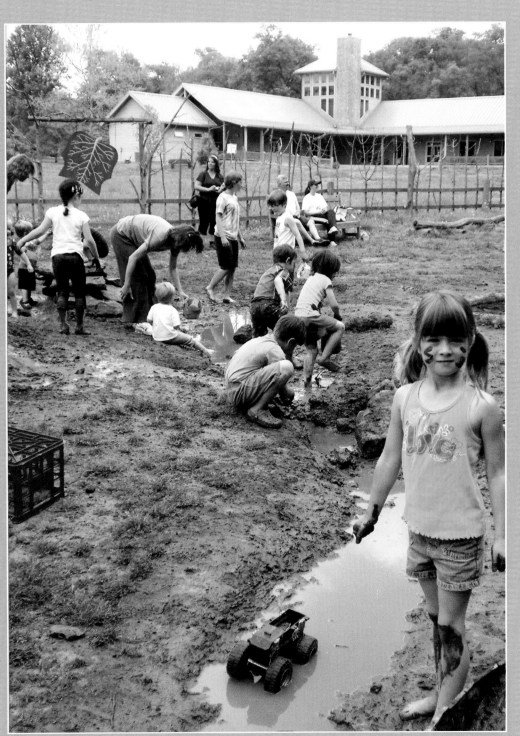

"The woods were my Ritalin. Nature calmed me, focused me, and yet excited my senses."

Richard Louv, *Last Child in the Woods: Saving Our Children from Nature-Deficit Disorder* (2005)

Nature-Play area at Warner Parks Nature Center. *(2012: Metro Parks Department)*

The land surrounding Percy Priest Reservoir features a buffer zone of trees and vegetation that aid reservoir water quality. *(2015)*

The approximately 250-acre Burch Reserve and adjacent Hill Forest, a state designated natural area, are located along Highway 100, adjacent to Edwin Warner Park. The master plan for the Burch Reserve envisions low-impact passive uses that provide a protected buffer to the old-growth Hill Forest.[13] *(Plan, 2011: Hodgson Douglas, courtesy of Friends of Warner Parks)*

The historic Mt. Olivet, Calvary, and Greenwood cemeteries feature 288 adjoining, or in the case of Greenwood, immediately adjacent, acres of walking paths that could connect to the local community. The cemeteries have beautiful mature trees, providing an escape from the industrial surroundings. *(2015)*

STRATEGY: *Identify and preserve existing open space in Davidson County as an environmental and educational resource for citizens and visitors. The primary vehicle is Nashville:* Naturally.

STRATEGY: *Conserve and/or restore a diversity of habitats for native plants and animals.*

STRATEGY: *Utilize open spaces that are not traditionally considered natural areas as assets, for example, historic cemeteries.*

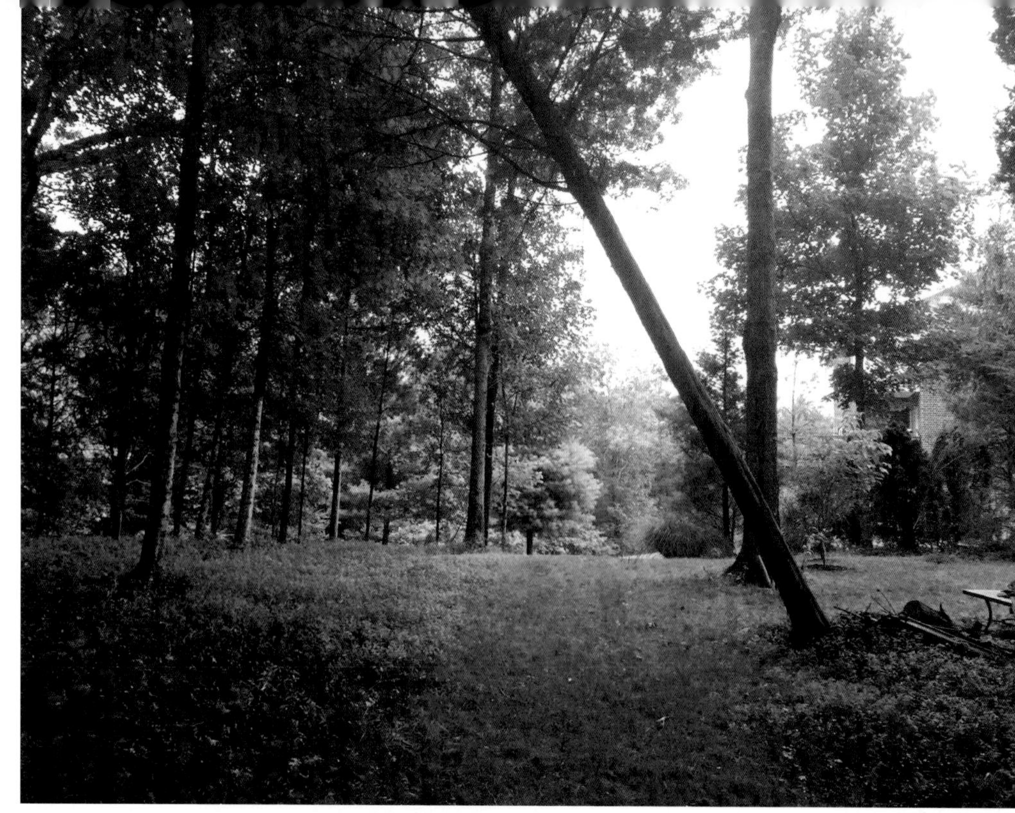

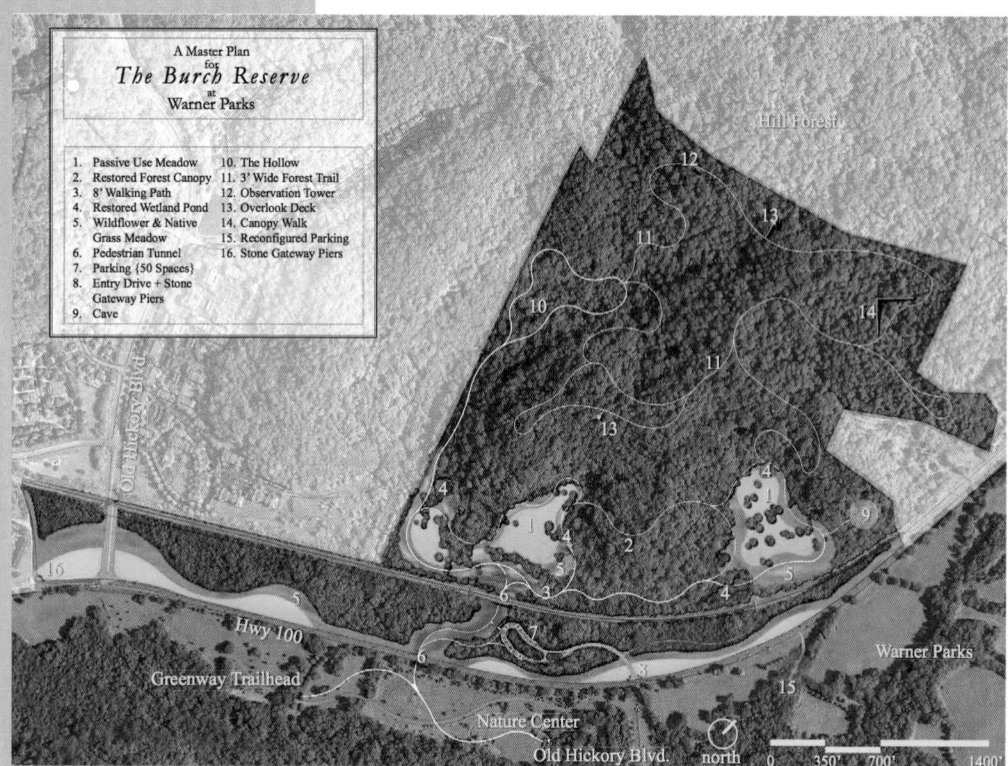

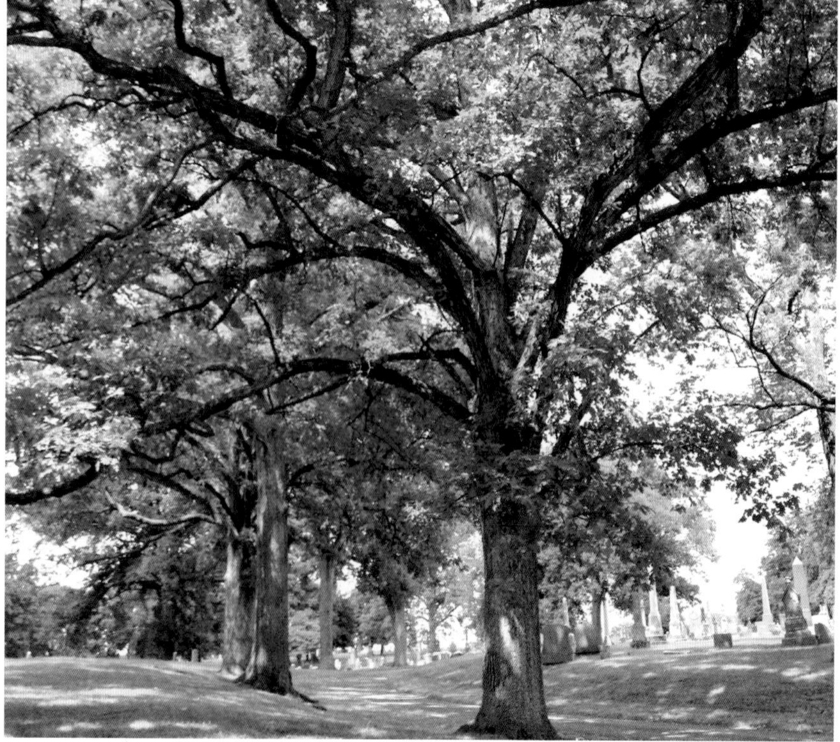

The Hill Forest

"In a nutshell, a [tree] harvest will ring a bell that can't be unrung." This sentence, at the conclusion of a dull analytical forester's report in 2005, changed the course of history for Friends of Warner Parks, Warner Parks, H. G. Hill Realty, and ultimately for Nashville.

The process to purchase land and preserve the viewshed to Warner Parks first began in 2002, when a group of concerned Friends of Warner Parks board members intervened in a real estate transaction and, with the support of the full board, made the commitment to purchase 35 acres on Highway 100 across from Warner Parks. Within weeks the group had committed to purchase a noncontiguous 87 acres, and the quest was on to raise the funds to pay for the land.

One issue surfaced time and time again: "What about the 75-acre strip bisecting the two parcels?" The 75 acres were a dogleg off a larger 175-acre parcel that was on the other side of the ridgeline and mostly fronted on Highway 70. Although Friends was interested in the property and valued the responsibility of land preservation, their interest and focus was Warner Parks, protecting the viewshed and habitat there. Until the H. G. Hill Realty Company, which owned the additional acreage, shared the forester's report. The Friends' mission and land acquisition responsibilities had just expanded.

The report was technical, but what it revealed was a 250-acre "old growth" forest nine miles from downtown Nashville. Friends of Warner Parks led the way, ultimately purchasing the land in 2009. The last previous time the property had changed hands was in 1910 when Horace Greeley Hill acquired it as the site for his home. According to Hill family lore, Horace's wife was not interested in living so far outside the city. Instead of selling the property, Hill retained it, purchasing an alternate home site.

Hill was an excellent steward. He declined timber company proposals to harvest the wood. When he decided to run cattle on the land, he installed wire fencing to keep them out of the woods. The land remained in the family and was responsibly stewarded until the 21st century, when family members finally decided to sell.

What is still known as the Hill Forest, now part of Warner Parks, is an intact habitat of mixed hardwoods—oaks, hickories, tulip poplar, and American beech—with the lowest branches more than two stories from the forest floor. Native grapevines are larger than a man's thigh. Sassafras trees are more than two feet around. There is not a single stump to indicate that a tree had ever been cut. Nor is there the choking plague of invasive exotics—such as privet, honeysuckle, or euonymus—that obstruct passage and smother forests throughout the region.

Instead, a lean bare understory allows your eye to wander up and down the steep hillsides, counting the trees and watching the mammoth grapevines swoop and twist in arabesques. The only urban sound is an occasional train, and you are embraced by the power and majesty of the trees.

—JULIA LANDSTREET
former executive director, Nashville Civic Design Center

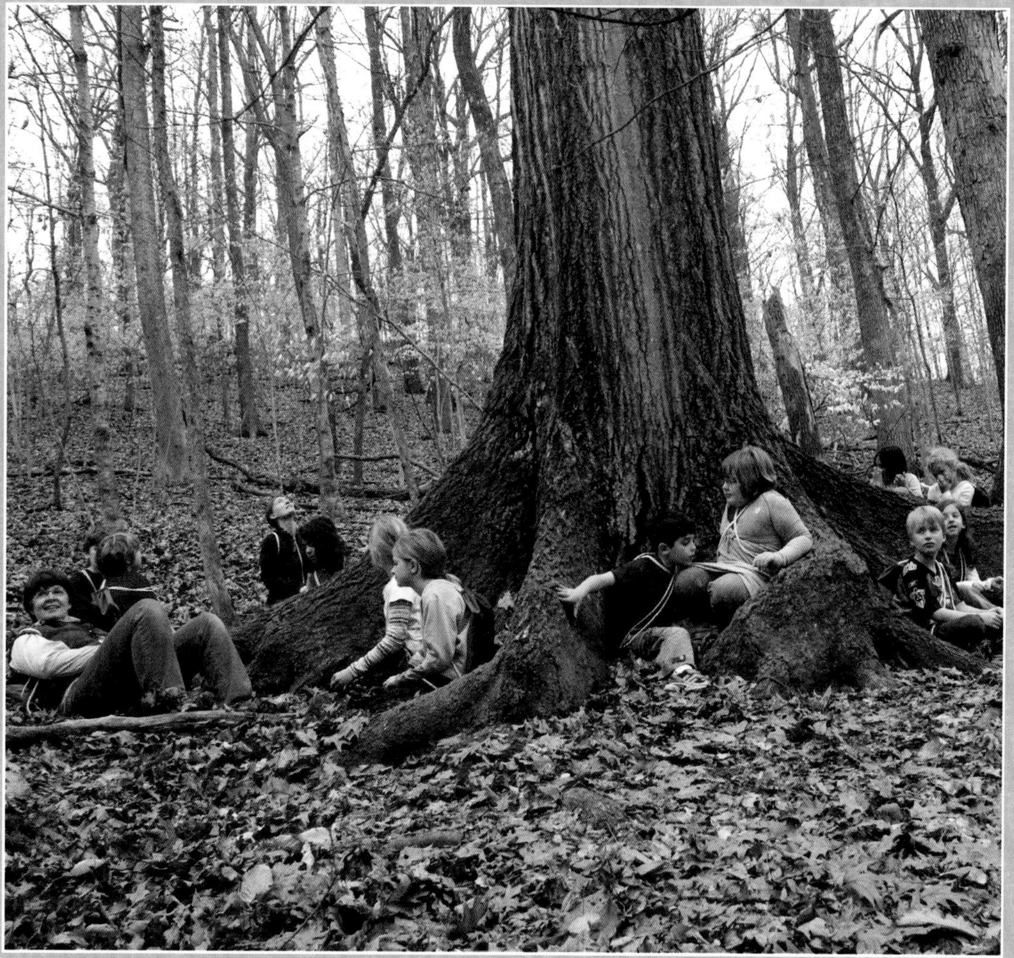

"Look deep, deep, deep into nature, and then you will understand everything better."

Albert Einstein, letter to Margot Einstein (1951)

Naturalists from the University School of Nashville connect with a 350-year-old red oak in the Hill Forest in Edwin Warner Park.
(2011: Mary Entrekin Agee)

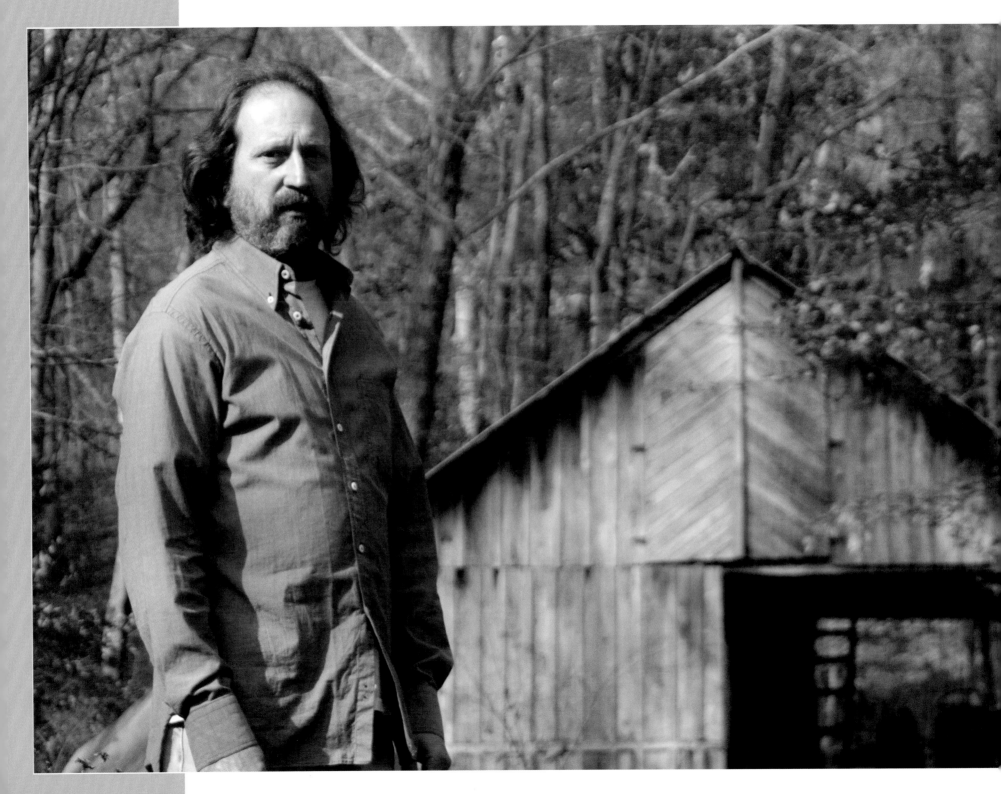

BARRY SULKIN

For environmental consultant and Scottsboro resident **Barry Sulkin,** 59, rural living is "the original model for healthy living." He contrasts "people jogging down West End Avenue, breathing fumes" with "hiking in the woods." Sulkin also points to the physical activity inherent in country life. "You cut firewood instead of lifting weights."

Food acquisition is a combination of trips to groceries outside the community—because "they don't grow Grey Poupon out here," Sulkin says—and the locally grown and raised. "For me to drive to the grocery in Belle Meade isn't a big deal. Once I leave my driveway it takes about 10 or 15 minutes, probably quicker than in many parts of town, with all the traffic. Most people out here that have jobs work in town, so it's on their way."

Sulkin's vegetables come from Bells Bend Neighborhood Farms, a cooperative of four properties lying in the Cumberland River bend south of the Ashland City Highway and thus south of Scottsboro. "I eat what I get in my weekly basket. We have around 100 Community Supported Agriculture (CSA) members, plus we sell to farmers' markets and restaurants." The farm also has pigs and plans to add cows next. "There's a chicken operation down in Bells Bend where I get eggs," he says. "Food is a major focus, an intentional effort by us to show the land in use as we were fighting development pressures."

Sulkin recalls "a while back, Metro's Planning Department wanted to rezone property here for commercial use, saying we didn't have enough goods and services. But the country is okay like it is, and people miss the concept that we live in the country on purpose."

Sulkin has been living on purpose on his 30 acres since 1978. Now that his daughter has grown up and moved away and his wife is deceased, he lives alone. That doesn't mean he's lonely. "Neighbors know each other," he says. "I credit the controversies for that."

The first controversy was the landfill threat. Then in 2005 it was Bells Landing, a so-called "conservation subdivision" that would have brought 1,200 residences to Bells Bend. Three years later it was May Town Center, a development proposal for a virtual downtown in the Bend: 10 million square feet of office space, 1.5 million more of commercial and 5,000 dwellings. The residents came together to defeat these plans. Sulkin predicts, "We're going to stay together, I think forever. We've seen what happens when you don't."

What happened was the widening of State Route 12, the Ashland City Highway bisecting Scottsboro / Bells Bend. "The road was two lanes and dangerous," Sulkin admits. "It needed to be improved, but [the highway engineers] got carried away. The original design was a parkway with a grass median, two lanes in either direction and then more grass or vegetation." When a few property owners complained that the median would prevent turning directly into their driveways, however, the engineers "just paved everything," he explains. "They made seven lanes of asphalt with curbs, gutters, and streetlights"—features of urban and suburban, but not rural roads. "A TDOT official told me it was built that way to encourage development, so they didn't have to come back later and add curbs and gutters as commercial and residential development grew," Sulkin says. "I said, 'That's not what we have planned out here.' The TDOT guy said, 'Well, that's just what we do.' So the people building the road had no concept of the community's plans, no thought of what the road would do to life around it."

What the widened road delivered was more traffic and "developers sniffing around here," Sulkin says. "We didn't get ahead of the road game. We're trying to stay ahead of the sewer game because sewers are the key to controlling growth. Once you put a sewer out here for one project, it's all over. You can't stop other people from tapping into it, just like a road." Advocates of keeping the community rural are "trying to work with the city, the Mayor's Office, and the Planning department, to pursue what we call agricultural zoning, which is done in other parts of the country, and a sewer-free zone," he says. "We need the city to embrace what we're doing out here, not just see us as the next place to put something."

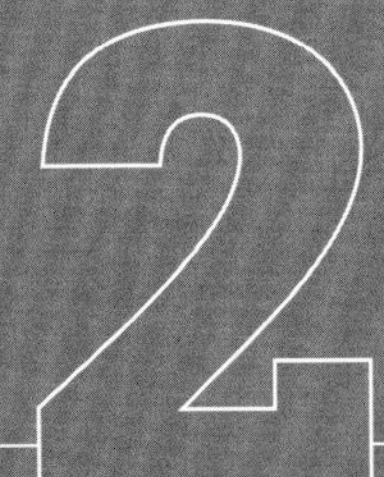

STRATEGIES

Strengthen the civic heart of rural communities.

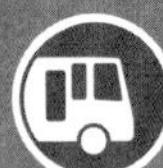

Encourage transportation alternatives to single occupancy automobile trips.

Create a safe network of pedestrian and bicycle paths connecting community resources.

Preserve and promote rural areas as sources for local food.

Incorporate a diversity of housing options while conserving rural areas and existing open space.

Create additional opportunities to connect regional parks and open spaces to surrounding communities.

Encourage conservation easements on privately owned open space.

Increase forestation in rural open space.

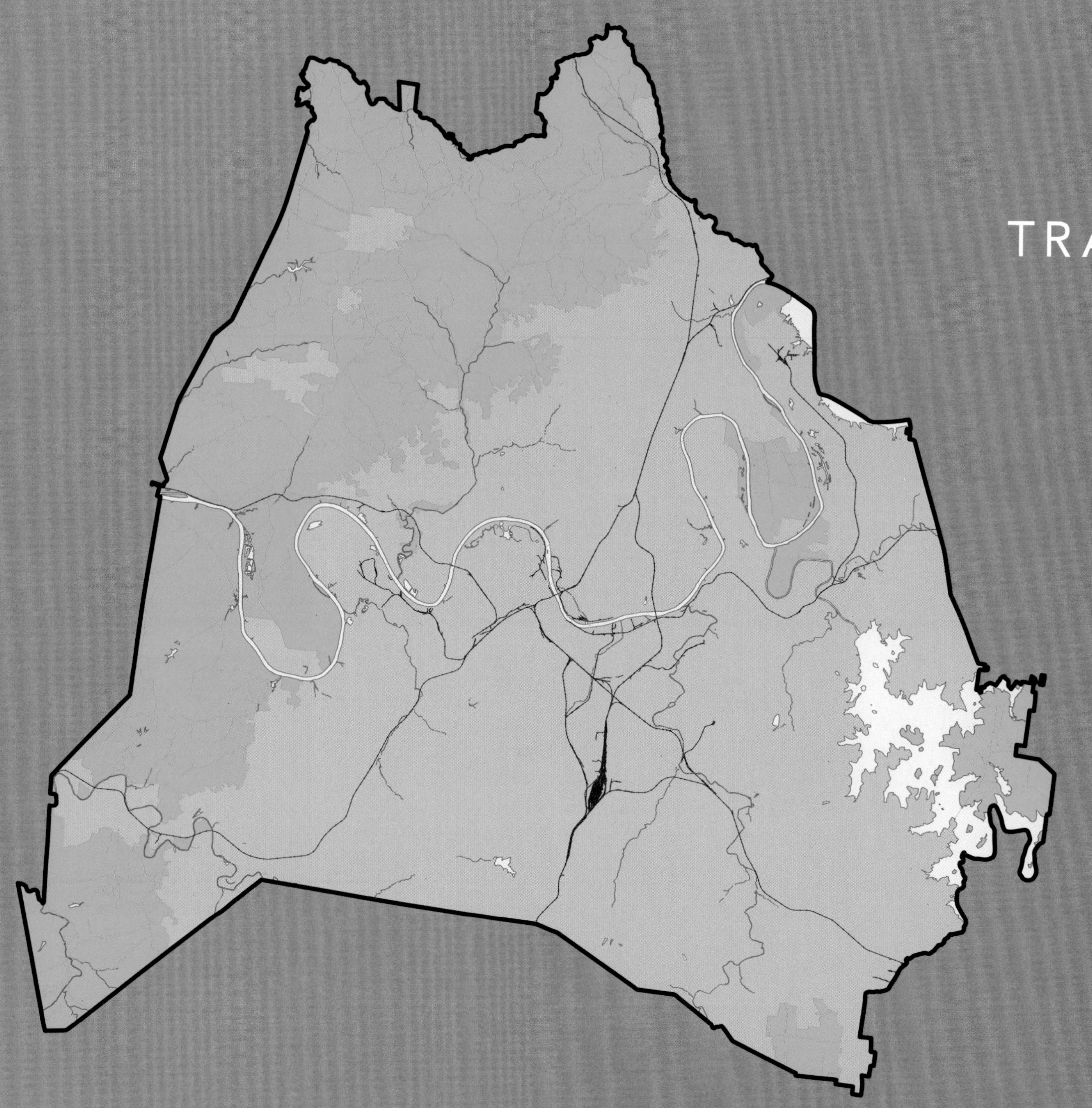

THE RURAL TRANSECT ZONE

Davidson County, with the rural zone highlighted. Note that rural zones lie in close proximity to suburban, and even urban, zones and are therefore not necessarily exclusively rural, just predominantly so. (Map, 2014: Metro Planning Department)

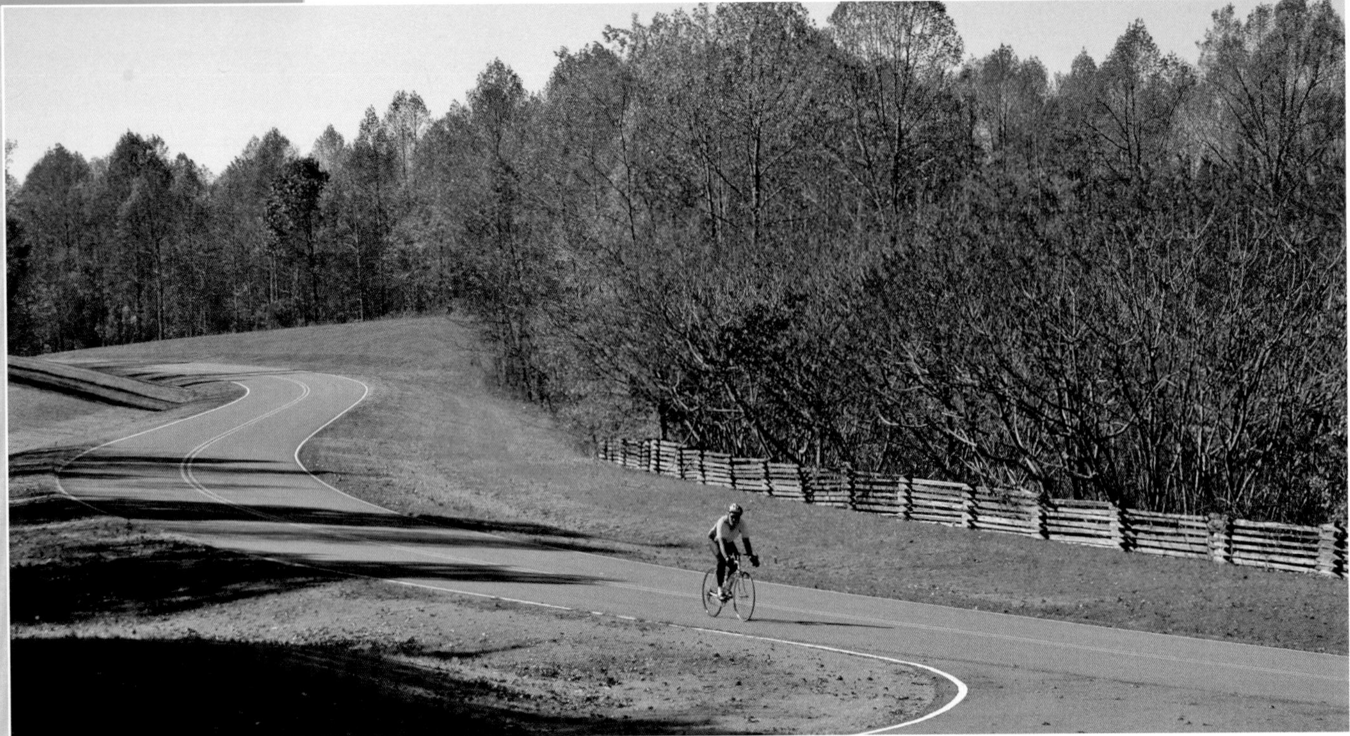

Natchez Trace Parkway.
(2010: Brian Phelps and Chris Whitis)

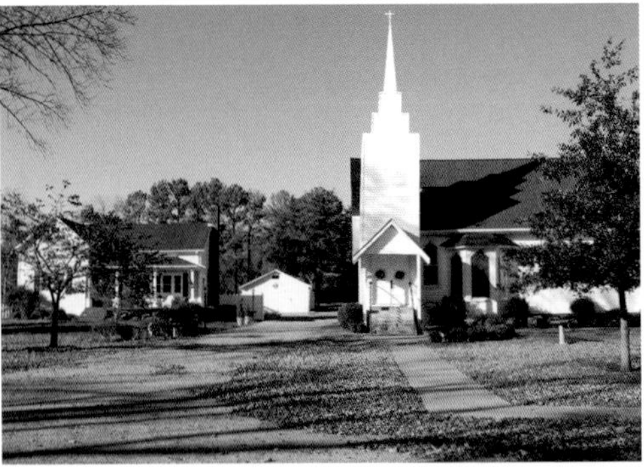

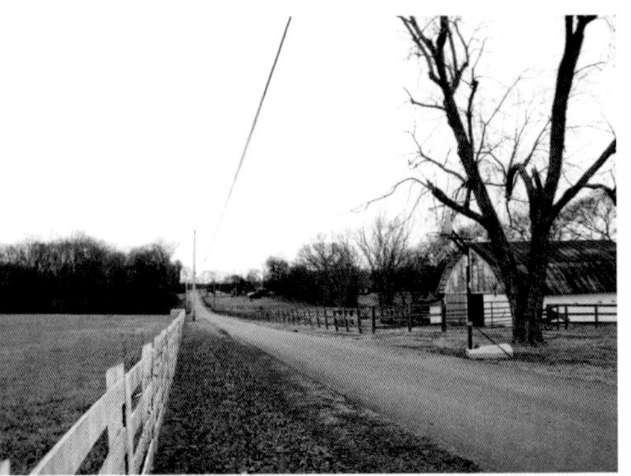

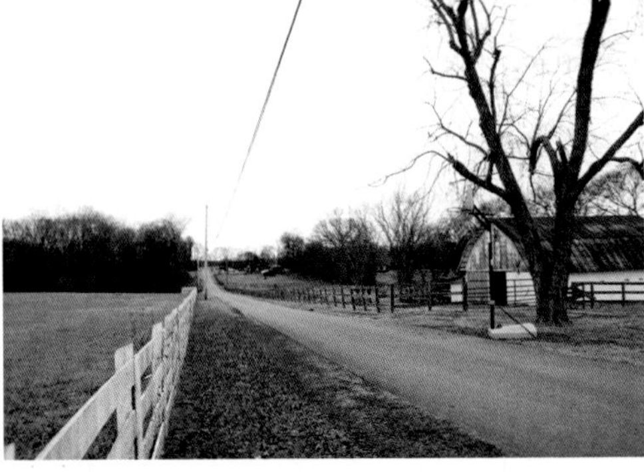

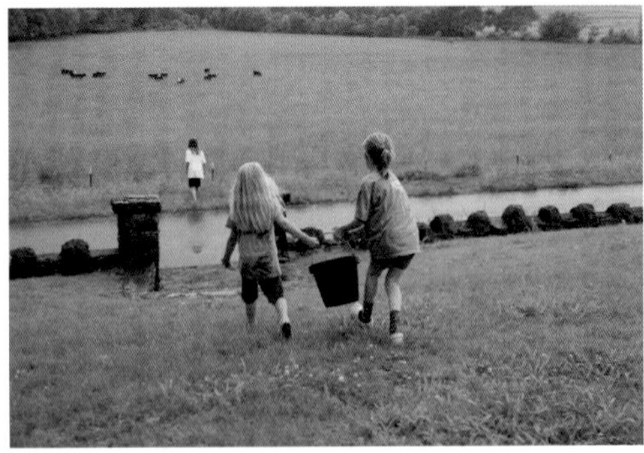

Right, top to bottom: Scottsboro United Methodist Church on Old Hydes Ferry Pike. *(2010)*

Farm on Neely's Bend Road. *(2012)*

Farm chores in Scottsboro / Bells Bend. *(2009: The Land Trust for Tennessee)*

COUNTRY LIVING

The pastoral tradition, which celebrates the agrarian lifestyle as free from the complexities and corruptions of city life, has had a long run in Western civilization. The ancient Greeks and Romans extolled the virtues of an idealized Arcadia, a theme that flowed outward from the Mediterranean basin during the Renaissance as the study of Classical texts spread north to Europe and the British isles.

When industrialization commenced in 18th-century England, intellectuals placed renewed emphasis on the spiritual values and independence of the rural life. In his 1802 "Preface to Lyrical Ballads," British poet William Wordsworth explained that he wrote of the rural landscape because there the "essential passions of the heart find a better soil in which they can attain their maturity."

Wordsworth's Romantic philosophy exercised a strong pull on Western thought when the United States became a nation. And the concept that human nature is best cultivated in our native earth has been a strong current in our culture ever since. Think Henry David Thoreau in his cabin by Walden Pond.

Today opportunities for rural living are much more constricted than they were for Thoreau. There are, however, pockets of space in Davidson County where open fields, forests, and free-flowing streams still hold sway. And a renewed interest in small-scale farming, local food sources, and open space preservation for environmental and recreational reasons has intensified the desire to keep these pockets rural.

Residents of these rural areas don't scorn the city. After all, many of them are dependent on the more populated sections of the county for employment, schooling for their children, and for goods and services. They merely prefer to live closer to nature than to neighbors and are willing to forgo the conveniences and develop the self-sufficiencies necessary to do so.

RURAL ZONE BASICS

For planning purposes, rural transect zones exhibit the following characteristics:

- **Sparsely developed**
- **Primary land uses are agriculture and low-density residential**
- **Limited commercial**
- **Wide spaces between buildings, except for hamlet-style developments**
- **Naturalistic landscaping and limited exterior and street lighting**
- **Roads typically two-lane with few intersections**
- **Low pedestrian and bike connectivity: few curbs, sidewalks, pedestrian crossings, or bicycle paths**
- **Minimal city services; many homes rely on wells and septic systems**[1]

In 2010, the US Census Bureau classified 118,643 acres in Davidson County—35 percent of the total land area—as rural land, with a population of approximately 24,900 residents.[2] But rural acreage is declining. The county lost over 45 farms totaling 9,000 acres between 2002 and 2007, the most recent year of the Census of Agriculture.[3] "We have lost a considerable amount of farms and acreage since then," says Audra Ladd of the Land Trust for Tennessee, an organization that works to preserve the state's natural and historic landscapes, "but there is no reliable quantification of this loss."[4]

SHAPING HEALTH IN THE RURAL TRANSECT ZONE

ANALYSIS AND STRATEGIES

In 2011, Mayor Karl Dean released the city's first open space plan, Nashville: *Naturally*. The plan aims to protect 22,000 acres over the next 25 years, including 10,000 acres of floodplain. Much of the focus of the preservation plan, logically enough, falls on areas within the rural transect zone, particularly on flood-susceptible land in the bends of the Cumberland River.[5]

In accentuating the health positives and mitigating the negatives of rural areas, therefore, planners, developers, and residents should consider strategies that preserve the rural, open character. Development options to meet the needs of residents—needs such as food resources, senior housing, and economic opportunities within the community—should be appropriately scaled and sited to not provoke future over-development. Strategies should be consistent with the fiscal limitations of government's public service provision to low-population-densities. Frequent MTA bus service, pocket parks, community recreation centers, and paved sidewalks, for example, are financially unrealistic. Infrastructure appropriate for higher-population-density communities, such as curb-and-gutter roads, street lighting, and sewers, should be avoided.

> The richest (prime) soils are in the bends of the Cumberland, Harpeth, and Stones Rivers. These are the areas that should be prioritized for agriculture use.
>
> —Nashville: *Naturally* (2011)

NEIGHBORHOOD DESIGN AND DEVELOPMENT

✓ *Left:* Adaptive reuse of historic structures into local business and restaurant in Whites Creek, Tennessee. The building on the left was at one time a bank. *(2012)*

✓ Leipers Fork. *(2010: Brian Phelps and Chris Whitis)*

✓ Pedestrian crosswalk at Leipers Fork. *(2010: Brian Phelps and Chris Whitis)*

✗ *Center:* Intersection of Old Hickory Boulevard and Whites Creek Pike. *(2012)*

✗ Derelict filling station at the corner of Old Hickory Boulevard and Whites Creek Pike. *(2012)*

Top right: Scottsboro Community Club. *(2011)*

✓ Health-Promoting

Historically, the small amount of commerce in rural communities has occurred in central locations, such as primary crossroads. These sites contain the potential to become true neighborhood centers.

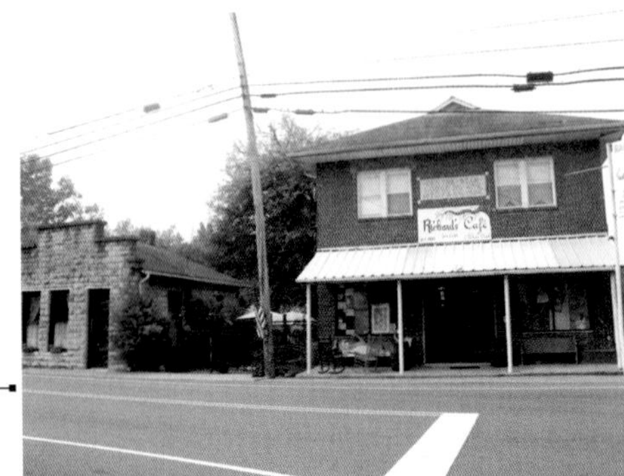

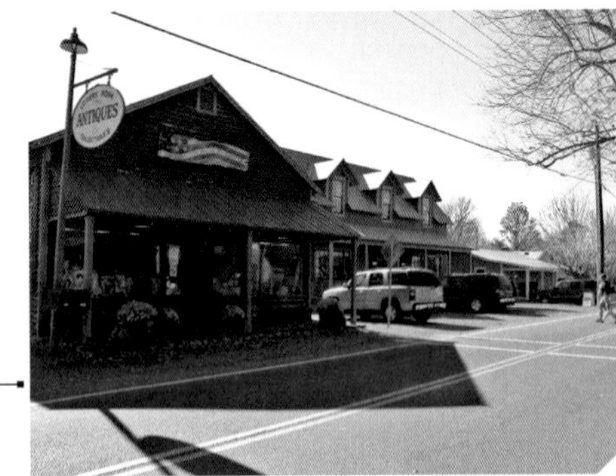

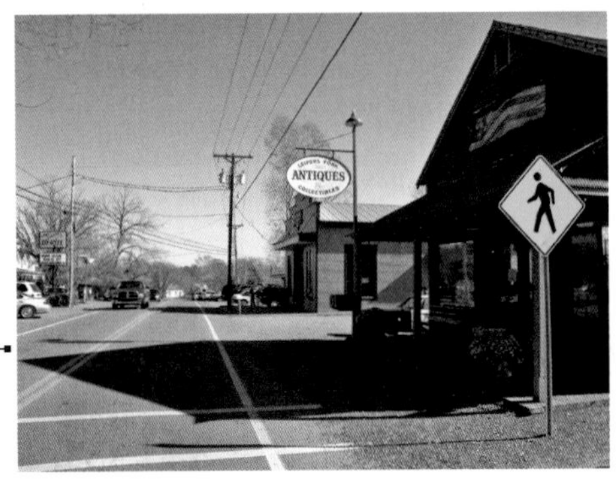

✗ Health-Defeating

Commercial centers in rural areas are underdeveloped. Residents must drive outside the community for basic needs, and fully mixed-use centers with a residential component are rare.

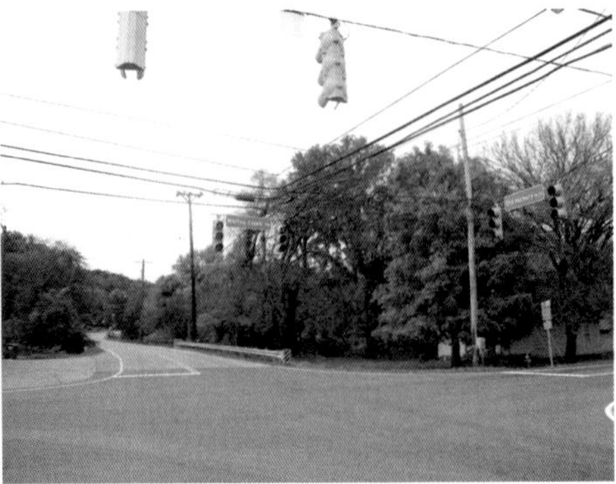

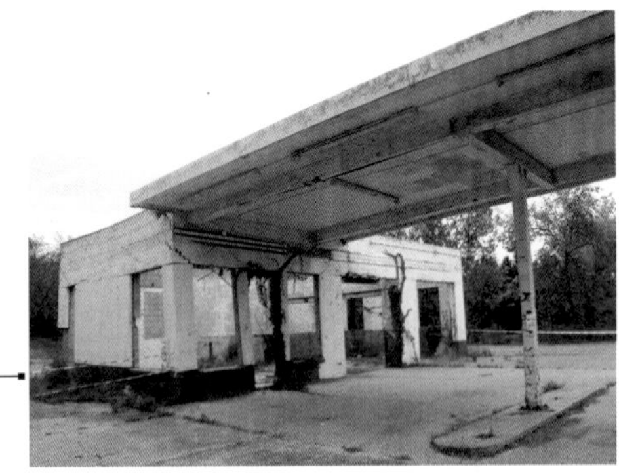

STRATEGY: *Create rural hamlets. Metro Planning's land-use policies encourage compact, small-scale, mixed-use neighborhood centers in rural communities. These should serve basic needs—a bottle of milk, a tube of toothpaste—and thus provide a destination to walk or bike to, increasing activity levels and reducing drive time for shopping outside the community.*

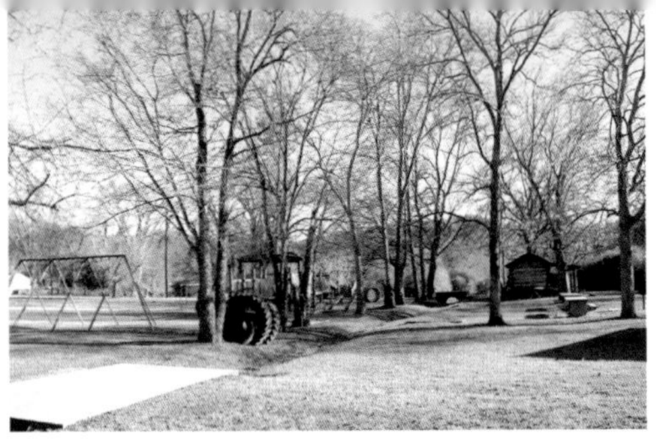

The center's residential component could house young people unable to afford larger properties and elderly residents ready for downsizing and a more walkable environment. Commercial elements could provide jobs within the community.

Neighborhood centers could also contain social space for community interaction. A place for residents to gather for meetings, meals, and celebrations need not necessarily be sited directly in the community's center, however. An adjacent location on more expansive grounds could offer space for playgrounds, picnics, and playing fields.

There is no one-size-fits-all model for the rural hamlet. Each should reflect the particular community's character and, to be successful, serve its specific needs and interests. Instead of generic chain store centers, the development of a rural hamlet should focus on incubating independently owned businesses, with features such as shared hazardous waste drop offs for mechanics and beauty parlors, for example.

Vacant properties located in the immediate vicinity of a rural community's center should be redeveloped to strengthen the center's economic and social viability. The form of the redevelopment, however, should reinforce rather than erode rural character. *The Visioning Workshop for Robertson County: Preserving Rural Open Space and Revitalizing Historic Town Centers* suggests "incentives to developers to follow architectural, landscape, scale and walkability guidelines."[6] The adaptive reuse of old structures—such as those found in Peeler and Bells Bend parks—offers opportunities to add amenities without altering architectural integrity.

✗ Health-Defeating

The rural transect's low population and building densities mean less pavement for roads and fewer vehicles on them than in more developed areas. The expected result would be lower vehicular emissions that contribute to air pollution. According to a Brookings Institution report, however, rural residents pollute more per capita than urban dwellers.[7]

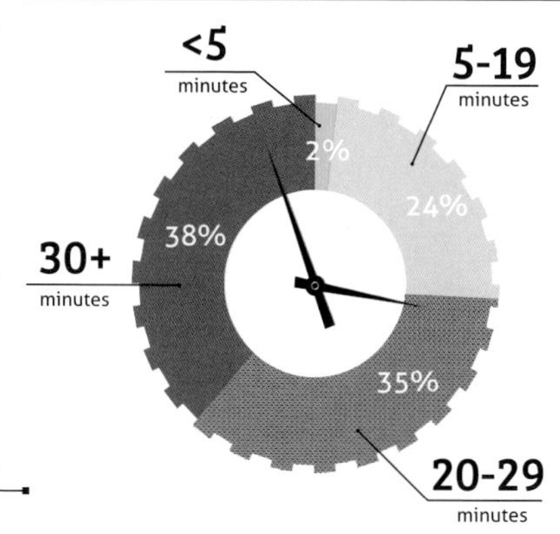

Rural residents are car-dependent due to the scarcity of public transportation. Bicycle infrastructure is also lacking. Roads built with wide shoulders can accommodate cyclists, but the distance between destinations and perception of lack of safety are inhibiting. Bike paths in parks lack connectivity to a wider system and thus are recreational in nature and not part of a transportation network.

Limited destinations within close proximity to homes compels travel outside the community to access groceries and other retail, as well as medical care, employment, schools, etc. The lack of alternative transportation options erodes the ability of the aging to continue living in their homes once they are no longer able to drive.

STRATEGY: *Encourage vehicle pools. Traditional public transportation is not economically viable in rural communities due to the lack of sufficient riders. Alternatives to the private car, therefore, must be scaled to smaller groups with shared needs to make them financially and functionally feasible.*

Rural communities with adequate numbers of daily commuters can organize car and van pools through the Regional Transportation Authority's database and the Franklin-based, nonprofit TMA Group. People with disabilities may apply for the Metro Transit Authority's AccessRide. Park-and-ride lots for cars and bicycles in areas with public transit stops could facilitate transit use.

✗ *Left:* Average commute time to work from rural transect zones in Davidson County, according to the US Census Bureau's American Community Survey. *(Information graphic, 2013: Ashley Nicole Johnson)*

Below: VanStar. *(2011, Debbie Henry, The TMA Group, www.vanstar.com)*

The Vanpool

Vanpooling is designed to work for communities and corridors with long distance commute patterns not served by traditional transit. Through vehicle sharing, rural residents have an affordable transit option to access job centers.

Ridesharing also broadens the workforce reach of employers. A large company in a rural community with a small population can use vanpools to bring in talent from urban areas. Urban-sited companies can extend their recruitment to rural areas where transportation costs used to be a barrier.

The development of vanpool and rideshare transport solutions, through programs administered by government and nonprofit agencies, fits neatly into the culture of small rural towns. A vanpool is built "by the people, for the people." Riders choose departure times, pickup and drop off locations, and routes. And some customers, after going through approval and training processes, become drivers themselves, minimizing costs. Vehicles, insurance, maintenance, and the web-based management portal are provided by TMA to each group for a small per mile charge. AAA estimates that the fully allocated cost for a person driving alone to work is 50 cents a mile, a vanpool rider approximately one tenth of that.

In Middle Tennessee, over 80 vanpool routes operate daily. These pools connect rural communities to employment centers, most with direct service. Vanpools can be implemented in less than two weeks and are financially sustainable.

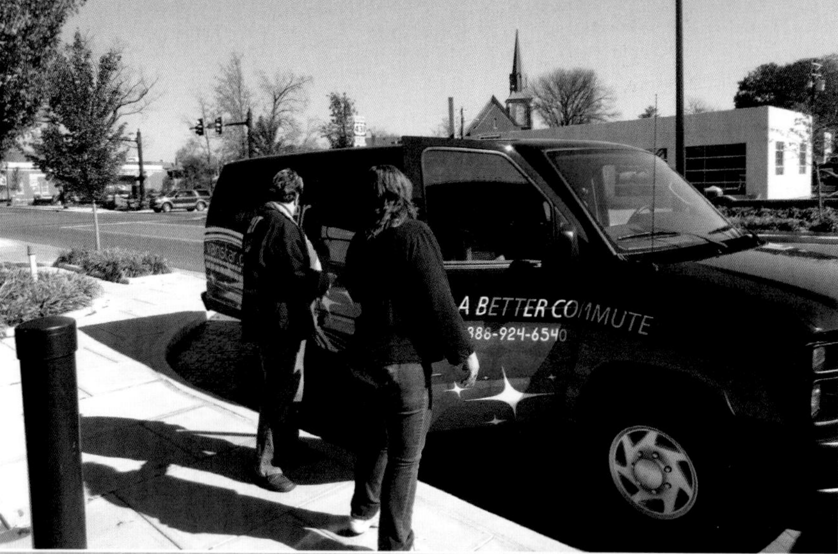

In Middle Tennessee, where commutes are long and traditional transit infrastructure is still being developed, vanpools can fill the void and provide rural communities with the transit connections they need.

—STANTON HIGGS
former business development and operations director, The TMA Group (Transportation Management Association)

WALKABILITY AND PEDESTRIAN SAFETY

✓ Health-Promoting

The abundance of open fields and forests in the rural transect zone presents great pedestrian potential. Residents on large parcels can walk on their own land, and neighbors can exchange walking rights. The regional parks within rural communities contain walking and biking paths.

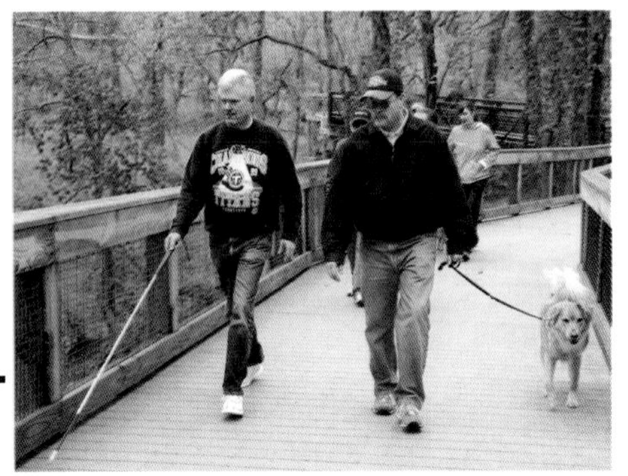

✓ Stones River Greenway *(2008: Gary Layda)*

✗ Health-Defeating

The rural zone lacks public pedestrian infrastructure. Wide spacing between dwellings makes paved sidewalks financially unfeasible. Rural arterials and subsidiary roads are not typically designed to accommodate pedestrians. The shoulders on some roads offer space for walkers, but many lack this amenity, and high vehicular speeds create safety issues. Crosswalks are rare, even at signalized intersections.

Paths on public lands are self-contained and used for recreation; lack of connectivity to a wider network constricts their viability as a transportation option. The creation of a pedestrian network would involve easements on private land that establish a limited form of public access to private open space. In Great Britain, Switzerland, and the Scandinavian countries, common law enshrines an ancient "right to roam" tradition of public paths on private lands, but this has not been an American custom.

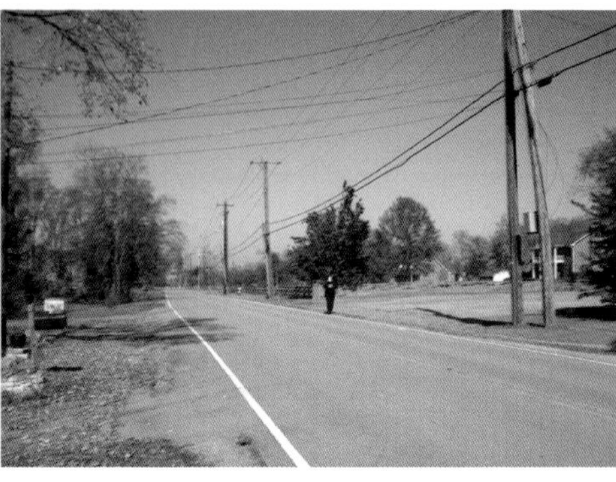

✗ *Right:* Pedestrian walking along Neely's Bend Road. *(2012: Jeffrey Bond, Vanderbilt University)*

STRATEGIES: *Ensure pedestrian safety for roadways and multi-use paths. Add safety features, such as crosswalks, signage, and medians at prominent intersections, to provide safe passage across main thoroughfares.*

Multi-use paths for pedestrians and cyclists along main roads can serve as both recreational and active transportation corridors. Such paths can be designed using pervious materials—compacted gravel, mulch, or short-mown grass—more in keeping with rural character.

Off-road primitive paths could be accomplished through a variety of alternative financing mechanisms. Examples of nongovernmental sources include funds from foundations and materials grants from corporations like Home Depot and Lowe's. Volunteer labor from the hiking community could help bridge a project's realization.

Shared-use agreements between Metro government and private landowners could speed the implementation of a pathway network by avoiding costly land acquisition. By granting easements, property owners can also offset their federal income tax burden for a set number of years.

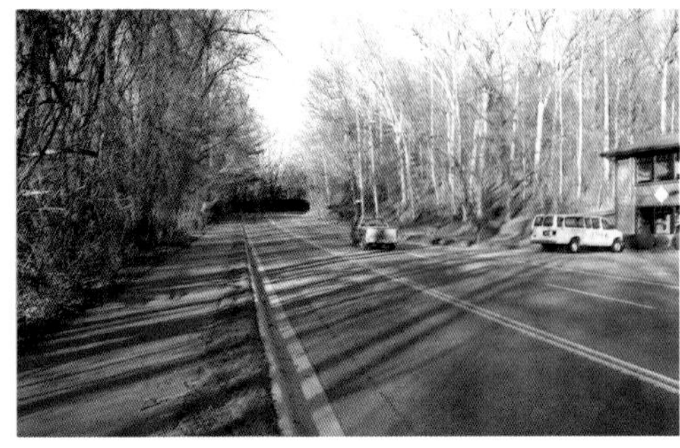

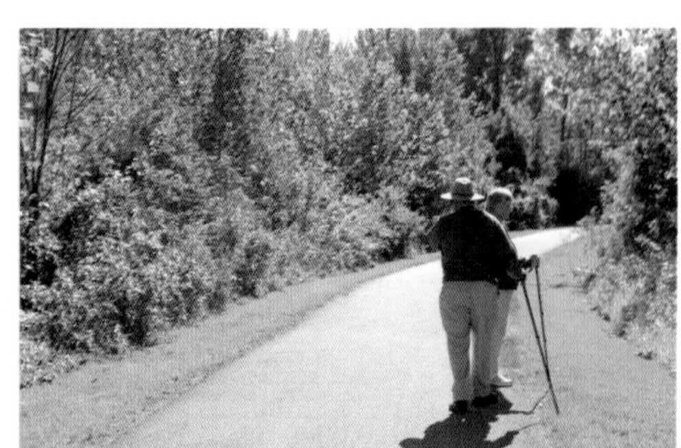

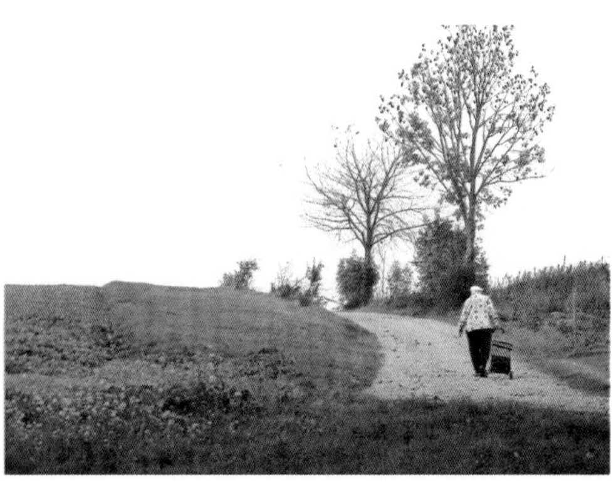

Rural multi-use corridor. Note the grass divider between vehicular road and ped/bike path. Paths physically separated from roadways, while less dangerous for walkers and cyclists than using road shoulders, are not the safest option for rural areas because of their close proximity to motorized vehicles. *(2008: Metro Planning Department)*

Center: Shelby Bottoms Greenway. Here the path for pedestrians and cyclists is completely distinct from the surrounding road system. *(2012)*

Right: Senior walking along a footpath through privately owned farmland, connecting various public parks and community centers in Zurich, Switzerland. *(2009)*

FOOD RESOURCES

Health-Promoting

Virtually all the farmland in Davidson County lies within the rural transect zone. This zone is thus the logical source for local food. Since the relaxation of strictures against farm stands by the Metro Council in 2012, these agricultural lands also contain the potential for residents and visitors from throughout the county to buy fruits and vegetables directly from farmers. Large lots also give households the opportunity to grow their own food in family gardens.

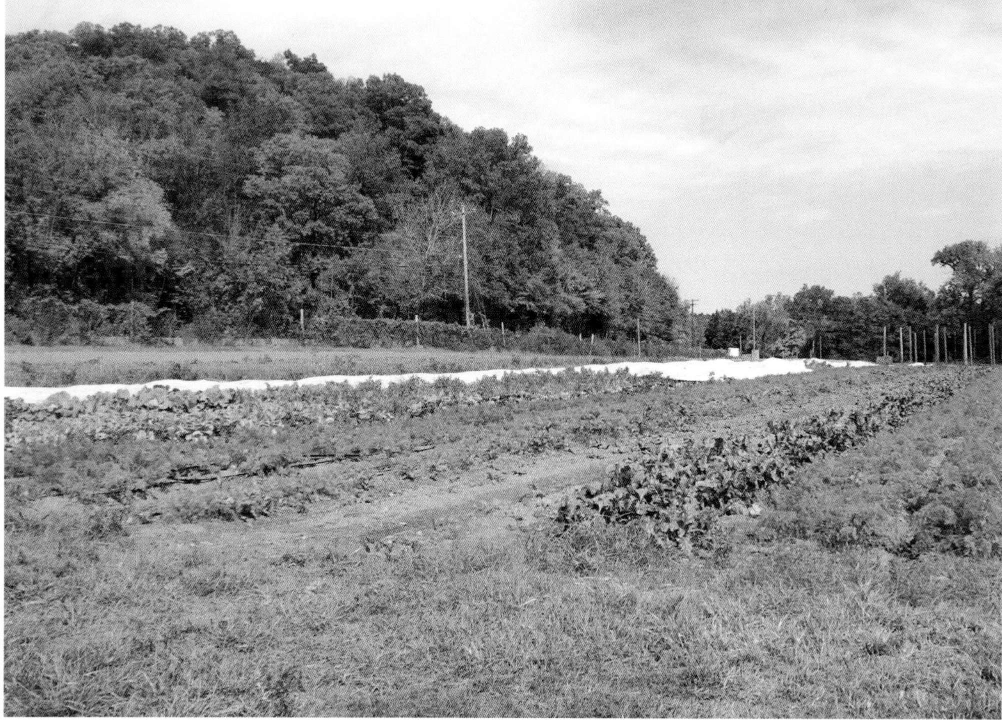

Sulphur Creek Farm, a Bells Bend Neighborhood Farm. (2012)

The Food Hub

Imagine a quaint farmers' market set in a church parking lot or public park on a Saturday morning, with local vendors selling their wares to strolling families. As picturesque as this view of local agricultural business is, the Saturday market model is inherently limiting. One-day-a-week markets do not address the busy work schedules of customers wanting to buy fresh food, and many larger and bulk buyers, such as schools and restaurants, are cut out of the farmers' market business.

According to the US Department of Agriculture's (USDA) Economic Research Service, local food sales through all marketing channels in the United States were estimated to be $4.8 billion in 2008 and were projected to climb to $7 billion by 2011.[8] To best promote this growth, the model needs to grow and adapt to the needs of local agribusiness and bulk buyers. A more permanent environment used to store, process, and distribute agricultural goods could propel the businesses of smaller farmers and increase the availability of local food.

A regional food hub, defined by USDA as "a business or organization that actively manages the aggregation, distribution, and marketing of source-identified food (products primarily from local and regional producers) to strengthen their ability to satisfy wholesale, retail, and institutional demand,[9] addresses many of these needs. Not only can the food hub serve as a retail center for individual customers, it can have a centralized distribution infrastructure for wholesale customers, such as schools and restaurants.

Recent studies reported in the *Journal of Consumer Affairs* show that in the US we waste about 40 percent of all edible food.[10] A shared community kitchen within a food hub could help reduce producer-side waste by turning "seconds," less attractive or blemished goods, into value-added products like jams and canned food, bringing more products to market and helping to balance sales outside of the growing season.

Other benefits of developing a food hub include the combination of financial resources for physical facilities, insurance, and marketing. Dependable source-identification and branding would simplify buying choices for all consumers. The central physical facility could be an agricultural learning and training center serving as a small farm and food business incubator, offering training in food safety, farming practices, and business development.

—LAURA WILSON

chef, formerly of Grow Local Kitchen, Nashville Farmers' Market

Health-Defeating

A basic fact about food: what we don't grow or raise ourselves, we must buy. In the rural transect, buying entails driving outside the community if the consumer desires healthier foods than the highly processed products sold in small convenience marts. Full service groceries depend on larger populations than are found in rural communities.

STRATEGIES: *Cultivate new market approaches. In designing their developments and in merchant recruitment, developers of rural neighborhood centers should recognize the increased demand for locally grown and artisanal foods among Nashville consumers. Setting aside space in a center's parking lots on a seasonal basis for farm stands, pop-up farmers' markets, and CSA drop-offs would increase foot traffic, as well as establish a central location within the community for farmers to market their products and residents to buy them.*

Nashville also needs investment in facilities—such as canneries, dairy processing, and butchering facilities—that turn raw agricultural products into finished goods for local sale.

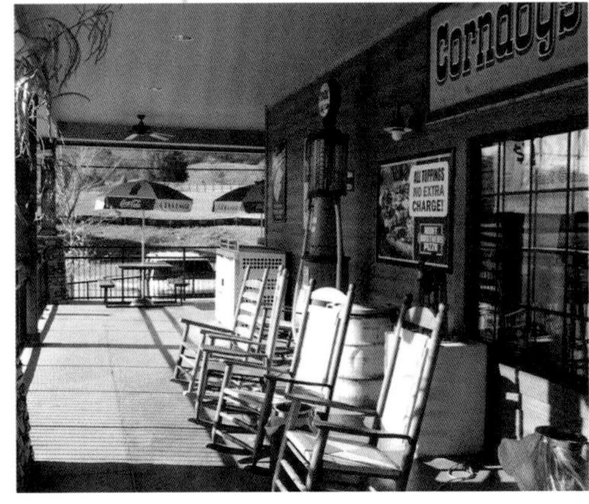

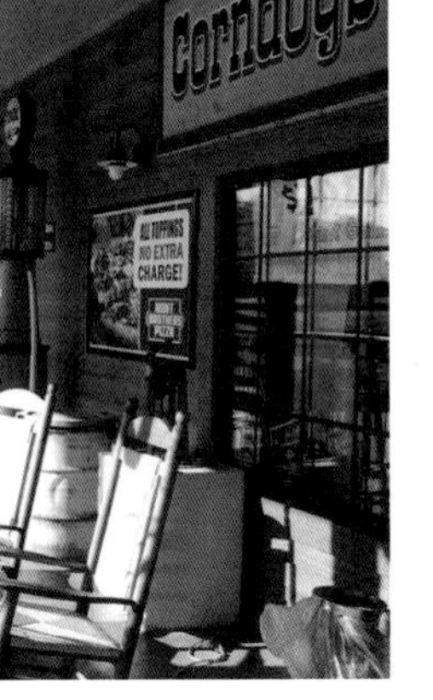

Lewis Country Store is a gathering place for Scottsboro / Bells Bend residents. But the store does not carry local fresh foods, even during the seasons when the fields in the surrounding community are producing them. *(2011)*

BOX:
Farm stand, Green Door Gourmet, Hidden Valley Farm, River Road, Nashville. *(2012: Gary Gaston, NCDC)*

Barn Dance event at Sulfur Creek Farm. *(© 2012: Alan Messer, alanmesser.com)*

Green Door Gourmet, Hidden Valley Farm, River Road, Nashville. *(© 2012: marylindsay photo)*

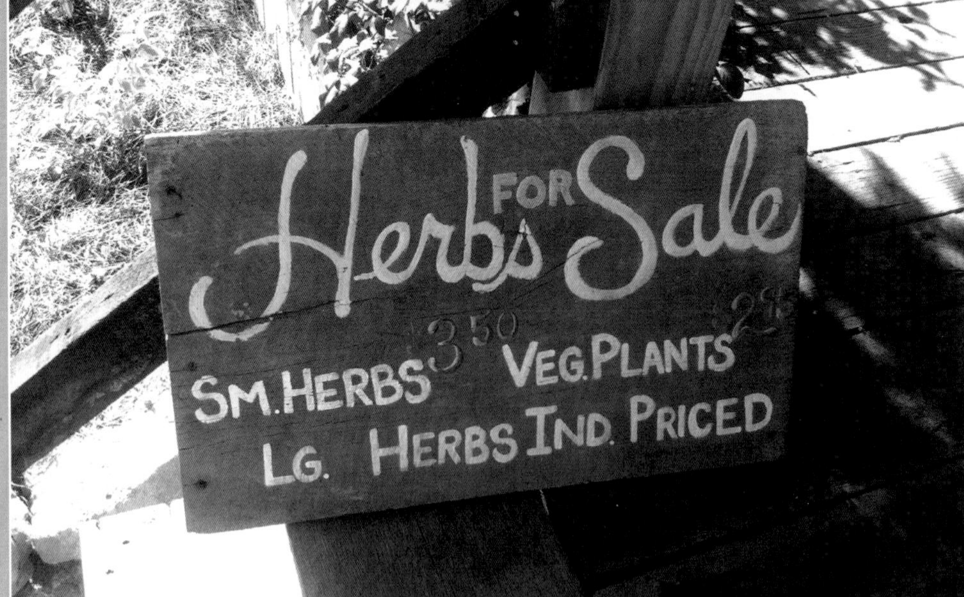
Herbs FOR Sale
SM. HERBS 3.50
VEG. PLANTS
LG. HERBS IND. PRICED

Agritourism

Small farms operate with thin profit margins, making it difficult for farmers to survive on agriculture alone. Leveraging the scenic rural setting and the direct experience of growing and harvesting food brings some farmers out of the red ink. Enticing suburban and urban folks with special activities to come out and enjoy the farm—and pay for the experience—is called agritourism. And it's a burgeoning business on Middle Tennessee farms.

Nashville's Green Door Gourmet hosts a fall festival with pumpkin carving, hayrides, and picnics and has built a hall for receptions, parties, and live music. Garden clubs come on-site for lectures on heirloom plants and school groups learn about plants, bees—and square dancing. Sylvia Ganier, proprietor, draws on her culinary roots for tour-and-taste events featuring chef-prepared samplings and local cheeses.

Bells Bend Neighborhood Farms supplement income from farm products with dinners, a Hops Fest and Barn Dance, and a tomato fest. Eaton's Creek Organics in Joelton presents a fall farm-to-blanket BYOB gourmet dinner on the grounds. Homeplace Farm in Antioch offers a pumpkin patch, hayrides, and pick-your-own produce.

—AMY ESKIND, NCDC

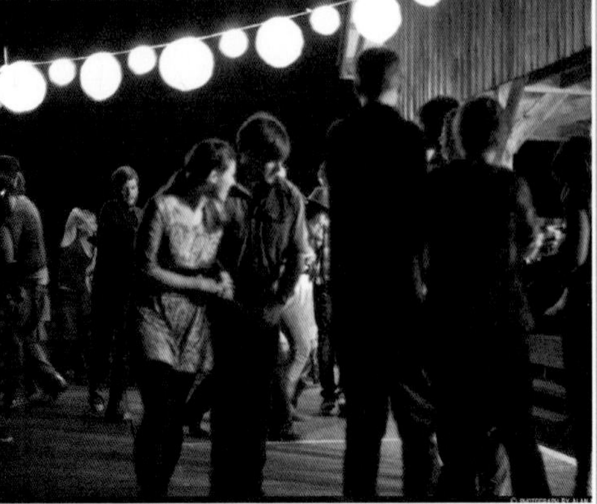

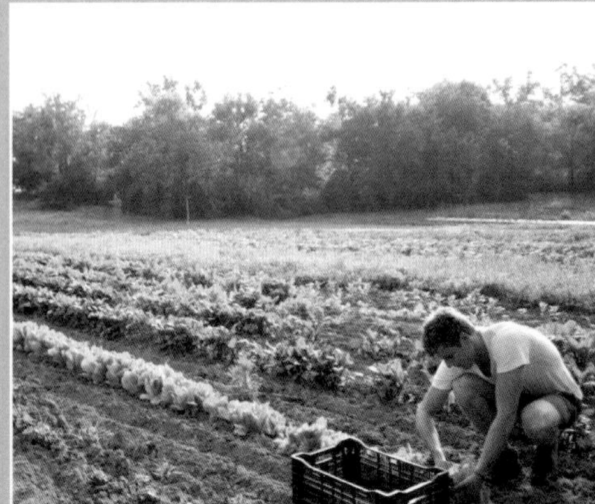

HOUSING

✕ Health-Defeating

Housing stock in the rural zone is generally single-family homes in a pattern of very low density. But rural communities need a broader range of housing types. Rural residents who want to downsize and/or drive less may find it hard to stay in the community as they age. Young adults who grew up in rural areas may not be able to afford a first-time home in the country.

Affordability in housing is usually tied to small units on small parcels of land. The construction of such housing in rural areas is most feasible and appropriate in neighborhood centers so as not to violate rural character.

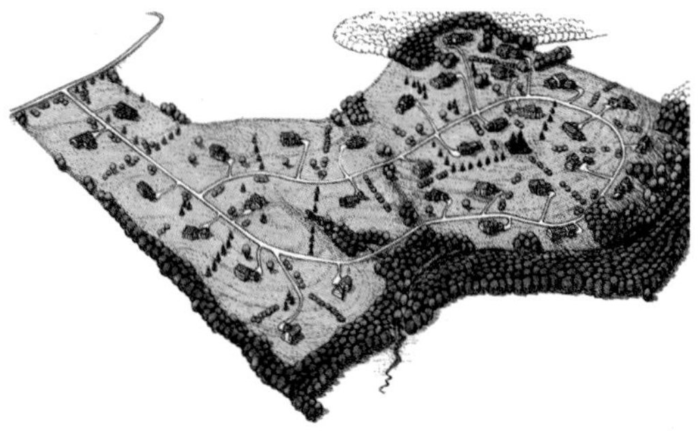

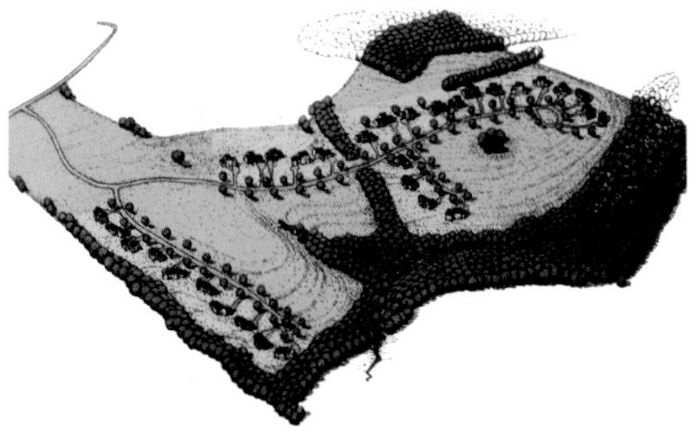

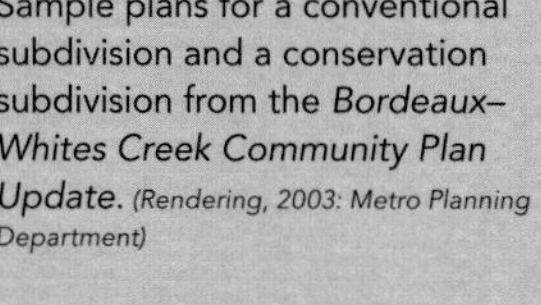

Sample plans for a conventional subdivision and a conservation subdivision from the *Bordeaux–Whites Creek Community Plan Update.* (Rendering, 2003: Metro Planning Department)

STRATEGY: *Promote conservation design. Diverse housing stock can be achieved in rural areas without resulting in sprawl through the design of compact residential plans known as "conservation developments." Such designs maximize housing units on a small piece of land and offer alternative and diverse housing options for the community while minimizing loss of open space. If properly located in neighborhood centers—rural hamlets—and appropriately designed, conservation development enables a community to create lower-cost housing and increase age and income diversity while retaining rural character.*

There are, however, caveats to this approach. The introduction of sewers into a rural community currently relying on septic systems could open up the whole area to more intense development, replacing rural with suburbia. This could only be prevented by the establishment of sewer-free land-use zoning beyond the boundary of the conservation development. And the increase in population, if on a large enough scale, could trigger the widening of roads, another infrastructure change that could severely erode rural character.

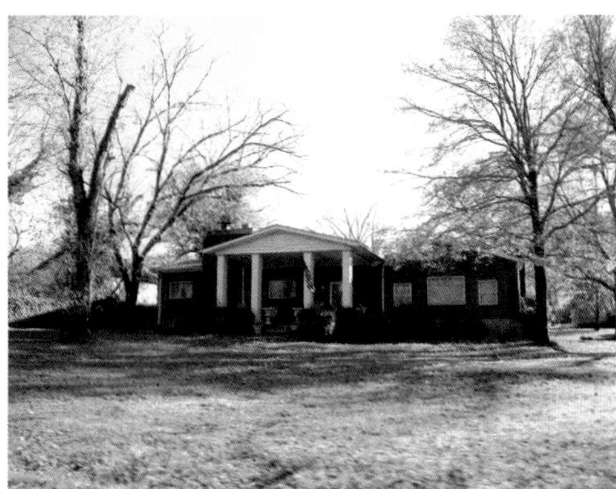

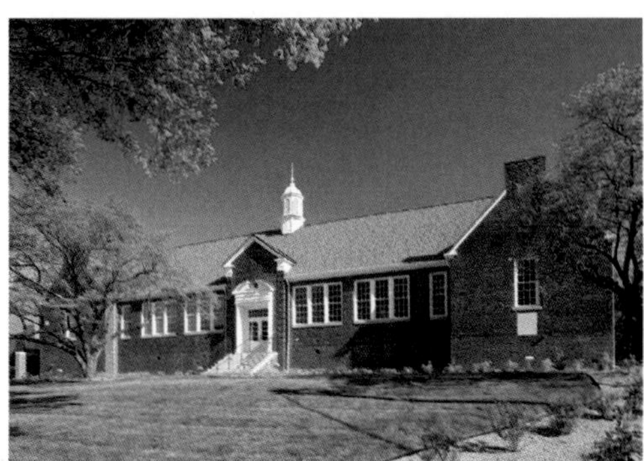

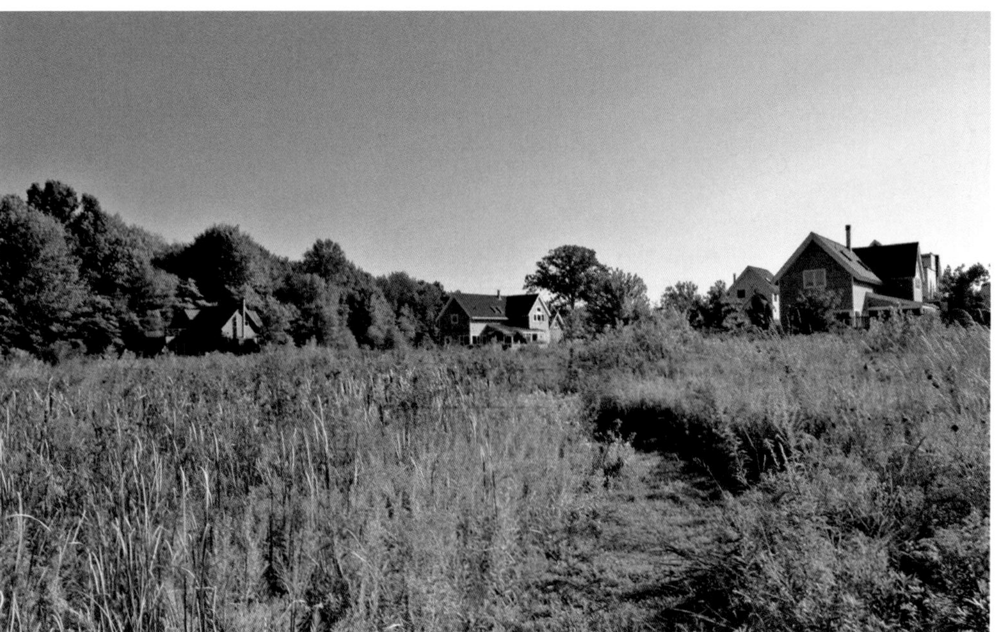

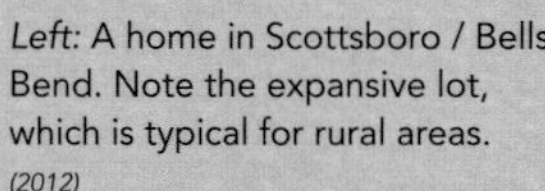

Left: A home in Scottsboro / Bells Bend. Note the expansive lot, which is typical for rural areas. (2012)

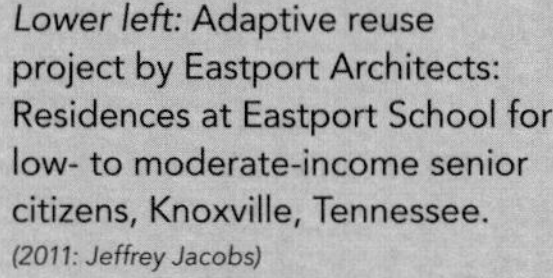

Lower left: Adaptive reuse project by Eastport Architects: Residences at Eastport School for low- to moderate-income senior citizens, Knoxville, Tennessee. (2011: Jeffrey Jacobs)

Lower right: Example of an existing conservation subdivision. Tryon Farms, Michigan City, Indiana. (2010: Brian Phelps and Chris Whitis)

PARKS AND OPEN SPACE

✓ Health-Promoting

A main benefit of rural living is access to large areas of private and public open space. Private single-family residences typically sit on very large lots, so owners literally live in an open space context. (Property in Davidson County zoned agricultural requires a minimum lot size of five acres per dwelling unit (AG) or two acres per unit (AR2a).)[11]

In addition, several of Davidson County's large regional public parks are located in rural areas: Bells Bend (808 acres), Beaman (1,688 acres), and Peeler (650 acres) parks. Rural public parks are not only beneficial for local residents, but are assets for the whole county—and beyond. According to the Smart Growth Network, the potential of rural parks to lure more urban dwellers "out to the country" should not be overlooked.[12] Such parks can generate lodgings, restaurants, and shops that cater to outdoor tourism. Rural parks can thus contribute to efforts to preserve these transect zones as open space.

Trees are a defining physical feature of rural communities and play a vital role, as the "lungs and filters of Nashville," in improving countywide air and water quality and mitigating the heat island effect of more developed areas. The Metro Tree Canopy Assessment reports on the existing tree coverage and identifies potential areas in the county for increasing it. The county's rural and natural transect zones, as would be expected, have the most extensive tree canopy, with areas reaching to almost 67 percent coverage.[13]

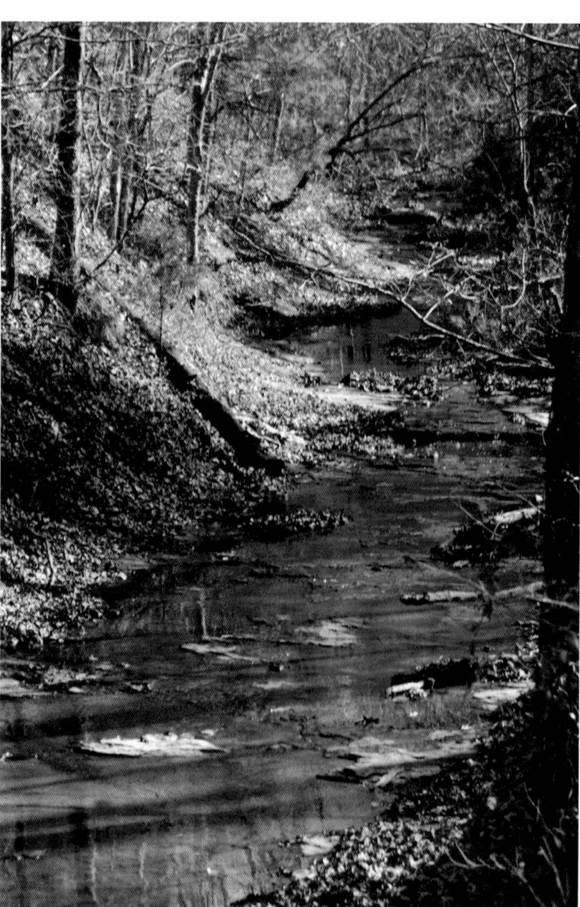

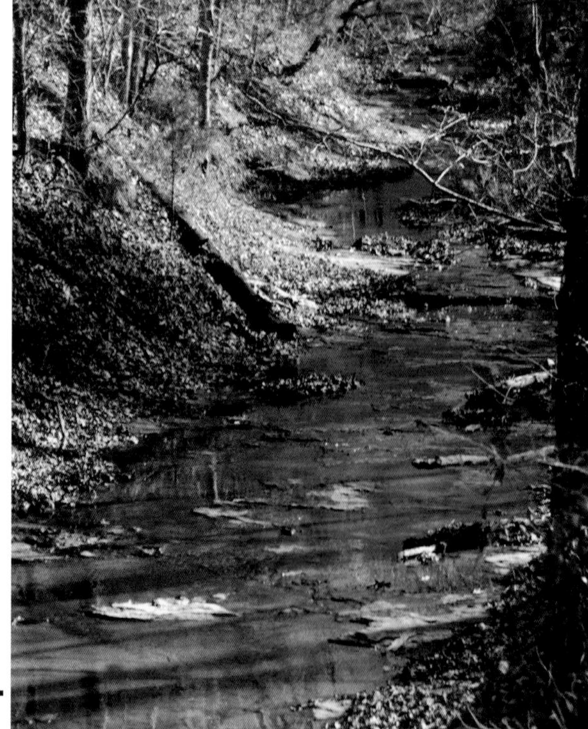

✓ Beaman Park. Ponds, streams and creeks are recreational assets in rural areas. *(2012)*

X Health-Defeating

With the exception of the rural zone's regional parks, which are accessible primarily by private vehicle, open space in rural areas is privately held. This abundance of undeveloped private land should not be considered a substitute for public open space.

STRATEGIES: *Incentivise easements and tree planting. Some property owners in rural areas have placed conservation easements on their acreage through the Land Trust for Tennessee. Such easements keep private land undeveloped in perpetuity while providing tax benefits to owners. This tool for preserving open space should be vigorously pursued in Nashville's rural transect zone.*

Increased forestation in tree-deficient rural areas could offer benefits to the county as a whole in the absorption of air pollutants, carbon sequestration, and reduction of water runoff. Large-scale tree planting by Metro government in rural areas, however, is neither practical nor economically viable. Incentives for tree planting by landowners of rural property would be more feasible.

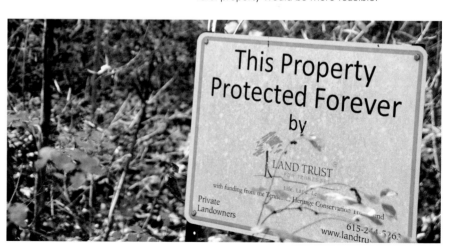

Property conservation signage on private property, Scottsboro / Bells Bend. *(2012)*

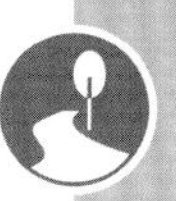

Nashville's existing tree canopy by transect zones. Darker green represents denser coverage. *(Map 2013: Metro Public Works Department)*

metro tree advisory committee

Tree Canopy by Transect

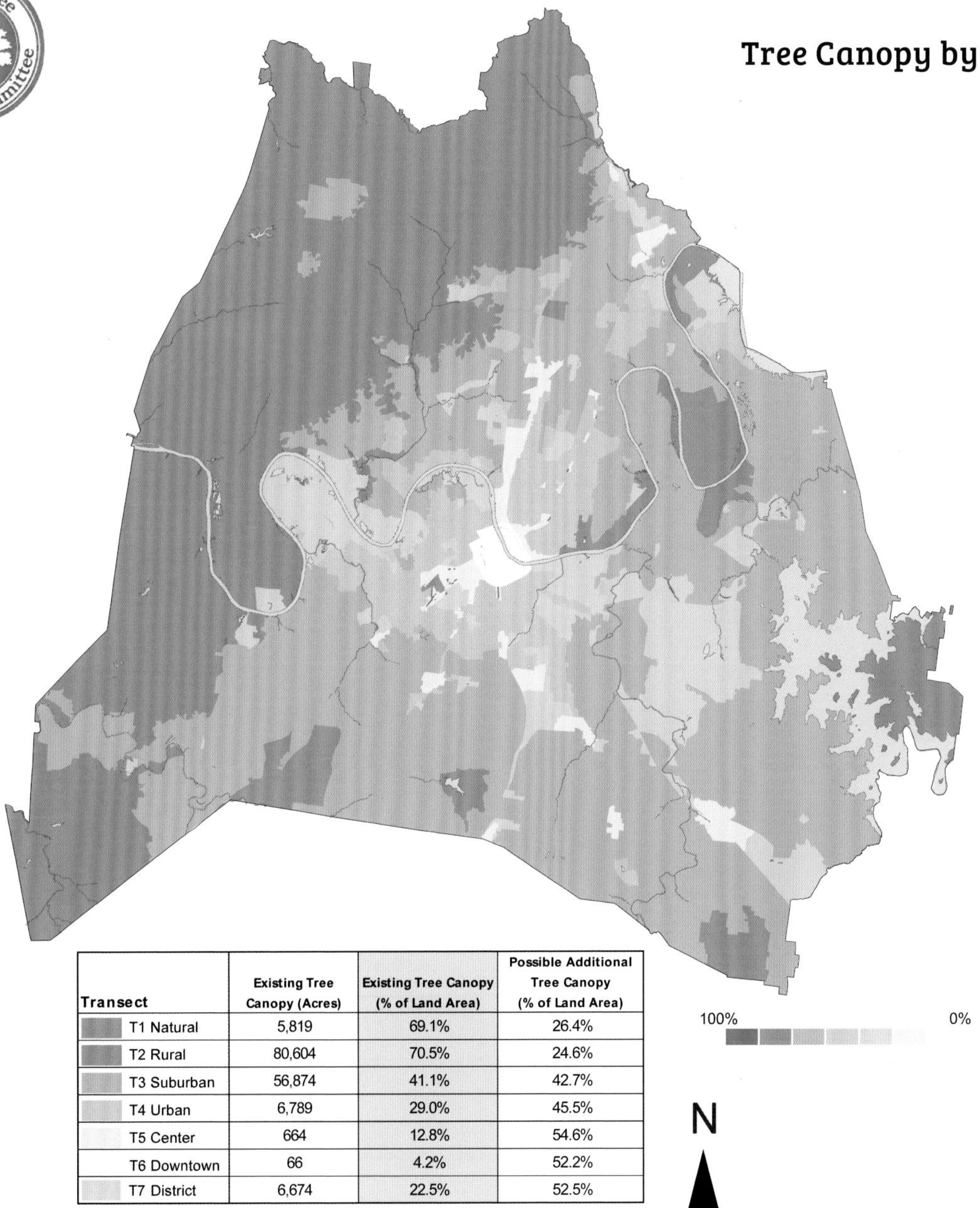

Transect	Existing Tree Canopy (Acres)	Existing Tree Canopy (% of Land Area)	Possible Additional Tree Canopy (% of Land Area)
T1 Natural	5,819	69.1%	26.4%
T2 Rural	80,604	70.5%	24.6%
T3 Suburban	56,874	41.1%	42.7%
T4 Urban	6,789	29.0%	45.5%
T5 Center	664	12.8%	54.6%
T6 Downtown	66	4.2%	52.2%
T7 District	6,674	22.5%	52.5%

100% 0%

N

CASE STUDIES

NEELY'S BEND AND SCOTTSBORO / BELLS BEND

Davidson County's rural areas share agricultural and low-density residential land uses. Individual rural communities, however, vary in their socio-economic conditions and available resources. The case studies on Scottsboro / Bells Bend and Neely's Bend illustrate how these distinctions among rural communities require different strategies to improve the health of residents.

The communities of Scottsboro / Bells Bend and Neely's Bend are rural enclaves within the urban/suburban context of Nashville. These are places where you can watch eagles soar, horses graze—and canoe to downtown. Both owe their relatively undeveloped state to their lack of accessibility and infrastructure. These lacks have historically been determined by their geographies and topographies.

Bells Bend and Neely's Bend are peninsulas inscribed by deep bends in the Cumberland River. Neither "bend" has a bridge across the river to provide easy ingress and egress for vehicles. While Scottsboro / Bells Bend is bisected by the wide arterial of Ashland City Highway, subsidiary roads are narrow and curving. Access to the southern and rural end of Neely's Bend is two lanes. The large areas of floodplain in the "bends" and the steep slopes of Scottsboro, which lies on the western edge of the Highland Rim, have also inhibited development.

The feasibility of development in Scottsboro / Bells Bend and Neely's Bend, whether urban or suburban in nature, has always depended on the construction of bridges, wider roads, and city sewer. And community residents who advocate the preservation of rural character have come to realize that such infrastructure would enable the destruction of what they want to conserve.

While similar in many physical characteristics, Scottsboro / Bells Bend and Neely's Bend differ significantly in their demographics. These demographic disparities suggest other distinctions between these communities. For example, very few people rent housing in Scottsboro / Bells Bend or are financially burdened by housing costs (households are considered financially burdened when more than 30 percent of monthly income is spent on rental or mortgage costs), and there is a low percentage of vacant housing. In Neely's Bend, on the other hand, almost ten percent of the occupied households are burdened by housing costs.[14]

Definition of Family / Non-family

Family = Contains at least two people related by birth, marriage, or adoption. Family households are of two types:

- **Married** = When a married couple is considered the householder
- **Other** = When a single man or woman is considered the householder and lives with other family

Non-family = This may be one person living in a household or multiple people who are not related to each other.

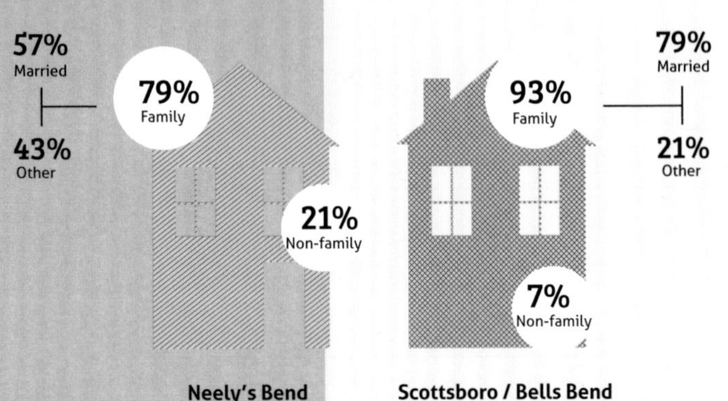

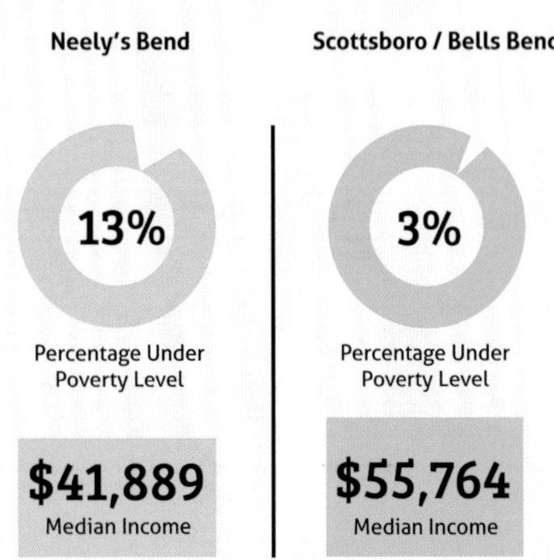

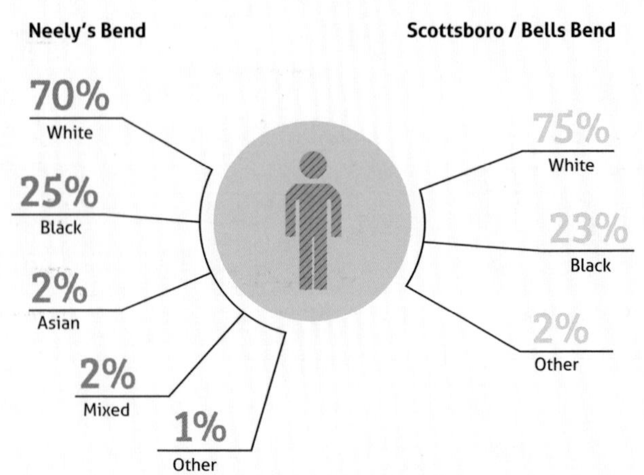

Information graphics, 2013: Ashley Nicole Johnson

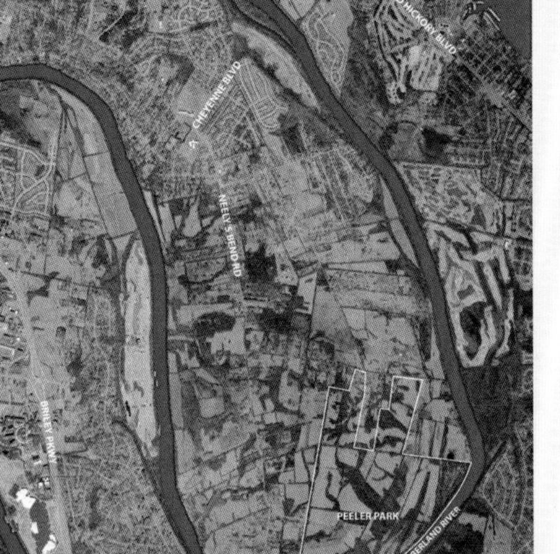

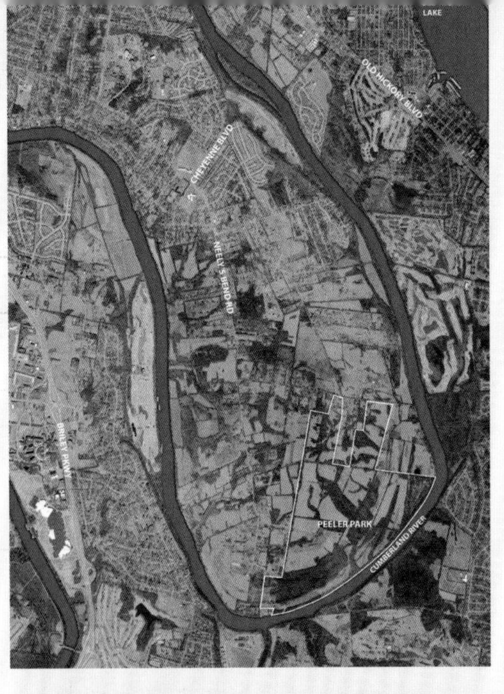

Case study locations. *(Diagram over map, 2012: Samuel Barringer, NCDC)*

Top right: Aerial image of Neely's Bend. *(2012: Metro Planning Department)*

Lower right: Aerial image of Scottsboro / Bells Bend. *(2012: Metro Planning Department)*

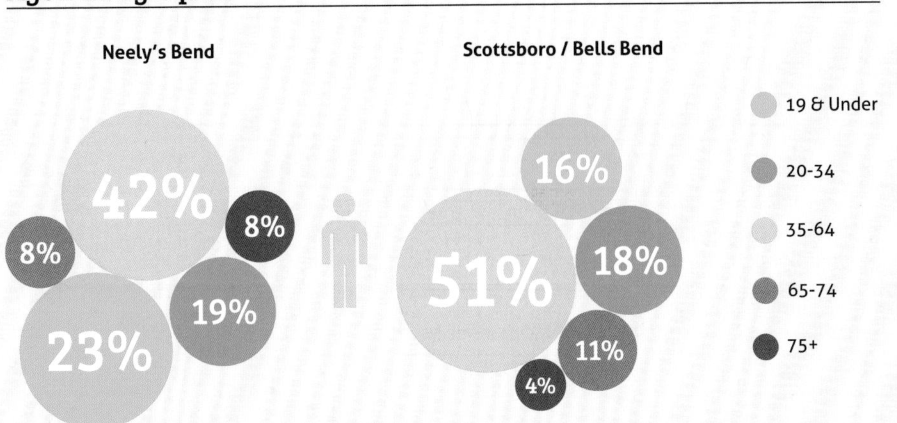

Demographic data from the US Census Department's 2010 American Community Survey (5 year estimates). At the time of research for this publication, the 2010 dataset was the most current data available. For the case studies, neighborhood boundaries were identified and data was then collected from the census tracts that best corresponded to those geographic boundaries.

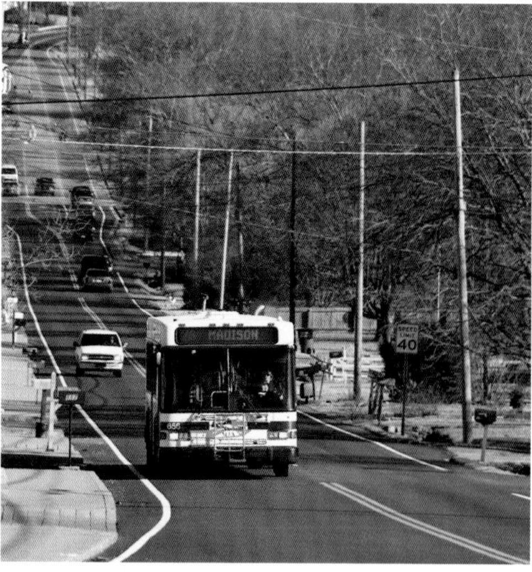

Left: Neely's Bend Road has an hourly bus service from 5:00 a.m. to 7:00 p.m. that connects the homes and schools in the community to Gallatin Pike in Madison. This successful connector service, which regularly exceeds 7,000 passenger trips a month, weaves its way throughout the community, connecting residents to the frequent bus service along Gallatin Pike. On the pike both local buses and a Bus Rapid Transit (BRT) line travel to and from downtown Nashville. The connector on Neely's Bend Road is important to the two percent of the Bend's workforce that lacks access to cars. *(2011)*

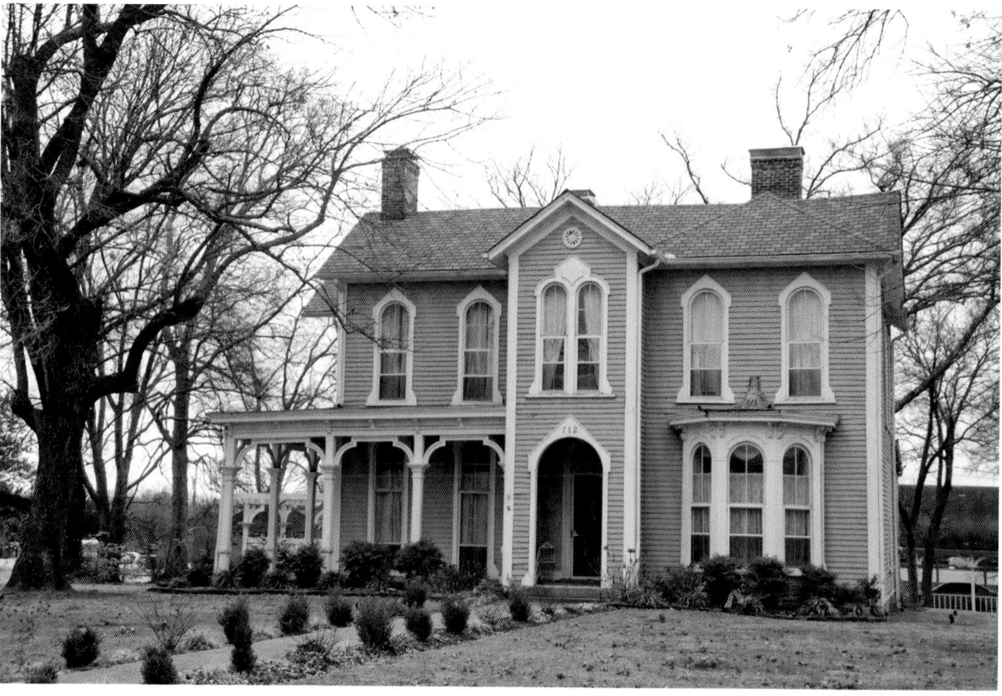

Top right: Idlewild. Italianate home built in 1874. *(2012)*

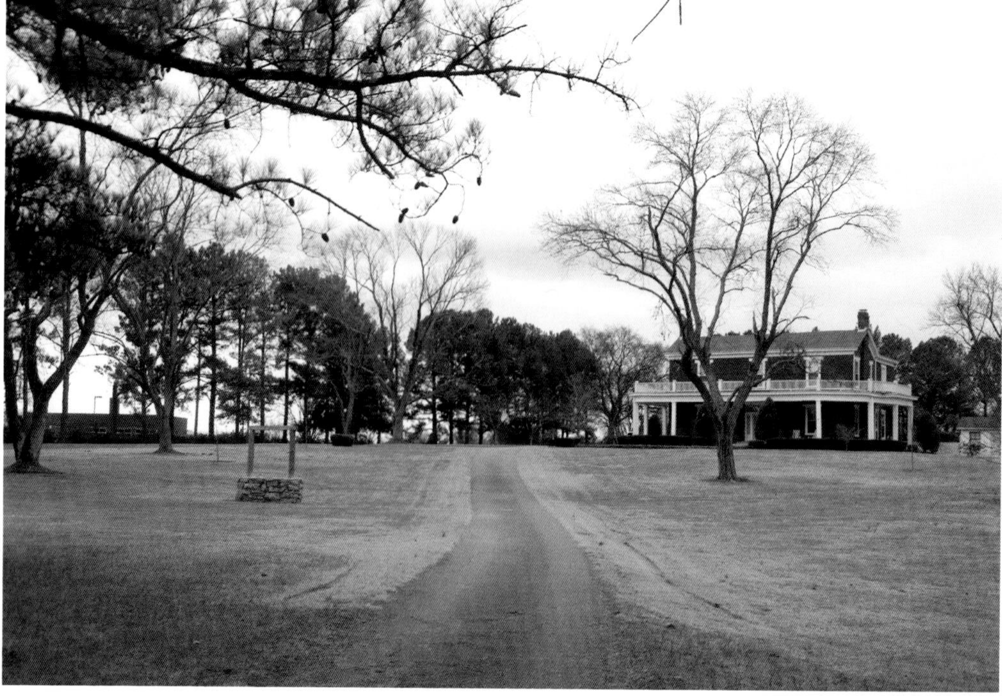

Lower right: Through the trees at 1248 Neely's Bend Road stands the Gee house, all that remains of an antebellum Cumberland River farm. The one-story wrap-around porch in the Colonial Revival style was added in the early 20th century. *(2012)*

NEELY'S BEND

A drive down the six-mile, two-lane Neely's Bend Road is a journey backward through the history of Nashville development. You start at Gallatin Pike, whose crush of cars and welter of big boxes and strip shops, with their cacophony of signage, all testify to the pike's status as one of Nashville's major arterials. Heading south into the Bend, you pass by 1950s and '60s subdivisions intermixed with later infill housing—the kind with names like "Candlewood" and "Kimbolton." Occasional relics of the 19th century—large houses on expansive grounds such as the Italianate Idlewild (1874) and the Gee House (1839)—recall the time when all of the Bend was farmland. Once past the cluster of Neely's Bend elementary and middle schools, lots grow in size, then pastures appear. The road terminates at Peeler Park.

Neely's Bend is named for William Neely, who arrived in 1779 with the group of settlers led by James Robertson.[15] They established Fort Nashborough near where the Metro Courthouse now stands for protection against the Native Americans, who had traditionally used the land for hunting and trapping and resented encroachment by

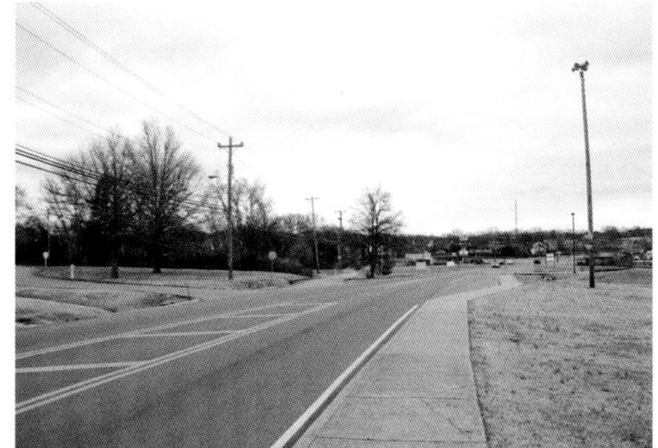

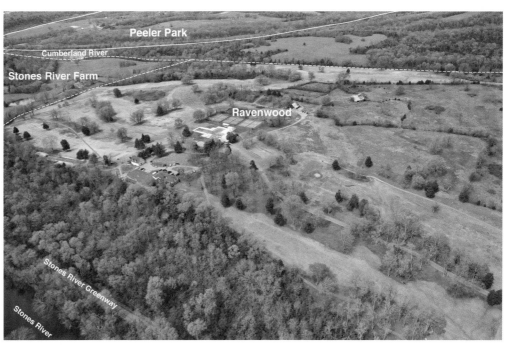

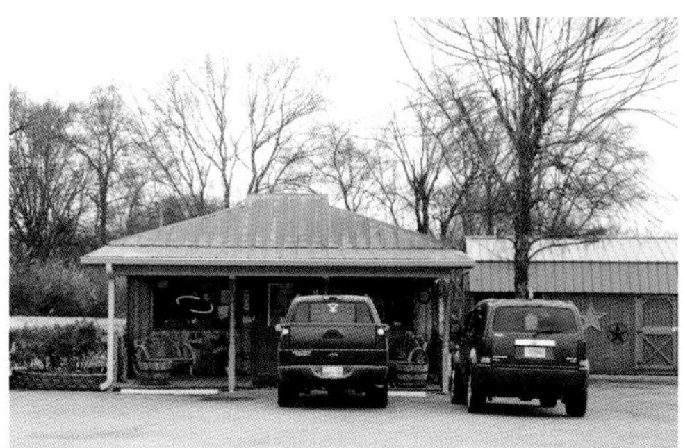

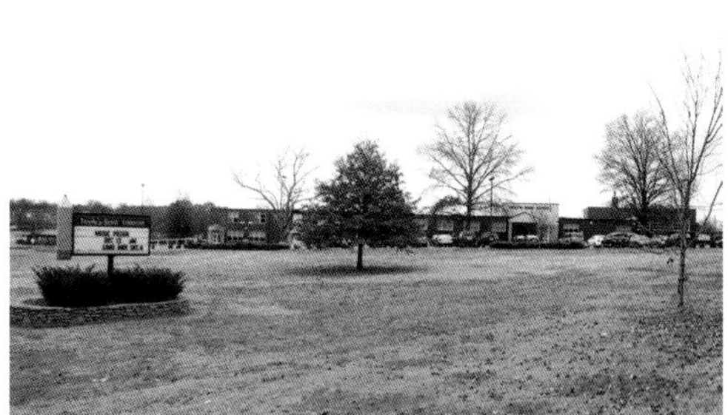

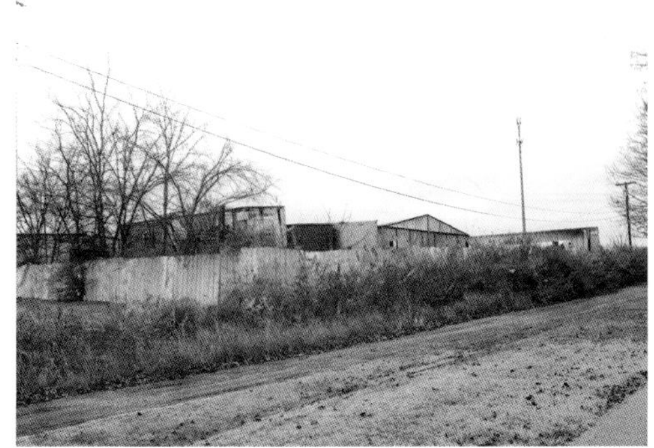

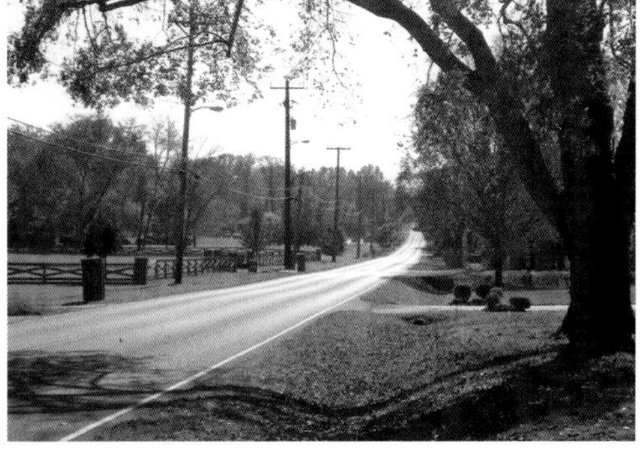

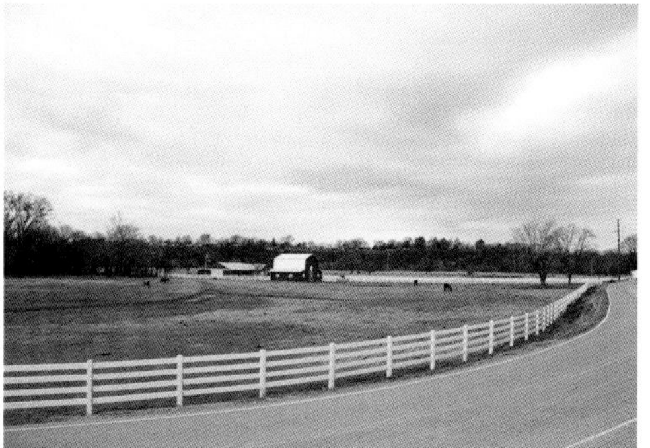

Left, from top: The rural character of the Bend becomes stronger past the intersection of Neely's Bend Road and Cheyenne Boulevard. While this intersection itself is not located within the rural transect, it is zoned for mixed-use development and should be recognized as having the potential to become the neighborhood center for Neely's Bend. *(2012)*

Only two commercial properties currently stand at the Neely's Bend/Cheyenne intersection: a hair salon lies directly across the street from a gas station/convenience store that sells snacks, drinks, and a small number of canned and dried foods. *(2012)*

The Neely's Bend Elementary and Middle Schools occupy opposite corners of the Neely's Bend/Cheyenne intersection. Good sidewalks connect these schools to the surrounding streets and more densely populated areas in the northern part of the Bend. These sidewalks enable walking to school and to the neighborhood bus service, which terminates here. *(2012)*

A small junkyard occupies land in Neely's Bend along Nawakwa Trail, surrounded by suburban residential development. *(2009: Gary Layda)*

Top Right: Peeler Park can be seen at the top of this photograph. In the foreground (across the Cumberland River to the south) lie Ravenwood and Stones River Farm, recent acquisitions by Metro Parks. *(Aerial, 2012: Gary Layda)*

Center: Neighborhood character along Neely's Bend Road between Neely's Bend Church of Christ and Neely's Bend United Methodist Church. *(2012: Jeffrey Bond, Vanderbilt University)*

Center right: Riverview Farm sits on the southwestern tip of Neely's Bend. *(2012)*

white settlers. Neely and his family settled on a deep bend in the Cumberland River two miles east of the fort, where cattle could be contained by the surrounding waters. A spring and salt lick—originally called Neely's Lick and later Larkins Sulphur Spring—attracted game; the salt was also used to cure food. But there were dangers to living out on open land. William Neely was killed by Native Americans the following year.[16]

Neely's Bend was once, as Scottsboro / Bells Bend remains today, an entirely rural community. But some farmland was sold for suburban estates beginning in the late 19th century and, after World War II, for subdivisions. There is a diverse housing stock in the northern part of the Bend, with senior towers, multifamily housing, and single-family homes on smaller lots. There are still, however, over 2,800 acres of agricultural farm land in the southern end of the Bend.[17]

Recent community planning efforts in the form

of the *Madison Community Plan* encourage the maintenance of the rural character in the area, but also call for a walkable neighborhood center to provide for daily needs of residents.[18]

The main recreational amenity in Neely's Bend is E. N. Peeler Park, named for the man who farmed the land before its sale to Metro government in 1963. Metro land-banked the site, which appeared on a 1989 list of possible locations for a new landfill. Area residents organized to protect the land and created a new master plan in 1991. Metro's Parks and Recreation department began to develop trails in the park in 2007.

Today, Peeler Park, at 650 acres, is the largest park in this part of the county, offering a greenway for walkers and cyclists parallel to the river through forest and fields. Three miles of horse trails are off-limits to pedestrians and cyclists. A remote control airplane field attracts enthusiasts to the field clubhouse in the park. A boat ramp provides access to the river.

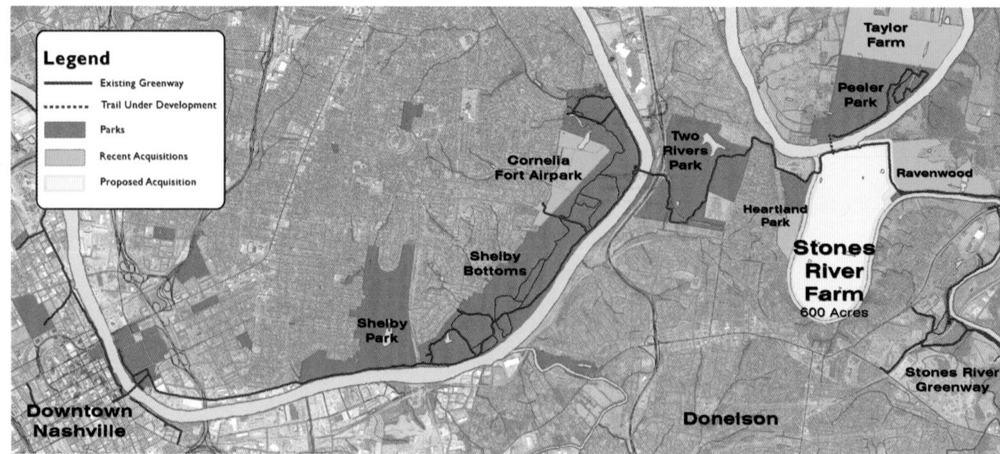

Map of recently acquired Stones River Farm with a proposed pedestrian bridge connection to Peeler Park. *(Map, 2012: Metro Parks Department)*

STRATEGIES:

- ***Create*** *a growth boundary to prevent further encroachment by suburban development into the rural areas of Neely's Bend.*
- ***Create*** *a mixed-use neighborhood center at the intersection of Neely's Bend Road and Cheyenne Boulevard.*
- ***Connect*** *the neighborhood center to Peeler Park via multi-use path along Old Hickory Boulevard.*
- ***Repurpose*** *existing structures in Peeler Park for park uses, such as a visitor/nature center.*
- ***Connect*** *Peeler Park via a pedestrian/bicycle bridge to the Stones River Greenway and the Donelson and Hermitage communities. Metro Parks is currently exploring the bridge's feasibility. Such a bridge would also connect Peeler to the 26-mile Music City bikeway, which runs through Shelby Bottoms all the way to downtown, and to Stones River Farm—acquired by Metro Parks in 2012—which will create a 1,500 acre nature preserve.*

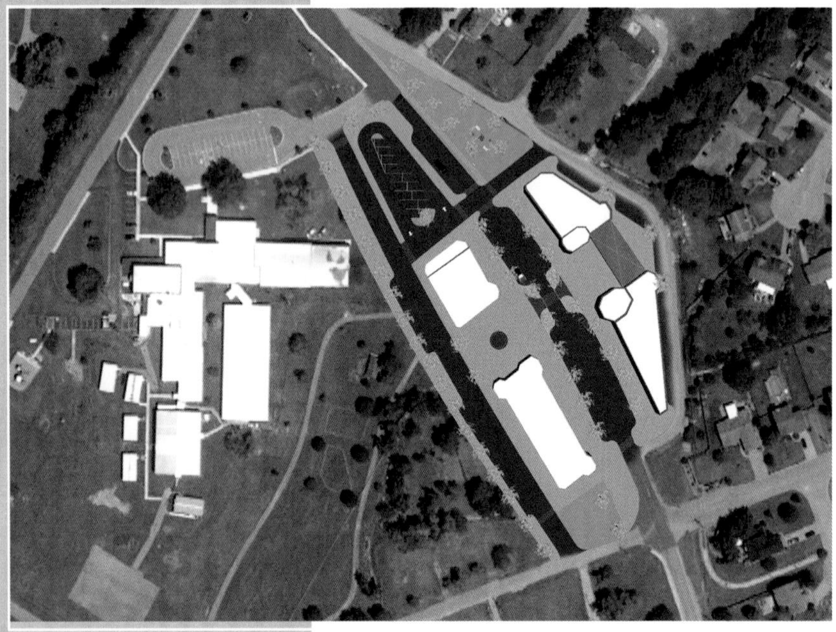

Below: Plan of intersection of Neely's Bend Road and Cheyenne Boulevard accommodates a mix of uses to create a walkable center for the community. *(Plan, 2013: Eric Hoke, NCDC)*

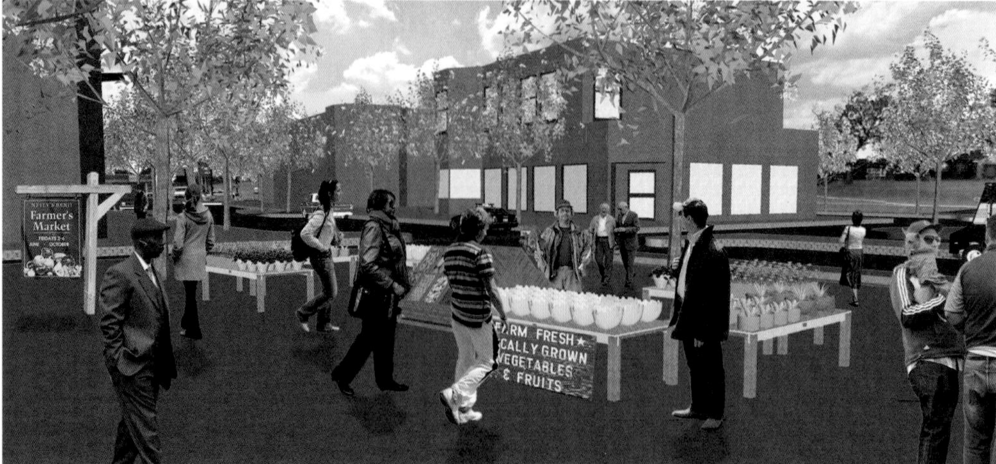

Right: Perspective view of Neely's Bend village center, with retail and office space on ground floors and residential above. *(Rendering, 2013: Eric Hoke, NCDC)*

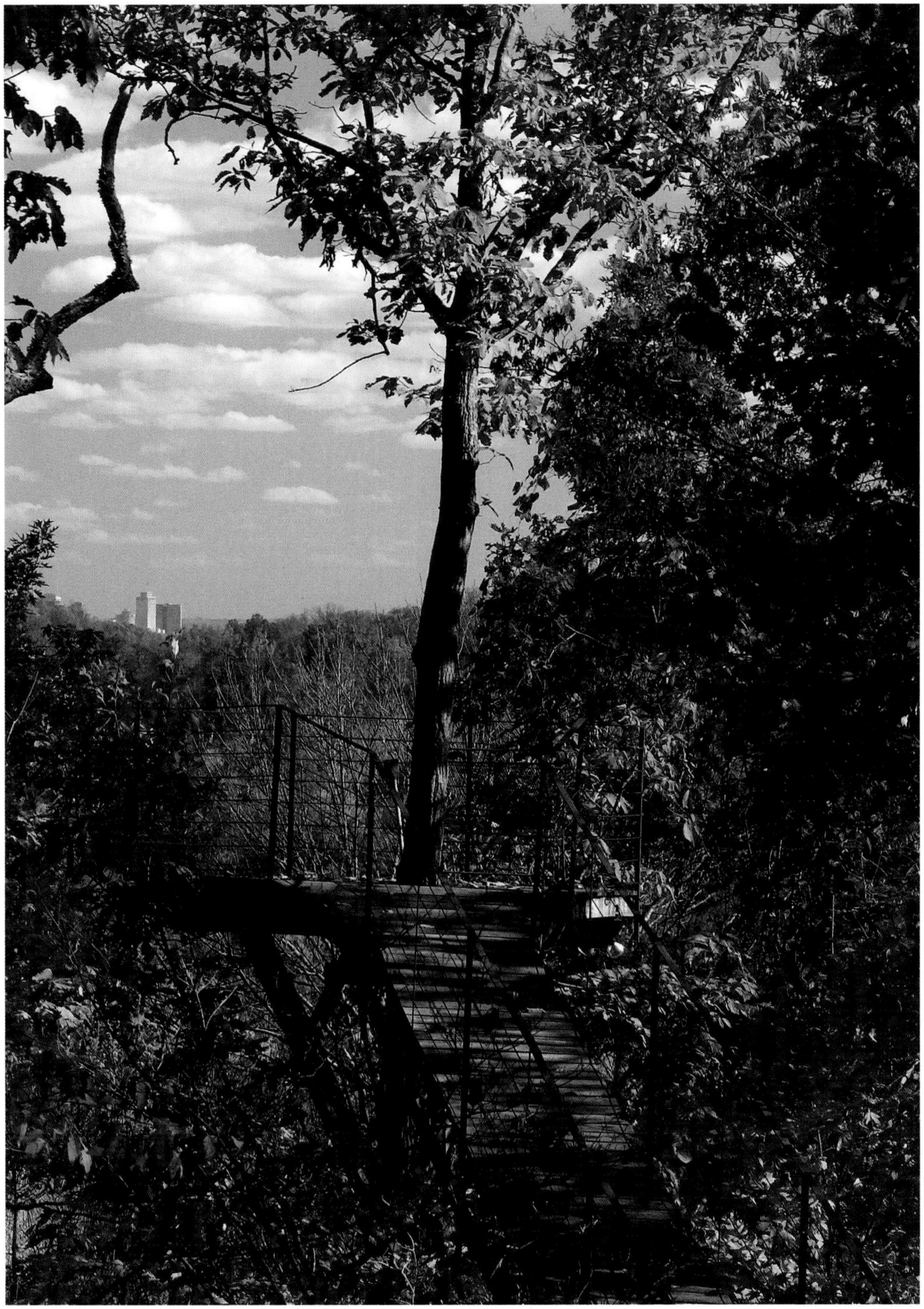

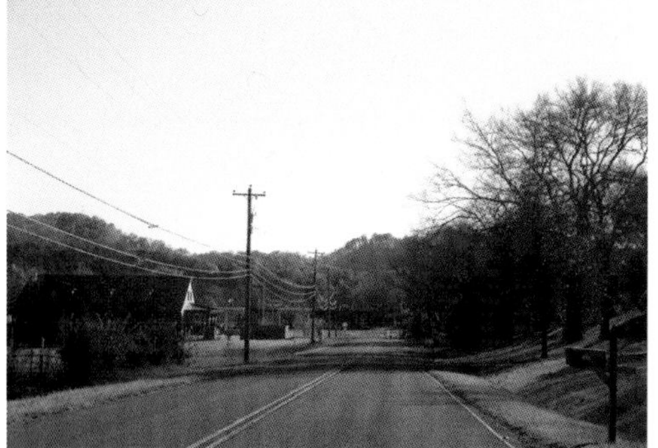

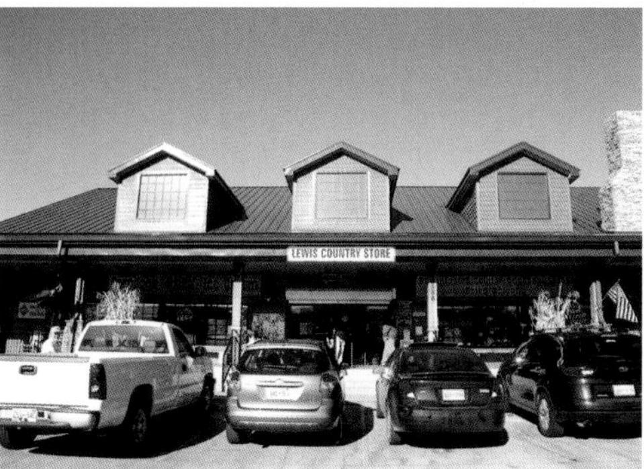

Left: A view of downtown Nashville from the Loiseau property in Bells Bend. *(2012: John Felts)*

Right: Bells Bend along Old Hickory Boulevard, near Ashland City Highway. *(2011)*

Lewis Country Store. *(2011)*

SCOTTSBORO / BELLS BEND

The Scottsboro / Bells Bend community is tiny—approximately 380 households on 13,400 acres.[19] But it features the largest remaining agricultural and forested landscape in Davidson County. Despite its proximity to Nashville's urban and suburban areas—you can see the downtown skyline five miles away from the higher ridges—Scottsboro / Bells Bend has stayed rural due to its lack of sewer and vehicular infrastructure. The Bend in particular is infrastructure-challenged, with only one way in and out. And that way, Old Hickory Boulevard, is two curvy, narrow lanes with minimal shoulders.

Thus even today the community is a place where homesteads can go back for generations, where gunshots ring out in deer season, and whooping cranes make a migratory stop.

Many natural markers of the land as well as manmade infrastructure bear historic family

Right: Land-use vision from *Scottsboro / Bells Bend Detailed Design Plan.* *(Map, 2008: Metro Planning Department)*

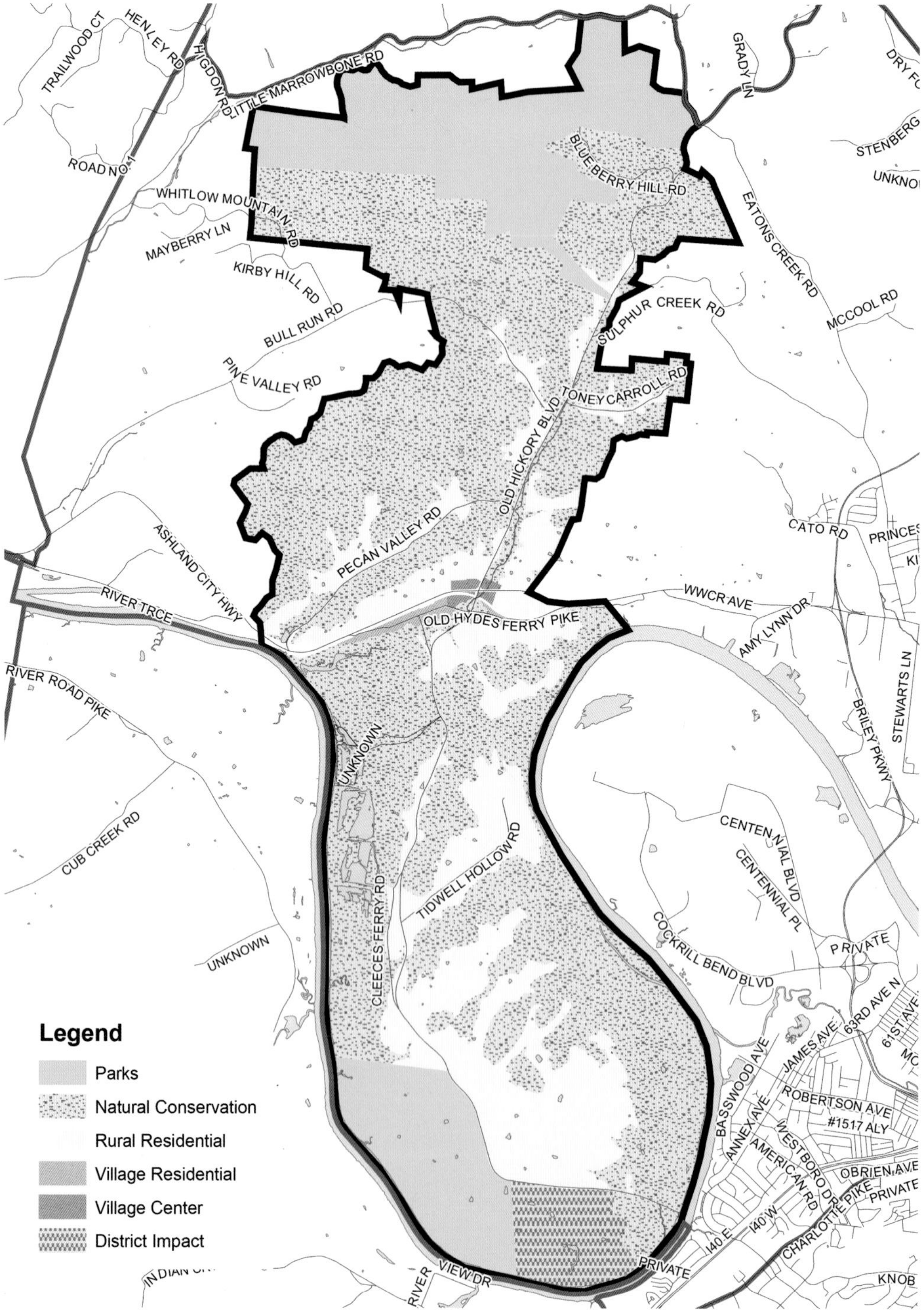

Below: The Wade School was built in 1936 by the Works Progress Administration, a New Deal agency established by President Franklin Roosevelt during the Great Depression. The school closed in 1999, then stood empty for 13 years. In 2012, the building was sold to MillarRich, which provides employment opportunities for adults with intellectual and developmental disabilities. The renovation of the structure, completed in 2013, was guided by faithfulness to the original school in the replacement of windows, light, tiles, and flooring. The following year, Old School Farm was established on land adjacent to the former school as a community supported agriculture nonprofit to offer education and employment to individuals with disabilities. *(2014: Joanna Mechan)*

"There's nothing else in Nashville like this: working farms next to outdoor recreation opportunities (kayaking, hiking, caving, birding, camping, biking), a network of blue ways, greenways, and primitive trails, private residences, archeological sites, and plenty of space for 'developments' that enhance and protect the natural resources and tourist opportunities."

—Minda Lazarov, Scottsboro / Bells Bend resident and community leader (2008)

Legend

- Parks
- Natural Conservation
- Rural Residential
- Village Residential
- Village Center
- District Impact

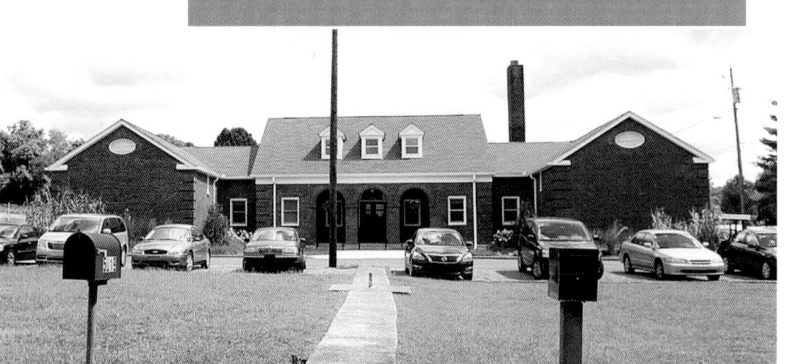

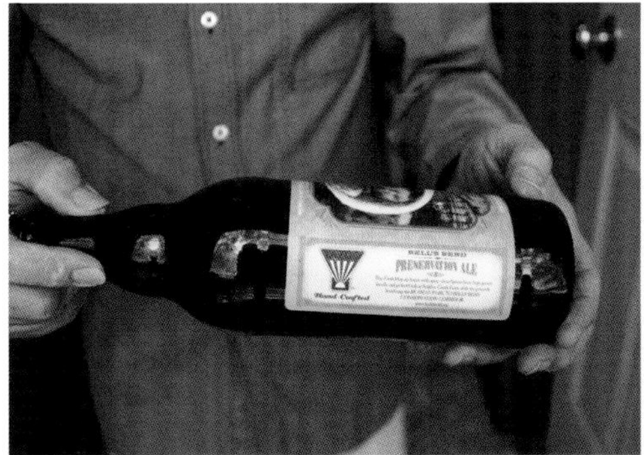

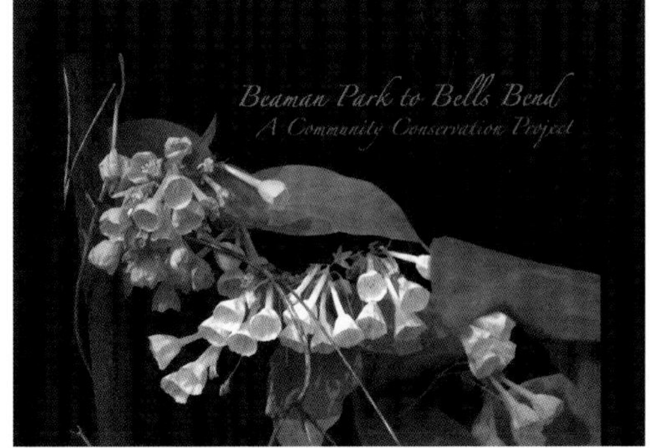

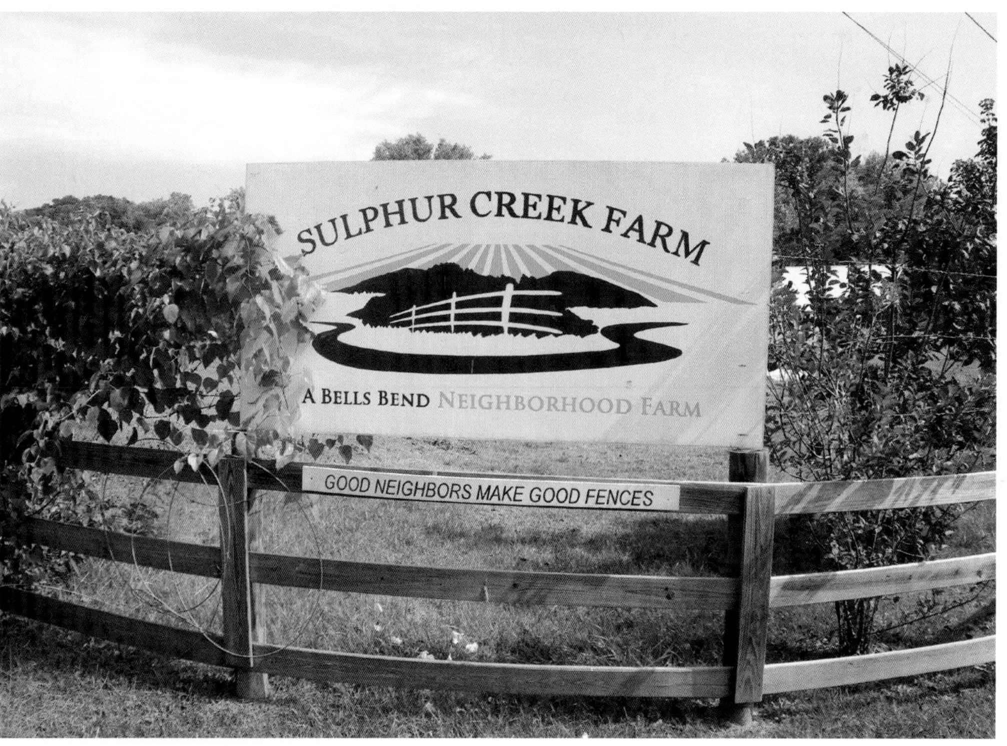

Left, from top: Nashville's Yazoo Brewery harvested hops from the Sulfur Creek Farm to create "Bells Bend Preservation Ale." (2012)

Cover image, *Beaman Park to Bells Bend: A Community Conservation Project.* (2007: Land Trust for Tennessee)

Right: Sulphur Creek Farm, one of the Bells Bend Neighborhood Farms that supply local foods to the West Nashville Farmers' Market as well as offer a CSA program and online market. The intent of the four-farm cooperative is to illustrate why farmland in Davidson County is worth preserving as a locus of sustainable agriculture and job creation. (2012)

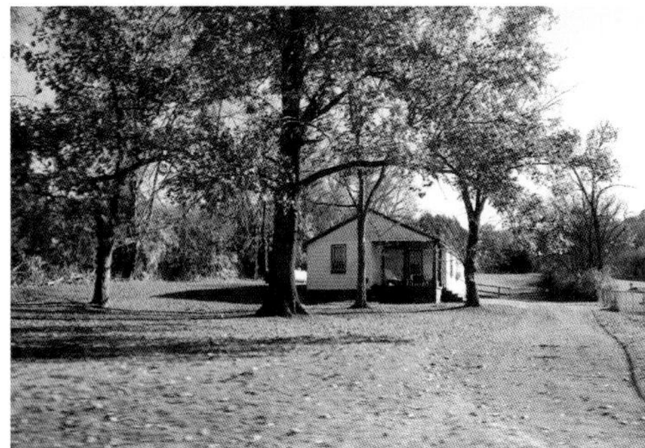

Vernacular housing in Scottsboro / Bells Bend. (2011)

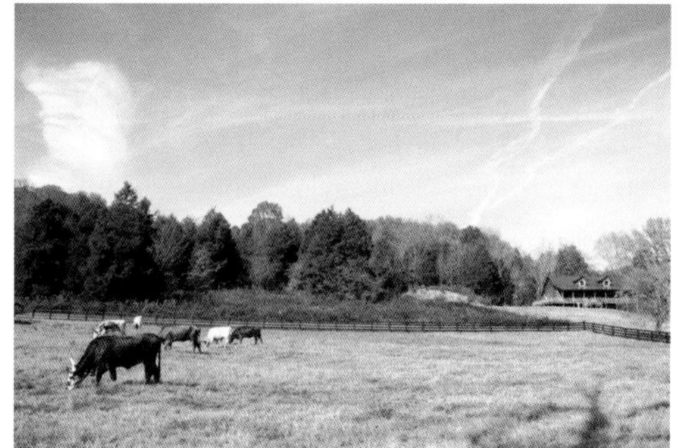

Cows grazing on farmland is still a common site in the Scottsboro / Bells Bend area. (2011)

names: Whites Creek and Hyde's Ferry Pike, for example. The river bend itself was originally known as White's Bend and later Bells Bend, after Montgomery Bell, like David Lipscomb an early landowner in the area. Farming came to the Bend in the early 19th century. In 1870 the Clees family began operating a ferry service to take people, and later cars, across the river.

The Lewis Country Store, which sits at the intersection of Old Hickory Boulevard and Ashland City Highway—four travel lanes and a turn lane, with urban lighting—is the commercial center of the community. Here people pump gas, buy convenience and deli food, and, on warm summer evenings, play fiddles and strum guitars on the front porch. The store is the sole commercial development in the center. Nearby civic facilities, such as the Scottsboro Community Club or the Wade School property lie on the other side of the highway, on a small lane off Old Hickory Boulevard.

In the *Scottsboro / Bells Bend Detailed Design Plan* for the area, community members envision a restaurant, coffee shop, music venue, and farmers' market for their village center.[20] The center could also offer housing of a hamlet scale.

The fertile bottomlands of Bells Bend once had large scale farming operations, but those declined in the latter decades of the 20th century. The approximately 8,000 acres of agricultural land, however, have the potential to produce a large percentage of Nashville's locally grown and raised food.

Community members have fought fiercely and successfully to prevent developments that would endanger the rural character they feel defines Scottsboro / Bells Bend. In 2009, Metro's Planning Commission failed to approve the zoning change

Left, from top: The wide Ashland City Highway, gas station of Lewis Country Store to right. *(2011)*

Pedestrian walking along Old Hydes Ferry Pike near the Scottsboro Community Club. *(2012)*

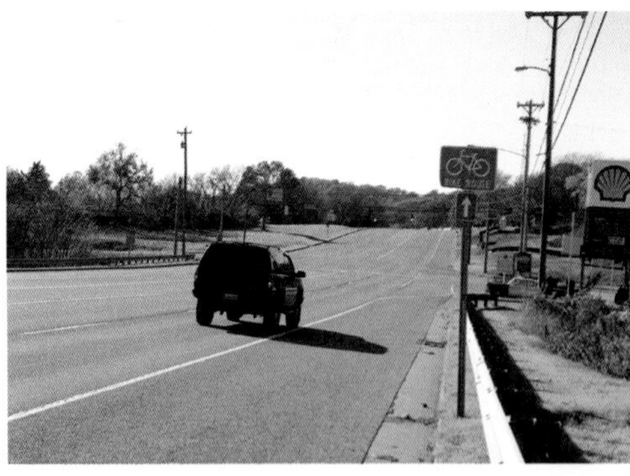

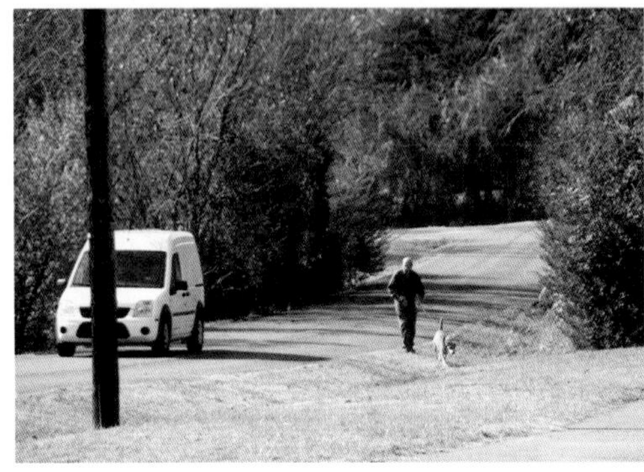

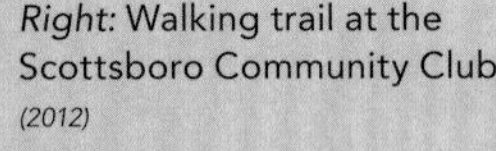

Right: Walking trail at the Scottsboro Community Club. *(2012)*

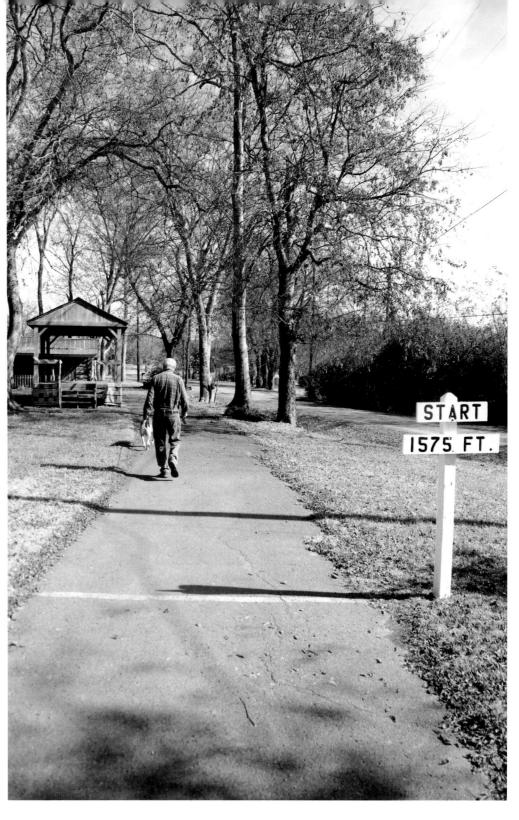

for the largest and most recent proposal, that for May Town Center—150 buildings and a workforce of 40,000. And the Nashville open space plan Nashville: *Naturally* (2011) identifies Scottsboro / Bells Bend as a "potential open space anchor."[21]

Nevertheless, Bells Bend remains an endangered species. In its report of 2012, the Nashville Area Chamber of Commerce's Redevelopment Task Force lists the 450 acres proposed for May Town among its potential "County Office Sites." This despite the fact that among the report's "minimum location requirements" is that land be "zoning correct" for office development, which Bells Bend isn't.[22]

In order to move beyond the "Just Say No" mode, community residents proposed an alternative vision for Scottsboro / Bells Bend that would preserve the existing natural and rural farming character. They articulated this vision in *Beaman*

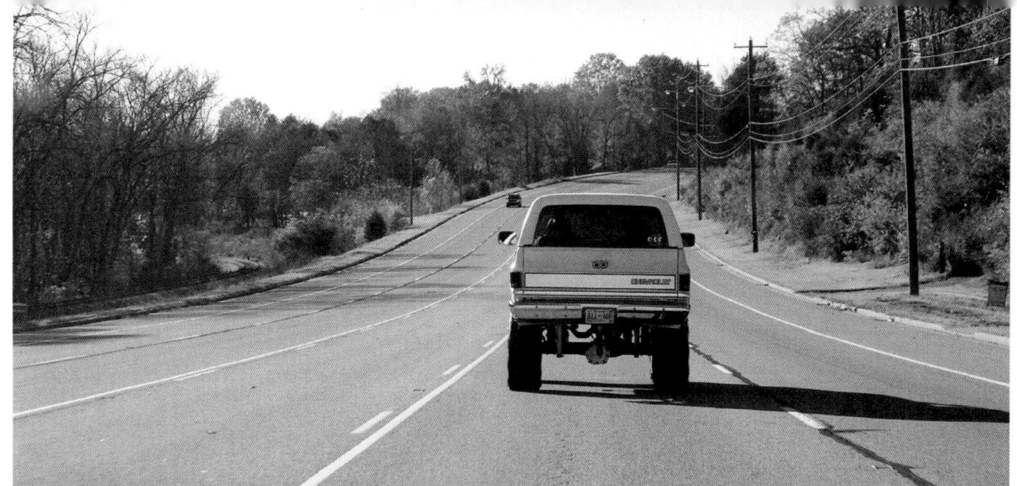

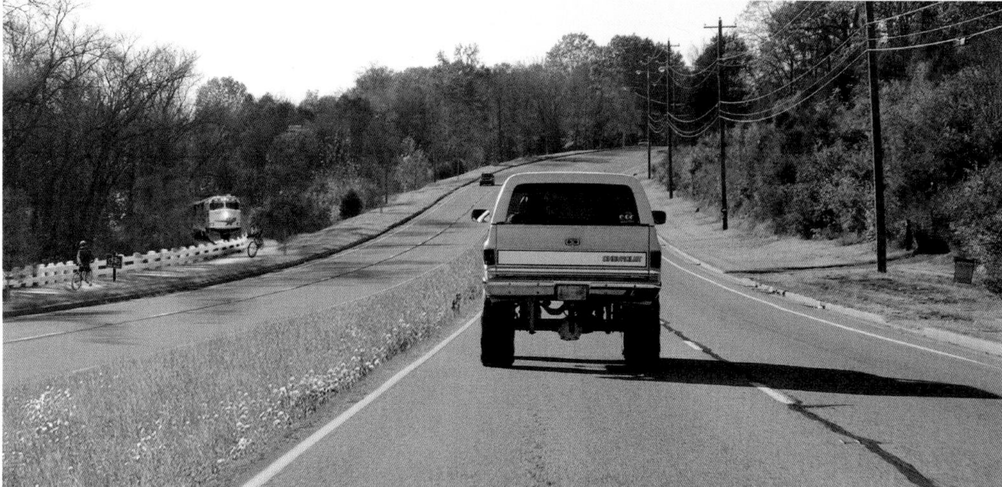

Left: Ashland City Highway before and after. Envisioned with a grass median, separated greenway, and shared freight / passenger rail routes. *(Vizualization, 2013: Eric Hoke, NCDC)*

Park to Bells Bend: A Community Conservation Project, a book that documents existing resources and creates a plan for a rural preservation district.

Scottsboro / Bells Bend has no bus service.[23] Car ownership is high and those cars travel many miles: in 2009 over 700 residents reported commuting between 20 and 90 minutes to work.[24] This statistic suggests a potential ridership for van- and carpooling.

Scottsboro has some shared bicycle lanes on Ashland City Highway, as well as along Old Hickory Boulevard south to the Cumberland River. Public Works' long-range plans call for dedicated bike routes connecting Bells Bend Park to Percy Priest Dam, which can be used for recreation but lack the potential for alternative transportation.[25]

Scottsboro / Bells Bend is home to two of the county's regional parks. To the north lies 1,688-acre Beaman Park; to the south is 808-acre Bells Bend Park. There is also a mini-park that houses the Scottsboro Community Club. The club has a 1,575-foot walking trail, swings and seesaws, a baseball backstop, a horseshoe pit, music stage, outdoor bbq smokers, and picnic tables. The potential for communitywide use here is strong. The club, however, is situated off a secondary road, with no clear connectivity to the nearby neighborhood center or surrounding homes. Directional signage and a multi-use path connecting the club to Ashland City Highway could enhance usage.

STRATEGIES:

- ***Strengthen*** *the community center of Scottsboro with a hamlet-style development that features a mixture of uses and a diversity of housing types that fit the character and scale of the community. Any such development should be accomplished without the extension of sewers to the surrounding area.*
- ***Perform*** *a "road diet" on Ashland City Highway. Reduce right of way to four lanes (two in each direction) with a planted median.*
- ***Establish*** *a multi-use pathway parallel to Ashland City Highway along the rail corridor from Nashville to Ashland City. Long-range plans for this freight corridor call for implementation of the Music City Star passenger service between downtown and Clarksville with stops in midtown Nashville and Ashland City.*[26]
- ***Connect*** *Bells Bend Park to Beaman Park via a bike lane along Old Hickory and multi-use paths utilizing private property easements.*

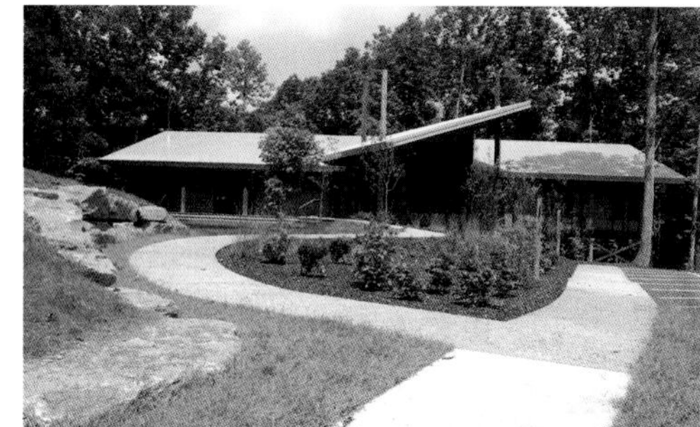

Beaman Park Nature Center. *(2008: Gary Layda)*

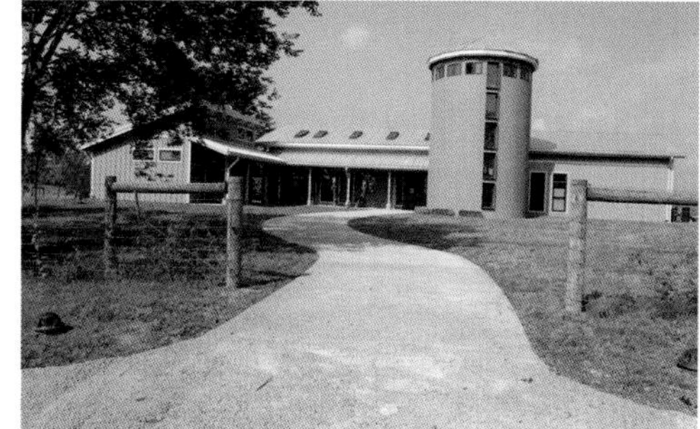

Bells Bend Outdoor Center. *(2008: Gary Layda)*

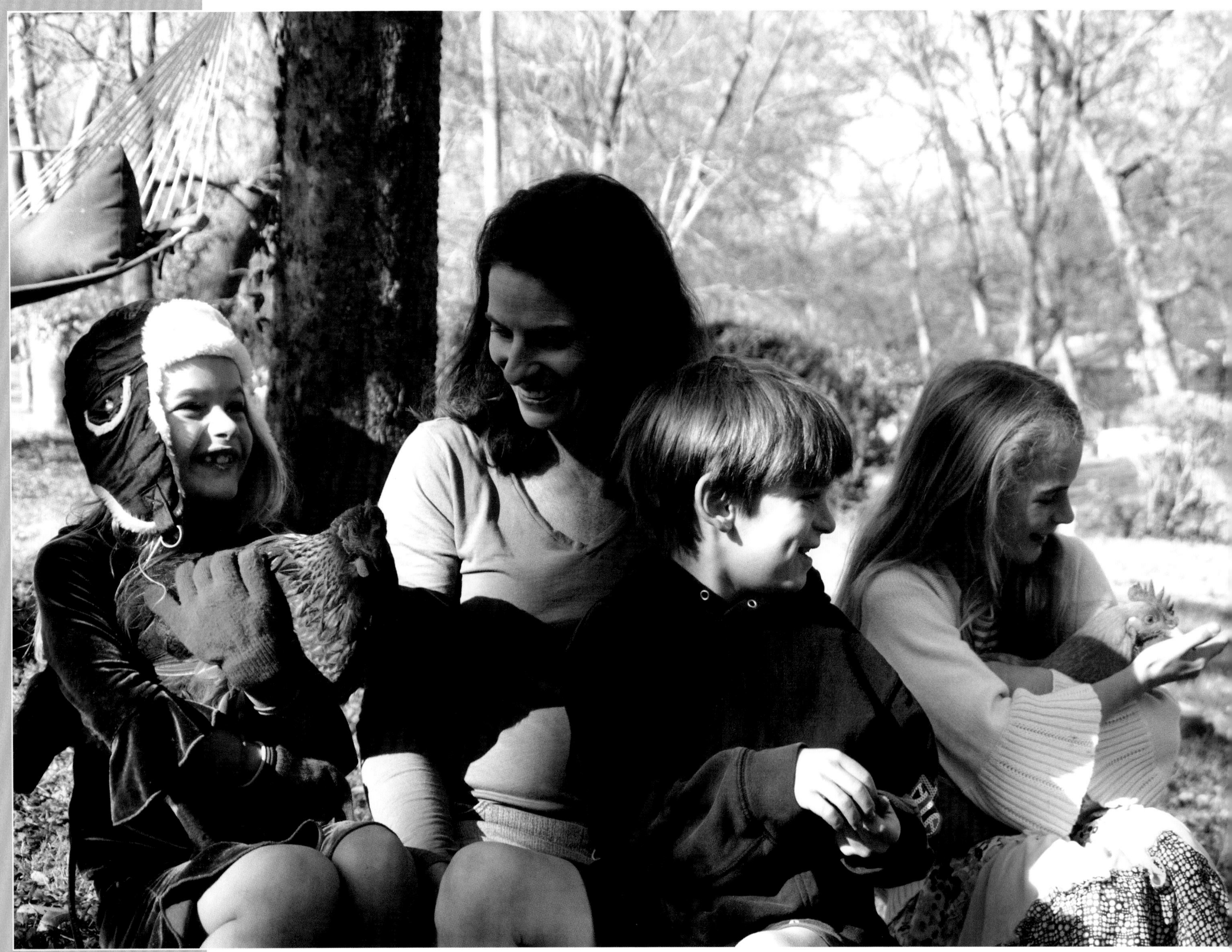

JENNIFER GENTRY

Jennifer Gentry, 43, had enjoyed urban life in the historic precincts of East Nashville, especially the easy access to the Shelby Bottoms Greenway and the Turnip Truck organic market. But after a sojourn in Boston, Tennessee, with her husband, and the addition of three children, the family needed larger quarters.

So six years ago the home school parent, master gardener, and triathlon coach moved out Gallatin Road to suburban Madison. The rationale was more space for the money and land for a garden in a location just a short drive from her old neighborhood.

"We don't particularly care for the 1950s ranch-style houses in Madison," Gentry says, "but we like the quality, affordability, and land. It's also convenient. My husband works near the airport and he can get there in 10 minutes. We can also drive to downtown very quickly."

Note that Gentry says "drive" and not "ride." Her family has two cars and travels in them almost exclusively. She appreciates the frequency of the new BRT line on Gallatin Road (every 15 minutes), but says, "we haven't utilized it" because of the expense. "If we go to the downtown library by car, I might pay two or three dollars to park. Even with the cost of gas that's less than the bus."

The car-dependence of suburban life can be a particular challenge for the numerous Madison residents who are the original owners of their homes and have lived there for decades. "Our neighbor across the way is in her mid-80s and her husband is 90-something, so I can see how difficult it is when you don't drive," Gentry says. "I'm not sure what services are available for them."

What's not available to the Madison population at large is a coherent system of sidewalks. "More and more people in my neighborhood are walking and running, but a lot of streets don't have sidewalks," Gentry says. "I'm always on guard, ready to jump off the road if I have to."

There are other safety issues. When out running Gentry has been chased by dogs and witnessed drug deals in Cedar Hill Park. She would prefer to have a greenway in Madison, but for now she drives out of the neighborhood to Shelby Bottoms.

The bicycle as a mode of transportation and/or recreation also has its issues. Gentry says she "would love" if her family could bike the mile to Amqui Station, a recently rehabbed 1910 train station that's now a civic landmark, museum, and meeting space, "but there's not enough room for the kids to ride safely on the road. Drivers go 45 mph and there's a hill and a curve, making it treacherous."

If Gentry's transportation options are limited, so are destinations close to home. She wishes for more shops "so we can support Madison instead of always going to East Nashville." Gentry thinks that the catalyst lies in housing. "We need to have types of housing that attract younger, single people who have more disposable income."

For food, Gentry drives or grows her own. Staples come from Kroger, although she says the produce at the Madison branch of the chain is far inferior to that at the Inglewood Kroger. "Turnip Truck in East Nashville has bulk food items at a good price," she notes. "And while it's not organic, the Madison Inglewood Market has good fresh produce at a great price. For anything fancy, we drive 11 miles to the Publix in Hendersonville."

Gentry's backyard garden produces tomatoes, zucchini, squash, sugar snap peas, peppers, blueberries, raspberries, and blackberries in season. "When you buy raspberries at the store you pay a fortune and they don't taste anything like the raspberries you grow," she says.

Gentry also started a community garden two years ago on the grounds of the public library branch in Madison with a grant from the Greater Nashville Association of Realtors. "We bought $500 worth of fruit and nut trees," she says proudly. "We have mulberries, but it will be five years before most of the trees start producing. We want everyone to come and pick berries."

Gentry hopes that the library and the FiftyForward center in Madison will offer gardening and nutrition classes. She sees the garden project as a way to bring the people together. "The community tends to be divided socio-economically," she says. "But the library is well utilized by a diverse cross-section of the community, and it's a great way to reach kids."

Although Madison has recently gained a new fire station, with a new police station on the way, these can hardly be expected to provide the public gathering places that Gentry sees as central for curing the isolation of life in the suburbs. "There's no real opportunity for interaction with people unless you already know them," she says. "I'm acquainted with the people living in the houses I can see from my house, and that's it. There isn't a sense of community; it's more a bunch of individuals. Sidewalks would help people meet each other," she says. "But what we really need is a coffee shop."

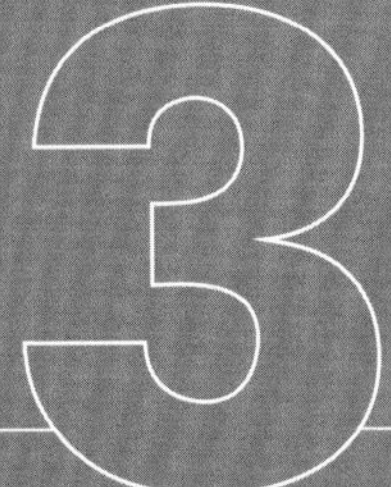

STRATEGIES

Strategically connect housing to schools, goods, services, and transportation.

Retrofit aging shopping centers—dead malls and strip malls—located along historic pikes, arterials, and collector roads to create mixed-use developments.

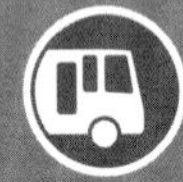

Increase the availability of community connector transit route services. These bus routes deliver passengers to and from bus transit stops on major roadways to central locations on secondary streets.

Utilize road diets and complete streets policies to incorporate additional sidewalks, crosswalks, and bike lanes.

Connect schools to their surrounding communities via sidewalks, greenways, or multi-use, nonvehicular paths; locate new schools near existing infrastructure: roads, sidewalks, bikeways, mass transit.

Enable access to existing food resources with better connectivity to surrounding communities.

Focus infill housing along commercial corridors to help preserve the character of existing neighborhoods and create a larger ridership pool for mass transit.

Integrate a variety of housing types, sizes, and prices in new developments.

Increase active transportation access to mini-parks, community parks, and community centers.

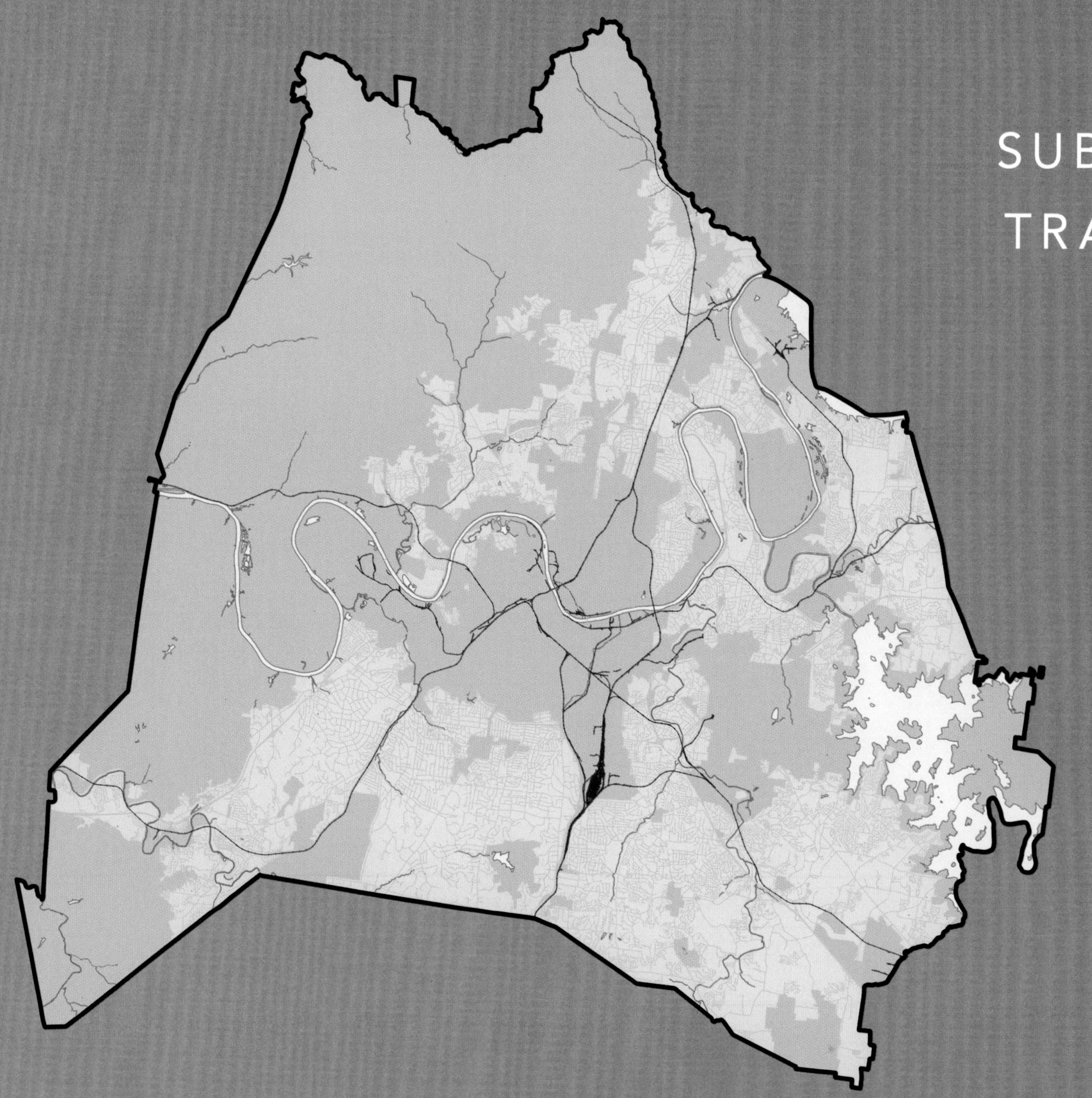

THE SUBURBAN TRANSECT ZONE

Davidson County, highlighting all areas in the suburban transect zone. Note that the suburbs consume the majority of land in the county. (Map, 2014: Metro Planning Department)

SUBURBAN

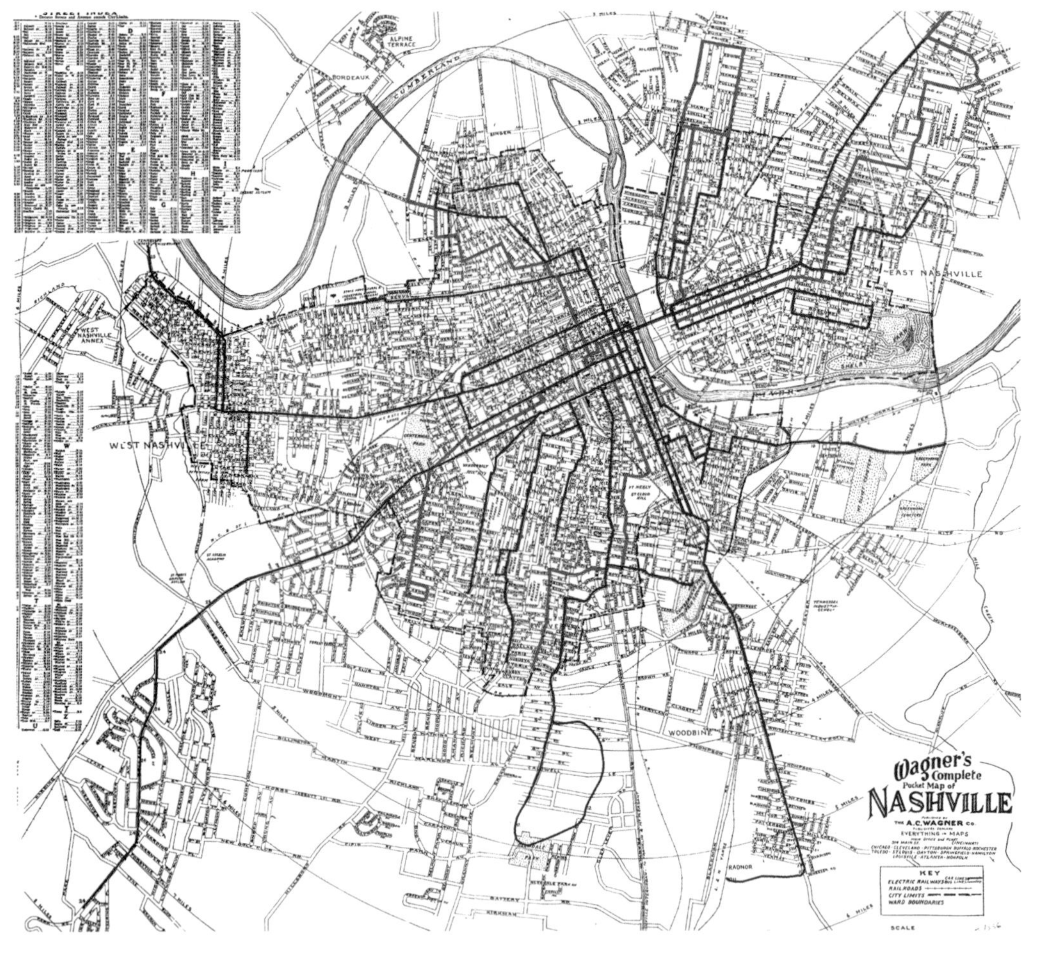

The streetcar lines at their peak. Note how fine-grained the routes are within the city—enabling people to walk to stops from their houses—and how far the lines reach into less populated territory. *(Map, 1927: Wagner's Complete Pocket Map of Nashville)*

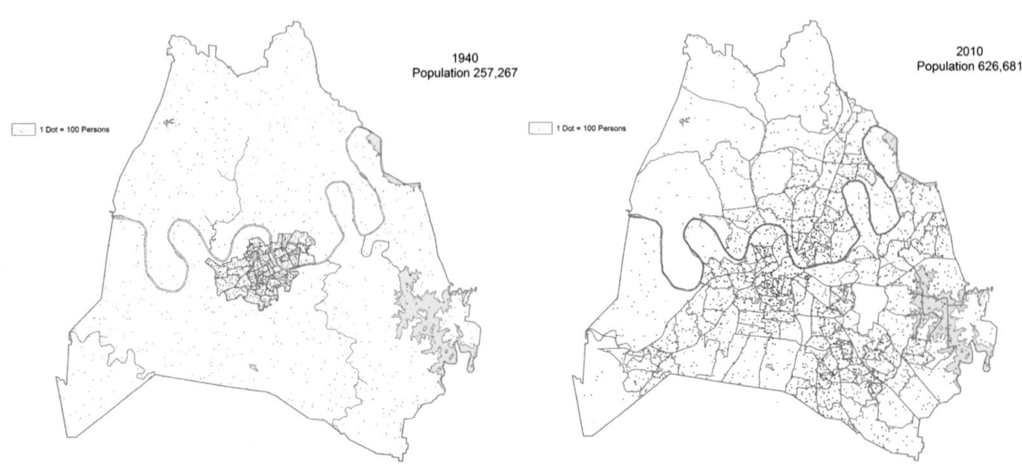

Maps of Nashville's settlement patterns in 1940 and 2010. Compare the dense clustering of the population in 1940 with the sprawl 70 years later. *(Map, 2012: Metro Planning Department)*

"The children themselves, before they get access to a car, are captives of their suburb, save for those families where the housewives surrender continuity in their own lives to chauffeur their children to lessons, doctors, and other services that could be reached via public transport in the city."

David Riesman, *Abundance For What?* (1964)

SUBURBAN LIVING

In the 21st century the suburbs often get a bad rap. Thus the online *Urban Dictionary,* a slangy compendium created by volunteers, defines "suburb" as "a mind-numbingly dull place located on the outskirts of a larger, and probably more interesting, city. Completely devoid of culture, activities, black people, good coffee, independent business and pedestrians."[1] This may be disregarded as the smug slur of a publication whose title alone indicates its bias.

Historian Lewis Mumford, however, is hardly less disparaging of what he calls "mass Suburbia." In *The City in History* (1961), Mumford warns: "The end product is an encapsulated life, spent more and more either in a motor car or within the cabin of darkness in front of a television set."[2] Since then our screens have proliferated and the "crabgrass frontier," peopled by "desperate housewives," has spawned the "asphalt nation" and "the geography of nowhere."

Suburbia is more complex and varied and has more amenities and a longer history than its critics acknowledge. The suburbs to which Mumford and the urban hipsters refer are the post-World War II version, with their segregated land uses and car dependency. But the nation's first suburbs were enabled by public transportation. Initially Nashville's streetcars were drawn by mules and provided service roughly two miles from the city center. The conversion of the transit system to electricity in 1888 opened up territory farther afield.

The people who rode the trolleys into the suburban fringe had valid reasons for wanting to live in a more sylvan setting. Increasing congestion, air blackened by the soft coal used for heat, and the lack of proper garbage disposal and safe drinking water all made the central city an unhealthy and unlovely place.

The neighborhoods that sprang up surrounding the downtown along the streetcar lines were

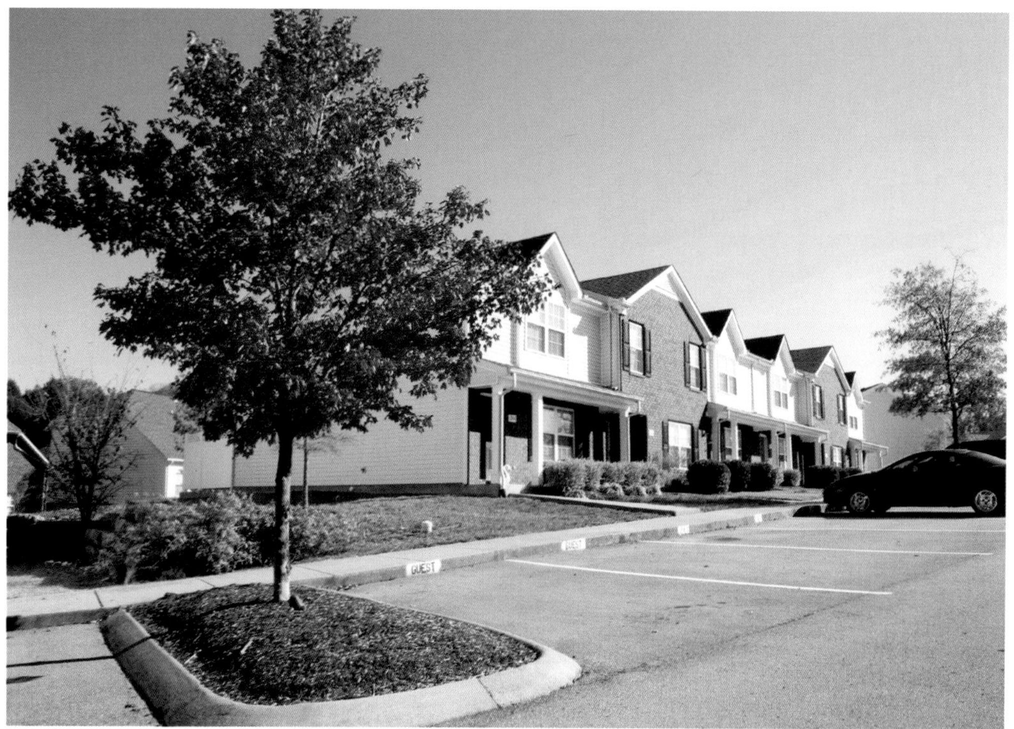

Townhomes in the Woodland Pointe neighborhood near Percy Priest Lake. Note how cars receive up-front treatment. *(2012)*

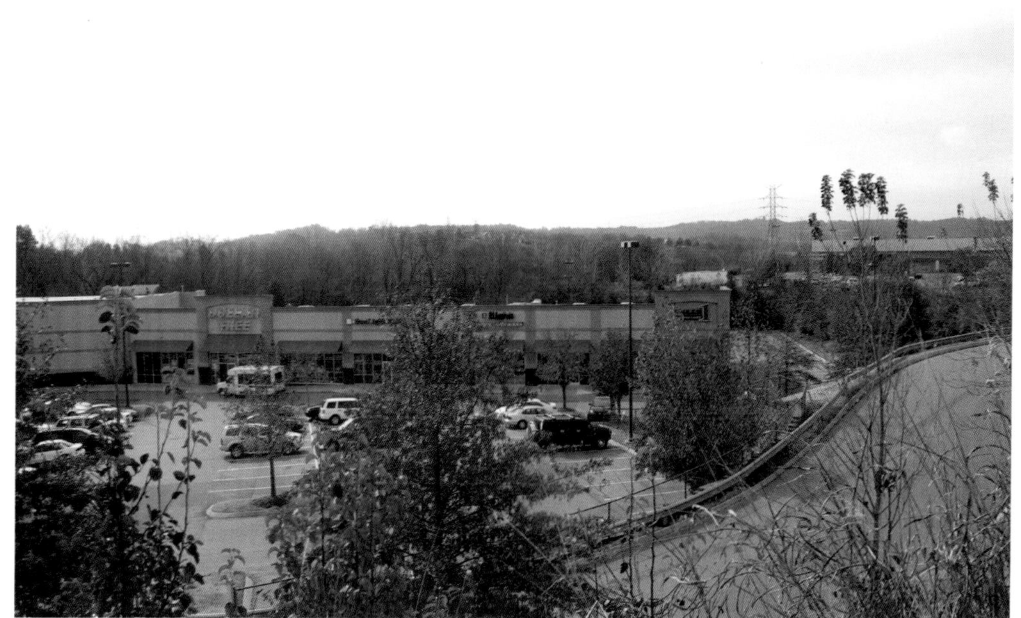

Typical suburban retail strip mall in Bellevue. Buildings are set back from the main road and clustered around large surface parking lots. Vehicular access is privileged and pedestrian connections are poor. *(2012)*

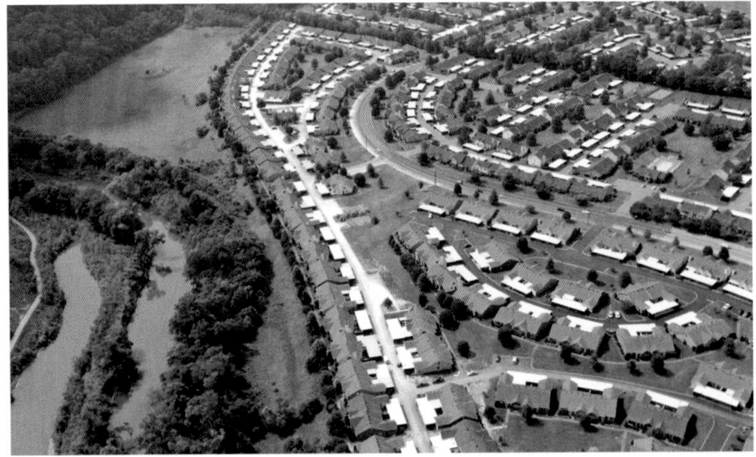

Left: Aerial view of River Plantation neighborhood, Bellevue. Development of this "garden-style" condominium project near the Harpeth River began in 1972. The massive flooding of the river in 2010 severely impacted the development. *(2011: Gary Layda)*

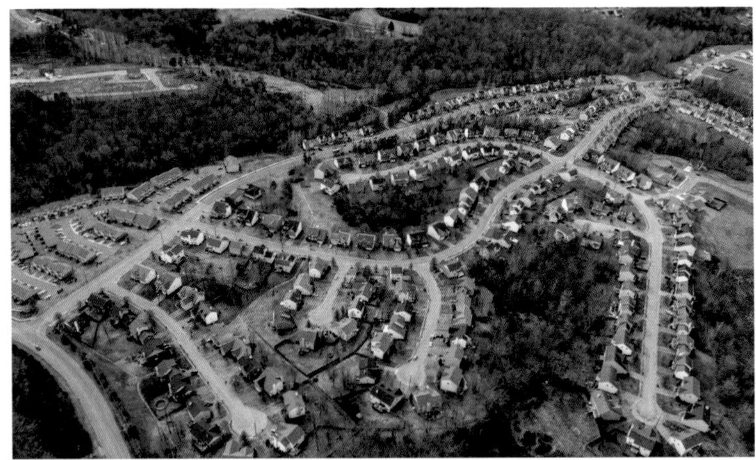

Right: Suburban cul-de-sacs lack both pedestrian and vehicular access to nearby roadways, neighborhoods, institutions, and commerce. *(2013: Gary Layda)*

reasonably compact and walkable, because residents traveled on foot to and from the stops as well as to schools, churches, and shops. Later suburbs were planned around the automobile as the primary form of transportation, replacing the streetcars and leaving the landscape of Nashville forever changed.

From the late 1940s onward, suburbanization consumed vast tracts of rural land, as well as government infrastructure budgets for all the sewer lines and roadways. The result was decline in the urban areas, both economically and in the physical condition of buildings, which now seemed poor investments.

The people who moved outward were "exchanging decaying urban neighborhoods for a brand new house, a green lawn, and new schools and stores." And their low-interest mortgages were frequently underwritten by the federal government.[3] By the 1960s, another motive emerged. "Many white suburbanites also left the city out of an unspoken fear of blacks," writes historian Don Doyle in *Nashville Since the 1920s*. It was "an effort to maintain social distance by creating more physical distance between the races at a time when the legal barriers to racial segregation were crumbling."[4]

The suburban migration seemed to be a move into economically and physically healthier terrain—populated by the middle class, with cleaner air and all the grass and trees. But the long-term results have been otherwise. "In reports and studies of the 1950s, '60s and '70s, Nashville's planners warned that the low-density development patterns of the suburbs would make the provision of services to these areas prohibitively expensive, dilute the level of services in the traditional neighborhoods, and make it all but impossible to establish an efficient and economically feasible mass transit system for Metro Nashville," writes Christine Kreyling in *The Plan of Nashville*.[5]

In areas where land uses are compartmentalized—commerce segregated from residences—where lots are large, sidewalk-less cul-de-sacs feed into wide arterials, schools and churches sit on large campuses surrounded by car storage, and each business has its own parking lot, driving is a way of life.

In addition, the increased suburbanization of jobs "obstructs transit's ability to connect workers to opportunity and jobs to local labor pools," states a 2012 report by the Brookings Institution.[6] In an analysis of data from transit providers in the nation's 100 largest metropolitan areas, the Middle Tennessee region ranks 92, with only 49.4 percent of its jobs in areas with public transit service. And the share of the region's population that can reach a job by transit in 90 minutes is 15.6 percent.

Another 2012 study explored the impact of residential density on miles traveled and fuel consumed and found "moving a household from a suburban to an urban area reduces household annual mileage by 18 percent." The study also discovered "a lower neighborhood residential density induces consumer choices toward less fuel-efficient vehicles."[7] It's unclear why suburbanites prefer more gas-guzzling cars, although one could hazard a guess that those more frequently in road-warrior mode feel the need for heftier armor.

Increasingly clear are the health consequences. All the cars create congested streets, which engender air pollution and stressful commutes. The people in those cars are sitting, not walking. Basic exercise thus is not an incidental part of daily life but a discrete event—trips to the gym or park—that suburbanites must program into schedules already tight because of all the time spent sitting in cars.

Nashville is clearly not going to abandon its suburbs, nor scrape them and start over. What we must do is reshape them.

SUBURBAN ZONE BASICS

For planning purposes, the suburban transect zone exhibits the following characteristics:

- **Single-family residences predominate in low to moderate density patterns**
- **Condominium and apartment complexes, in the suburbs that permit them, are frequently clustered adjacent to major roadways**
- **Typically, though not necessarily, suburbs are commuter communities**
- **Many amenities, including retail, food, entertainment, and commercial facilities. These are located in malls, commercial strips, and stand-alone lots, none of which are easy to access other than by car**
- **Access to institutions such as churches and schools primarily via automobile**
- **Increasing congestion on arterials and major collector roads.**
- **Limited public transportation**[8]

The approximately 127,225 acres of suburban land in Davidson County represent 37.6 percent of the county's total land area. More people—409,810—live in the suburban transect zone than in any other zone of the county. The level of density is 3.2 persons per acre. (The smaller urban transect zone has a density of 5.4 persons per acre.)[9]

SHAPING HEALTH IN THE SUBURBAN TRANSECT ZONE

ANALYSIS AND STRATEGIES

Given that the suburban transect zone is the most extensive in the entire transect of Nashville and that more people currently live in suburbia than in any other zone, it is important to shape healthier suburban communities as we prepare for growth over the next 20 years.

The key challenge is the car-dependency inherent in the suburban form of development of the last 60 years. Reducing the need to drive will require denser residential development in selected locations, primarily along the arterials and collector streets, to enable a larger ridership pool for mass transit, thus increasing transit's financial viability and frequency of service. The installation of a more complete system of pedestrian and bicycle infrastructure is also necessary. Integrating a mixture of land uses can reduce the distance between destinations and encourage residents and workers to walk and cycle to meet the needs of daily life rather than drive to large-scale pods of commerce.

"Meet me at the …?"
This question was posed to residents of Madison during a community workshop presented by the Nashville Civic Design Center that focused on the topic of "livability." Those attending had no clear answer. Many suburban communities lack a defined center or a sense of place. Recent efforts to retrofit suburbs seek to create these types of civic gathering spaces surrounded by a mix of uses.

—Nashville Civic Design Center, The Livability Project: Building More Livable Communities *(2011)*

✓ *Top left:* The addition of a sidewalk has improved conditions for pedestrians along Abbott Martin Road, but these walled-off neighborhoods lack "eyes on the street," thus inhibiting these communities from becoming truly socially connected to surrounding residents. *(2013)*

✗ *Top right:* Homes with rear elevations along Abbott Martin Road. Metro Planning's new subdivision regulations discourage these double frontage lots that turn their "backs" to the primary public right-of-way. *(© 2012: Google)*

✓ *Center left:* Lenox Village offers sidewalks on both sides of the street. Note that a planting strip separates walkers from cars to increase perception of safety. A departure from convention in 2001, this pedestrian infrastructure is now required for all newly constructed subdivisions. *(2012: Brian Phelps and Chris Whitis)*

✗ *Center right:* Reelfoot in Donelson, an older suburban neighborhood with no sidewalks. Note also the overhead utility lines, now required to be underground. Burying lines reduces power outages from events such as ice storms and presents a better curbside appearance. *(2013)*

✓ *Bottom:* Cottage-style housing within the Lenox Village neighborhood: small lot, shared-wall housing that frames open space. In current regulations, residential lots are generally required to have street frontage, but provisions have been made for fronting onto a common open space with vehicular access from a rear alley. *(2012)*

✓ Health-Promoting

Some private suburban developments offer residents recreational amenities such as sidewalks, pools, walking trails, gyms, and golf courses.

Metro Planning's new land-use policies encourage mixed-use development along suburban road corridors. The department's updates of its subdivision regulations[10] over the last decade have been intended to counter "conventional development planning" and correct suburban residential sprawl. Revisions in 2006, and further amendments in 2011, created the following examples of how regulations are being used to create greater connectivity and pedestrian safety.

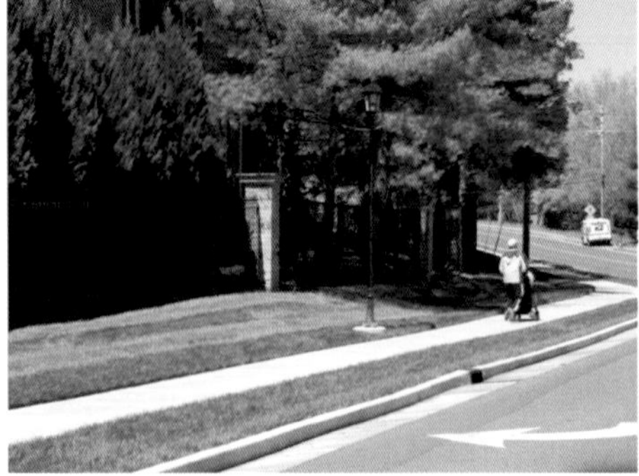

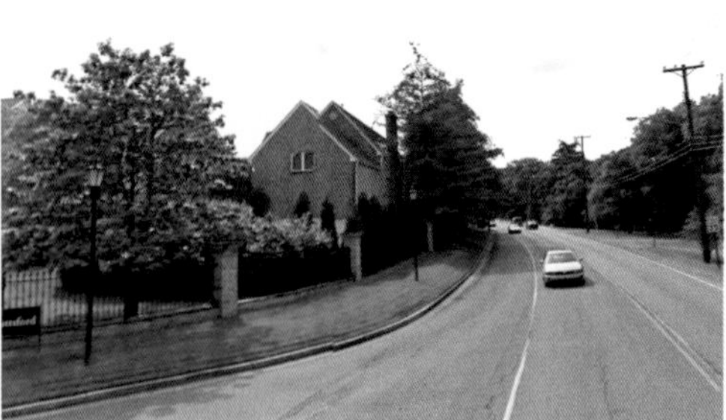

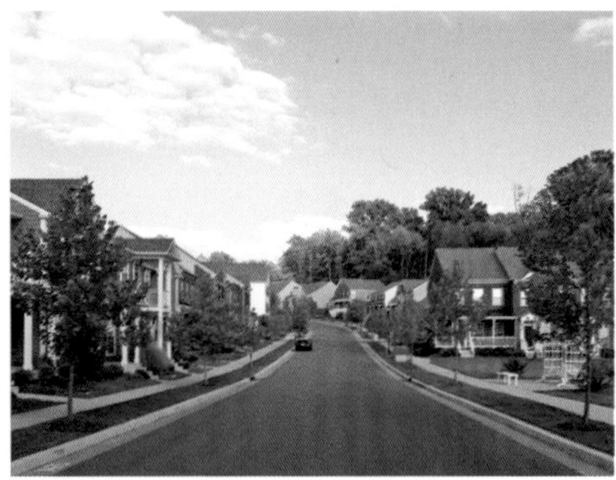

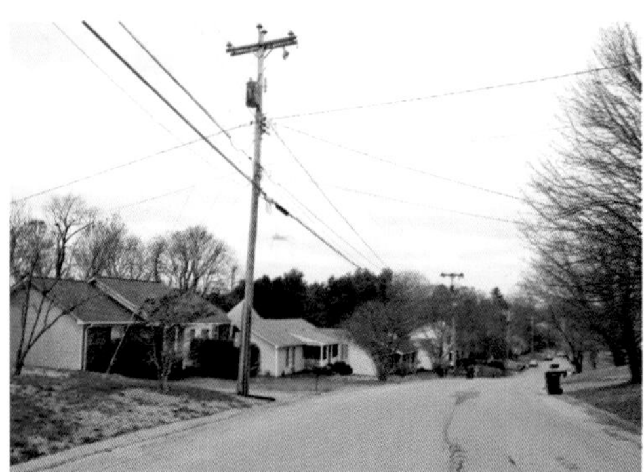

Additional new subdivision regulations include:

- ✓ Direct access from subdivisions to arterial and collector streets is limited to avoid excessive curb cuts on major roadways. Curb cuts put pedestrians on sidewalks in conflict with turning vehicles. Numerous curb cuts also increase turning incidents, which slow vehicular traffic.
- ✓ Requirements for pedestrian and bicycle easements, as well as facilities such as bike racks. Specific locations are recommended by the *Strategic Plan for Sidewalks and Bikeways* or an adopted Community Plan.

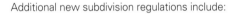

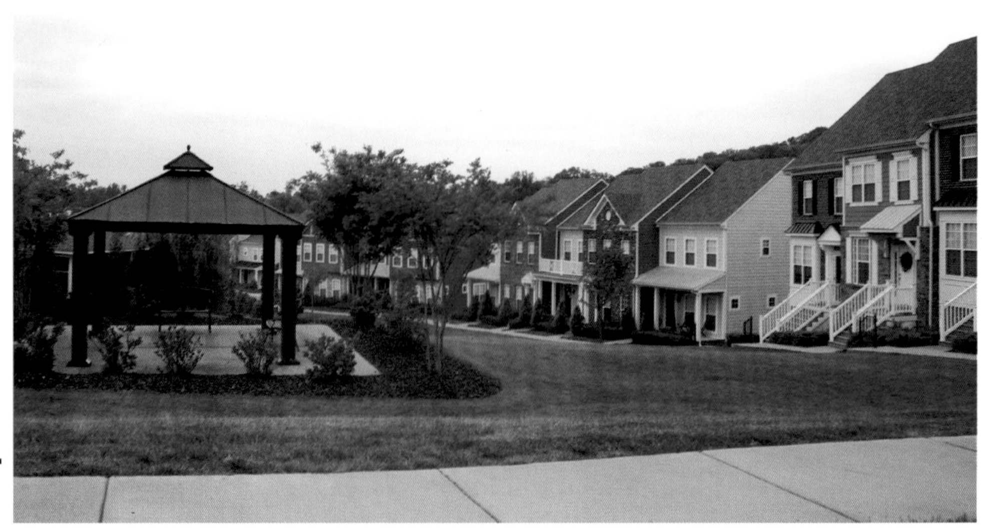

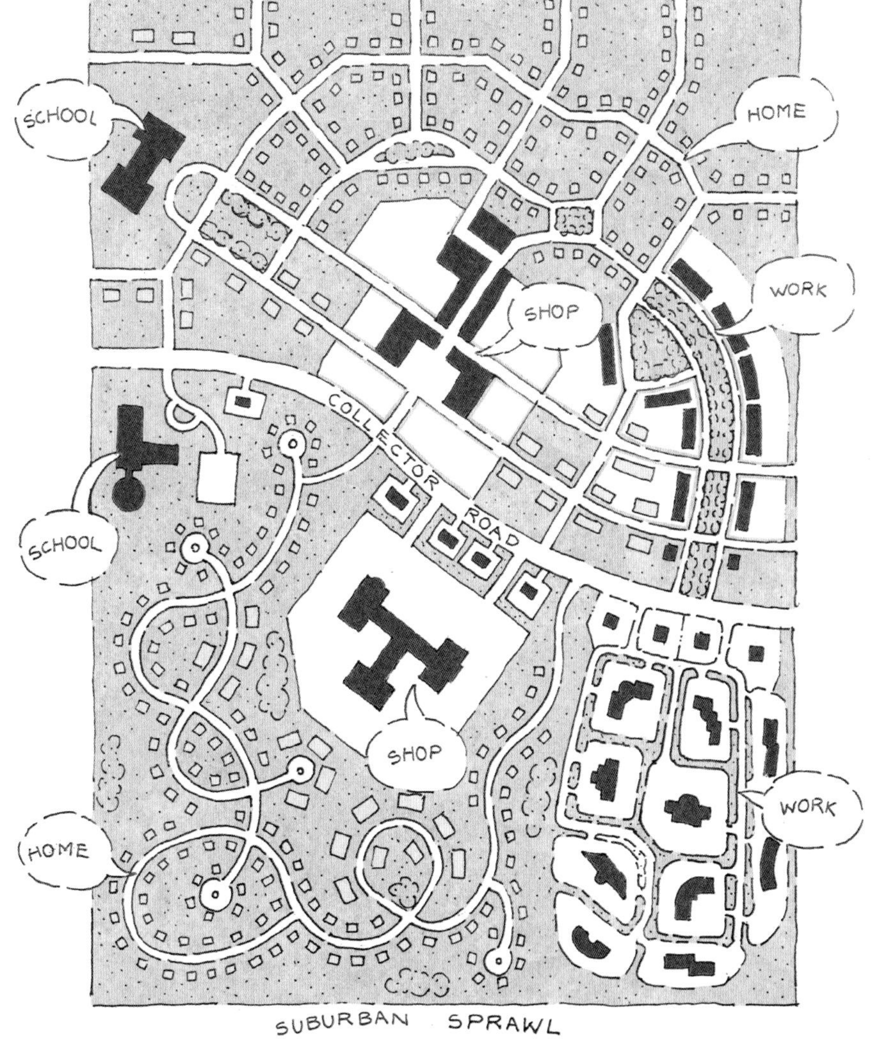

✗ Health-Defeating

Deliberate separation of housing from other land uses. As a result, residents, especially those seeking to walk or bike, are poorly connected to the wider community and must depend on cars for transportation. Those without the ability to drive or the means to own a car have few or no transportation options.

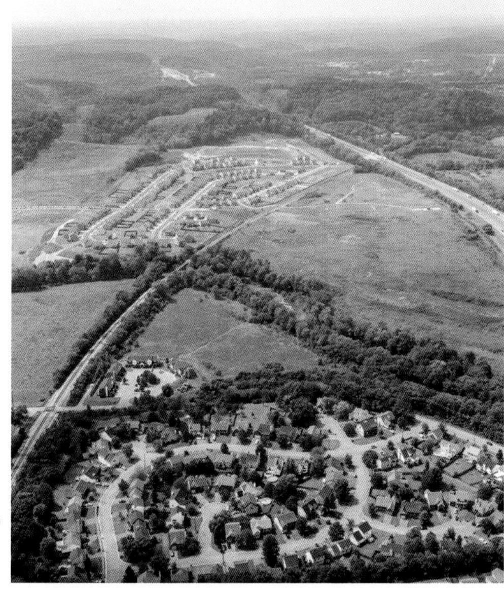

Traditional Neighborhood Design vs. Sprawl Development: in the traditional design, note the network of streets that connect the various land uses and provide many access points into the neighborhood. In the sprawl design, on the other hand, the housing component has few ingress/egress points and lacks direct links to the stand-alone pods dedicated to commerce and school. *(Illustration, © 2010: Used courtesy of Duany Platter-Zyberk & Co.)*

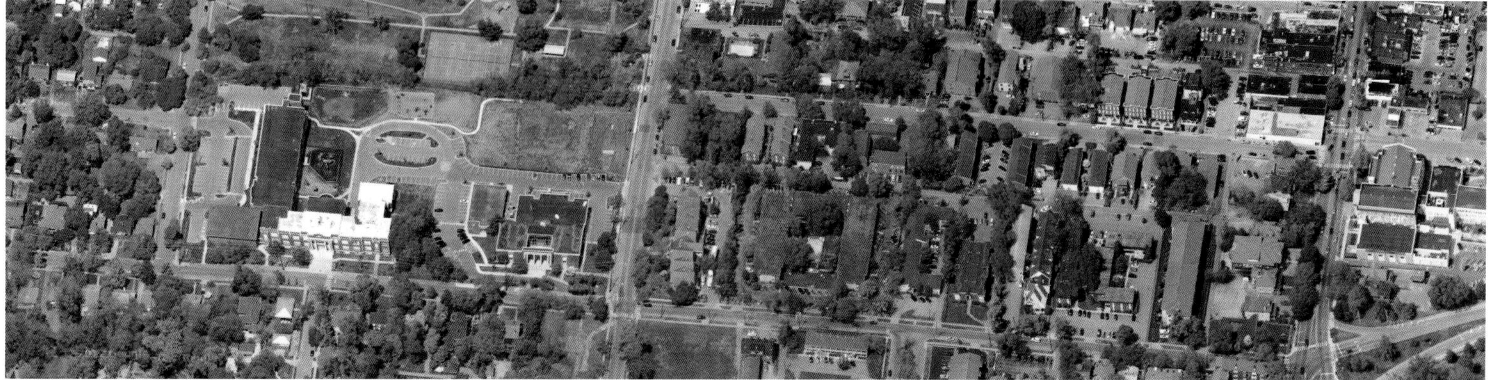

✗ *Left:* Aerial image of suburban development in Bellevue. *(© 2011: Google)*

✓ *Bottom:* The traditional neighborhood design of the Belmont-Hillsboro neighborhood. *(© 2012: Google)*

STRATEGY: *Retrofitting suburbs is the concept of directing growth to existing suburban areas by means of infill and redevelopment to prevent additional sprawl and consumption of remaining rural land. The benefits are the preservation of open space and the reduction of costs to government because the infrastructure already exists. In retrofitting, the emphasis should be on the mixture of land uses, including residential with smaller scale commercial, and on providing street and sidewalk connections to surrounding neighborhoods and commerce.*

Significant economic redevelopment opportunities may be found all along our arterials, especially in "dying" shopping centers, malls, and outdated big box stores. "The belief that the commercial-only arterial is best must be rethought in favor of concentrated commercial nodes linked by higher density mixed-use corridors," writes Rick Bernhardt, Metro Planning director, in his 2005 essay, "Reforming the Arterials." "There is much more property along our arterials zoned for commercial use than can be economically sustained. And the amount of existing arterial commercial development—in the form of the big box and the strip mall—cannot be supported under today's economic realities."[11] This is even truer now, with the escalation of online shopping.

Increasing the density of development along the historic pikes and arterials that are now mostly commercial will create a larger ridership pool for public transit while protecting existing neighborhoods served by local streets.

STRATEGY: *Facilitate the evolution of mixed-use neighborhood centers.*

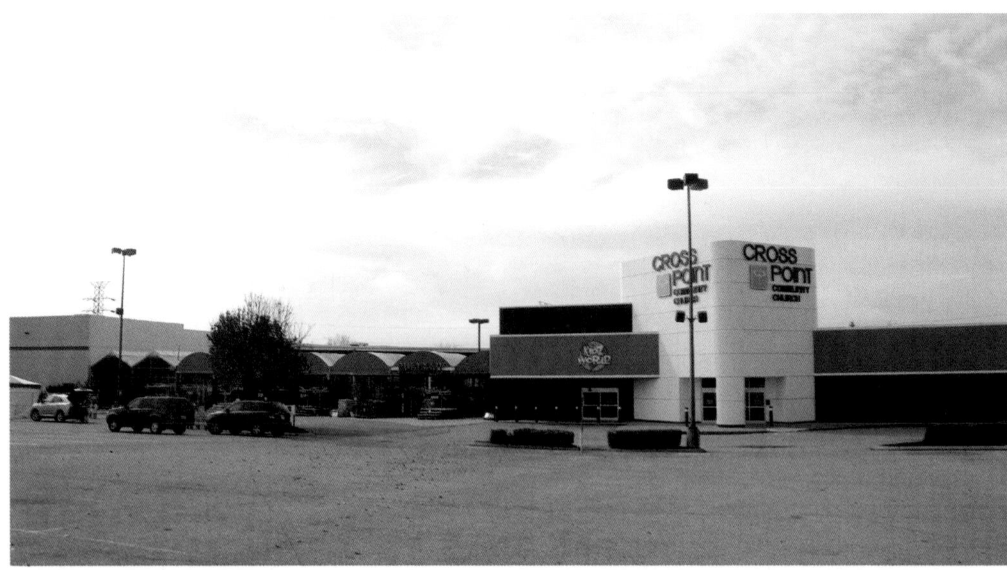

Big box reuse as a community church in Bellevue. The adaptive reuse of outdated retail structures activates spaces that would otherwise be vacant. Infill in the vast acreage of parking around these structures would increase densities; a mixture of uses would enable residents and workers to walk to nearby destinations and public transit. *(2012)*

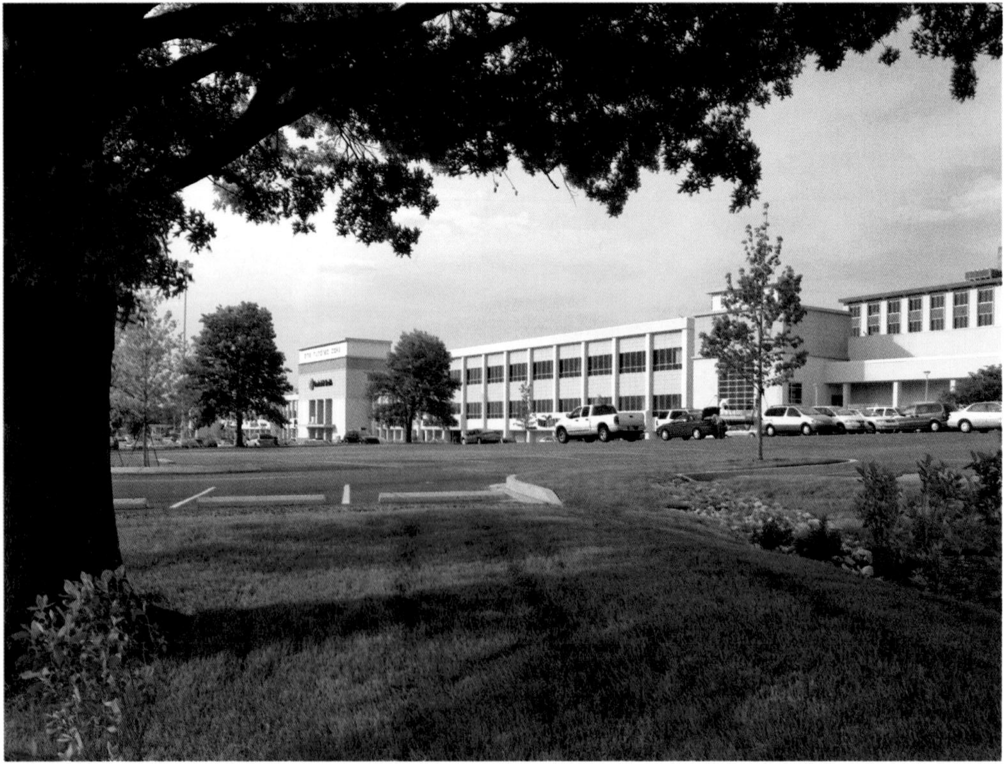

The 100 Oaks Mall, named after the estate it replaced, originally opened in 1968 as the state's first enclosed mall. By the late 1970s, the mall had lost many of its major anchors, including JCPenney, and closed for the first time in 1983. The mall endured three "dying" periods before its most recent revival that introduced a new concept for rehabilitation through diversification of its uses. In 2007, plans for its renovation were spearheaded by the announcement that Vanderbilt University would become the main tenant, leasing over 400,000 square feet for medical office space. The entire site was overhauled and is now a successful example of renovating and greening a dead mall site. *(2010: Gresham Smith & Partners)*

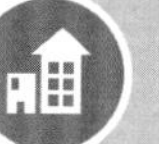

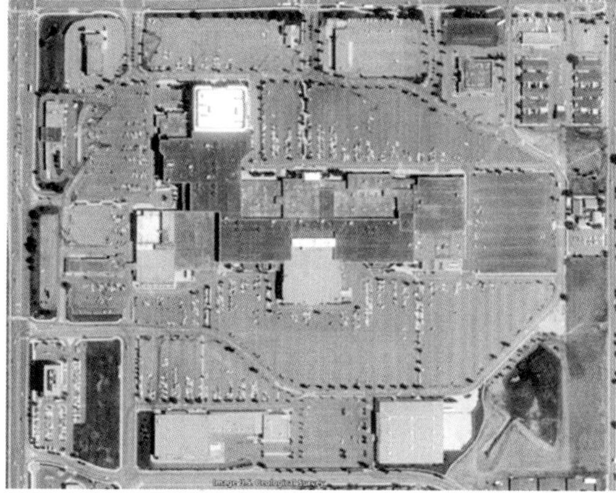

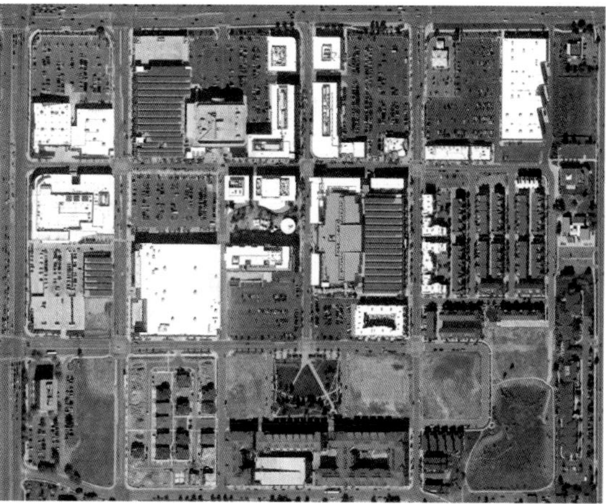

Left: Aerial view of Villa Italia, another former estate carved up for a mall in 1966 and located in the suburban community of Lakewood, 4.5 miles southwest of Denver, CO. By the late 1990s this mall was considered dead, and plans began for its redevelopment. *(© 2003, Google)*

Right: Aerial view of Belmar, the new name for the redevelopment of the 104-acre Villa Italia site. Belmar created a new town center for the community—including new streets, shops, restaurants, offices, diverse housing types, and nine acres of open space—all connected to public transportation. *(@ 2012, Google)*

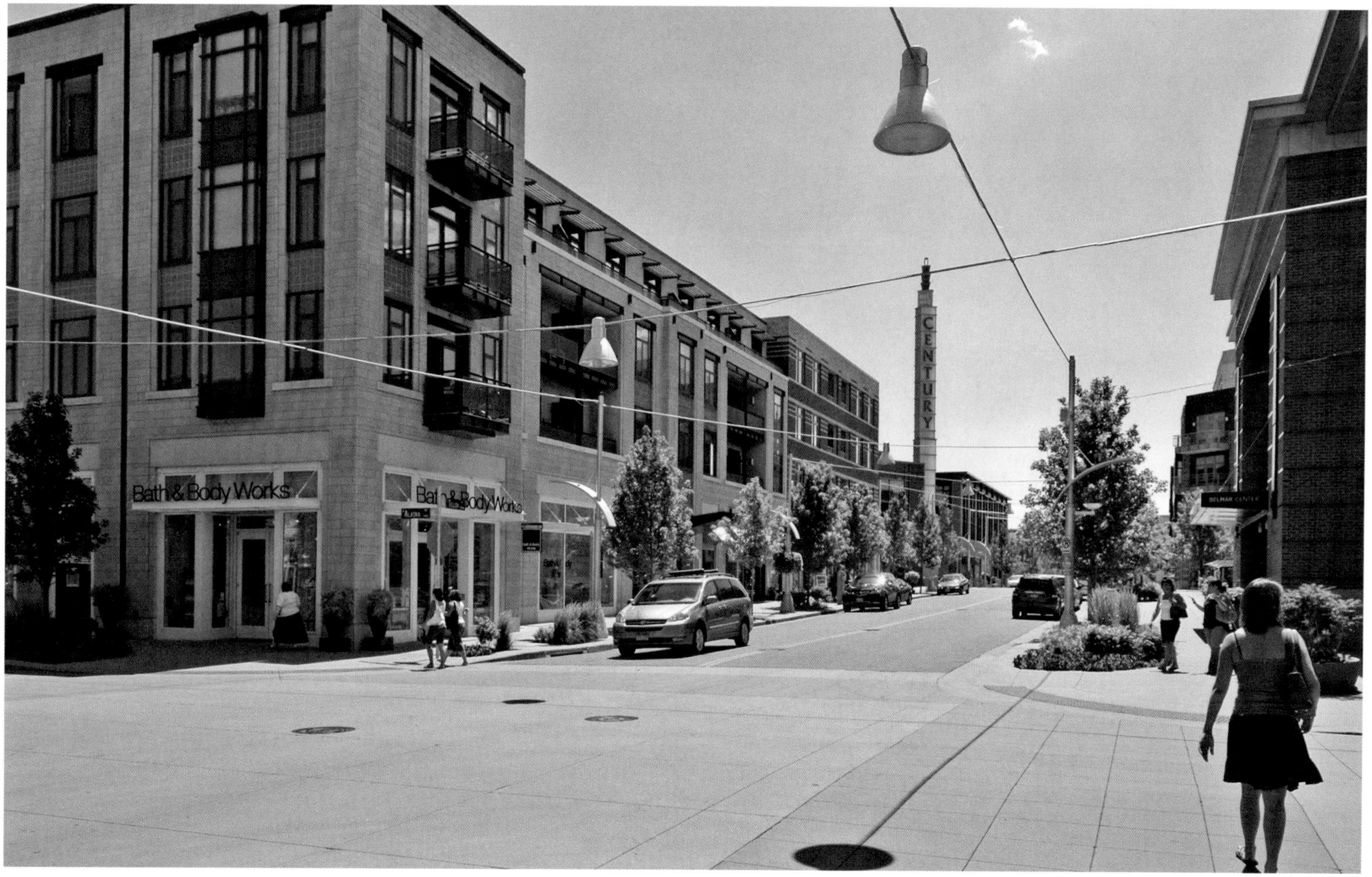

Today, Belmar is a vibrant and walkable mixed-use community. *(2010: Brian Phelps and Chris Whitis)*

Lenox Village

The cul-de-sac (French for "bottom of the sack") subdivision was envisioned as an antidote to cars—and strangers. The one-way in and out would eliminate through traffic, theoretically making streets safer for children. The street form also effectively restricts entrants into the subdivision, usually limited to single-family homes, to residents, their visitors, and service providers: lawn care guy, house cleaner, window washer.

But the defensive posture of the dead-end street goes back much further. In the walled cities of ancient and medieval times, many streets and lanes formed loops or terminated at the enclosure. Such street patterns were potential traps for enemies. Invading soldiers who plunged down a cul-de-sac after breaching the outer fortifications would find themselves with no through passage and, with luck, at a literal dead end.

The problem for inhabitants of the modern cul-de-sac is what's encountered when you get out of them—and you have to leave to acquire goods and services. The streets of many such subdivisions feed directly into a large arterial or collector roadway unsafe for walking or cycling. So residents must drive.

For an alternative model, meet Lenox Village. Built by Regent Homes and designed by Looney Ricks Kiss, the 208-acre site is Nashville's first full-scale "traditional neighborhood development," so-called because it mimics the form of streetcar suburbs laid out before the car was king.

Lenox Village's street grid is an interconnected hierarchy, with service alleys, sidewalks, and pedestrian passages between parcels. The widths of vehicular rights-of-way are limited to calm traffic. A mixed-use village center of 150,000 square feet bridges the primarily residential areas and the commercial corridor of Nolensville Road. Businesses share parking between daytime and nighttime venues to minimize asphalt. The retail and service mix—coffee and food shops, restaurants, day spa and pet spa, gym, dry cleaner, etc.—enables consumers to do at least some of their shopping on foot.

The village center also features small offices as well as multifamily housing and live/work units. Other housing types among the projected 1,200 to 1,400 units include single-family (attached and detached), and over-the-garage "carriage units." The variety acknowledges that the nuclear family no longer dominates the market and facilitates economic and lifestyle diversity among residents.

Lenox Village is compact and its buildings of a scale not intimidating to pedestrians. The compactness allowed the developers to dedicate a minimum of one acre of open space per 30 residential units. This open space includes the village green and mini-parks, a 15-acre greenway with a restored stream that's home to the endangered Tennessee crayfish, and wooded hillsides left undisturbed.

When construction of Lenox Village began in 2001, Metro's planners were already committed to reshaping policies to promotee infill and new development that was more urbanist and friendly to modes of transportation other than cars. But Nashville's subdivision regulations hadn't yet caught up to this approach. The Lenox developers, therefore, had to devise, with the assistance of the city planners, an urban design overlay, an expensive and time-consuming process. This form-based rather than land-use-based code enabled Lenox's neotraditional design.

The extra effort has not gone unrecognized. In 2002, Lenox Village received an award for overall design from the Middle Tennessee Chapter of the American Institute of Architects. Two years later, the Home Builders Association of Middle Tennessee awarded Lenox its Smart Growth award.

— CHRISTINE KREYLING

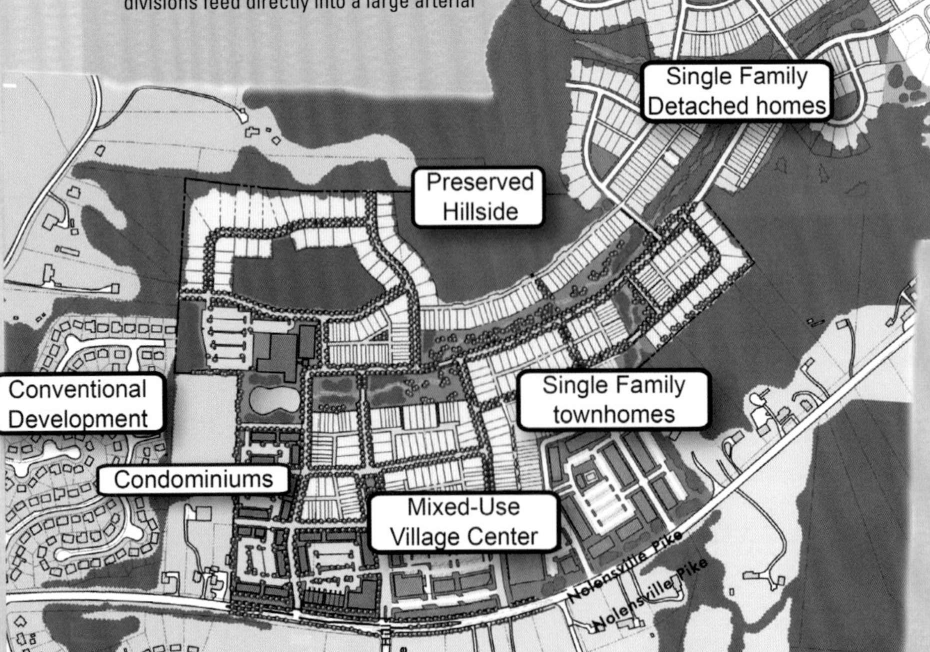

Lenox Village site plan. *(2001: Looney Ricks Kiss, Inc.)*

TRANSPORTATION

Health-Promoting

The addition of Bus Rapid Transit (BRT) and commuter rail to Nashville's public transit menu offers commuters alternatives to cars along the corridors served. BRT operates on Gallatin Road and Murfreesboro Pike, providing fewer stops and more frequent service than the regular lines on these roads, improved transit shelters, and digital signage that informs riders of approaching buses. The Music City Star, a commuter train, serves Donelson and Hermitage on its way from Lebanon to downtown.

Health-Defeating

Commute Time to Work

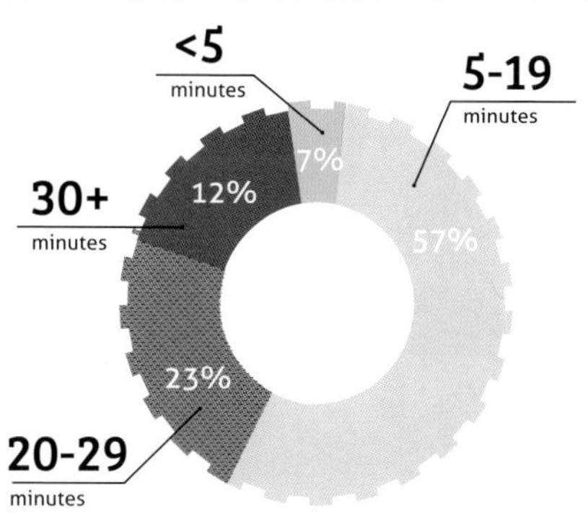

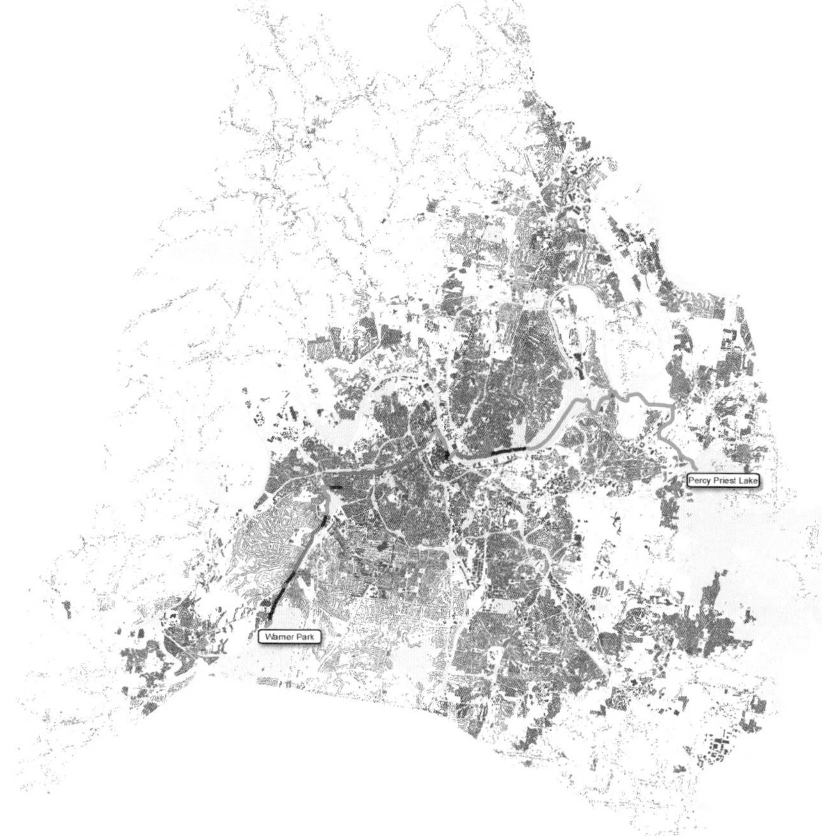

Map of the 26-mile Music City Bikeway. Green represents a multi-use path separated from cars; orange represents an on-street bike lane; and red represents locations where a bike and car share the outside lane.

The bikeway, connecting east and west Davidson County, is an active transportation option for commuters as well as a major avenue of recreation. *(Illustration over map, 2013: Eric Hoke, NCDC)*

Center left: Average commute time to work from suburban transect zones in Davidson County, according to the US Census Bureau's 2010 American Community Survey. *(Information graphic, 2013: Ashley Nicole Johnson)*

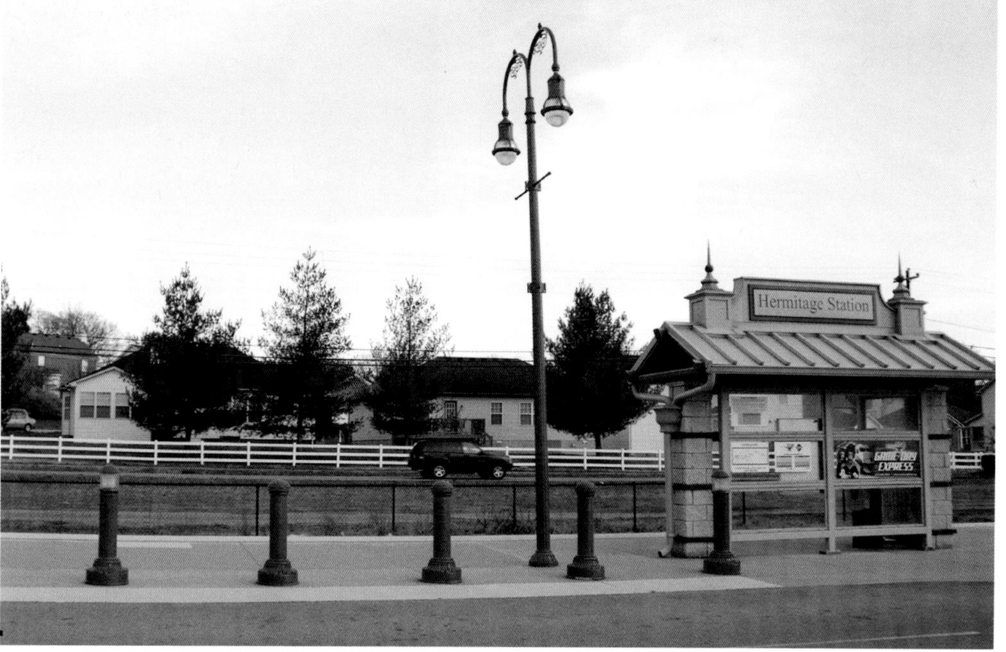

Music City Star Hermitage station. Note the proximity of suburban homes to the train platform. *(2013)*

The traditional suburban design focus on the automobile inhibits other forms of transportation, such as mass transit, walking, and biking. Statistics from the Federal Highway Administration (FHA) show that, in 2011, the citizens of Davidson County drove 21.75 million miles per day, an average of 34.7 miles per person. And each year Middle Tennessee commuters waste the most hours of any region—120—trapped in what a report by CEOs for Cities calls the "sprawl crawl."[12] Being stuck in traffic for all those wasted hours increases air pollution, stress, and the risk of hypertension and cardiovascular disease.

In suburban areas, which lack the grid street pattern that disperses traffic, congestion is especially acute. Among Metro Public Works' list of the top 20 busiest intersections, only two (21st Avenue South / Wedgewood Avenue and West End Avenue / Murphy Road) lie in the urban street network; the rest are in sprawlsville. The "winner" in the congestion contest: Nolensville Pike / Harding Place, with 76,000 cars per day.[13]

The reasons for suburban traffic congestion are rooted in development patterns that concentrate traffic on arterials, such as Gallatin Road, Hillsboro Pike, Harding Road, etc. Despite the fact that these roads are expected to carry a heavy load of traffic, however, Metro has zoned these roads almost entirely commercial.

Quick and efficient traffic flow occurs when cars stop infrequently. Commercial areas, however, induce frequent stops, slowdowns, and turns as drivers access parking lots. That each business typically has its own parking, immediately adjacent, increases the amount of turning. Recurrent curb cuts for all these parking lots erode sidewalks, if they are present at all, and force intrepid walkers into conflict with cars. Vehicular mobility reduced to a crawl undermines efficient mass transit. Thus the focus on cars has created a roadway system that is dysfunctional for all forms of transportation.

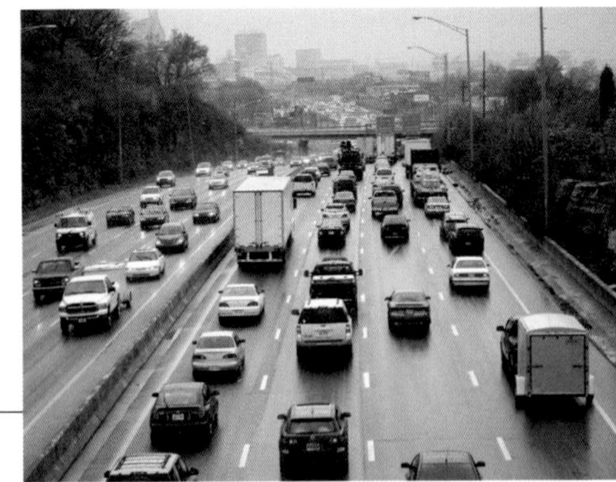

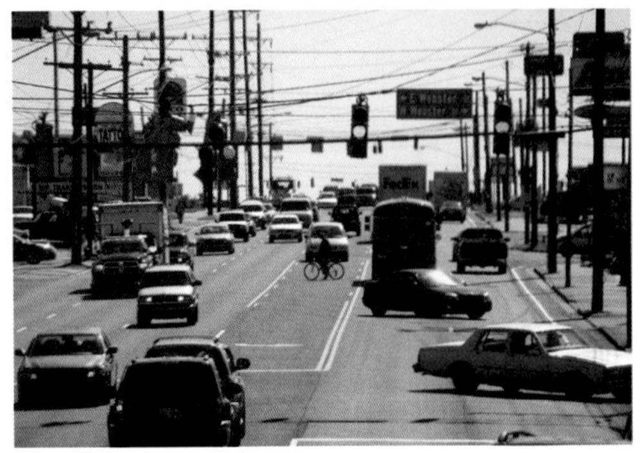

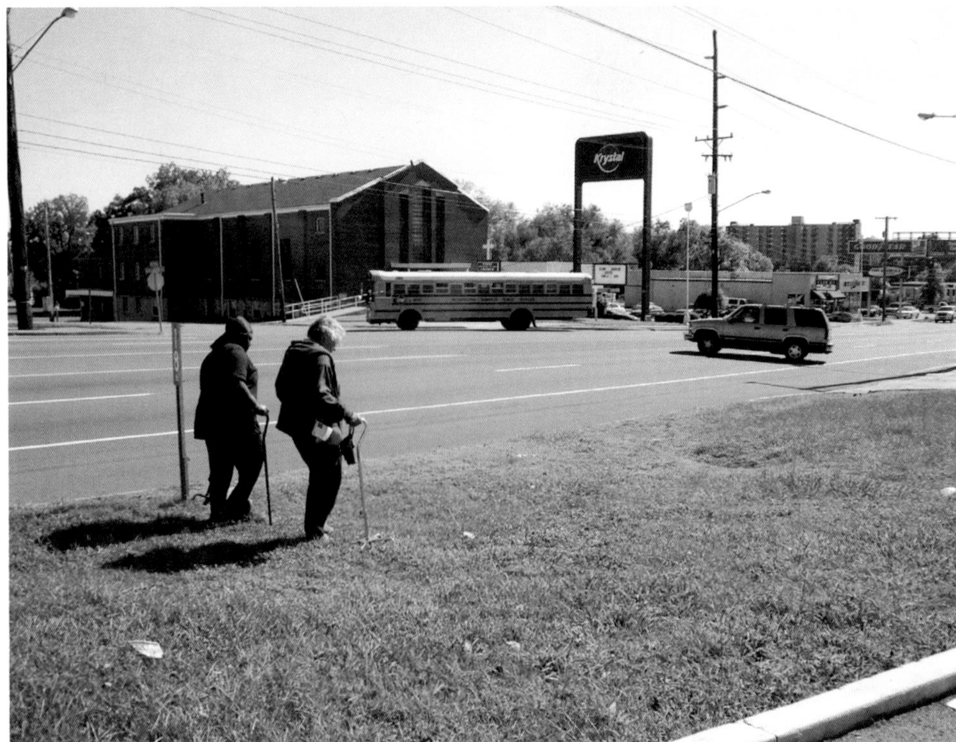

Left top: Traffic congestion on I-40 west of downtown Nashville. *(2012: Metro Planning Department)*

Left bottom: Traffic congestion on Gallatin Pike in Madison. *(2011)*

Right: Madison's lack of adequate pedestrian infrastructure makes it difficult for seniors and people with disabilities, as well as those who cannot afford a car, to easily access transit and nearby commercial and institutional facilities. *(2011)*

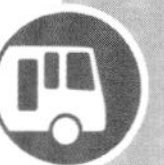

STRATEGY: *Enable independence from the automobile. Suburban communities require alternatives to car travel to reduce air pollution, driving related stress, and vehicular accidents, while allowing people the opportunity to become more active—ultimately improving their health and saving money. The American Public Transportation Association estimates that households can save an average of $10,000 per year by giving up one car and taking public transportation. The savings come from the elimination of fuel and maintenance costs, vehicle depreciation, and insurance premiums.*[14]

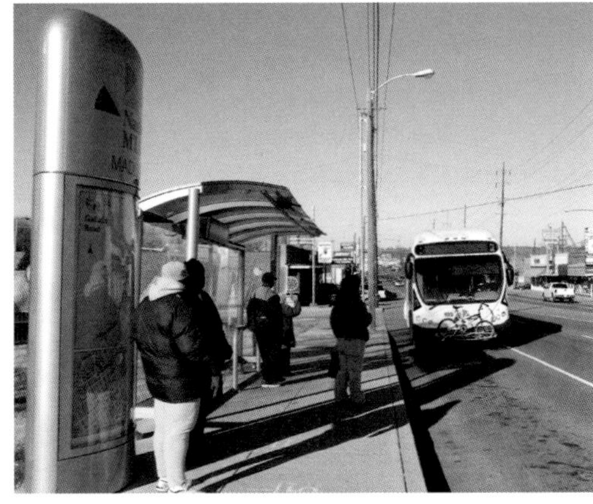

BRT stop on Gallatin Pike in Madison, complete with modern shelter and digital displays. Such amenities improve the visibility and perception of public transit. Note that the bus is equipped with a bike rack. *(2011)*

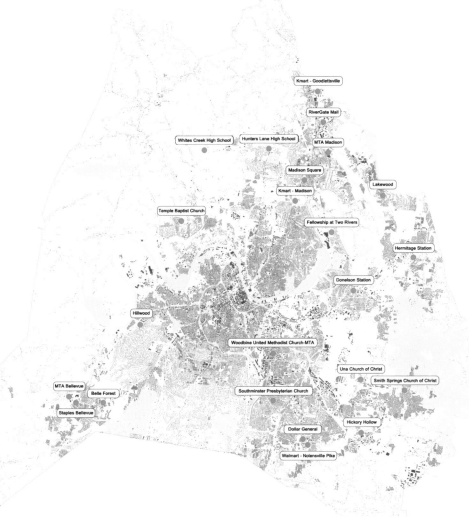

Map of Park and Ride Facilities. Metro currently operates 23 park and ride locations in Davidson county. Partnerships with shopping centers, churches, and schools exploit large swaths of underutilized parking lots and remove cars from roads during peak travel hours. *(Map, 2015: Eric Hoke, NCDC)*

Create viable transportation alternatives for the large number of suburban commuters by increasing public transit services (routes and frequency) between suburban communities and primary employment areas. The low-to-moderate density of residences and the arterial focus of the road pattern in the suburban transect zone, however, do not lend themselves to a fine grain of transit lines. More park-and-ride areas throughout the county is one option for enhancing ridership, which would enable better commuter service. These lots can be shared with facilities that do not fully use their parking during peak commuter hours, or installed on vacant land that can be banked for future high-density, mixed-use development.

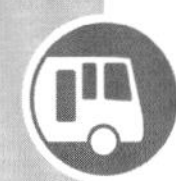

It is important to point out, however, that many car trips are not generated by commutes to work. Shopping, dining out, going to the gym, delivering children to and from day care, school, and extracurricular activities, and other errands occupy a significant amount of American travel time. The 2009 National Highway Travel Survey concluded that over 79 percent of all trips are not work-related. Of those, 28 percent are 1 mile or less, 40 percent are 2 miles or less, and 50 percent are 3 miles or less.[15] With the FHWA's defined bikeable distance at 5 miles or less, most trips can be accomplished by alternative means to the personal vehicle.

Thus prying people out of their cars also depends on increasing public transit service and active transit amenities—more sidewalks and bike lanes—*within* the community. Bus "connector" routes collect people at key locations—schools, medical clinics, senior towers—on secondary roads and deliver them to and from the main MTA lines located along the major pikes. The Madison connector is a successful example.

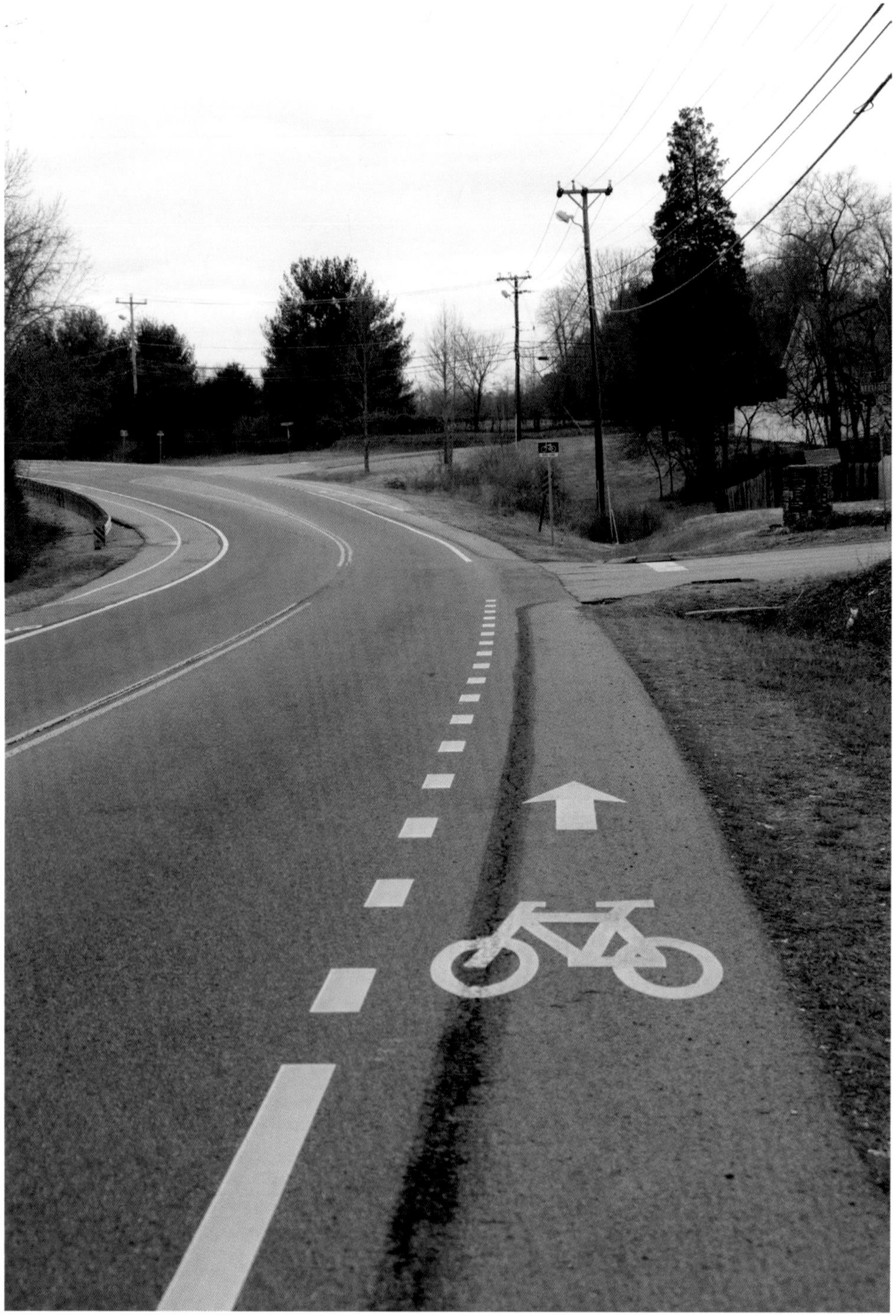

Bike lane on Bell Road in the Donelson community. The dotted line indicates where autos are permitted to enter the lane for turning. The excess shoulder space on many suburban roads can be converted into bike lanes by removing the rumble strip and striping. *(2012)*

Neighborhood route on Neely's Bend Road in Madison connects to frequent BRT service along Gallatin Pike. Here the connector picks up passengers at a Skyline Medical Center facility. *(2011)*

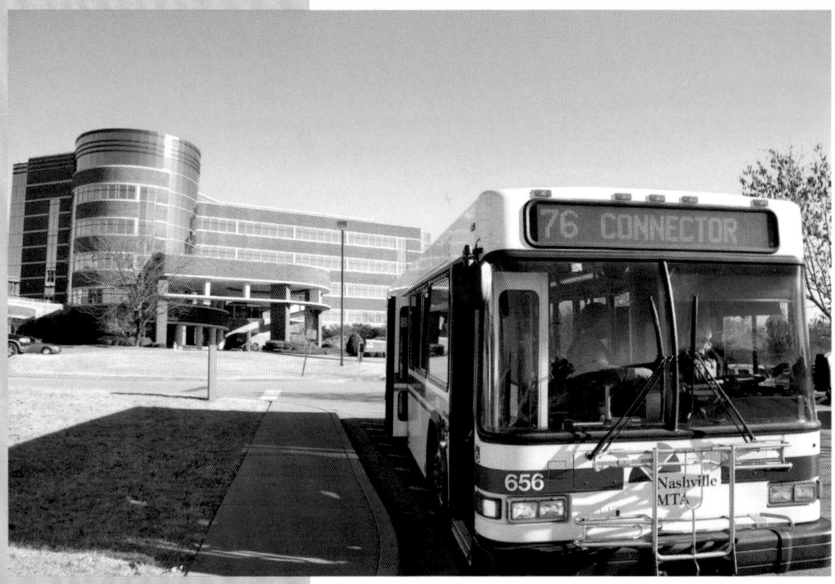

Just Saying No to the Car

After more than 50 years of relentless increases in the number of miles driven by Americans, this trend finally appears to be ebbing. The reason: the nation's young.[16]

- From 2001 to 2009, the annual number of miles traveled in cars by those aged 16 to 34 decreased from 10,300 to 7,900 miles per capita, a drop of 23 percent. (Source: National Household Travel Survey, Federal Highway Administration).
- From 2001 to 2009, the number of miles traveled as passengers on public transit by this same age group increased by 40 percent.
- In 2009, 16- to 34-year-olds took 24 percent more bike trips than in 2001, despite a 2 percent shrinkage in the size of the age group as a whole.
- In 2009, those aged 16 to 34 walked to destinations 16 percent more frequently than in 2001.
- From 2000 to 2010, the percentage of 14- to 34-year-olds without a driver's license increased from 21 percent to 26 percent.[17]

Clearly the transportation preferences of generation Y are different from those of older generations. The change has to do with higher fuel costs, the impacts of technology, and lifestyle preference.

In 2011 it cost over twice as much to fill up the car tank, on average, as it did in 2001(in 2011 dollars). While gasoline prices fluctuate, no one expects them to revert to the cheap per-gallon prices that enabled the addiction of previous generations of Americans to automobiles.

What the 16- to 34-year-olds are addicted to is technology, about which they are most savvy. The desire to stay constantly in touch via smartphones, tablets, and laptops is less compatible with piloting an automobile than with alternative transportation modes. Social media has become a replacement for some car trips. For safety considerations, an increasing number of states are outlawing texting—and even the use of hand-held cell phones—while driving. In 2011 the National Transportation Safety Board recommended banning cell phone use entirely while driving.

Bus and rail riders, on the other hand, can talk, text, and work their laptops without risking their own—or anyone else's—lives. In addition, websites and smartphone apps providing real time transit information make public transit easier to use and facilitate bike and car sharing (e.g., Zipcar) services in the cities that have them. A recent contest by *The Atlantic Cities,* an online publication, found that bike lanes, car sharing, and real-time transit arrival clocks ranked in the top eight of reader preferences for their city.[18] On the local level, Transit Now Nashville, a nonprofit organization, is currently working with MTA to develop a real-time mobile app to alert any smartphone to the whereabouts of any MTA bus.

The generation that's come of age in the 21st century is the most "wired" in history. But their choice of where to live is a reversion to traditional urban form. They are buying or renting condos and lofts in the urban core or returning to the streetcar suburbs once occupied by their grandparents and great-grandparents or to new ones with a similar urban design form and connectivity pattern. According to a recent survey by the National Association of Realtors, "America's youth are rejecting sprawl in favor of walkable, mixed-use neighborhoods with good access to public transportation." Residential developers and realtors are taking note. A recent infill project near the Brookside neighborhood on Nashville's west side, "Greenway Glen," uses the home sites' proximity to the Richland Creek Greenway and the Music City Bikeway as branding tools.

The shift away from sprawl is due to changes in suburban life, both actual and perceptual. Living in the suburbs was once considered a declaration of independence from the noise, congestion, and close quarters of urban living. And the cars that took us back and forth from town to the ranch house were the machines of freedom.

The automobile was marketed—and still is—as the vehicle of personal mobility. In a Ford commercial of the 1950s, a housewife laments, "I was practically a prisoner in my own house" in the suburbs during the day, when her husband took the car to work. Now that they are a two-car family, she declares, "I'm free to go anywhere, do anything, see anybody I want." She concludes, "Why be stuck with one expensive car when you can have the fun and freedom of two fine Fords?"[19]

Today, of course, she'd be stuck in traffic on the increasingly congested roadways of the suburbs. And she probably wouldn't solely be a housewife, because she'd be holding down a job, in part to pay for her car, its insurance, and maintenance.

What generation Y is increasingly seeking is freedom *from* the car. For them true freedom is the ability to choose among transportation options. They can't do this easily in the auto-dependent suburbs. So they are setting up house in the urban core or neighborhoods built before the car was king.

The implications of this change in attitude on transportation planning are obvious, as the authors of *Transportation and the New Generation* state: "Policy-makers and the public need to be aware that America's current transportation policy—dominated by road building—is fundamentally out-of-step with the transportation patterns and expressed preferences of growing numbers of Americans. It is time for policy-makers to consider the implication of changes in driving habits for the nation's transportation infrastructure decisions and funding practices, and consider a new vision for transportation policy that reflects the needs of 21st century America."[20]

—CHRISTINE KREYLING AND RON YEARWOOD
NCDC

Health-Promoting

Trips taken on foot enhance physical activity, opportunities for social interaction, and air quality (by decreasing the amount of car-generated exhaust). Metro has made progress on constructing and improving sidewalks, pedestrian crossings, and traffic calming measures to aid pedestrian safety.

New subdivisions in Nashville are now required to have sidewalks on both sides of the streets. Greenways, where available and connected to existing infrastructure, offer safe walking and cycling paths. Newly elected mayor Megan Barry pledged to update Metro's *Strategic Plan for Sidewalks and Bikeways.* Metro Public Works' website (*mpw.nashville.gov/IMS/Sidewalks/InteractiveMap.aspx*) features an interactive map of the county showing existing and planned bikeways, sidewalks, and greenways.[21]

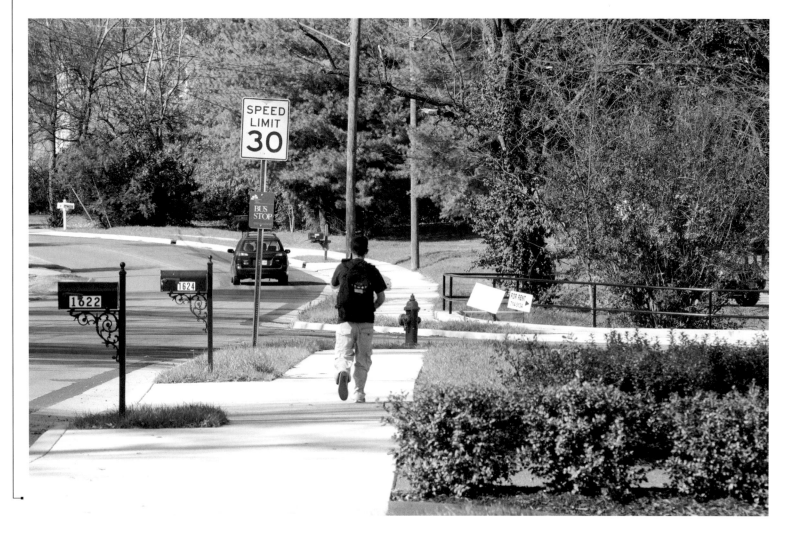

New sidewalks installed along Glen Echo Road connect residents to Green Hills' shopping centers and other public facilities. *(2012: Gary Layda)*

X Health-Defeating

Post-World War II suburbia's focus on the automobile as the primary means of travel has created a hostile environment for pedestrians. Suburbanites who do walk, bike, or wait at bus stops on the arterials are vulnerable to injury because of proximity to fast-moving traffic.

Local culture has reinforced the supremacy of the car on the roads. Drivers often ignore pedestrians in clearly marked crosswalks or the "walk" signs at signalized intersections. When cars and pedestrians or cyclists do come into contact, cars inevitably win. Slowing cars down, however, improves the pedestrian's chance of nonfatal injury. A car striking a pedestrian at 40 mph results in death 85 percent of the time, whereas the same car traveling at 20 mph only has a five percent chance of killing someone.[22]

Lack of connectivity is a problem. While sidewalks do exist in some locations, they are often discontinuous, hindering a suburban resident from walking on a sidewalk from home to schools, parks, shops, and services.

Pedestrian crossings are often inadequate or absent, even at major intersections. Main corridors are encumbered with heavy traffic and lack such pedestrian infrastructure as mid-block crossings and refuge islands for safe crossing of multi-lane roads. Transit stops are frequently not aligned with pedestrian crossings and sidewalks.

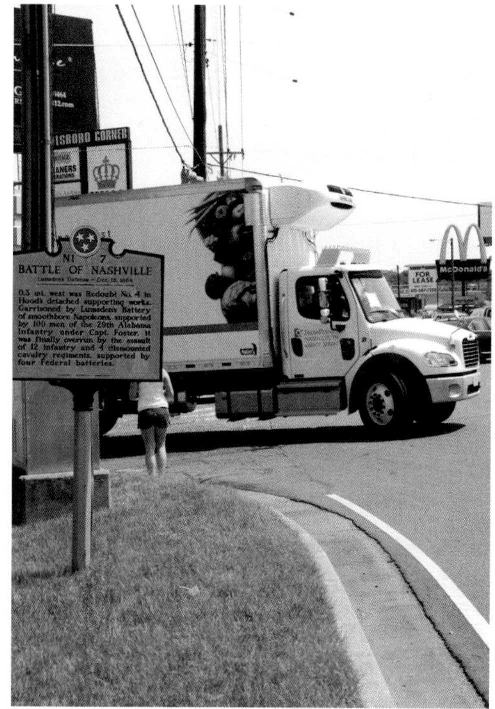

X An embattled pedestrian on Hillsboro Road in Green Hills. *(2012)*

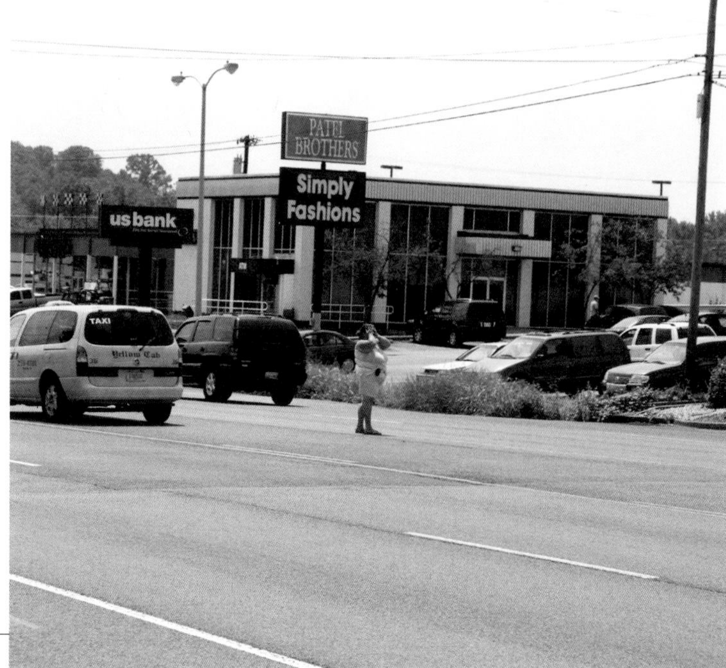

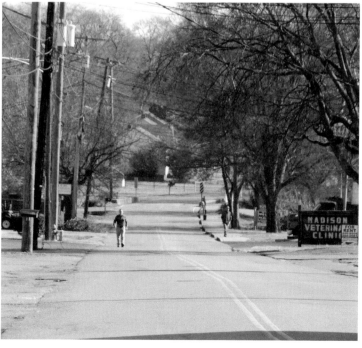

X *Left:* Woman crossing Nolensville Pike where a large retail grocery center exists, but without safe pedestrian crosswalks. The nearest signalized crossing is a quarter of a mile in either direction. *(2010)*

X *Right:* Pedestrians walking along a street in Madison. Note the abrupt termination of the sidewalk. Pedestrians, cyclists, and children at play often use streets in subdivisions with low traffic volume, because many do not have a complete system of sidewalks. *(2012)*

STRATEGY: *Make it safe and convenient to walk. Increase opportunities for incidental exercise and fewer car trips through the installation of an active transportation infrastructure connecting residential subdivisions to each other and to community-based amenities.*

Connect existing sidewalks around schools or in subdivisions to public transit stops, parks, and daily destinations via new sidewalks or greenways. Public Works already prioritizes the installation of sidewalks around existing schools within a two-mile radius.

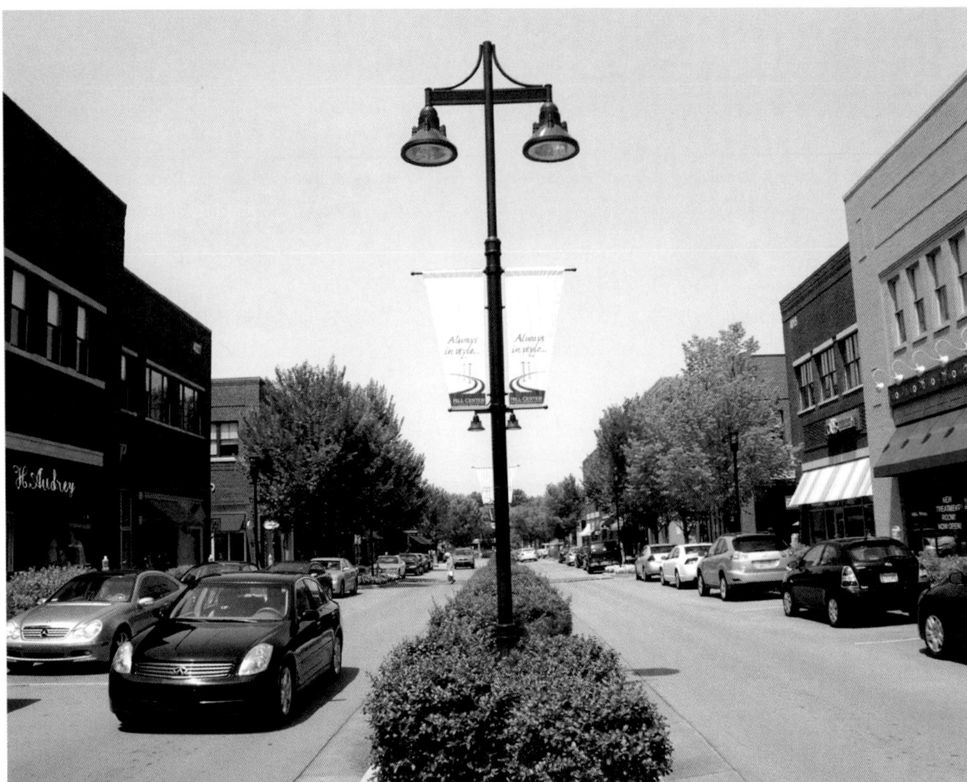

Right: The Hill Center in Green Hills provides a safe and pleasant pedestrian experience, with stop signs at crosswalks that are distinguished by special paving and a median that allows walkers to pause as traffic dictates when crossing the street. The center also promotes a "park once" strategy. Shoppers entering by car can park on the street or in a garage, shop at the numerous stores within the center, and return to their cars when finished. *(2012)*

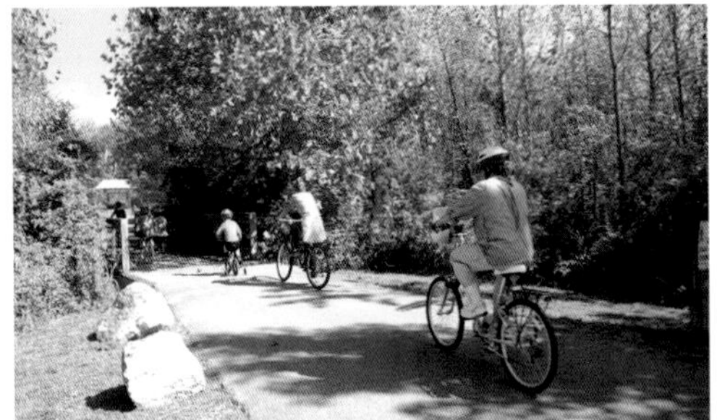

Left: Family biking in Shelby Bottoms greenway. This greenway features trailheads in several neighborhoods. Metro officials should work with neighborhood organizations and homeowners' associations to provide community access to public parks and greenways. These paths can be enabled through easements or by integration into the right-of-way. *(2012)*

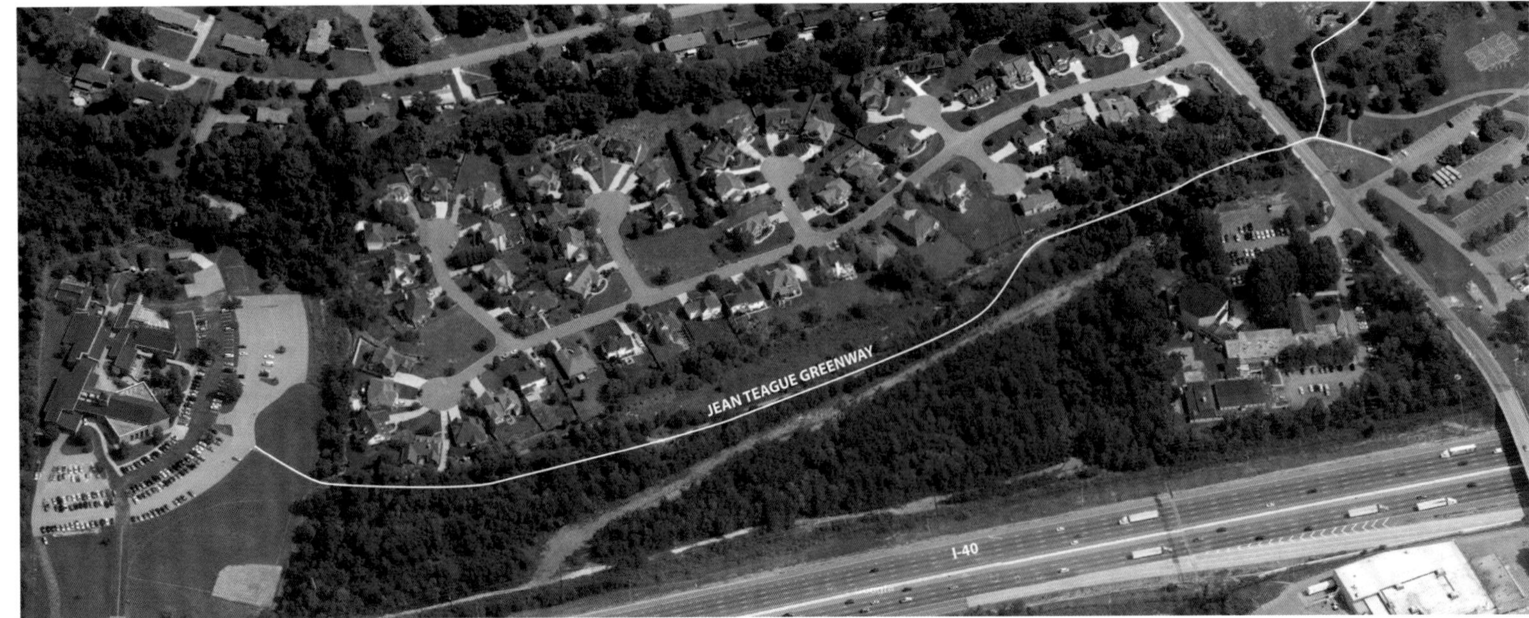

Jean Teague Greenway in Knoxville offers a good example of a greenway along the back of a conventional cul-de-sac suburban neighborhood that offers residents connectivity to the larger greenway system in the city, as well as two churches, a YMCA, and a park. *(© 2012: Google)*

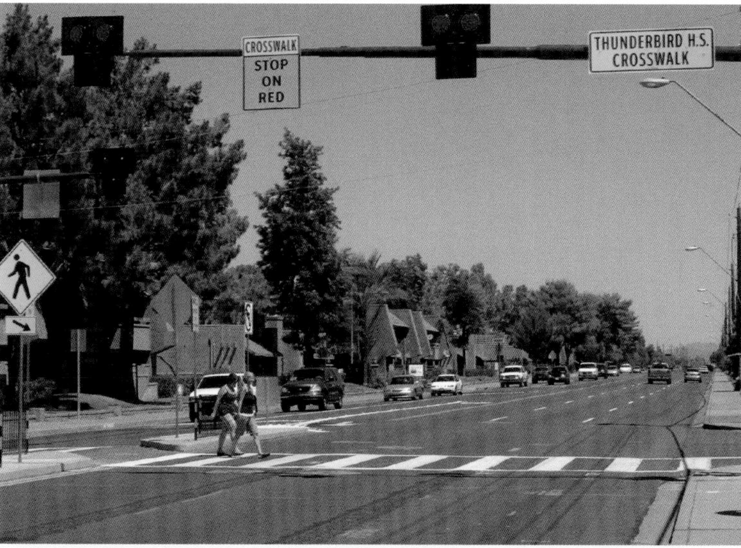

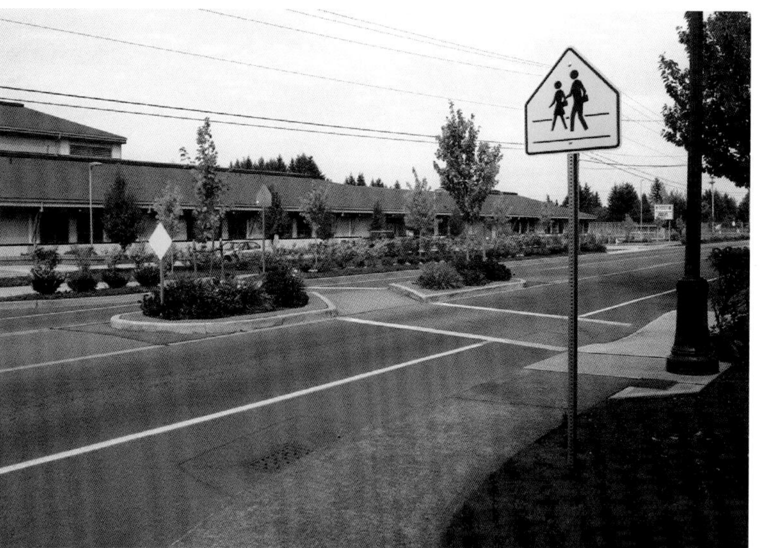

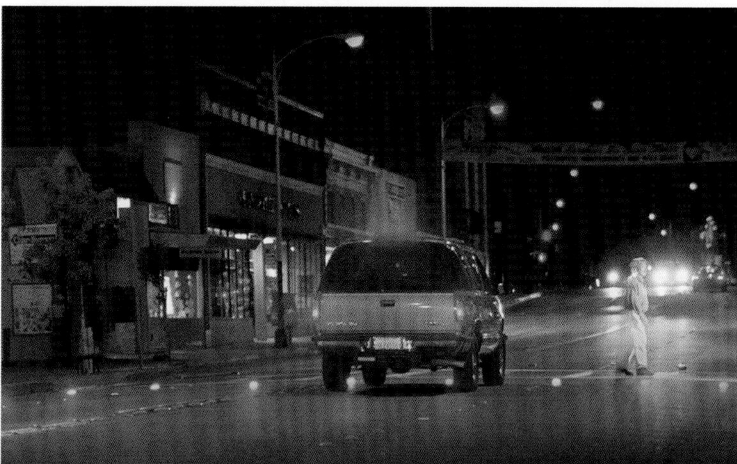

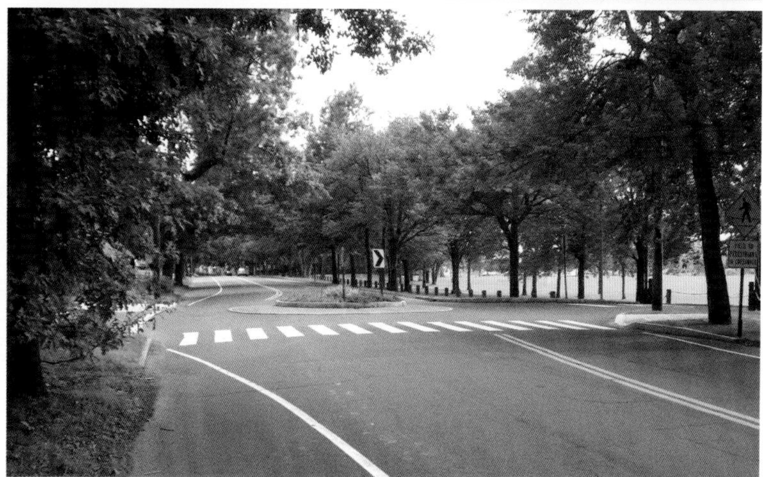

Top and Middle: Examples of features enhancing safe crossings, especially necessary on the wide and busy pikes. Pedestrian refuges—mid-right-of-way (ROW) islands—allow walkers to pause safely when traffic is heavy or a signal changes to "don't walk." Clearly marked crosswalks, pedestrian signage, and human-scaled lighting on active transport routes increases the safety of walking and cycling. Auto-focused lighting is not an acceptable substitute. Traffic calming interventions such as roundabouts inhibit vehicle speed. *(2009: pedbikeimages.org; photos taken by [clockwise from top left] Mike Cynecki, Dan Burden, Dan Burden, Tom Harned)*

TRAIL RULES

TWO WAY TRAFFIC

SPEED LIMIT 15

STAY TO THE RIGHT
NO MORE THAN TWO ACROSS

SIGNAL WHEN PASSING
SAY "ON YOUR LEFT"

DOGS ON 6' LEASH
SCOOP THE POOP

Walkers and bikers share paved paths in greenways, which can be hazardous when bikers travel at high speeds. These greenway signs are intended to enhance safety. When bike traffic volume warrants, separate paths for bikes and pedestrians should be constructed. *(2012: Metro Parks Department)*

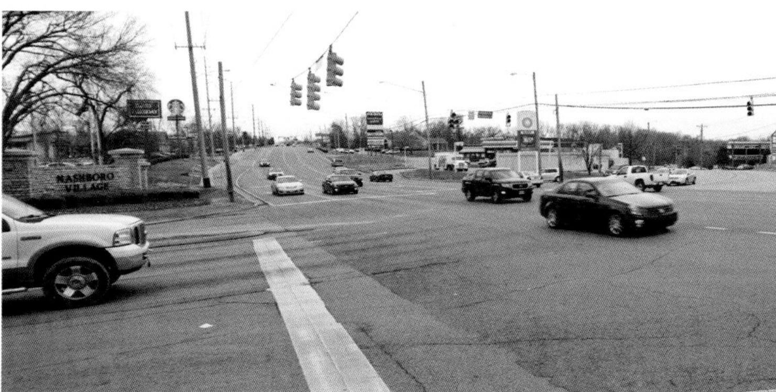

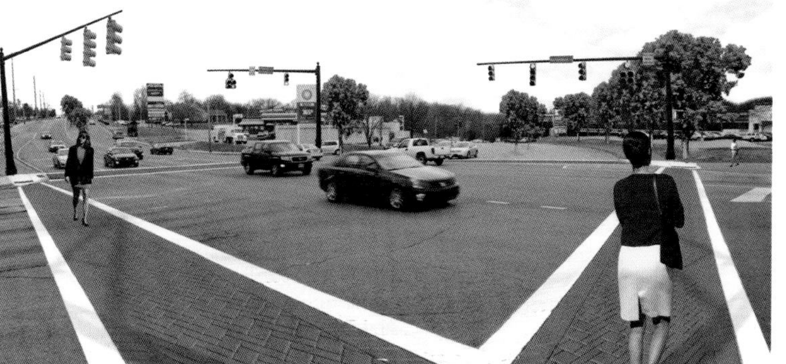

This wide intersection on Murfreesboro Pike lacks pedestrian crosswalks. Illustration shows how minor enhancements can improve pedestrian safety and connectivity. *(2013: Ron Yearwood, NCDC; Visualization, 2013: Eric Hoke, NCDC)*

Nolensville Elementary School recently installed bike racks on a shared, nonmotorized path leading to nearby suburban neighborhoods. *(2009: Leslie Meehan, Metro Planning Organization)*

The Henry L. Maxwell Elementary School in Antioch is sited on a two-lane street with no pedestrian access to its surrounding neighborhoods. Parents from these communities must wait in long traffic lines to drop off their kids, even though they live within a short walk. The addition of auto-free paths would provide an alternative to the automobile. Note: existing sidewalks are shown in orange, proposed multi-use paths in green. *(© 2012: Google; Illustration, 2013: Eric Hoke, NCDC)*

Helping Dick and Jane Walk to School

Historically, the neighborhood school served as the center of a community. This was especially true in urban areas, where walking or biking to school was a daily ritual for students from first grade to graduation. The morning and afternoon commute served not only as social bonding time for kids with their neighbors, but also offered daily exercise needed for growing muscles and bones and healthy body weight.

Fast forward to current times. Less than 15 percent of all school trips in this country are made on foot or bike (compared to almost 48 percent in 1969).[23] The reasons are several: some local, some manifestations of national trends and events.

The formation of Metro government in 1963 merged city and county public education. Although children in the city schools lived in neighborhoods that enabled walking, "the county schools weren't the same," says former Mayor Bill Purcell. "These schools served much bigger geographical areas, some largely rural."[24] The county schools were never designed, therefore, to be walkable. When these rural areas filled up with subdivisions, and the schools had to be expanded or replaced, the form of

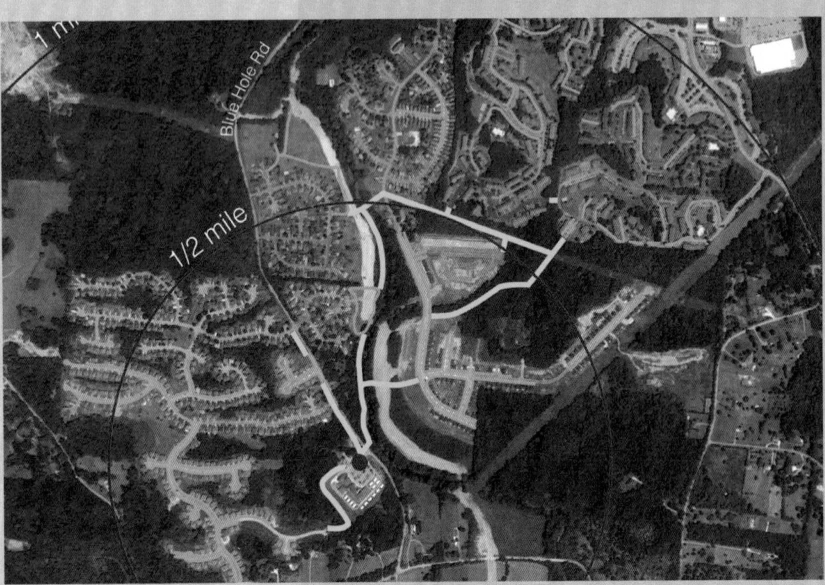

the newly minted suburbia didn't encourage walking.

Beginning in the 1970s, court-ordered busing to overcome residential segregation and improve the racial equality of education put children on buses that often carried them far out of their neighborhoods. Consolidation, which merged schools and centralized their management as a means of increasing fiscal efficiency, also compelled students to travel farther to access their education. Newly constructed schools were larger and sited on sizeable campuses in areas of student growth—new suburbs—characerized by lower density, fewer sidewalks, and a cul-de-sac layout pattern that forced children to travel on roads with lots of vehicular traffic. "We'd love to build in areas where kids can walk, bike, or ride public transit to school," says Joe Edgens, former executive director of facility services for Metro Nashville Public Schools (MNPS) and currently a consultant to the system. "But that's not where the kids are, where the growth is."[25]

The recent focus on school choice in public education also undermines the concept of the neighborhood school. Parents now may select from a menu of magnet, enhanced option, and charter schools as well as themed academies. If they choose a school other than the one for which their child is zoned, they must provide transportation, which frequently means a private car. All these factors have eroded the ability of children to walk or bike to school.

According to MNPS, 45,000 of its 81,000 students travel on a school bus. MNPS has the 29th largest pupil transportation department in the country, spending $250,000 per day to operate 549 school buses. Busing is offered to students in K–8 who live 1.25 miles or more from school; for high schoolers the threshold is 1.5 miles. Those who live closer or opt not to take the school bus can get to school by walking, biking, public transit, or automobile. MNPS says it issues 1,200 Metro Transit Authority bus passes per month. Unfortunately, however, too many students travel by car.

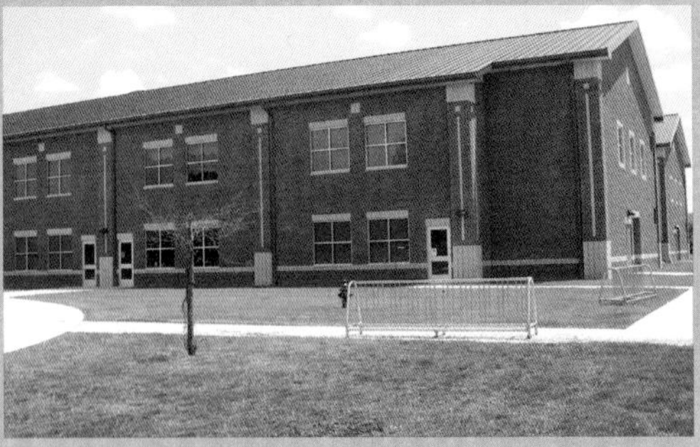

The result is increased traffic on Nashville roads, creating congestion for all commuters. The amount of time parents spend as chauffeurs reduces their work and leisure time and requires them to sit more and exercise less. Waiting in drop-off lanes delays parents, and engines idling outside schools taints air quality. For the students, commutes in buses or in the car with mom or dad impinge on their ability to get the doctor-recommended 60 minutes of daily physical activity.

Commuting in cars is, of course, not the only reason for a sedentary lifestyle. Students' preoccupation with electronic media is also a significant factor. But walking or biking to school would provide some physical activity as part of daily life as opposed to participation in organized extra-curricular activities. And while nearly a third of all elementary school students participated in Nashville's Walk to School Day in 2012 according to MNPS, far fewer walk to school regularly. Parents cited three reasons most often: It's not safe. There's too much traffic moving way too fast on adjacent roads. Sidewalks and crosswalks are inadequate.

While the cause for parents' fears is rooted in car-centric suburban development patterns, MNPS school siting regulations can, if unintentionally, contribute to this problem. These regulations were adopted in 1992, when the state ceded such requirements to local jurisdictions. According to the current rules for new schools, these are the siting requirements:

- Elementary schools: campus of five acres plus an additional acre per 100 students. Note: newer elementary schools serve almost 800 students.

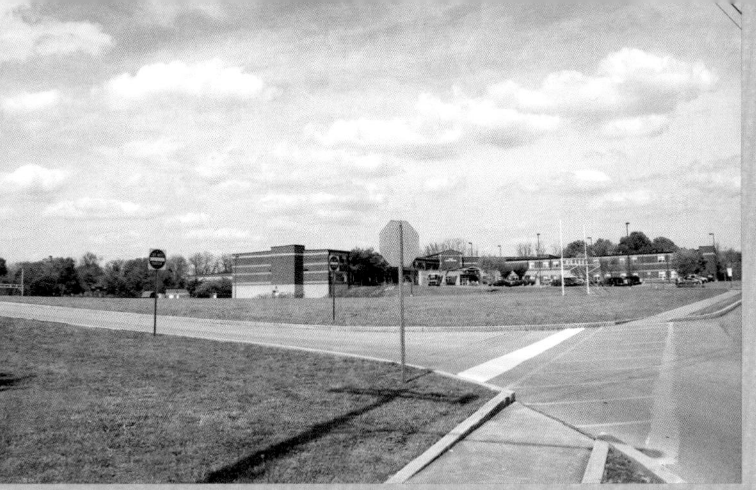

Left: Recent installation of sidewalks that connect suburban neighborhoods in south Nashville to the nearby Croft Middle School. Note that separated path, crosswalk, and signage provide added safety features for pedestrians. *(2013)*

- Middle schools: campus of 10 acres plus one per 100 students. Note: newer middle schools have almost 800 students. Location must be on a collector street.
- High schools: campus must be 15 acres plus an additional acre for each 100 students. Note: the largest high school has 2,250 students, with the average well over 1,000 students. Location must be at the intersection of two collector streets or a collector and an arterial roadway.

The basic campus size required plus the greater numbers of students served by newer schools, which adds to the mandated acreage, requires large tracts of land that are difficult to find. Thus MNPS may have to acquire property in locations less than desirable from a walkability perspective. The Planning department, after discussions with MNPS, has prepared a draft of legislation to relax campus minimum-size requirements. "We support that; campus size could be smaller," Edgens says "And they're not appropriate for more urban areas."

The directive that middle schools and high schools must be built on the city's wider and more heavily trafficked roadways is an accommodation to the school's vehicular traffic. And major roads may offer access to public transit. Such a location, however, also discourages walking and biking due to safety issues. The consequence: today's children are the most sedentary generation in the nation's history, with only one in three children participating in daily physical activity.[26]

While cost constraints and the promised economies of scale are used to justify large schools on less expensive, previously undeveloped land, such locations can carry costs of their own in terms of infrastructure. In particular, roads may need to be widened, signals and sidewalks added.

For existing schools, especially elementary and middle schools, it is necessary to increase connectivity to surrounding suburban communities by means of sidewalks, crosswalks, bike lanes, and greenways. A 2012 study reports that when kids utilize active transportation, they concentrate and perform better in the classroom.[27] The market also recognizes the value of active transportation infrastructure. A 15-city survey by CEOs for Cities found that neighborhood property values were higher in areas with more walking infrastructure. Community-centered schools can also be catalysts for public and private investment in the area.[28]

STRATEGIES:

- *Develop specific strategies to increase walkability for existing suburban public schools through collaboration among MNPS, parents of students, and Metro departments such as Planning, Public Works, and Parks.*
- *Metro should require developers to work with MNPS and Metro's planners and public works staff to build necessary roads and a complete sidewalk system before granting approval for new subdivisions. An impact fee for subdivision developers, as exists already in Williamson County, could pay for the additional infrastructure.*
- *Incorporate collaborative, long-term planning (including ten-year growth projections) for new schools. Include relevant Metro departments in the discussion of site selection: Planning, Health, Public Works, Parks, and the Tennessee Department of Transportation.*
- *Perform a health impact assessment of proposed new school sites.*
- *Prepare a transportation cost-benefit analysis for sites that includes walkability and bikability, private vehicles, school busing needs, and public transit.*
- *Modify the new school site selection cost analysis to include costs to be born by Metro for widening roads, signalization of intersections and sidewalks, as well as those funds to be expended by MNPS. Fiscal calculation should also take into account the monies required for school busing.*
- *Increase shared civic uses. MNPS and Metro Parks already have many shared sites. School playgrounds and sports fields may also be used for public recreation during non-school hours. Sharing parking with neighboring facilities such as churches can reduce school campus footprint.*
- *Modify the zoning code to minimize parking lot requirements. Schools located near existing community infrastructure for walking, biking, and mass transit generate less car traffic.*
- *Request an active transportation plan from applicants to operate charter schools. Locate charter school incubators in areas that have active transportation infrastructure.*

—CHRISTINE KREYLING, GARY GASTON and AMY ESKIND, NCDC, and LESLIE MEEHAN, formerly of MPO; Tennessee Department of Health

FOOD

✓ Nashville Foodscapes works with property owners to create edible gardens on their home turf. This example in a suburban community in the West End area offers an alternative to the manicured, chemically treated lawn, while providing a significant number of vegetables for consumption. *(2012: Nashville Foodscapes)*

X Pedestrian walking along Murfreesboro Pike with groceries in hand. This portion of the road lacks adequate sidewalks and bus stop infrastructure. *(2013)*

✓ Health-Promoting

Suburban communities are generally well served by large-scale grocery stores. These stores are oriented toward car access, but their typical location on large commercial roads enables access by public transit.

Metro land-use policy allows community gardens, commercial gardens, and chickens (for most of Davidson County) on private lots. Suburban lots are frequently large enough for some food growing. The rise of food options such as CSAs offer alternatives to grocery stores for local produce.

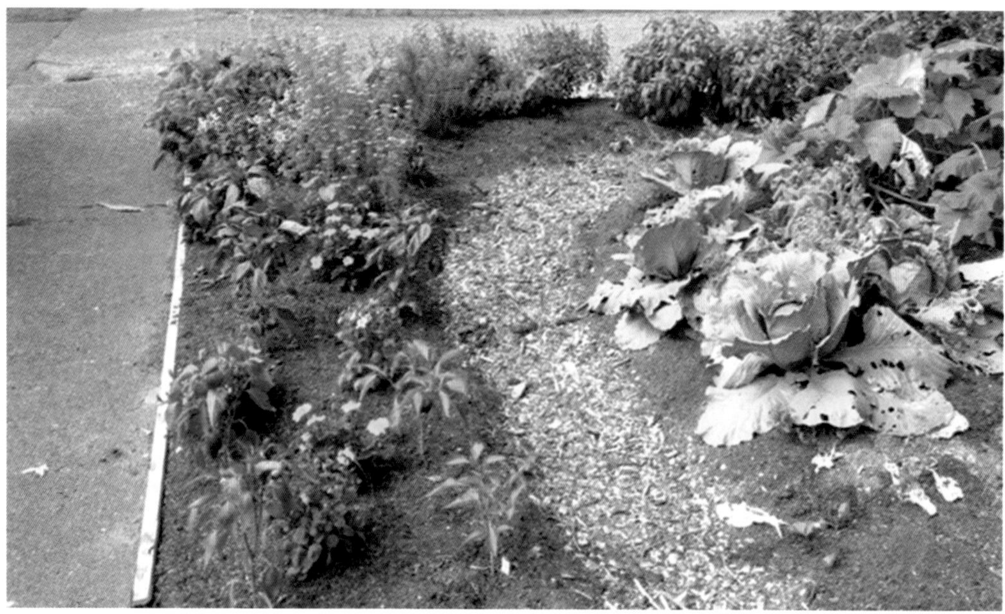

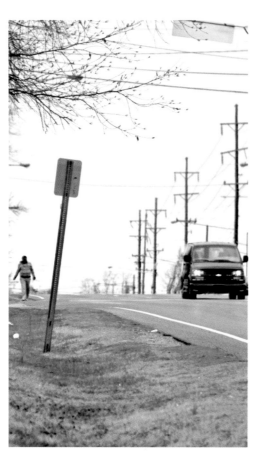

X Health-Defeating

Because residential areas are not well connected to commercial centers for foot or bicycle traffic, residents in most of suburban Nashville need a car to access food stores. Studies of "food deserts" (areas lacking access to affordable fresh foods) have been conducted in urban areas, but extensive studies for suburban areas of the county have not been completed. According to Dr. David Padgett of Tennessee State University, research shows that poverty is much more prevalent in the suburbs now than in past decades. It stands to reason that food deserts might be another ill normally associated with the inner-city that has migrated to the suburbs.

STRATEGY: *Increase access to healthy food options. Provide increased alternative transportation options to enable those without cars to access existing food stores along the commercial corridors. Strategies must be tailored to the specific suburban context.*

STRATEGY: *Conduct an analysis to determine levels of food insecurity in suburban areas. Areas that are determined to be food insecure should receive attention from Metro to increase access to fresh foods, with methods such as increased transit services, construction of sidewalk and multi-use paths, as well financial incentives that would help promote grocery store construction.*

STRATEGY: *Expand gardening options in suburban communities. Resources such as the Nashville Grown online interactive map (*nashvillegrown.org*) connect landowners to those wanting to grow food, often in exchange for a share of the produce.*

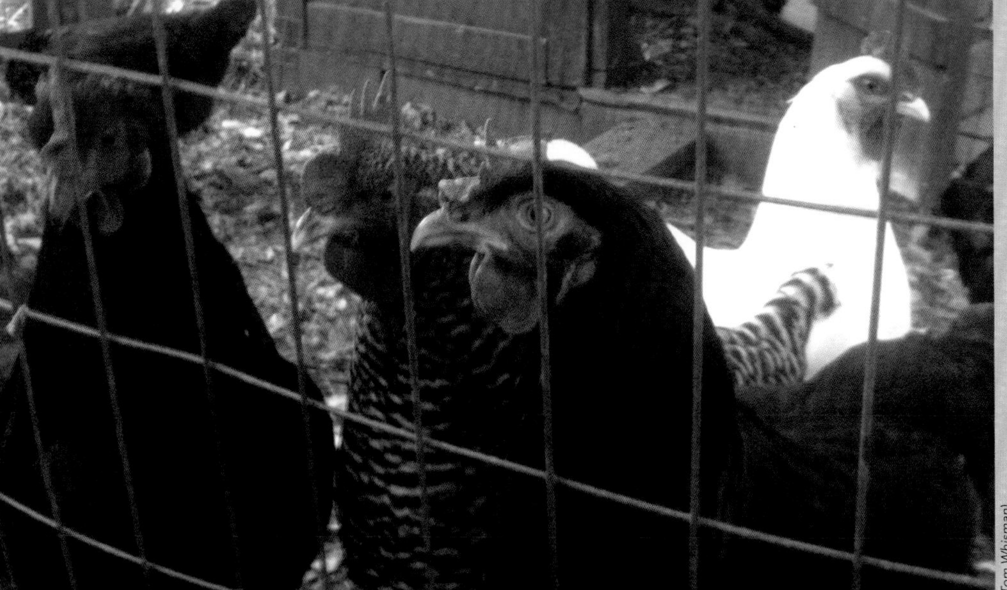
(2012: Tom Whisman)

Hens in the City

It was once common for Americans to keep farm animals "out back" of urban residences and those of the streetcar suburbs. And if there was a garden it was devoted to fruits and vegetables to supply the kitchen, not flowers. But as the backyard evolved into a place for leisure and recreation, perennials and patios displaced household agriculture.

A counter trend to eat locally, spurred in part by the obesity epidemic as well as fears about genetically modified crops and hormone-infested meat, has led to calls for the relaxation of zoning rules to allow the homegrown. In 2009, Nashville's Metro Council approved an ordinance to permit commercial and noncommercial community gardens. Three years later, the Council passed the so-called "chicken bill" to allow hens in residential zoning districts. Before the bill passed, raising chickens was forbidden to residents in the Urban Services District or to those within the outlying General Services District who lived on less than 5 acres.

Because the point of the bill is egg production, the breeding of chickens is not allowed: no roosters. Chicken slaughter on the property is also forbidden. The hens must be kept in a predator-proof enclosure, not in the front yard, and at least 25 feet away from an adjoining residence and 10 feet from a property line. The ordinance mandates that the enclosure and henhouse be kept clean and odor-free.

The "chicken bill" was written to expire March 1, 2014, to assess its impacts, a gesture to opponents worried about smell, noise, problems with neighborhood dogs and rodents, general unsightliness, and the difficulty of enforcing the rules for keeping chickens. To get passage, the pro-chicken forces organized as Urban Chicken Advocates of Nashville (UCAN), wore yellow, and appeared at countless Metro Council meetings for more than two years.

Eight Council districts originally opted out of the hen party, primarily in the southeastern part of the county. A month before the ordinance's expiration, the Council voted to permit chickens in all districts. Residents pay $25 to the Health Department for a permit and can house up to six chickens, depending on the size of the property (.24 of an acre or more for 6 hens).

— AMY ESKIND, NCDC, and CHRISTINE KREYLING

HOUSING

✓ Health-Promoting

A wide range of housing types, lot sizes, and prices are available in the suburban transect zone. Newer residential development forms include condos, zero-lot-line single-family homes, and planned communities that offer a diversity of housing, as well as cohousing proposals.

✗ Health-Defeating

Housing tends to be segregated by type, lot size, and price, with single-family homes dominant. Recent down-zoning in suburban residential neighborhoods—usually from duplex max to single-family only—were intended to preserve the quality—i.e., property values—and character of existing neighborhoods. Both segregation and down-zoning limit a resident's ability to age in place.

The down-zoning was an attempt to prevent the intrusion of out-of-scale or badly designed duplexes on scraped lots. Design guidelines are a solution that would still allow some increased density. The ability to create an additional residence on a lot—such as a loft over a garage—increases the diversity of the population and preserves the affordability of communities.

STRATEGY: *Diversify housing. The demographic for which the suburban transect zone was designed, the couple with children, no longer dominates the American housing market. Recent trends show a rise in single-parent households, couples without children, and those who live alone. The population bulge known as the boomers is reaching retirement age. If the suburbs are going to house these groups, they must offer more residential variety.*

Backyard hens. *(2013: Tom Whisman)*

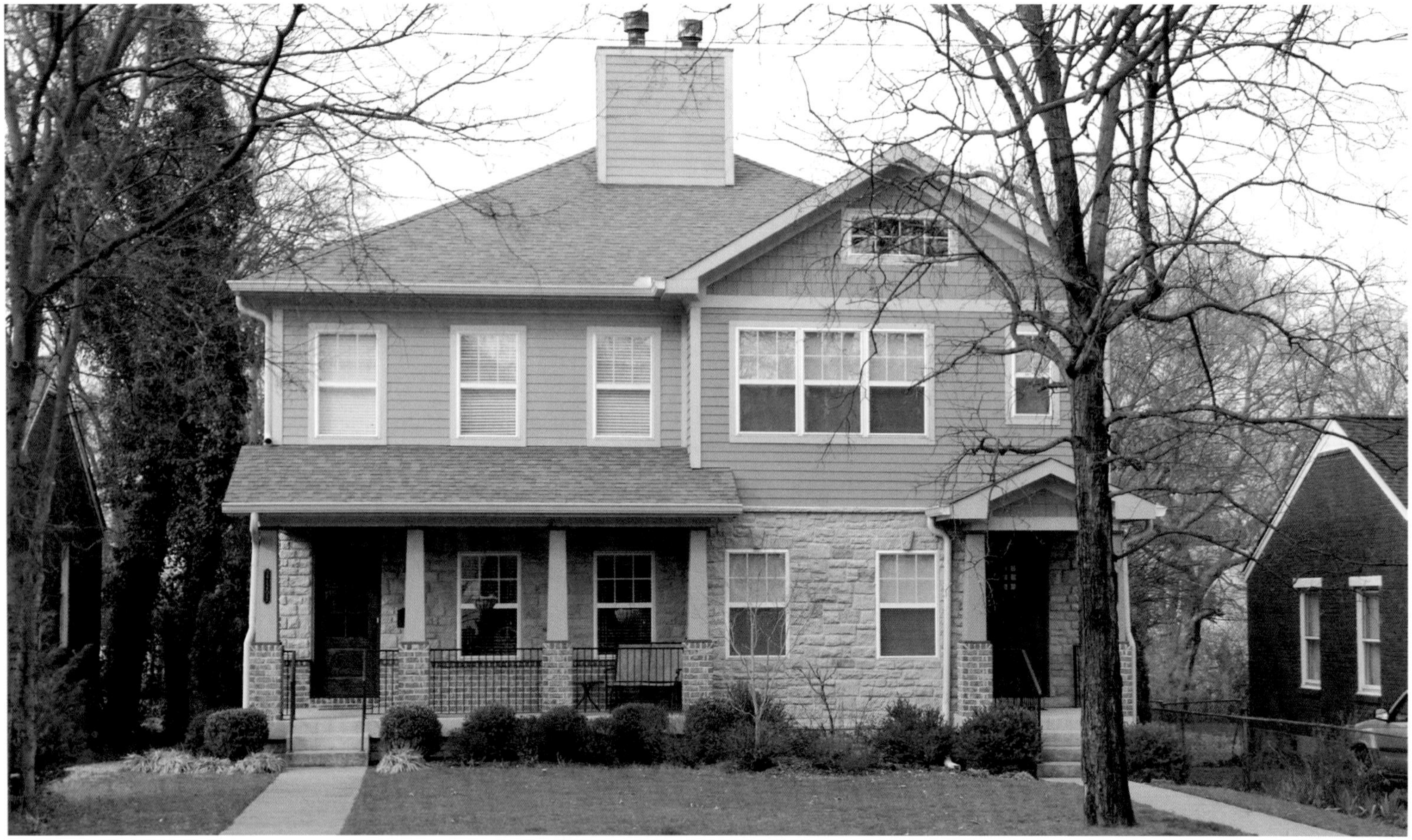

Example of a duplex in west Nashville with with a design that makes it appear like a single family home, and massing that complements the character of the existing neighborhood. *(2013)*

Accessory dwellings, such as this one on Forrest Avenue in East Nashville, are currently only permitted in districts with preservation zoning overlays. *(2013: Metro Historical Commission)*

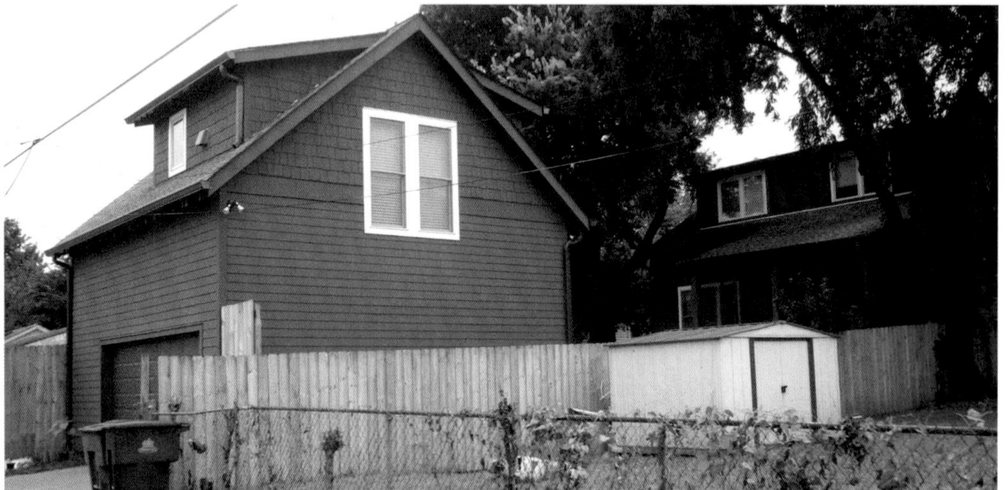

STRATEGY: *Suburban infill and new development should integrate housing for a variety of demographics, ages, and incomes. Design guidelines for duplexes, especially size limits, can prevent the erosion of community character. Allow accessory dwelling units throughout Davidson County. Enabling residents to live a lifetime in a neighborhood will increase neighborhood stability and cohesiveness.*

PARKS AND OPEN SPACE

✓ Health-Promoting

Low density housing usually correlates to significant private open space around individual homes. Subdivisions and apartment complexes may have shared open space, as well as recreational facilities such as tennis courts, pools, and walking paths.

Numerous regional parks and open space with sports-oriented amenities, such as baseball diamonds, basketball courts, and walking loops, are scattered throughout suburban communities. Some segments of the suburban zone, however, as in the southeast quadrant of the county, are underserved in this regard.

The presence of Old Hickory and Percy Priest lakes and the Cumberland River's winding path through Davidson County give many communities water access, in some places offering water-based recreation and walking trails.

The suburbs were designed with large lots, emphasizing private greenspace. Thus this zone lacks public open space on a neighborhood scale. The rains of May 2010, however, have provided an opportunity to create smaller-scale greenspace in suburbia.

The flooding engendered government buyouts of severely affected properties in floodways and floodplains. Metro has demolished the buildings acquired and is turning these areas into greenways, with plans to install walking trails and other recreational amenities. Park Terrace on Brown's Creek and England Park on Richland Creek are two examples of this approach. The long-term goal is to link these sites into Metro's larger greenway system.

✗ Health-Defeating

Existing open space is often not connected to surrounding neighborhoods by sidewalks, trails, bike paths, or public transit; therefore, a personal vehicle is required for access. Few pocket parks lie in close proximity to residences in the suburban transect zone.

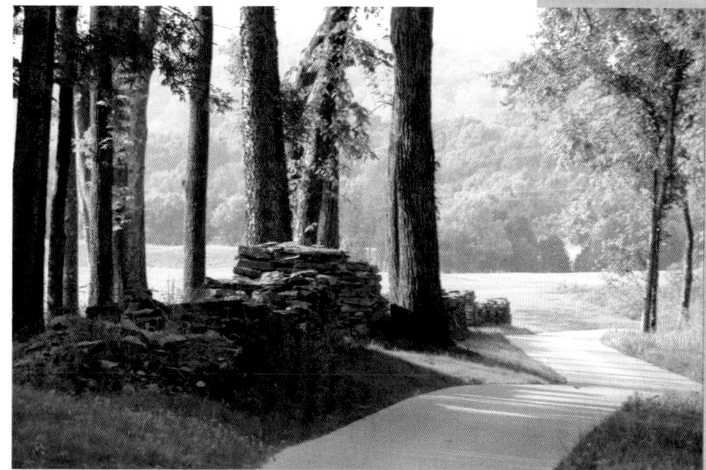

Top: Pedestrian pathway connects to homes in Franklin's Westhaven community. *(2012: Southern Land Company)*

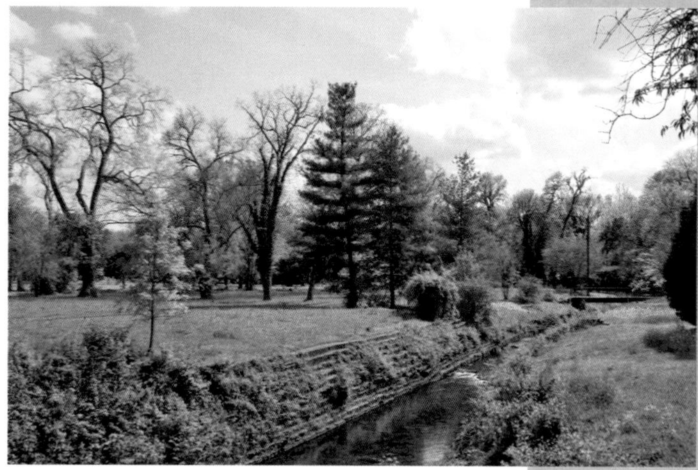

Land on Park Terrace that was flooded in 2010 and subject to the government buyout program. Metro plans to turn the area into a neighborhood park and greenway. *(2013)*

STRATEGY: *Increase interconnectivity and public neighborhood-scale greenspace. Improve connectivity between residential areas and existing open space and public recreational facilities.*

STRATEGY: *Prevent future development in floodplains. Metro still allows for some construction on land designated as in floodplains. This control should be tightened.*

The floods of May 2010 severely affected areas in the suburban transect zone, especially residential ones. This was due, in part, to the fact that before flood controls on the Cumberland River, developers had to be more aware of the potential for flooding. More recent suburbs were built on the land that was left, which was frequently located on steep slopes and in floodplains. The financial costs of the May rains and the environmental costs of future floodplain development are too steep to pay in the future. Preserving floodplain land as open space would provide the opportunity for more suburban neighborhoods to share it.

CASE STUDIES

BELLEVUE AND MADISON

As examples of suburbs developed in the second half of the 20th century, Bellevue and Madison share many characteristics: segregated land uses, commerce accessible primarily by car, the concentration of traffic on the major arterials, and a lack of active transportation infrastructure.

Both communities lie primarily in Metro's outlying General Services District, whose residents pay lower property taxes for fewer services. The Urban Services District, for example, receives garbage collection and streetlights. Both Bellevue and Madison are also plagued by dead or dying shopping centers and lack neighborhood centers.

There are also differences. Madison lies eight miles from downtown Nashville and became suburban in the 1950s. Its residential areas are more connected with each other. Bellevue, on the other hand, is 13 miles from the city center, experienced major suburban growth beginning in the 1970s, and contains many disconnected subdivisions and apartment complexes. Bellevue is more affluent than Madison, and has less access to public transit. Madison has a greater number of households that do not own a car, and therefore rely heavily upon the frequent transit services offered along Gallatin Pike.[29]

"What once had been a cow pasture then a golf course became an office park and eventually a movie theater."

Doug Underwood, *A History of Bellevue and Surrounding Areas* (1995), referring to the intersection of Belle Forest Circle and Hwy 70S in Bellevue.

Definition of Family / Non-family

Family = Contains at least two people related by birth, marriage, or adoption. Family households are of two types:

- **Married** = When a married couple is considered the householder
- **Other** = When a single man or woman is considered the householder and lives with other family

Non-family = This may be one person living in a household or multiple people who are not related to each other.

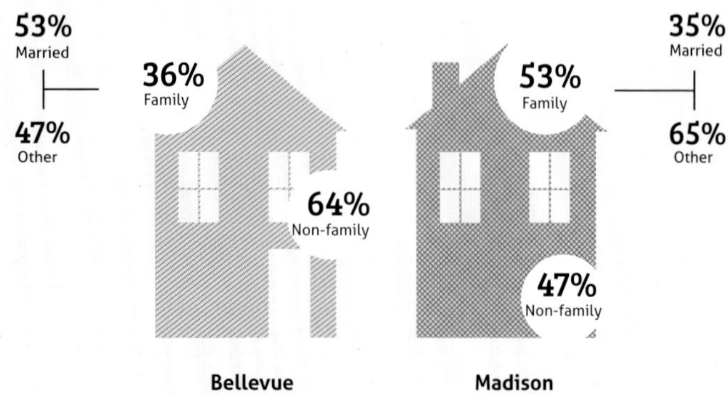

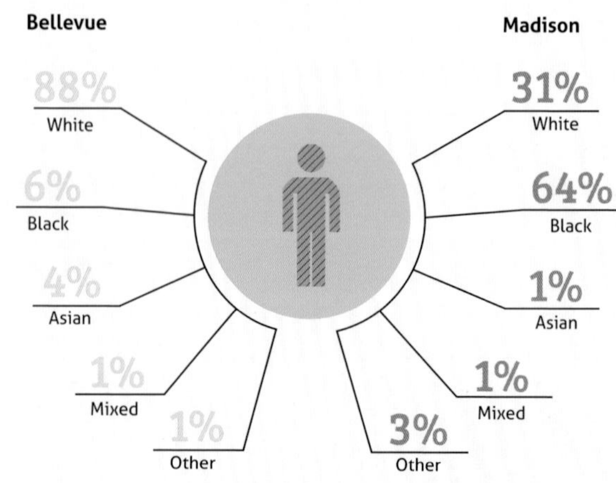

Information graphics, 2013: Ashley Nicole Johnson

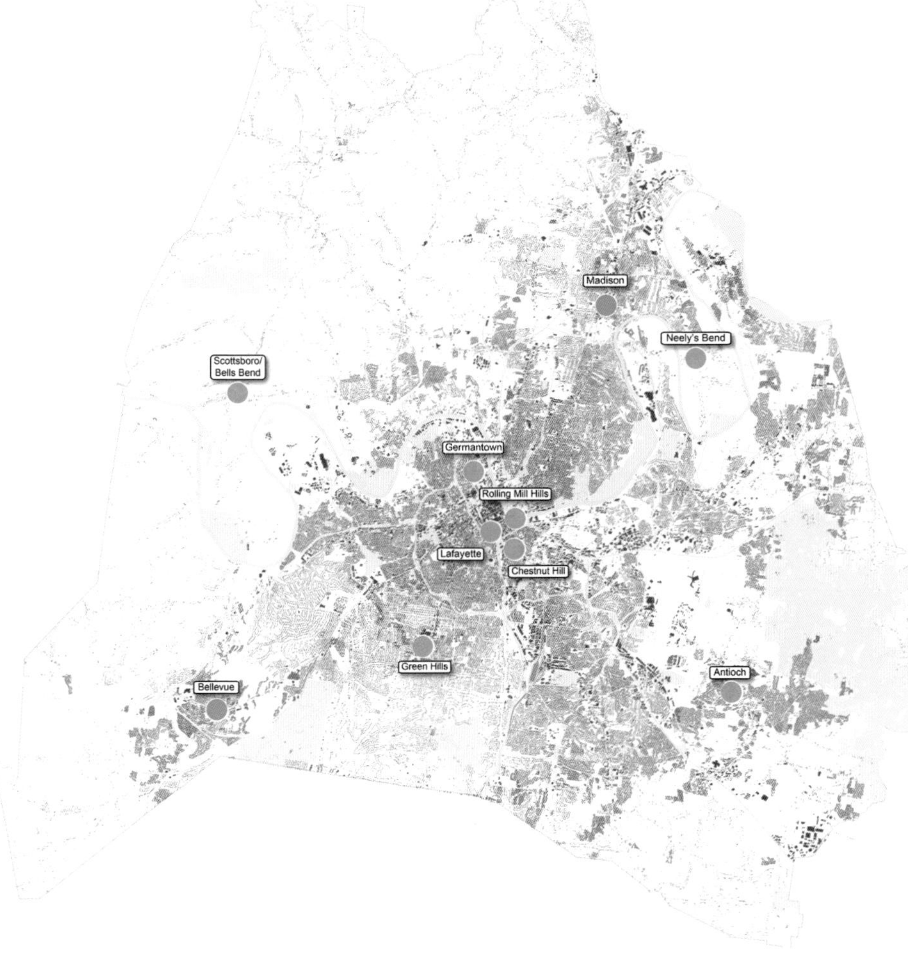

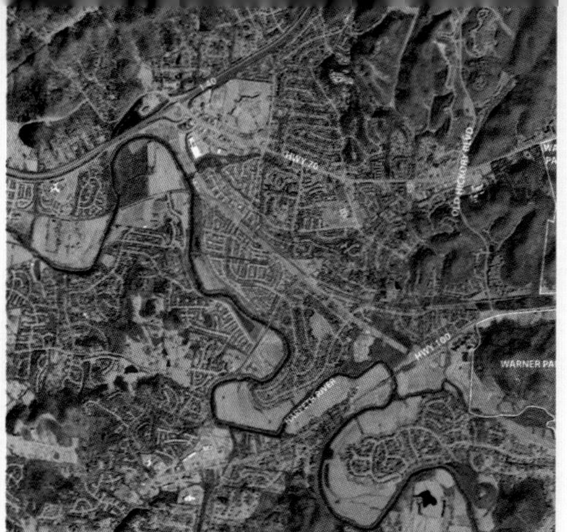

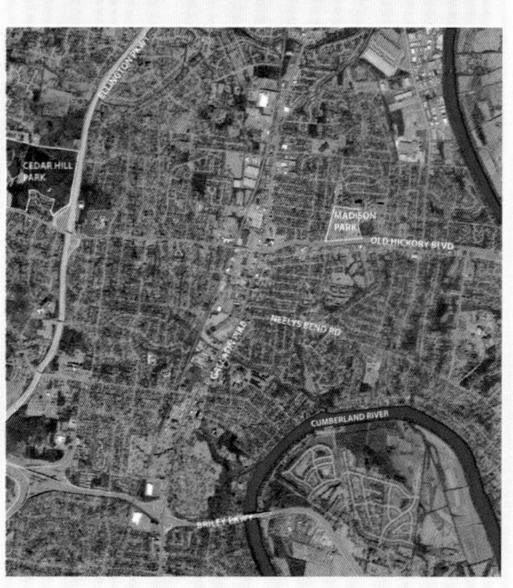

Left: Suburban focus areas, Bellevue and Madison communities. *(Diagram over map, 2013: Eric Hoke, NCDC)*

Top right: Aerial image of Bellevue area. *(2012: Metro Planning Department)*

Lower right: Aerial image of Madison area. *(2012: Metro Planning Department)*

Income

	Bellevue	Madison
Percentage Under Poverty Level	7%	23%
Median Income	$49,492	$35,967

Age Demographic

Age	Bellevue	Madison
19 & Under	21%	24%
20-34	24%	22%
35-64	42%	40%
65-74	6%	6%
75+	7%	7%

Demographic data from the US Census Department's 2010 American Community Survey (5 year estimates). At the time of research for this publication, the 2010 dataset was the most current data available. For the case studies, neighborhood boundaries were identified and data was then collected from the census tracts that best corresponded to those geographic boundaries.

BELLEVUE

The town was officially established in 1795 and named after the home of Revolutionary War veteran Adam DeMoss, a cabin called Belle Vue.[30] The earliest settlers established farms. The Newsom family built a mill along the Harpeth River, which winds through the community before ultimately joining the Cumberland River. Much of the land surrounding the river valley is characterized by steep slopes and ridges.

By the mid-19th century, a few merchants had established stores near the railroad tracks, which featured three stations: Newsome's Station, Bellevue, and Hicks Crossing. Locals could catch a commuter train that ran from Humphreys County to Nashville. The main road was Harding Road / Hwy 100, until the Memphis / Bristol Hwy / Hwy 70 South was built in 1927. The historic Natchez Trace—then still a dirt road, before its incarnation as a federal parkway—also ran through the area.

During Prohibition (1920–1933), gambling and bootlegging clubs flourished along Highway 70. Bellevue High School opened in 1931; electricity arrived in 1936. The heart of Bellevue was then at the intersection of Old Harding and Bellevue roads, where stood the Bellevue Market, including a post office and a blacksmith shop. As late as the 1950s Bellevue's hardware store, market, and post office existed largely to serve the needs of nearby farmers.

In 1963, the same year the governments of Nashville and Davidson County merged to form Metro Nashville, the Harpeth Valley Water District opened. That, and the arrival of I-40, made possible the suburban development of Bellevue.

Bellevue's transition from country hamlet to Nashville suburb became official in the 1970s when the US Postal Service changed the status of the town's post office, officially making it a branch of Nashville's. In 1980 the community's high school closed, due to countywide desegregation

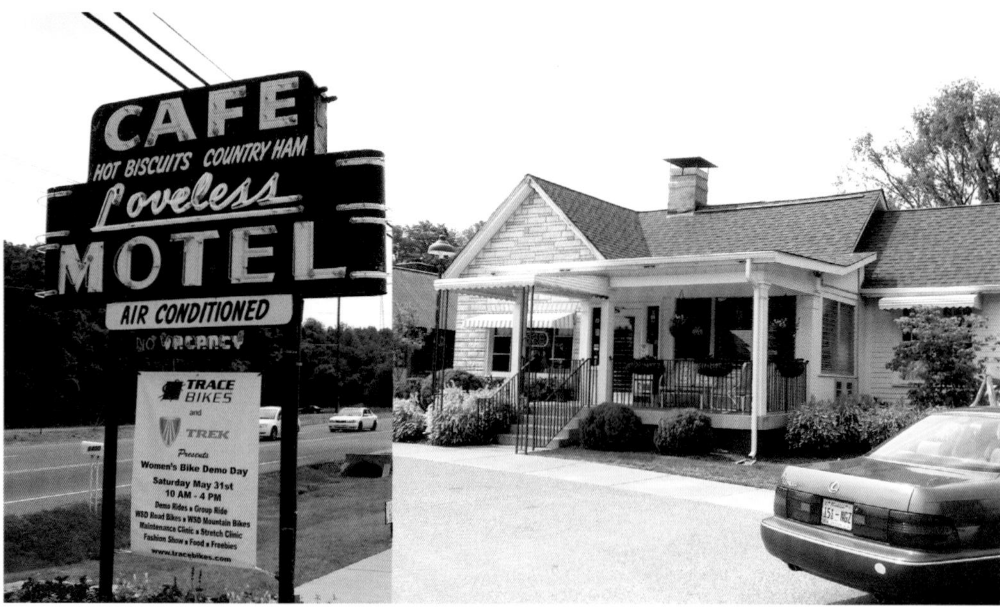

The Loveless Cafe on Highway 100 near the terminus of the Natchez Trace Parkway. In 1951 Lon and Annie Loveless purchased the Harpeth Valley Tea Room, added rooms for renting to travelers, and renamed it the Loveless Motel and Cafe. The motel ceased operations in 1985 and has been converted to retail space. The café still serves its signature country ham, fried chicken, homemade biscuits, and preserves. The Loveless Barn opened in 2009 and serves as a rentable event venue for weddings and parties. *(2012: Wikimedia Commons)*

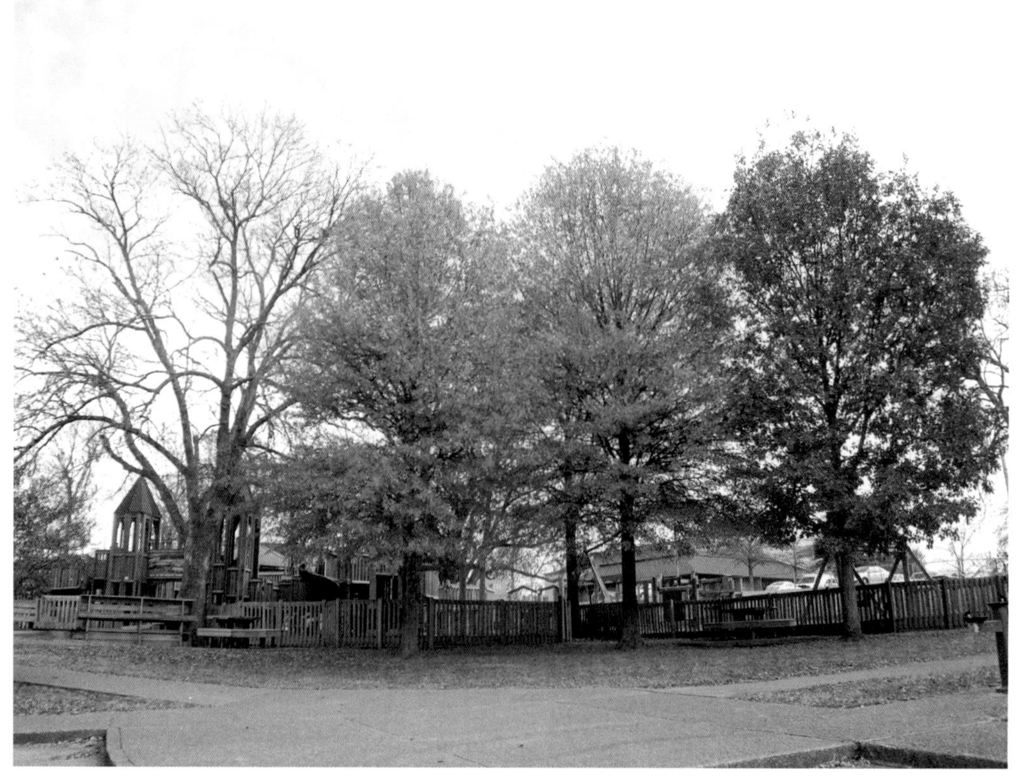

Bellevue's Red Caboose Park, built by volunteers in 1996. *(2012)*

and the resulting consolidation of schools.

The opening of the Bellevue Center Mall in 1990 was indicative of Bellevue's increasing suburbanization and close proximity to I-40. Like many regional malls across the country that suffered from the overbuilding of retail and the rise of online shopping, the Bellevue Mall gradually declined and finally closed in 2008.

A new, larger library for Bellevue opened in 2014; a new community center is still needed for the area.

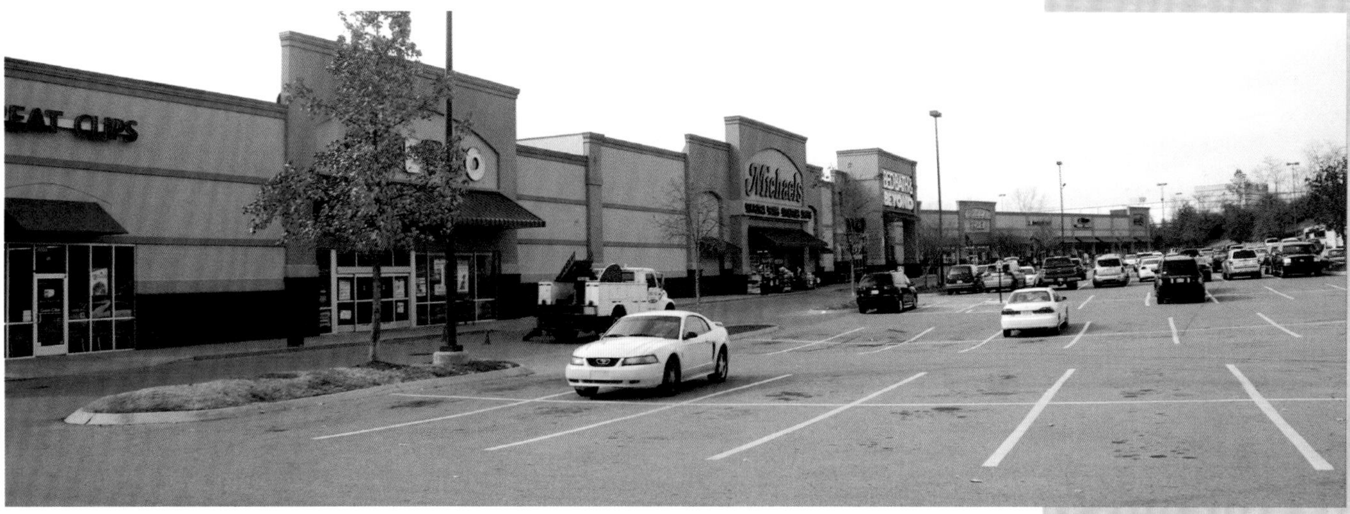

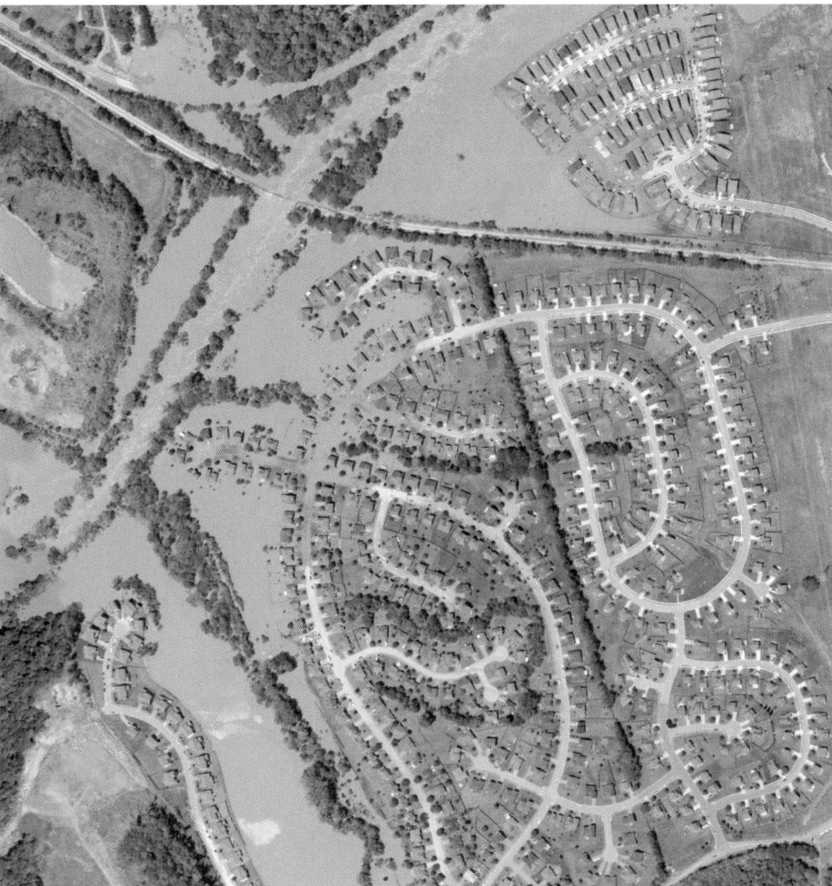

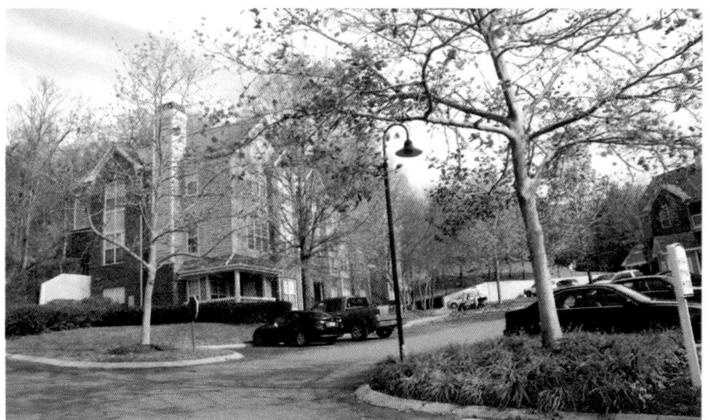

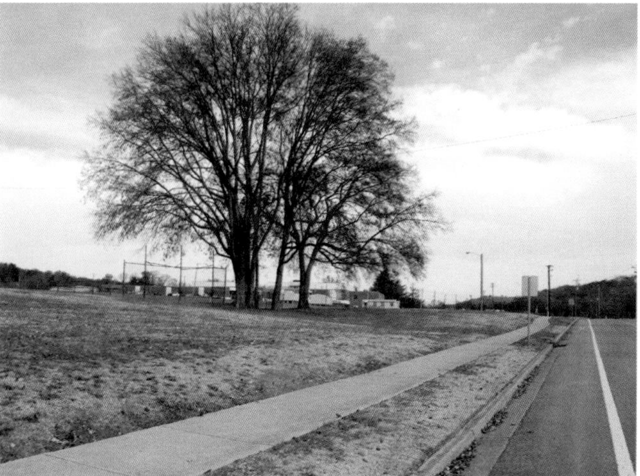

Above: Strip retail center in Bellevue set back from the road, with surface parking fronting the buildings. Pedestrian infrastructure is an afterthought or lacking all together, emphasizing the need for vehicular access. *(2012)*

Left: The Harpeth River that winds through the Bellevue community delivered much devastation during the May 2010 floods. *(2010: Metro Nashville)*

Center: Suburban apartment complex in Bellevue. Note how residences face parking, emphasizing the primacy of the car. *(2012)*

Bellevue Middle School is surrounded by residential neighborhoods within walking distance. The school grounds are adjacent to public transit stops for the MTA buses 24 and 5. Even though the school has sidewalks along its property borders, there are few connections to the surrounding community that allow children and parents to walk to school. *(2012)*

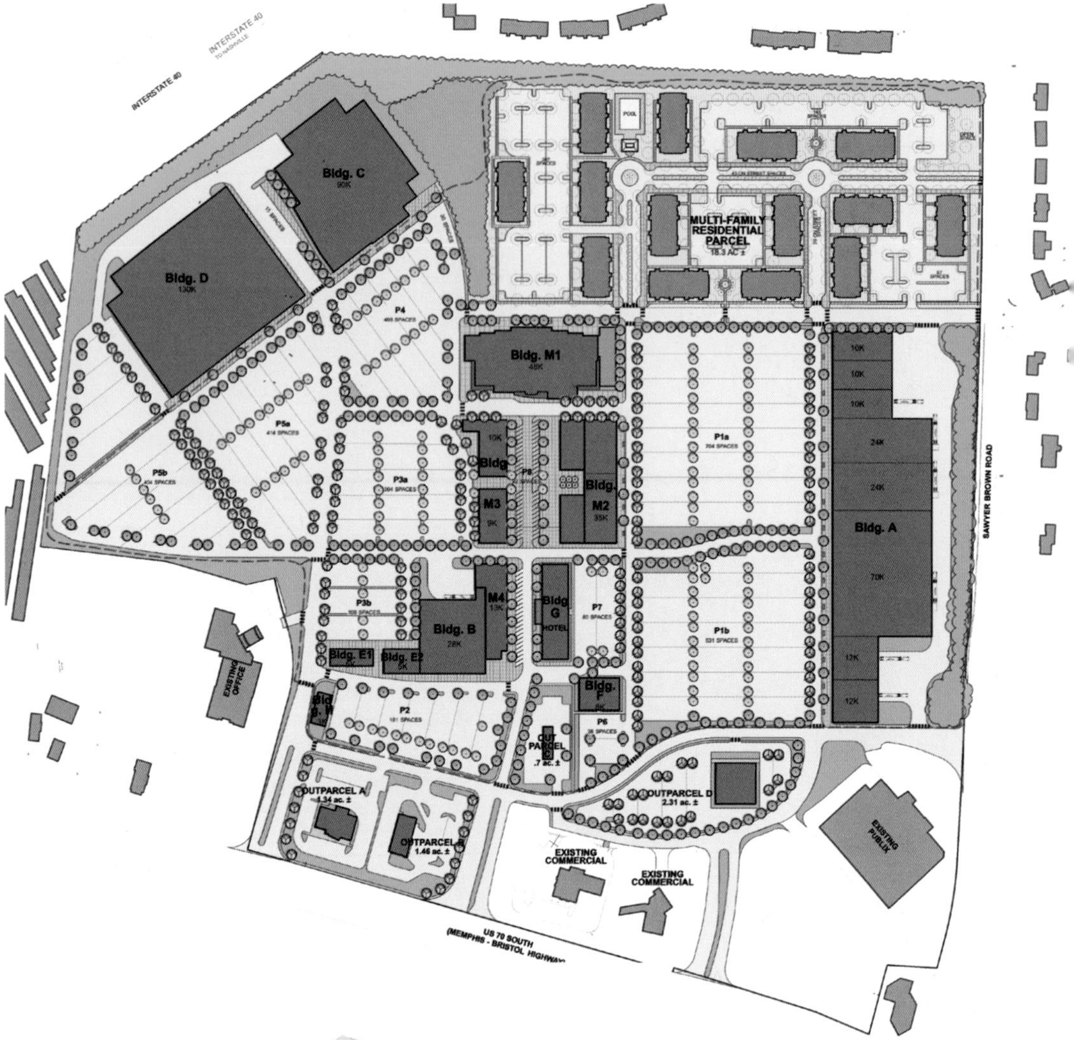

This proposal by Crosland for the defunct Bellevue Mall is similar to the developers' site plan for Providence Marketplace in Mt. Juliet and reflects a reworking of the Bellevue site that neglects most urban design principles, which could create a walkable community supportive of other alternative forms of transportation. Note in particular the typical suburban character, with big boxes dominant; the large amount of surface parking laid out in a manner to encourage people to drive between sections of the site; the parking fronting major roadways, which will erode the pedestrian experience at the edge of the site; the fragmentary nature of pedestrian connectivity. The proposal does include some multifamily residential in the NE corner of the plan, but the large, unvarying footprints of these buildings suggest that diversity among residents is not a consideration. This plan ignored a conceptual design done by the Metro Planning Department that would have created a pedestrian-friendly mixed-use center. *(Plan, 2012: Crosland Development)*

STRATEGY: *Implement a walkable, mixed-use, master-planned redevelopment for Bellevue that creates a civic center for the community. Uses could include retail, office, and a variety of housing (based on type, size, and price). Active transportation infrastructure should link the center to the surrounding neighborhoods.*

STRATEGY: *Link the many disconnected suburban neighborhoods and apartment complexes in Bellevue via sidewalks, greenways, and paved and unpaved trails to existing goods, services, schools, civic buildings, and public transportation.*

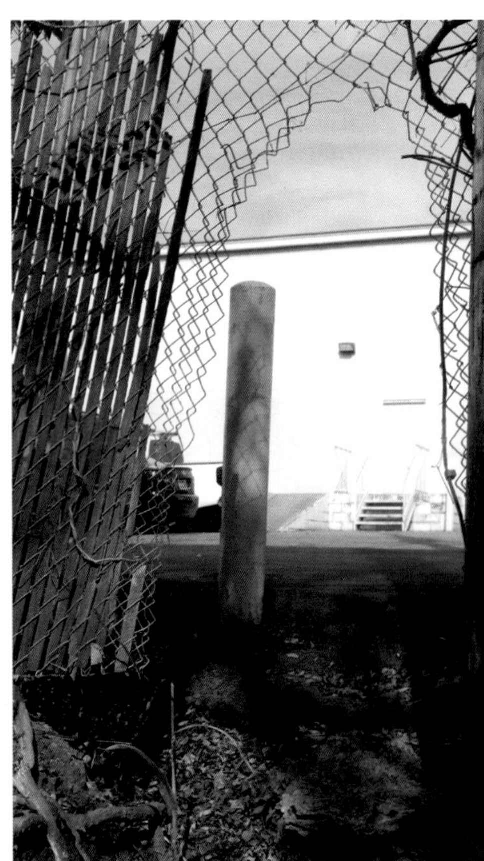

"Informal" connection made by pedestrians desperate to access a big box retail strip mall from the River Plantation community. Neighborhoods bordering shopping areas should be better connected to allow active transportation. *(2012)*

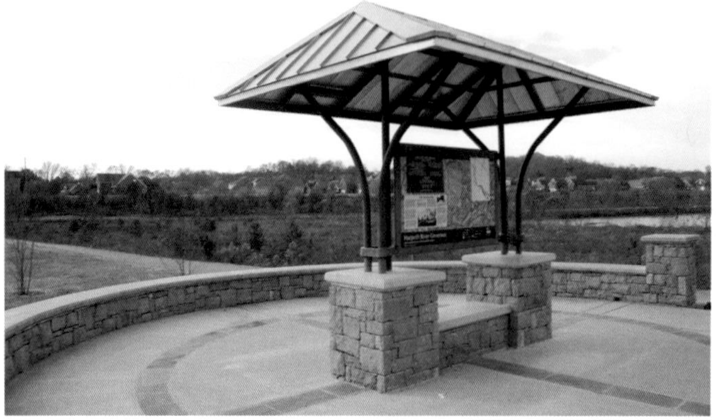

Right: Harpeth River Greenway in Bellevue. *(2012)*

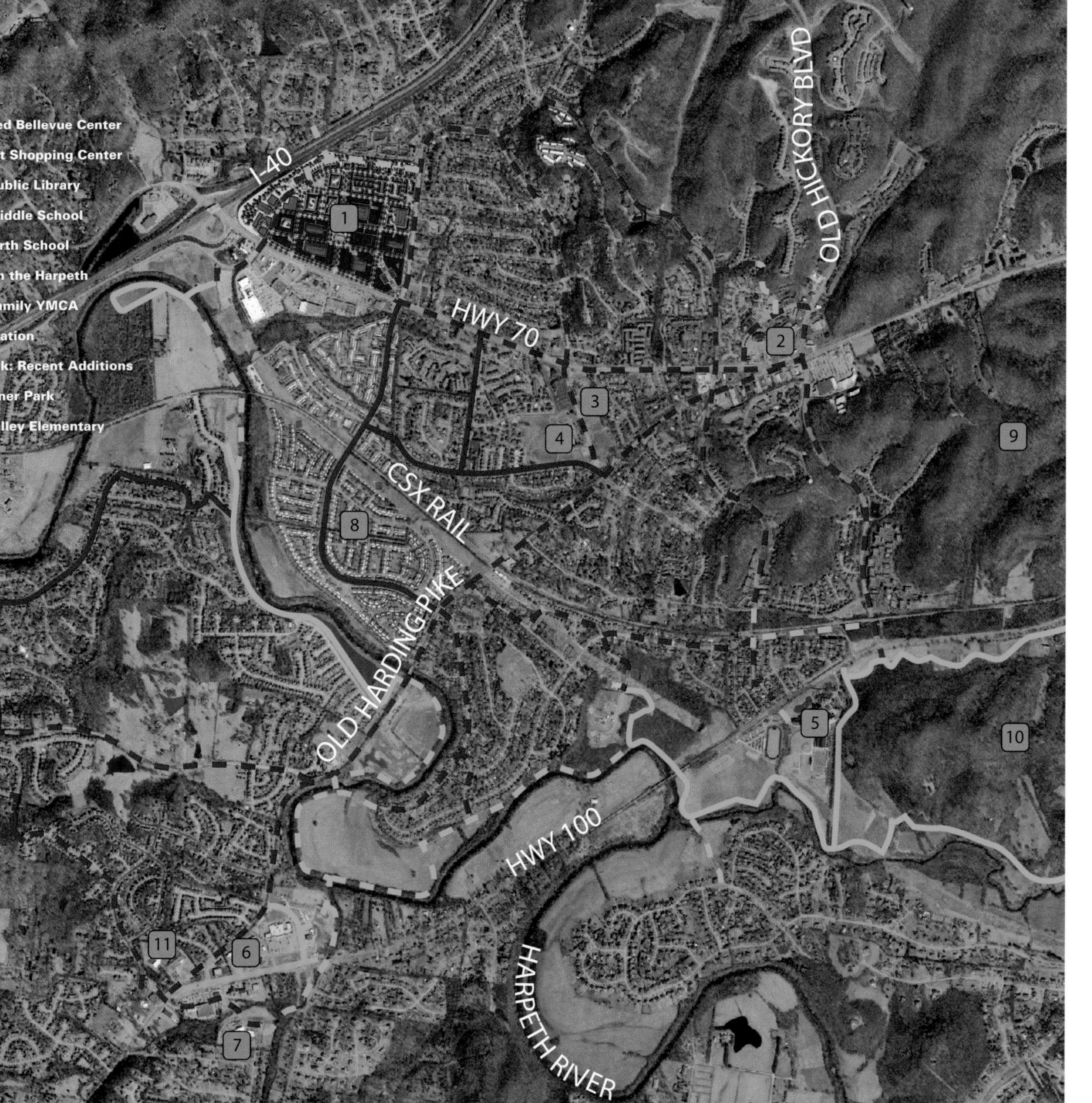

Existing and potential greenways and bikeways in Bellevue can serve to connect the community. Solid green lines represent existing greenways, dashed green represent potential ones. Solid red lines represent existing bike lanes, dashed red potential ones. (*Diagram over aerial photograph, 2013: Eric Hoke, NCDC*)

STRATEGY: *Improve multimodal infrastructure along Old Harding Pike to connect the commercial and civic areas in Bellevue.*

STRATEGY: *Preserve existing open space in Bellevue and expand the greenway network.*

STRATEGY: *Explore creation of a circulator bus service in Bellevue, similar to the successful route in Madison.*

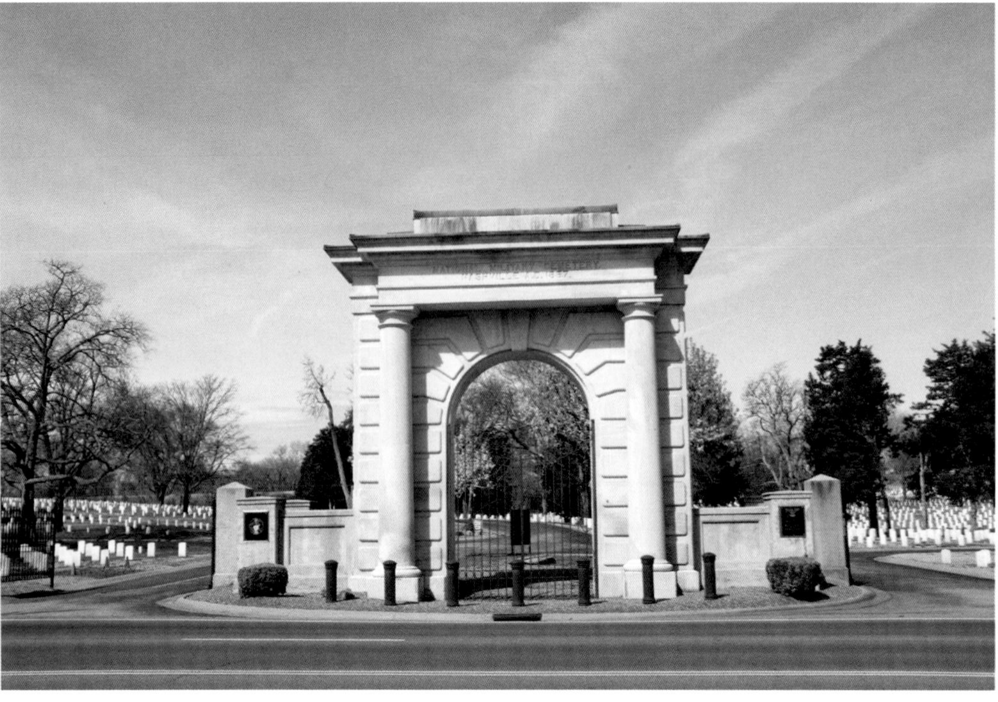

Nashville National Cemetery in Madison. Many soldiers from both the Union and Confederate forces died in the Battle of Nashville near the end of the Civil War. The dead of both sides were initially buried in City Cemetery. Part of the Craighead property, just across from Spring Hill Cemetery, was transferred to the United States in 1866 for use as a separate federal burying ground. The arched limestone gateway was erected in 1870 and is one of five monumental masonry archways constructed as entrances to the national cemeteries of the South. The cemetery is listed on the National Register of Historic Places. *(2013)*

MADISON

The first settlers approached the Central Basin of Middle Tennessee and what is now Nashville from the northeast, where Madison lies. Thus what is now Madison is the site of some of Nashville's earliest history.[31]

The community, which lies on the banks of the Cumberland River, was founded in 1779 and named Haysboro after a local landowner. There the Reverend Thomas Craighead, a Presbyterian minister and educator from Kentucky, established the Spring Hill Meeting House, the first church west of the Cumberland Mountains. Craighead is buried in the church's graveyard, the nucleus of today's Spring Hill Cemetery. Craighead's school, the first in the county and called Davidson Academy, later moved to Rutledge Hill and evolved into the University of Nashville.

Haysboro's port on the Cumberland lay at the tip of Neely's Bend. In 1800 the port was connected by a wagon road to the old Haysboro Road (now Gallatin Pike) leading to Nashville. By 1830 there were dwellings, including Craighead's Evergreen (razed for a Home Depot), a log store, and three stagecoach lines running from Nashville.

Among the second wave of families was the Stratton family. Madison Stratton bought up hundreds of acres of land and then successfully lobbied

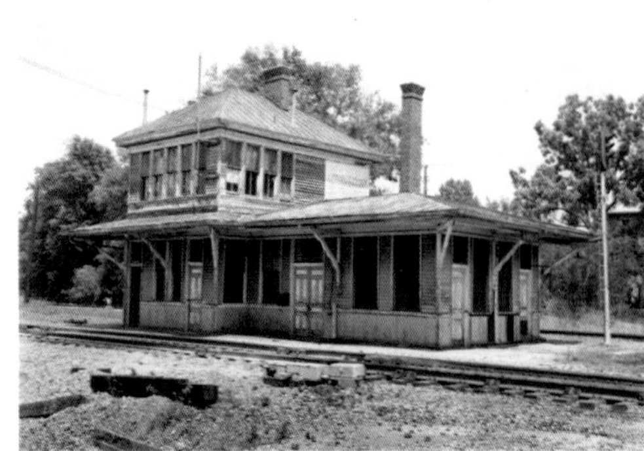

Left: Amqui Station in its original location. *(Date unknown: Courtesy of the Tennessee State Library and Archives)*

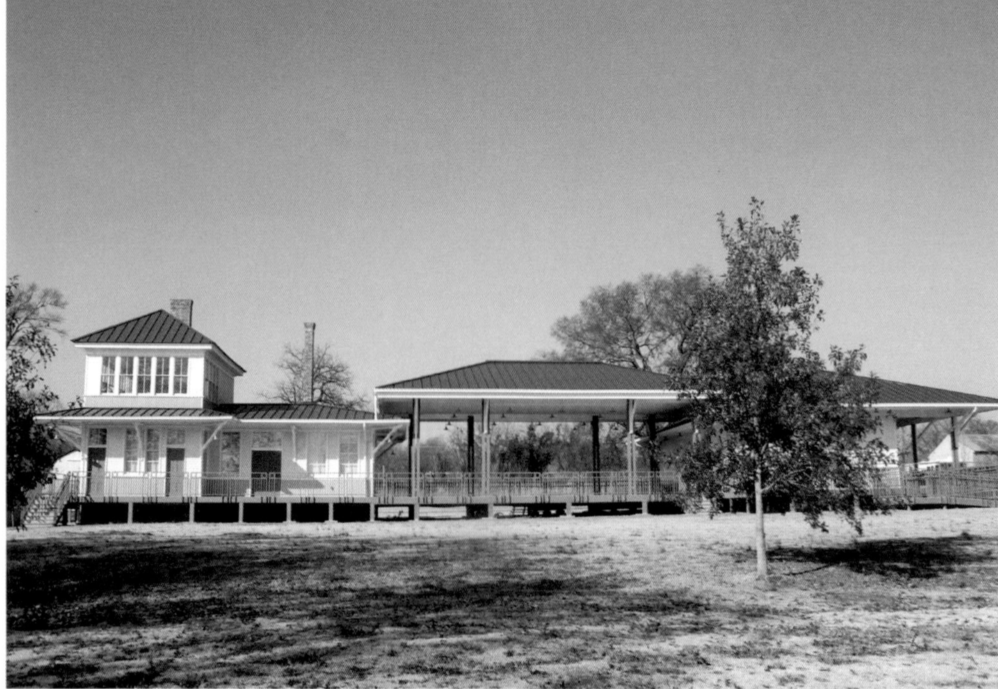

Right: Amqui Station and Museum today. *(2013)*

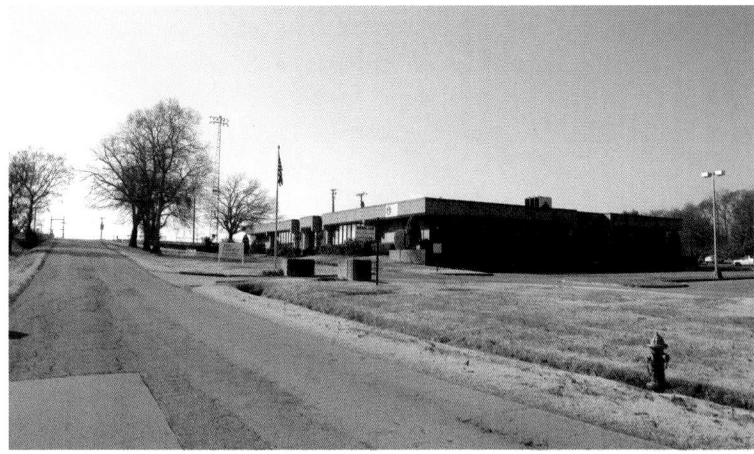

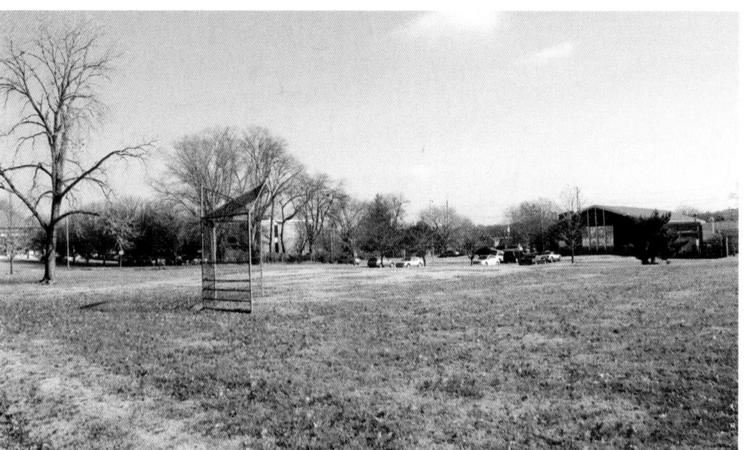

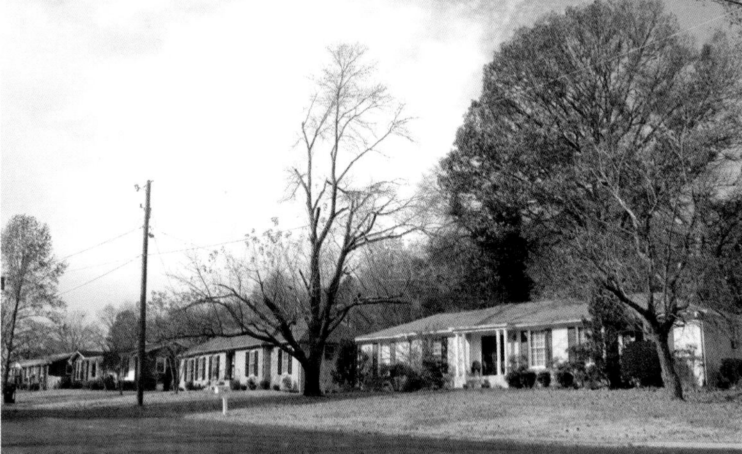

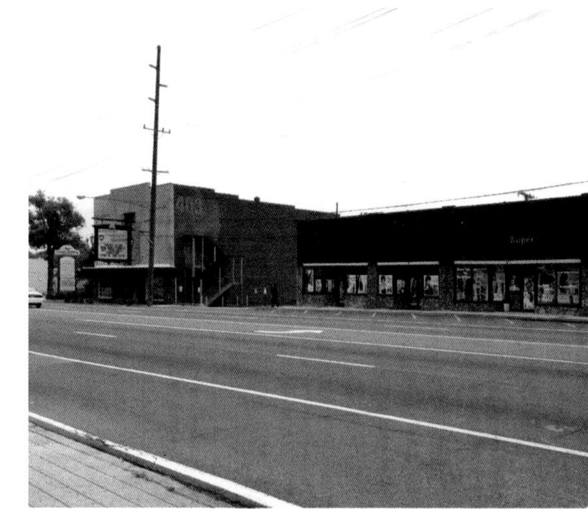

Top left: The Madison FiftyForward center. Note that, even though this is a community center for seniors over the age of 50, it lacks the infrastructure for those who can't drive a car. *(2013)*

Top right: A large open lot behind the Madison Public Library currently functions as a small park and baseball practice field. *(2013)*

Center left: Suburban residences in Madison typically have open lots with mature trees—and no sidewalks. *(2013)*

Center right: Image of buildings on Gallatin Pike in what was once the neighborhood center of Madison. The car-centric nature of residential and commercial development, in particular the construction of Madison Square Shopping Center, sucked the energy and economic viability from the town's traditional commercial center. Today, both town center and shopping center are struggling. *(2015: Gary Gaston, NCDC)*

for a railroad line through his property. Stratton sold land for a station and in 1857 the town was renamed Madison Station. By the early 1900s, "station" was dropped from the town's name.

Built in 1910, the station serviced 40 to 50 trains daily during its heyday. With the decline of rail passenger service, the station was abandoned. In 1979 singer Johnny Cash purchased the building, relocated it to his property in Hendersonville, and restored it to house his train memorabilia. Upon Cash's death in 2003, the structure was returned to Madison and opened as a museum and visitors center in 2010.[32]

In 1918, the United States government commissioned DuPont Engineering Co. to construct the world's largest gunpowder plant in neighboring Hadley's Bend. The Bend was linked to Madison, at first by a swinging bridge that in 1929—after flood damage—was replaced by a more stable structure. After World War I, DuPont built cellophane and rayon plants in what was now called Old Hickory. Workers from all over the country moved into Madison, generating new neighborhoods, banks, and businesses.

By 1950 Madison had grown to nearly 10,000 residents. The Madison Square Shopping Center opened in 1956 with more than a dozen stores. With the merger of city and county government in 1963, Madison became part of Metro Nashville.

Metro built the Madison branch library and Cedar Hill Park in 1977. A new library opened on Gallatin Road in 2000. Recent additions include a new fire station and police precinct. Madison is the only community in the suburban transect zone to have both neighborhood connector transit service and a BRT line connecting to downtown.[33]

Left, top and bottom: Before and after images of Madison's historic center. Note in the "after" rendering the enhanced streetscaping and pedestrian amenities, as well as re-apportioned lanes and parking spaces. *(2012: Ron Yearwood, NCDC; Visualization, 2013: Eric Hoke, NCDC)*

Right, top and bottom: Satellite views of Gallatin Pike and Madison's historic strip showing existing conditions and potential streetscaping with alternative parking scenarios. *(© 2012: Google; Visualization, 2012: Eric Hoke, NCDC)*

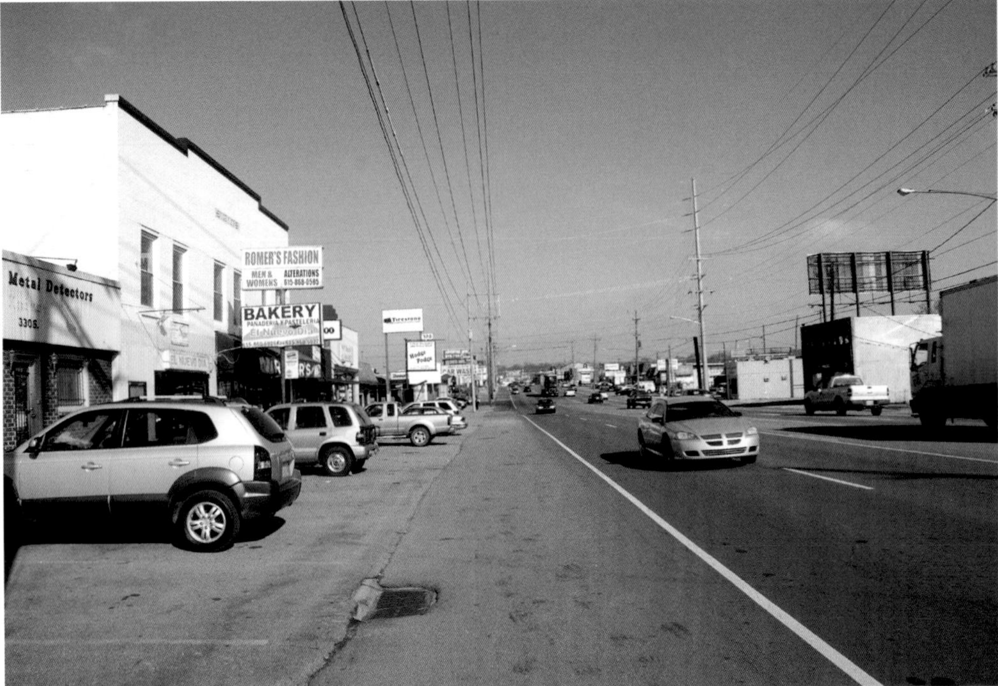

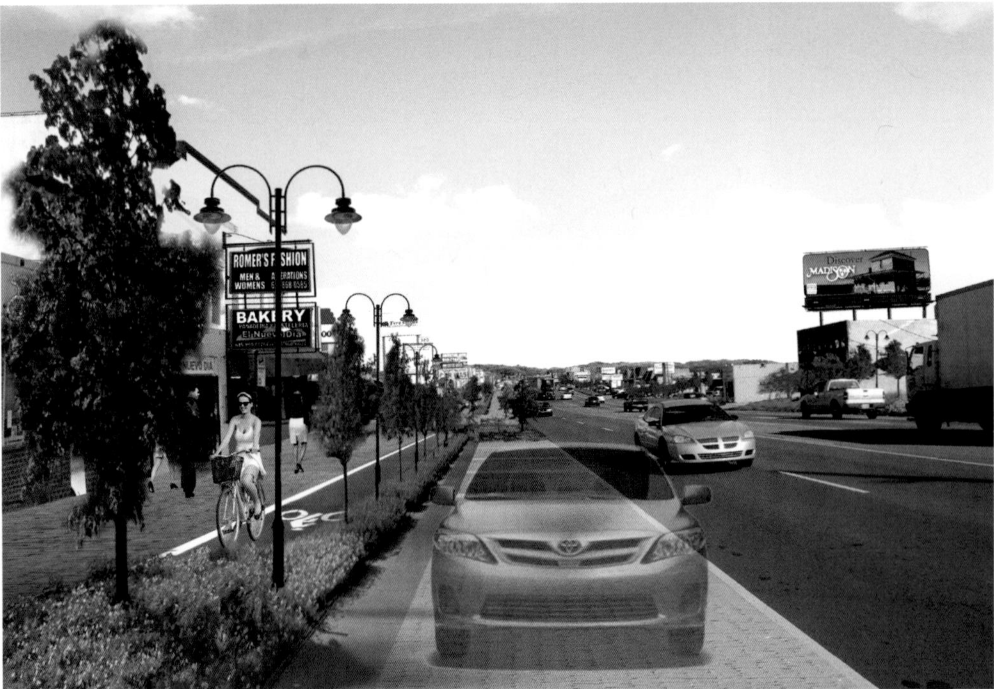

STRATEGIES: *Revitalize the historic Madison town center. Utilize the many plans and studies that have already been conducted in Madison, including the Metro Planning Department's* Community Plan Update, *Nashville Civic Design Center's* Livability Project, *the Metro Planning Organization and the University of Tennessee College of Architecture and Design's conceptual designs for Madison, and the Urban Land Institute's* Action Plan for Reinvestment and Revitalization in Madison.[34]

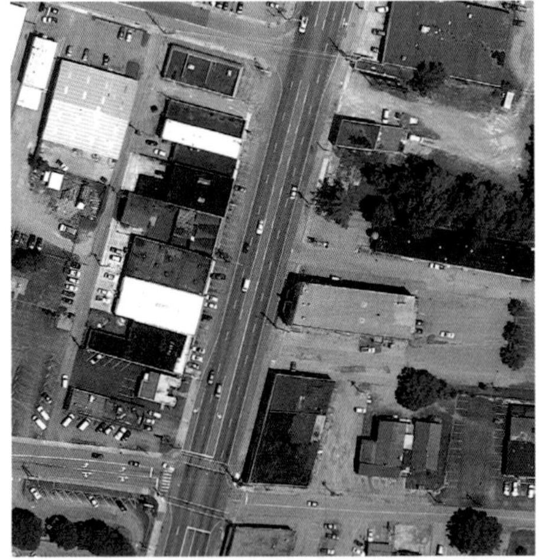

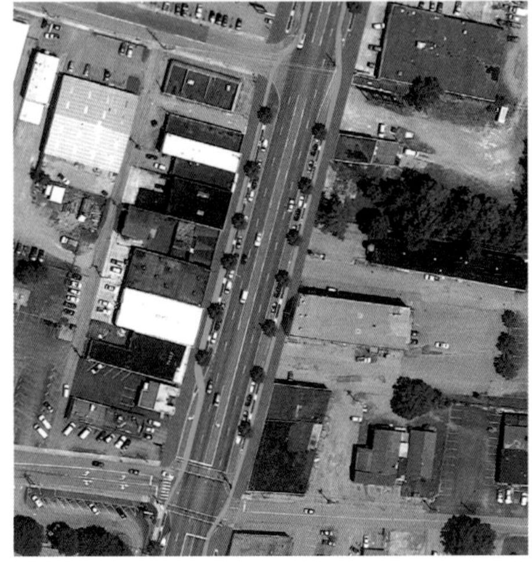

STRATEGY: *Retrofit the ageing Madison Square Shopping Center into a mixed-use development that increases density along Gallatin Pike.*

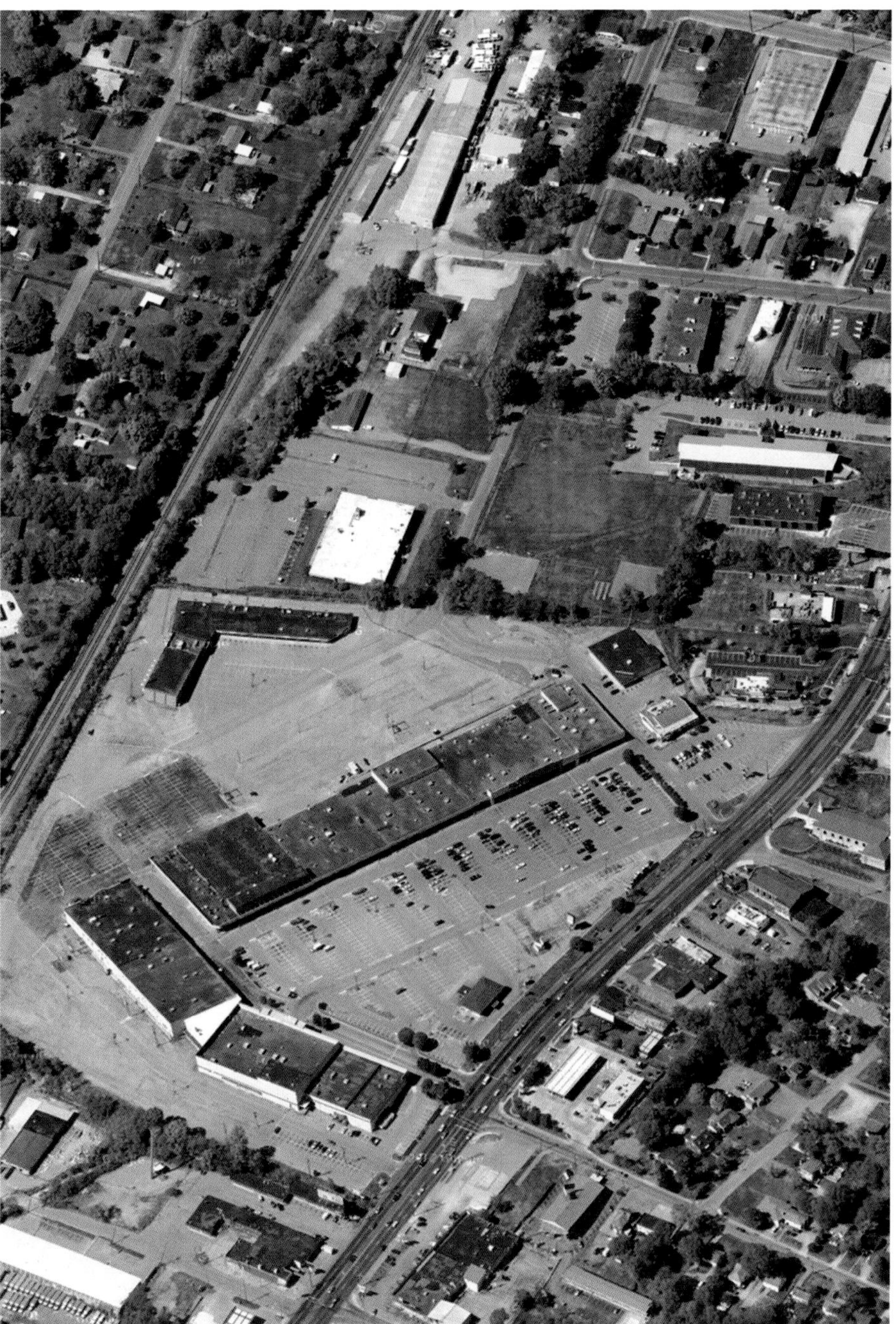

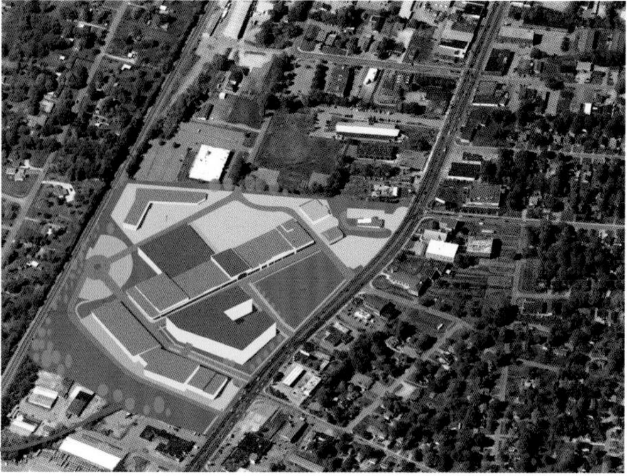

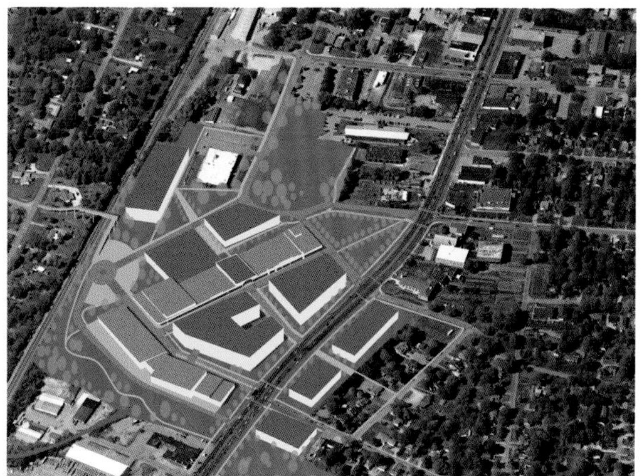

Bird's eye view of Madison Square Shopping Center along Gallatin Pike. The 33-acre site is home to an aging building that is surrounded by largely empty parking lots. *(© 2012: Google)*

Right: Phase 1 retains and renovates existing structures; incorporates a street grid into the former parking lots; and adds to the site new mixed-use construction, a parking garage, and green space. *(Visualization, 2013: Eric Hoke, NCDC)*

Phase 2 continues the site's buildout by incorporating more mixed-use features, for example: senior housing to complement the FiftyForward center, new developments across Gallatin Pike to help transform this stretch of roadway into a pedestrian-friendly town center, and a pedestrian bridge across railroad tracks that connects suburban neighborhoods to the new mixed-use center. *(Visualization, 2013: Eric Hoke, NCDC)*

STRATEGY: *Implement a pedestrian/bicycle network that connects the Madison and Cedar Hill Parks, Amqui Station, the Nashville National and Spring Hill Cemeteries, the Cumberland River, and Peeler Park in Neely's Bend to enable active transportation and recreational opportunities for residents.*

STRATEGY: *New development along Gallatin Pike should be transit-oriented in nature to make the best use of the existing BRT service: buildings constructed close to the street with parking located behind.*

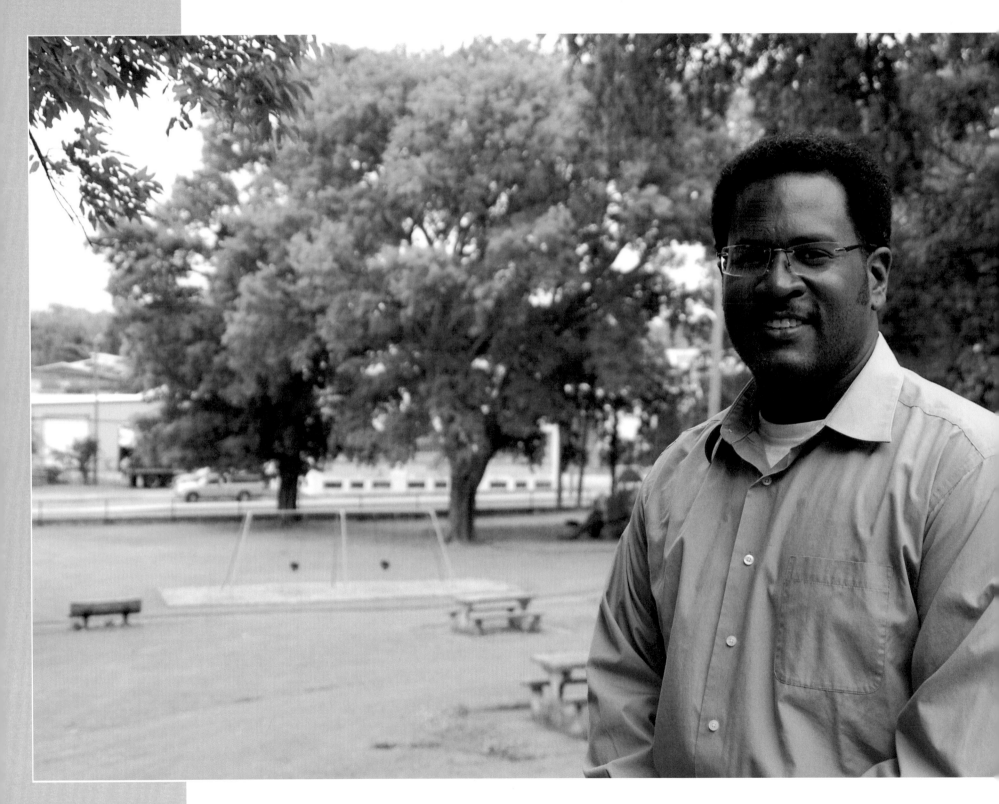

SAMUEL DION WHITE

Samuel "Dion" White, 44, is a Metro police officer who lives on North Hill Street in the historic Chestnut Hill neighborhood south of the central core.

For White, it's "the right spot. I'm not too far from downtown, and I'm not too close. I walk to church or I walk to the park to exercise. I'm used to footin' it. Living in the inner city, you have your challenges. But we have sidewalks."

Although the neighborhood is walkable, White usually gets in the car for his morning commute. He drives his 12-year-old daughter to school two miles away while on his way to work in the morning. "It takes me five minutes to get on the interstate," he says. And then he sits in traffic. "Everybody's coming downtown to go to work." Despite the slow-crawl frustration, White enjoys having the time alone with his daughter. "She could catch the school bus but I prefer to drive her, to mess with her, talk to her while we do the father-daughter thing," he says.

About one-third of White's neighbors don't own a car. Public buses regularly traverse the Chestnut Hill neighborhood, and many residents use the service. But taking the bus can be time-consuming. Passengers are delivered to the downtown hub and often must transfer to another line to get to their destinations. Still, White is glad to have the bus option in case his car breaks down. He'd like to see bike lanes that would enable him to cycle.

White can often be seen running on the paths in Louise and Rebecca Dudley Park after work. Diabetes is prevalent on both sides of his family, so he tries to stay fit and is careful about what he eats. He worries about others in the community who are not as diligent. "There's a lot of diabetes and high blood pressure in my community," he says. "People just have to change their lifestyle, do more exercise, eat right, not sit around watching TV. A lot of people just go to work, go home, and that's it. They feel fine, so they don't feel like diet and exercise are important, and that's what makes their health go down."

Fresh food isn't easy to come by in Chestnut Hill. Eddie's Cee Bee is the only grocery in the community, and White is not a fan. "The building looks rundown and the way they present the food doesn't look good to me," he says. White prefers to drive to Kroger or Walmart. "I have to drive 10 to 15 minutes to other neighborhoods to shop, but I don't mind it," he says.

Relatively new to the neighborhood are the Nashville Mobile Market, a rolling grocery store initiated by Vanderbilt University students that targets food insecure areas, and the community garden on two formerly vacant First Avenue lots. White has not yet taken advantage of either, but is considering purchasing a garden box. Residents supply their own soil and plants. "So many people came and got boxes, they had to get a lot on my street, too," he says. "They even have access for handicapped people."

Neighbors also get together at Dudley Park on Third Avenue South, which has served the neighborhood for a century. People walk dogs, children flock to the playground, youth football and soccer teams practice, and older boys play Frisbee. Grills and picnic tables are available for cookouts. "The majority of the time the park is a great place to be," says White. "On the downside, transients come there to drink." White would like to see the city update the playground equipment. "That'd be great for the kids."

Other parts of the neighborhood also need sprucing up. White wishes his neighbors would take better care of their property. "We have a lot of mulberry trees and they get diseases," he says. "Before you know it, they're rotten, branches fall down. When somebody's property is not maintained it just runs wild."

Some parts of the neighborhood are dotted with vacant lots, making the streets look rundown. "On my street alone there are about seven or eight empty lots," White says. "There are a lot of elderly people and when they pass away there isn't anybody to take care of the property. Sometimes transients use it and end up burning the house down trying to stay warm in winter. Then the city comes in and knocks the house down. If the city owns the lot they cut the grass once a month or whenever it gets high. With the privately owned lots, someone comes every now and then," he says.

Building on the vacant lots would make the community look better and reduce crime. "Abandoned lots give people a hiding place to do drug and prostitution deals," White says. Churches in the community have purchased some of the empty properties. "I noticed on First Avenue they're building condo-style houses. That's going to be nice to have in the neighborhood," he says.

Even though White is fully aware of urban blight in his surroundings, he would not live anywhere else. "There are issues in the community," he says. "People there, maybe they have a drug problem and they just gave up. We have a lot of prostitution and transients. Some apartments are rundown. In the inner city you're always going to have some issues, but my community, it's nice. It's home."

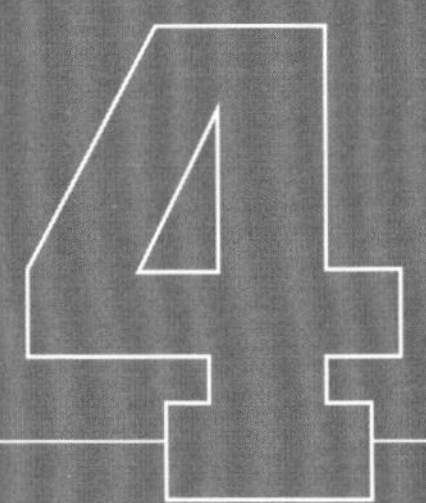

STRATEGIES

Strengthen urban form.

Promote urban infill development in existing communities and use the urban neighborhood form for new developments.

Make public transit more convenient by increasing the frequency of service and incorporating new neighborhood connector routes.

Utilize road diets and complete streets policies throughout urban areas.

Construct a network of bike lanes protected by bollards, curbs, or other buffers to reduce conflict with cars.

Increase pedestrian-accommodating infrastructure like sidewalks, crosswalks, human-scaled lighting, and signage.

Encourage access to fresh produce and nonprocessed foods in areas considered food deserts by promoting stores, pop-up markets, community gardens, and programs that provide healthy local foodstuffs.

Infill urban neighborhoods and commercial areas with new housing that promotes affordability through a variety of densities, types, and unit sizes.

Encourage community stewardship of existing and potential open spaces in urban neighborhoods.

THE URBAN TRANSECT ZONE

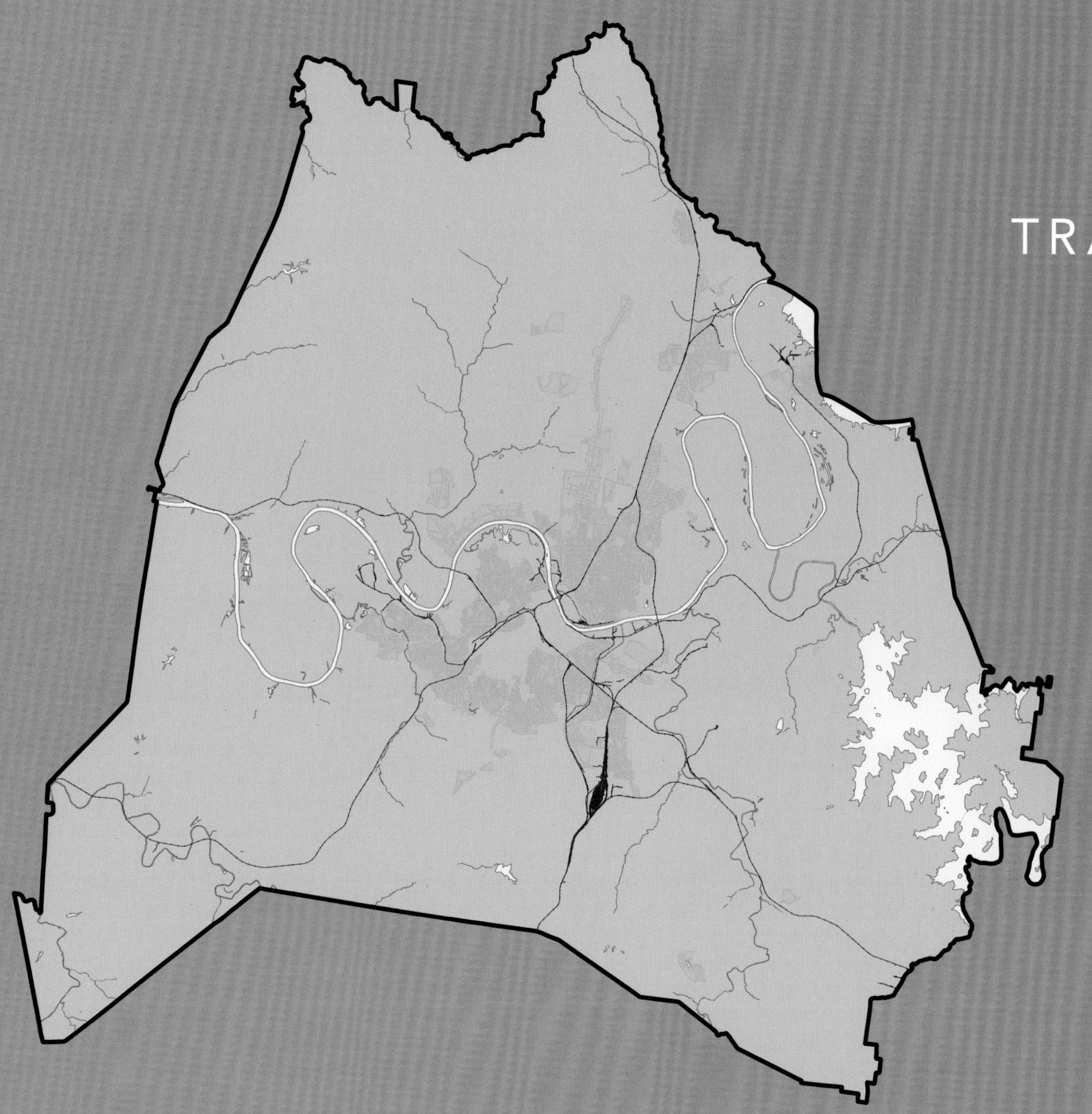

Davidson County, highlighting all areas in the urban transect zone. Note that the urban zone encircles the central core but does not include it; downtown is a separate zone of the transect. The urban zone includes the historic neighborhoods of Chestnut Hill, Edgehill, 12 South, East Nashville, Cleveland Park, Germantown, Salemtown, Buena Vista, Watkins Park, West End Park, Belmont-Hillsboro, Hillsboro-West End, and Richland-West End, as well as newer developments built in the traditional urban pattern.

(Map, 2014: Metro Planning Department)

URBAN

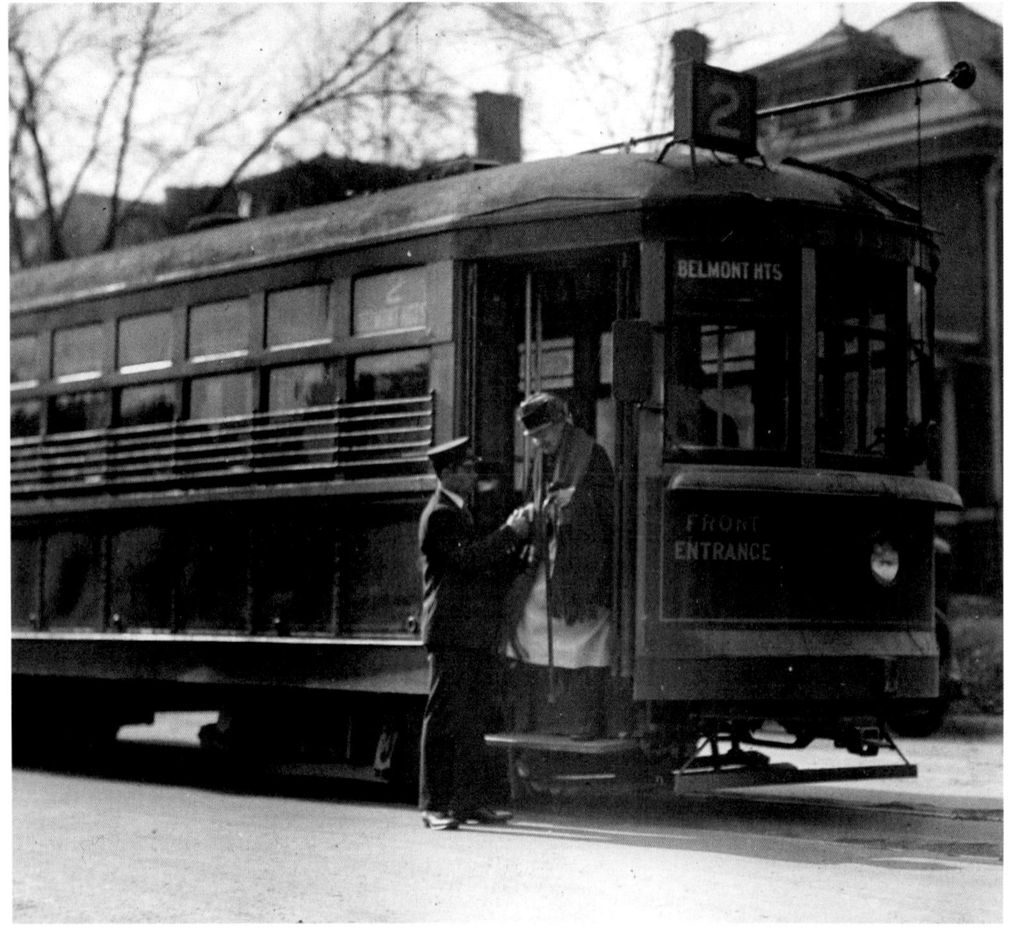

Historic streetcar lines, such as this one that ran down Belmont Boulevard, radiated from downtown to connect to the city's first suburbs. *(1920s: Metro Nashville Archives)*

URBAN LIVING

What a difference a few decades make. From the 1950s until the 1980s, the word "urban" usually found itself saddled with negative connotations. Thus the Urban Institute, founded in 1968 by a blue-ribbon commission appointed by President Lyndon Johnson to address problems such as decay, poverty, and crime thought to be endemic to the "inner city."

Today urban is a buzzword attached to all things millennial. A few examples:

- Urban Outfitters: clothing
- Urban Decay: beauty products with an edge
- Urban Home: furnishings
- Urban Airship: mobile marketing to the smartphone set

The neighborhoods in Nashville surrounding the central core have undergone a similar attitudinal shift. Once considered places to be avoided, especially after dark, these communities have in the last decade become the hot places to live, experiencing some of the steepest escalation of property values in Davidson County.

Ironically, the areas classified as urban on the transect map were originally intended to be anything but. This zone includes the first suburbs of Nashville's downtown, developed as residential refuges from the noise, filth, congestion, and disease of the city proper.[1] The suburban ideal was the antithesis of downtown dwelling: buildings in a park, with the greenery and fresh air that implied. This ideal was often literally realized. Land owners and developers who held financial interests in the trolley lines built parks at the ends of their lines to increase ridership and stimulate sales of the surrounding lots.

The form of these early suburbs was determined by the primary kinds of transportation available in the late 19th and early 20th centuries: the streetcar and the human foot. (The horse as a means of personal mobility—as opposed to commercial delivery—was too expensive for the average citizen.) The trolley lines ran on the main streets connecting these new neighborhoods to downtown. People walked to the stops as well as to local shops, schools, and churches integrated into the neighborhood fabric. Lots were relatively small, typically 50 to 60 feet wide and 150 feet deep, and connected by a network of streets with sidewalks.

Single-family homes of various sizes predominated, frequently with front porches that encouraged socializing among neighbors. Backyards were functional spaces dedicated to growing fruits and vegetables, raising chickens, and washing and drying clothes. Alleys provided access for garbage haulers and coal delivery.

A newer form of transportation, the automobile, spelled the decline of the street car suburbs. While the older neighborhoods could accommodate the car, the suburbs, built on a massive scale in the years following World War II and to which the middle class migrated, were designed around it. The resulting development patterns—low density residential, few sidewalks, backyard patios rather than front porches, economic and land-use segregation, acres of parking surrounding large pods of commerce—are distinct from those of the streetcar era and are what we today define as "suburbia."

The form of the ideal urban neighborhood offers many opportunities for integrating physical activity with daily life. Residents can walk or cycle to a grocery, branch library, coffee shop, restaurant, transit stop, or park. The possibility of "aging in place" is greater due to the diversity of housing types.

From an economic efficiency standpoint, urban development patterns make more sense than suburban ones. Services such as trash and recycling pick up and mail delivery, as well as infrastructure for water, sewer, and utilities, are cheaper and easier to provide and maintain if they serve five houses per acre rather than one. A recent study by Smart Growth for America pointed out the positive impact denser urban communities have on city tax rolls on a per acre basis.[2]

The Middle Tennessee region is expected to add over a million new residents by the year 2040.[3] The logical—and health-inducing—way for Davidson County to accommodate its share of this population is by embracing the urban development patterns of our city's earlier years. By incorporating denser, pedestrian-friendly development into underutilized land within its urban and suburban communities, Nashville can grow its tax base, enhance the effectiveness of public transportation, and provide services more efficiently to more residents.

National preference trends support the urban form of redevelopment. A 2011 survey by the National Realtors Association found that 58 percent of respondents favor neighborhoods that have stores and other businesses within walking distance of houses to a housing-only community that requires driving to access goods and services.[4] These trends are reflected in US Census

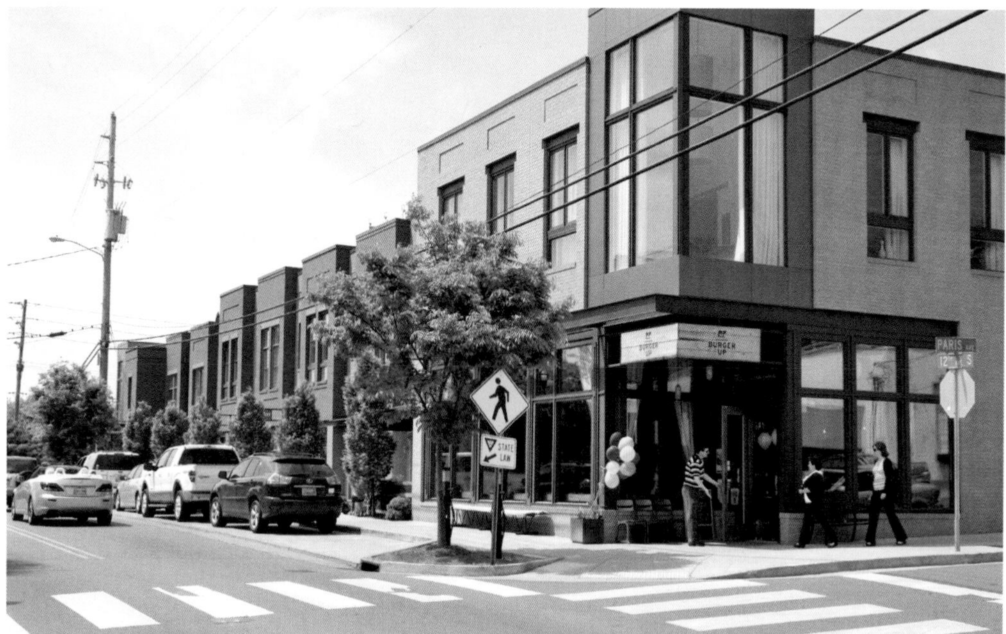

A 1997 streetscaping plan that emphasized walkability sparked the transformation of a moribund section of 12th Avenue South into the vibrant 12 South neighborhood. Rehabs of existing structures and new infill have created a community that attracts both locals and people from across Nashville.[5] *(2010)*

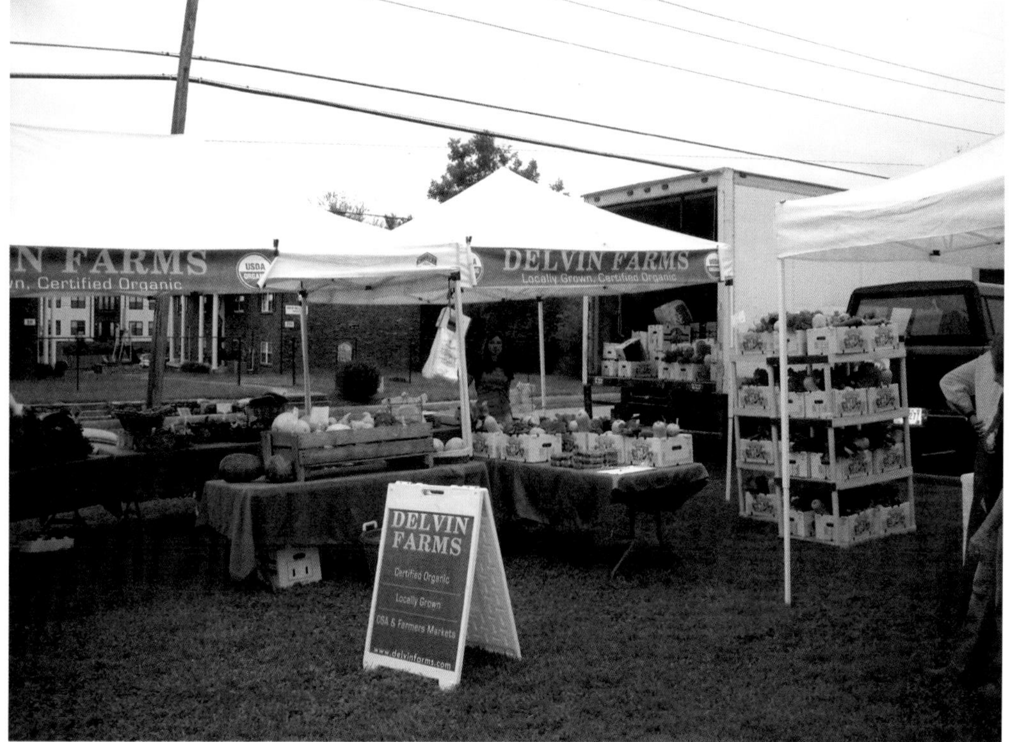

The East Nashville Farmers' Market is one of many pop-up markets across the city that are open during peak growing season (May to October), with vendors selling a variety of local fresh fruits, vegetables, meat, dairy, and artisanal goods to the local community. *(2013: Amy Delvin Tavalin)*

Bureau data released in June 2012, which show that urban growth is surpassing suburban growth in more than half of the country's largest cities, a marked shift from the past century.[6] In Nashville, urban population increases have almost caught up with suburban growth: from July 2011 to July 2012 urban areas grew by 1.2 percent versus 1.5 for suburban ones.[7]

The change in lifestyle preferences, especially among the young millennials and retiring boomers, has fueled this shift in the tide of growth and resulted in safer and cleaner urban areas with more amenities in the form of restaurants and retail.

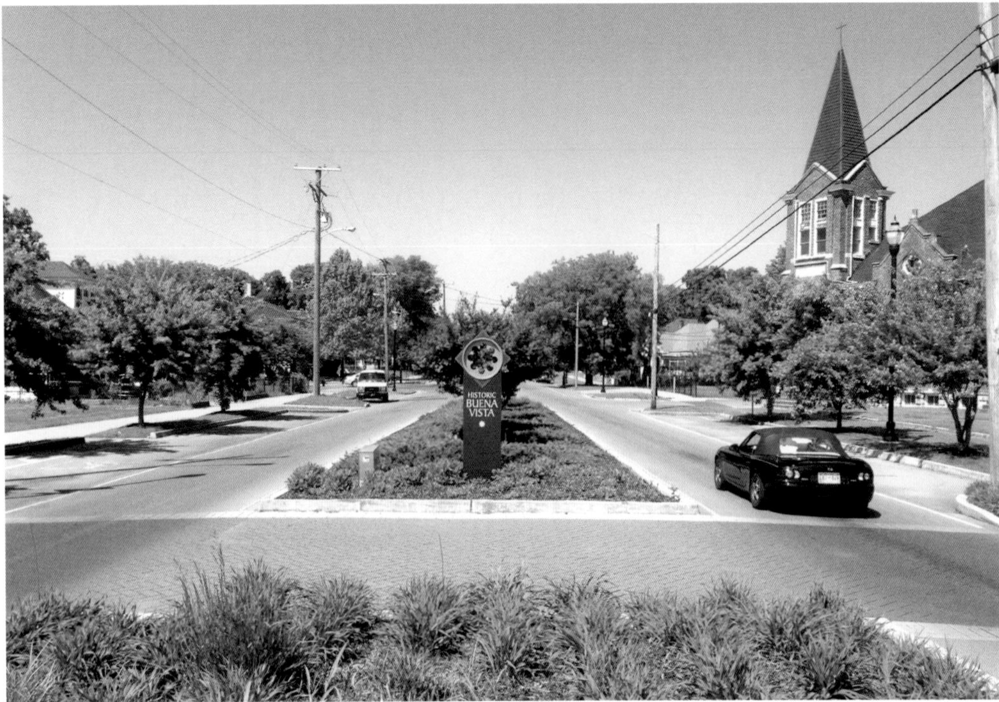

Gateway signage marks the entrance to the Historic Buena Vista neighborhood in North Nashville. Streetscape improvements such as the crosswalk, median, on-street parking protected by sidewalk "bulbs," and planting strip between street and sidewalk increase walkability and were made possible by a federal Community Development Block Grant that featured extensive neighborhood participation. *(2013)*

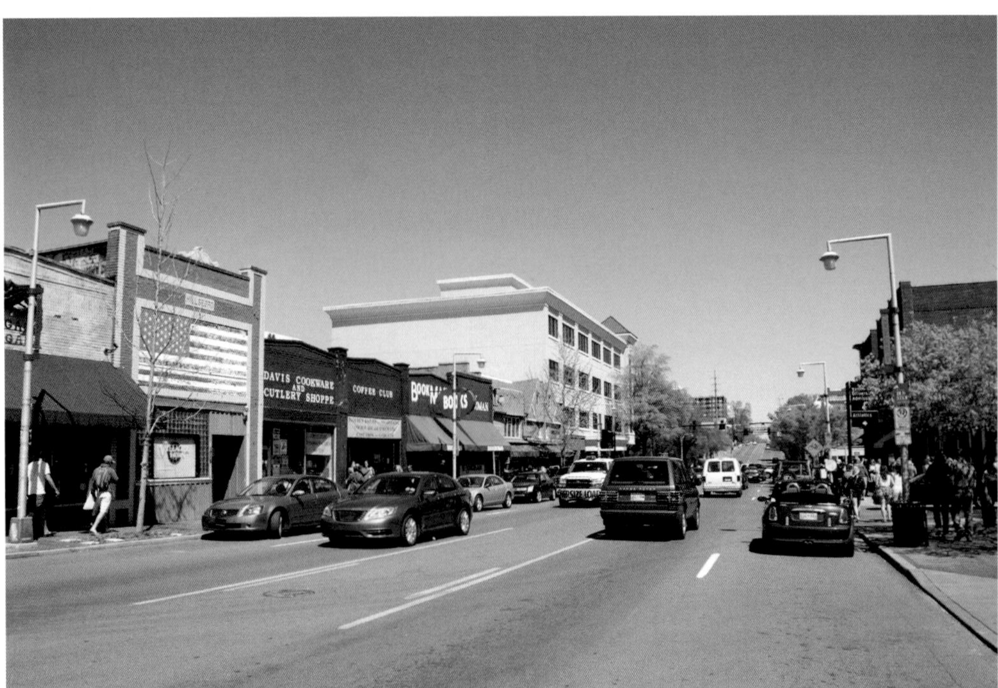

Hillsboro Village is a mixed-use neighborhood commercial center, with the ongoing addition of residential units over the shops. The Village's retail, restaurant, and arts offerings attract a diversity of patrons due to its close proximity to Vanderbilt and Belmont Universities and the Vanderbilt Medical Center. *(2013)*

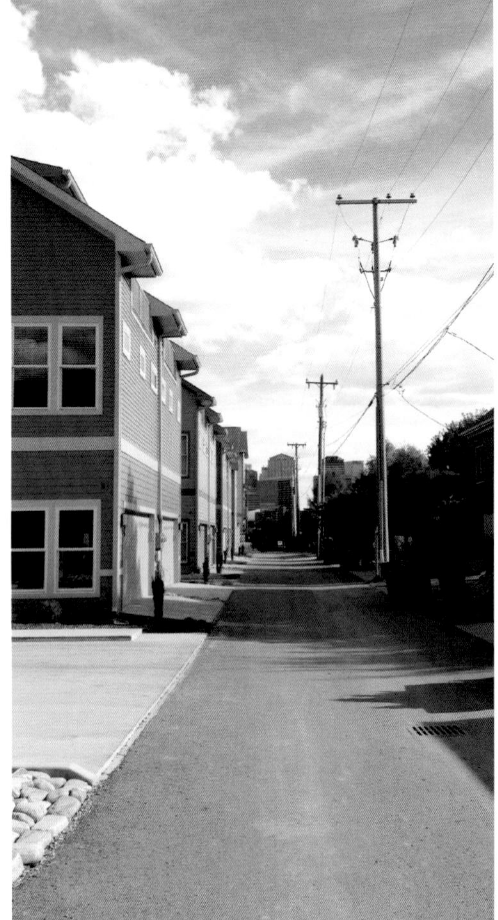

Right: This alley in Germantown contains residential units above garages, which increase neighborhood density without fundamentally altering architectural character. The use of the alley for utility infrastructure, trash and recycling bins storage and pickup, and parking restricts these necessary but mundane functions to the "back of the house." *(2013)*

URBAN ZONE BASICS

For planning purposes, the urban transect zone exhibits the following characteristics:

- **Development patterns and population of greater density than those in suburban and rural zones**
- **Intermingled land uses**
- **Multiple housing types, sizes, and prices that enable socio-economic and age diversity (residents can age in place)**
- **Convenient access to public transportation**
- **Walking distance to neighborhood commerce**
- **Good pedestrian and bike connectivity**
- **Active and passive open space and recreational facilities**[8]

According to 2010 US Census Bureau statistics, the urban transect zone in Davidson County has an estimated population of 136,423 residents—21.8 percent of the county total[9]—and contains 25,245 acres, or 7.5 percent of the land area. By way of comparison, the suburban transect zone contains 65.4 percent of Davidson's County's population on 37.6 percent of its land.

The 2010 census shows 5.4 persons per acre residing in the urban zone, with a trend toward greater densification. Urban infill development increased in Nashville from just 6.1 percent of the total housing construction between 2000 and 2004, to almost 11 percent between 2005 and 2009.[10]

SHAPING HEALTH IN THE URBAN TRANSECT ZONE

ANALYSIS AND STRATEGIES

If Nashville is to grow over the next 20 years in a manner that is economically and environmentally sustainable, the city will need to develop more compact commercial and mixed-use residential areas that are walkable and connect easily to mass transit. Traditional urban design is the model for this type of development, not only for infill in the urban zone, but also for underutilized properties along the historic pikes in the suburbs.

"The heart that pumps life into a metropolitan region is the urban center. But a healthy heart requires nurturing. Citizens must collectively develop a vision grounded in the natural, cultural, and historical attributes we all value. Then we can establish a course that shapes our environment—the fabric of buildings, landscapes, streets, and roads—along livable and sustainable lines."

—Christine Kreyling, on the opening of the Nashville Civic Design Center, 2001

Health-Promoting

The grid of streets in urban areas is inherently more pedestrian friendly than the suburban cul-de-sac / arterial combination. This is in part because an interlocking network offers multiple ways to get from place to place, so walkers and cyclists can choose less busy thoroughfares. The grid also slows vehicular traffic.[11] Stop signs, signals, and crosswalks, trolleys or buses pausing to discharge or take on passengers, cars slowing at intersections to turn at right angles, drivers scouting for an on-street parking space, all serve to equalize the playing field for walkers.

Other urban design characteristics also encourage walking. The small lot sizes typically found in urban areas better enable the minimum density necessary to support local retail and public transit. The mixture of land uses, with corner stores, neighborhood commercial centers, and housing over retail, enables daily necessities like food, shops, and jobs to be located nearby. Dwelling in close proximity promotes interaction among neighbors, increasing the social health of communities.

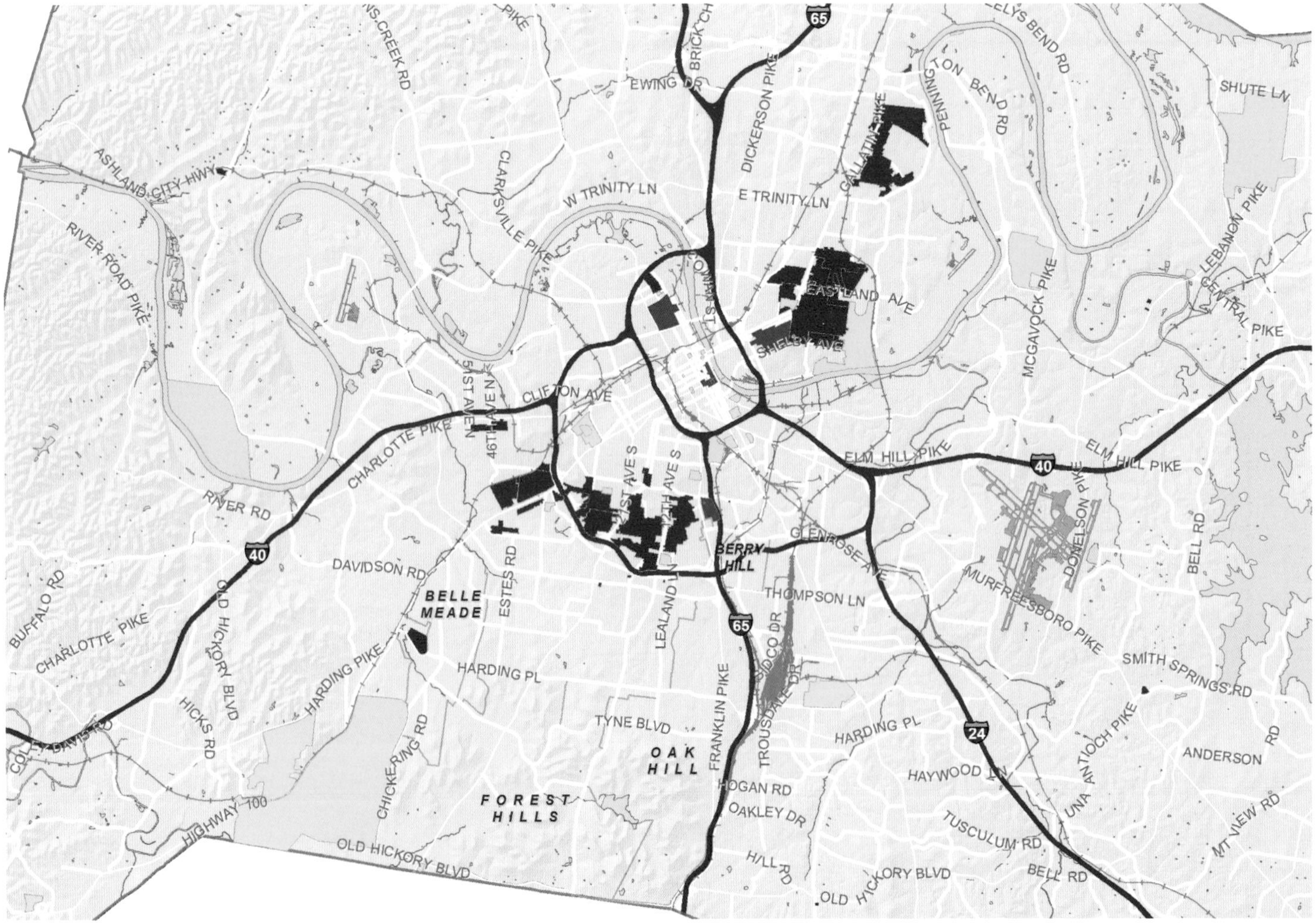

Preservation zoning overlays are planning tools used to protect the historic architectural character of Nashville's neighborhoods by managing growth and change through a public design review process. Nashville currently has eight historic preservation districts (blue), which have the strictest standards, and 18 neighborhood conservation districts (red). Virtually all of these are located in the urban transect zone. Nashville also has 46 individual landmarks (yellow).[12] *(Map, 2016: Metro Historical Commission)*

Who Knew?

When the preservation movement in Nashville began to gather momentum in the latter 1970s, those of us involved thought what we were about was saving buildings. We saved a landmark by preventing the destruction of the Ryman Auditorium; then we expanded our focus to include whole districts.

Edgefield was nominated to the National Register of Historic Places because of its fine collection of Victorian and early 20th-century architecture and in 1978 became the city's first historic zoning district. Its residents chose to submit to restrictions on the exterior design of restorations and new construction in order to halt demolitions and so-called "remuddlings." Other historic neighborhoods soon followed suit.

In 1984, however, the Metro Historical Commission conducted a survey of those living in such neighborhoods to determine the issues they saw as central to their communities. At the top of their list: absentee landlords, paltry enforcement of zoning and code regulations, crime, lack of neighborhood services, and the redlining by banks that denied property owners access to funds for rehab and renovation. "Historic preservation" was rarely mentioned.

It was then that we, the city's official preservationists, realized that saving buildings was not enough. As I wrote in an essay for *The Plan of Nashville,* the survey made "blindingly clear" that "true neighborhood preservation happens only when the entire environment is healthy."[13]

History makes this point obvious. What had reduced these neighborhoods to their eroded state was a philosophy-turned-public-policy that saw in the automotive suburb the ideal lifestyle. Derelict and demolished architecture in the former streetcar suburbs was just one of the results. For decades, city and business resources had been focused on the newer suburbs. Passive neglect and active practices damaged those neighborhoods that didn't qualify for this description.

Beginning in the 1930s, the relatively new tool of zoning was applied in a way that punished neighborhoods with a mixture of land uses. If an area had some commercial or industrial properties, all of it was zoned for those uses, ignoring the fact that many of these areas were primarily residential. For example, indiscriminate industrial zoning in the largely residential blocks now known as Germantown meant that, if a house burned, it couldn't be rebuilt, and industries incompatible with housing could move in, resulting in instability.

After World War II, banks made loans that the federal government insured to finance new houses—but not to purchase old ones. Whole sections of town were subsequently redlined.

As the older neighborhoods began to decline, they became the repository for agencies serving those in trouble and in need, concentrating social ills. Now blighted, these neighborhoods became the targets of the well-intentioned but draconian program of urban renewal, which renewed no "urb" but enhanced the blight. Blocks of older buildings were demolished. In their place came small houses of low resale value and vacant lots. Superblocks of public housing became warehouses for the poor. Interstate highway construction blasted through economically and architecturally fragile sections of the city, dividing neighbors from one another and destroying communities.

Inner-ring neighborhoods became identified with crime and other slum-inducing conditions. Inevitably, the desire for escape from such ills led to more sprawl. The central core was in danger of being ringed by slums.

Still there was no real attempt from the top by city or business leaders to reverse the downward spiral. The effort began from the bottom up in the 1960s by a small group of neighborhood citizens—Belmont-Hillsboro comes particularly to mind—concerned with unfair housing practices, abuse of power by the Board of Zoning Appeals, condemnation of properties for Vanderbilt University expansion, lack of design standards, and the planning of I-440, recalling the damage that highway construction had done elsewhere.

Then in 1975–1976, the Metropolitan Historical Commission (MHC) carried out an analysis of 23 older neighborhoods and published it as *Nashville: Conserving a Heritage*. The study was launched with a seminar hosted by Mayor Richard Fulton and entitled "Sales Opportunities in Older Neighborhoods." Invited by the mayor, bank presidents and prominent realtors attended. For the first time, the label "historic" began to be applied to these collections of structures.

The 19th- and early 20th-century architecture—its variety in styles and sizes, its affordability—was definitely a draw for the renewal of interest and investment. But the transformation of the once-deteriorating urban core into thriving multigenerational communities hasn't happened just because of the historic buildings, important as they are. The virtues of urban form itself must be credited.

In conversations with Rick Bernhardt, executive director of Metro's planning department, he has pointed to the national resurgence in urban neighborhoods as driven by the lifestyle preferences of two generations. Aging boomers want to downsize, reduce car dependency, and have walkable and bikeable access to libraries, parks, shops, medical care. Those known as gen Y or millennials seek easy access to friends, food, entertainment, and jobs; their focus is on quality of life and on connecting with others their age, not on commuting.

Sidewalks, small lots, proximity to a mix of services and land uses, and variety in house styles and sizes help to satisfy those drives. Those same design features, so typical in older neighborhoods and generally missing in newer suburban development, also offer some, if not all, answers to societal health problems related to a lack of physical activity.

When I realized in the 1980s that neighborhood preservation inevitably called for attention to the health of the whole neighborhood environment, I defined health in terms of economic well-being, the maintenance of properties, responsible owners, and safety. I wasn't thinking about the physical health of a neighborhood's citizens. Today residents of Nashville's increasingly desirable historic neighborhoods probably aren't consciously choosing to live in them for reasons of physical health, either.

Yet the increasing awareness of the role the physical design of a community can and does play in its residents' health adds yet another to the many reasons to preserve and enhance the older neighborhoods that enrich Nashville.

—ANN ROBERTS

former executive director, Metro Historical Commission

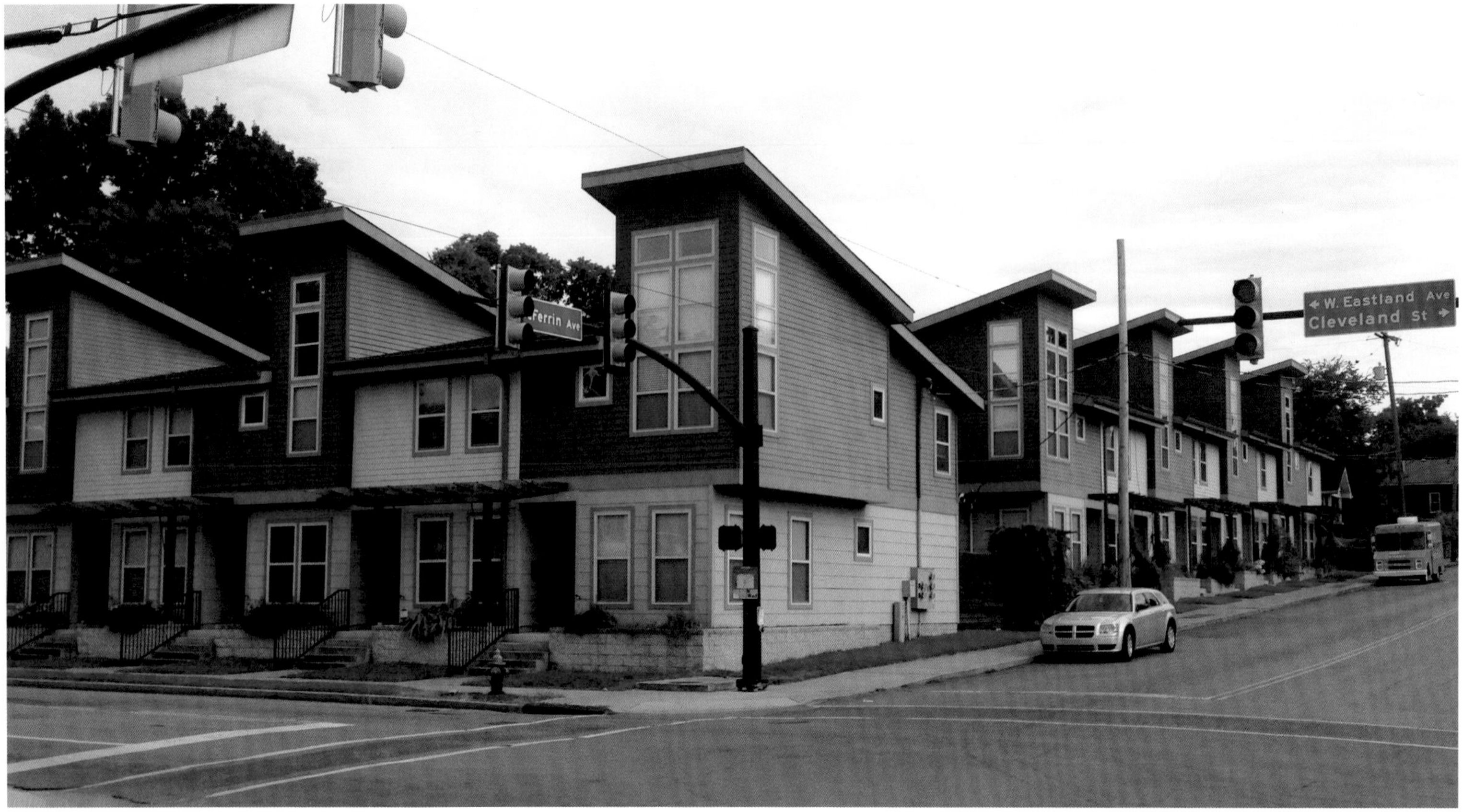

This 2007 residential infill project in Northeast Nashville contains ten workforce units and three affordable units. The 0.6-acre site was formerly a vacant lot on one of the neighborhood's commercial corners and lies at the intersection of two collector streets (West Eastland and McFerrin Avenues) and within walking distance of a Gallatin Road bus rapid transit (BRT) stop. This degree of density—the average would be 22 units per acre—supports a high level of transit service. *(2013: Gary Gaston, NCDC)*

✗ Health-Defeating

Light, noise, and air pollution occur in urban neighborhoods located adjacent to interstates and commercial corridors and centers. Noise pollution has become a particular issue for residents living near outdoor venues featuring special events and music.

STRATEGY: *Strengthen urban form. Continue the intensification of redevelopment within existing urban neighborhoods and plan for new neighborhoods in appropriate locations within the suburban transect zone that utilize the urban form. (Lenox Village is an example of a neighborhood built in the suburban zone that is considered urban in form.)*

In *Visualizing Density,* authors Julie Campoli and Alex S. MacLean state, "Depending on the extent of the developed area and road network, densities of fewer than six units per acre are often too high for the cars-only approach, but too low to support alternatives, resulting in a transportation limbo between urban and rural."[14] And according to the "Transit-Oriented Development Fact Sheet" published by the Capitol Regional Council of Governments, "the absolute minimum residential density required to support regular, on-street bus service is about 6 to 8 units per acre, on average, for a transit corridor. For express bus service with exclusively pedestrian access (i.e., no park and ride facilities) minimum average densities for the corridor should be about 15 units per acre."[15]

Nashville still has a way to go to reach these thresholds. In East Nashville, considered one of the city's most urban communities, the standard lot size is 50 feet by 150 feet, yielding an average density of 5.8 units per acre. Thus the need exists for greater density infill along arterials, collector streets, and larger parcels in existing urban neighborhoods.

STRATEGY: *Revitalize aging urban industrial and commercial areas with a mix of uses to create vital civic centers for surrounding communities.*

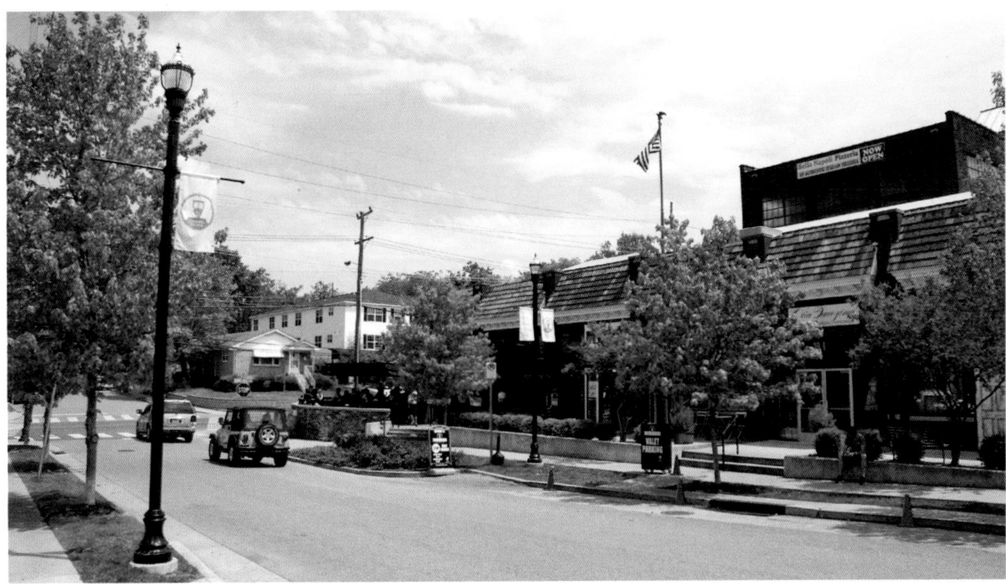

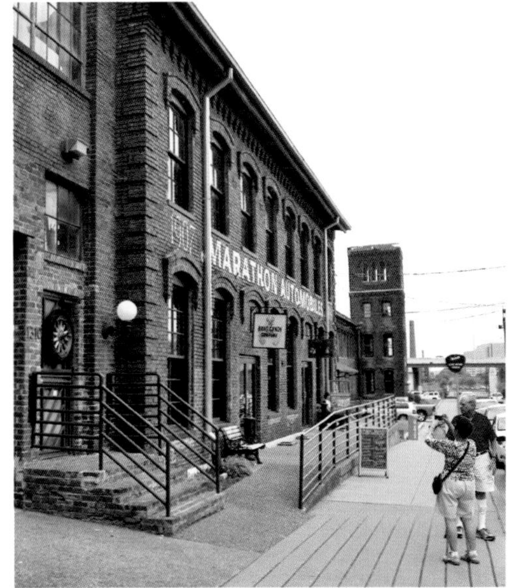

Left: Edgehill Village, a 1920s era complex of eight buildings, originally housed the Whiteway Cleaners and Laundry, a commercial steam laundry. In 2005 the renovated site reopened as a mixed-use destination containing shops, restaurants, residential lofts, and office spaces. Note the streetscaping , with pedestrian-scale lighting and a planting strip between sidewalks and street, which make it more pleasant to walk. (2013)

Right: Marathon Village, which lies slightly north and west of the downtown core, infused new life into a decaying neighborhood isolated by the construction of I-40. This historic 1907 warehouse, formerly home of Marathon Motor Works, now houses a variety of tenants with a strong focus on arts and music. (2013)

STRATEGY: *Provide a variety of neighborhood opportunities for physical activity and social interaction that accommodate residents of all income levels and ages.*

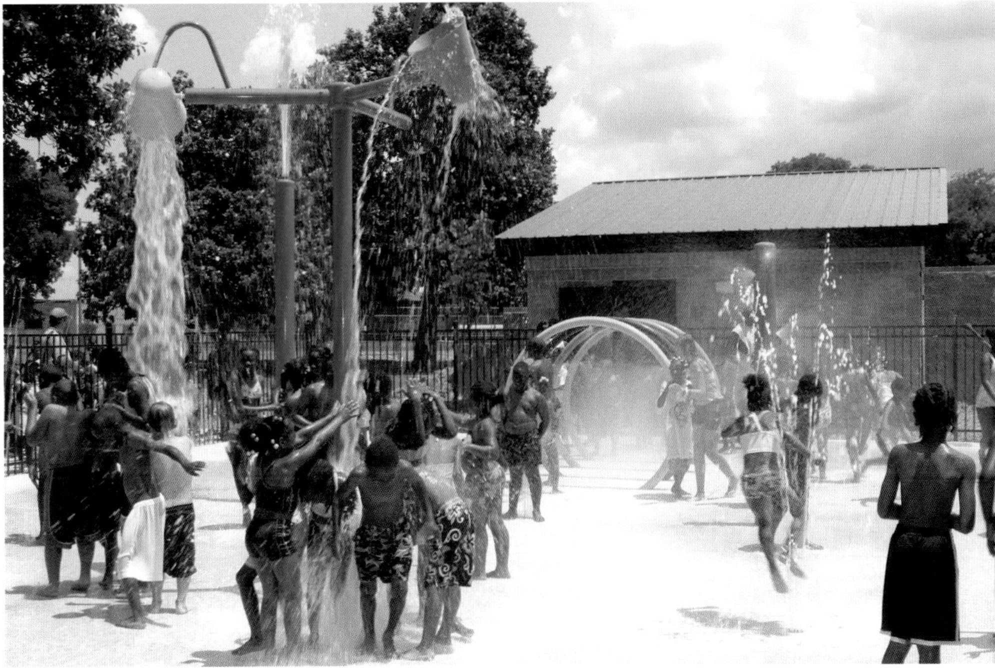

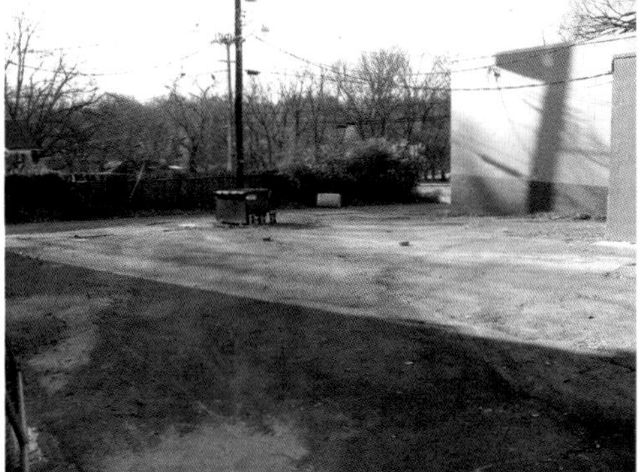

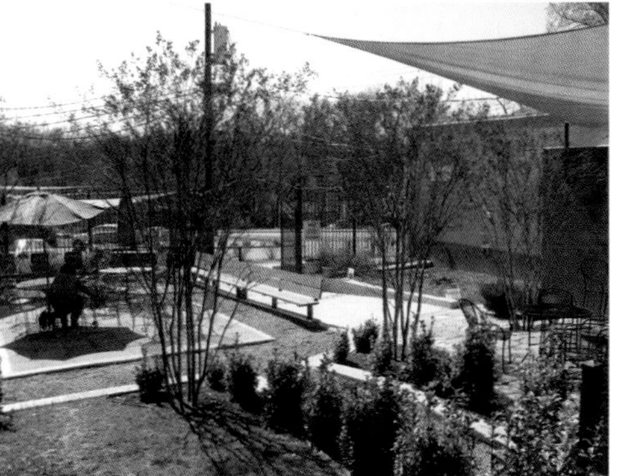

Left: Watkins Park provides an interactive "sprayground" for kids who live in the surrounding neighborhoods. (2005: Gary Layda)

Right: In 2007, the intersection of Riverside Drive and McGavock Pike in the Inglewood neighborhood began to see significant redevelopment. A strip of buildings on the southeast corner was rebranded as Riverside Village, with renovated buildings occupied by a new independent pharmacy and a handful of small, local restaurants and boutiques. The former parking and delivery area at the rear became a courtyard and community garden—with seating for restaurant patrons, a water fountain for dogs, and chess tables—and a casual gathering place for art shows, musical performances, and other community events.

Before, the underutilized backside of an aging strip mall. **After,** the same space repurposed. (2006 and 2008: Dan Heller)

The IDEA Hatchery, a commercial infill development on a vacant lot near Five Points, was conceived to spur retail activity in East Nashville by offering small (168 to 320 square feet), affordable spaces for start-up businesses. Even before opening in 2011, the complex had a waiting list of entrepreneurs interested in setting up shop. Note how the new construction respects the setback of the historic building next door. *(2013: Bret and Meg McFadyen)*

Center: The Shoppes on Fatherland in East Nashville provides inexpensive spaces that are filled with local businesses. A covered open-air hall offers a place for community special events complete with public restrooms. *(2013: Kate Cauthen, Native)*

Right: A mixed-use infill development in the Cleveland Park neighborhood in Northeast Nashville features retail on the ground floor and affordable housing units above. *(2015: Urban Housing Solutions)*

Lower right: In March 2015 Metro Nashville received a Cities of Service Award, which Mayor Dean dedicated to The Nashville Green Alley Project to place rain gardens in the Nations neighborhood of West Nashville. *(2015: Cumberland River Compact)*

STRATEGY: *Create opportunities within neighborhoods for new businesses, public event and meeting spaces, and residential housing.*

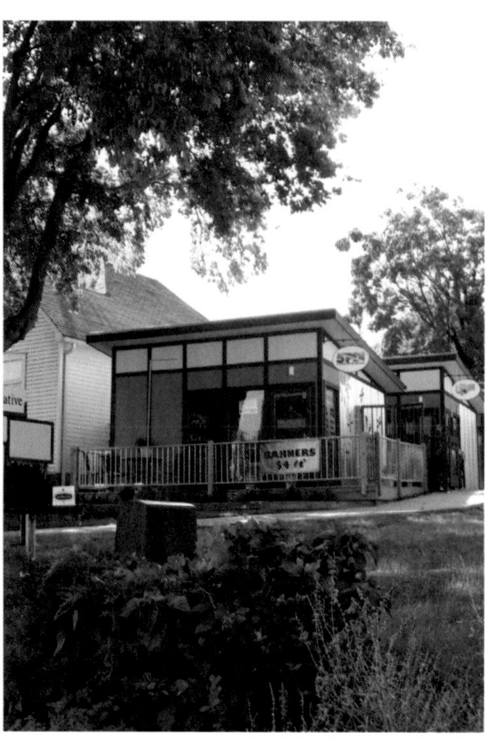

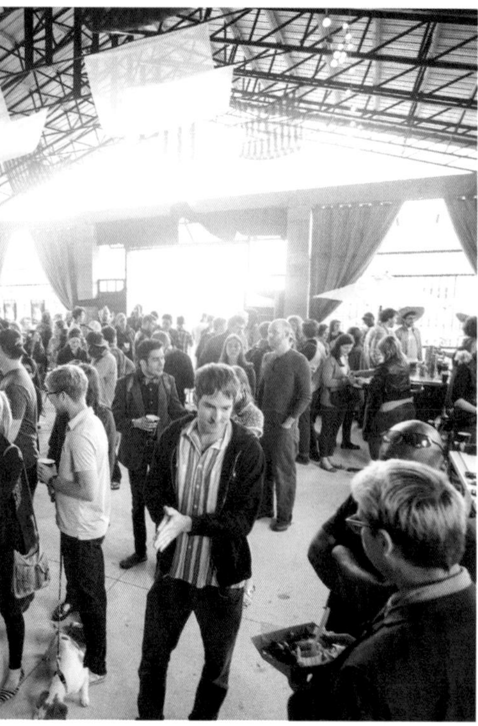

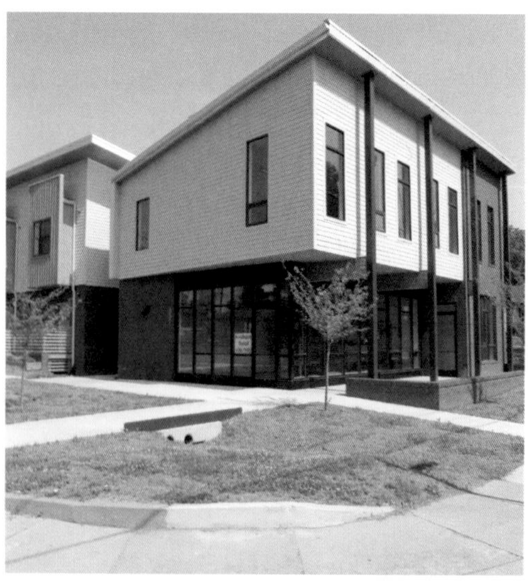

STRATEGY: *Design and implement a network of "Living Alleys" for Nashville's urban areas. Such alleys can become avenues to greater residential density and feature green infrastructure to mitigate runoff, which can contribute to water pollution.*

In the United States, cities such as Chicago and San Francisco have developed alley programs that focus on converting these service corridors into streets hospitable to residential and social uses. Ten years ago the city of Vancouver in British Columbia launched a pilot program for "greening" several of its alleyways to transform them into multipurpose lanes.

As Brian Hutchinson reported in Vancouver's *National Post,* "Asphalt paving was removed and replaced with "structural grass," rigid plastic honeycomb cells sprinkled with ordinary lawn seed and nurtured into green swaths. Concrete strips were embedded on two sides, creating a durable driving surface. Permeable brick pavers were installed in driveways and at the lane way entrances; these allow rainwater to infiltrate between their joints and into the ground, reducing runoff, the bane of municipal storm sewer systems. The grassed lane ways are cooler than asphalt in summer and they don't emit the dreaded "off-gassing."[16] These alleys-turned-lanes have become living quarters and places where neighbors socialize.

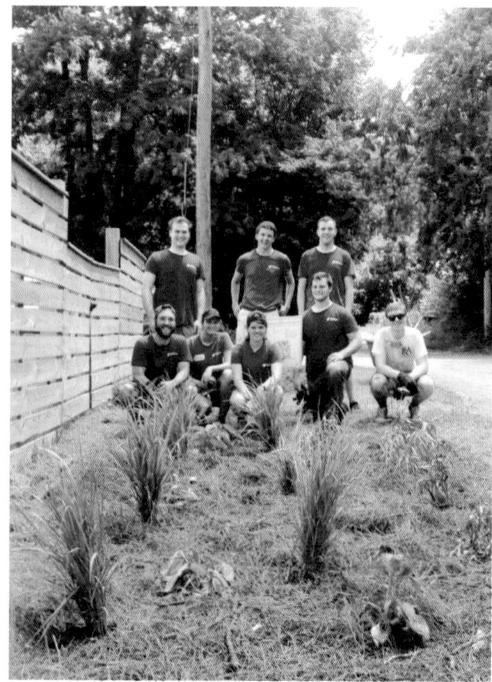

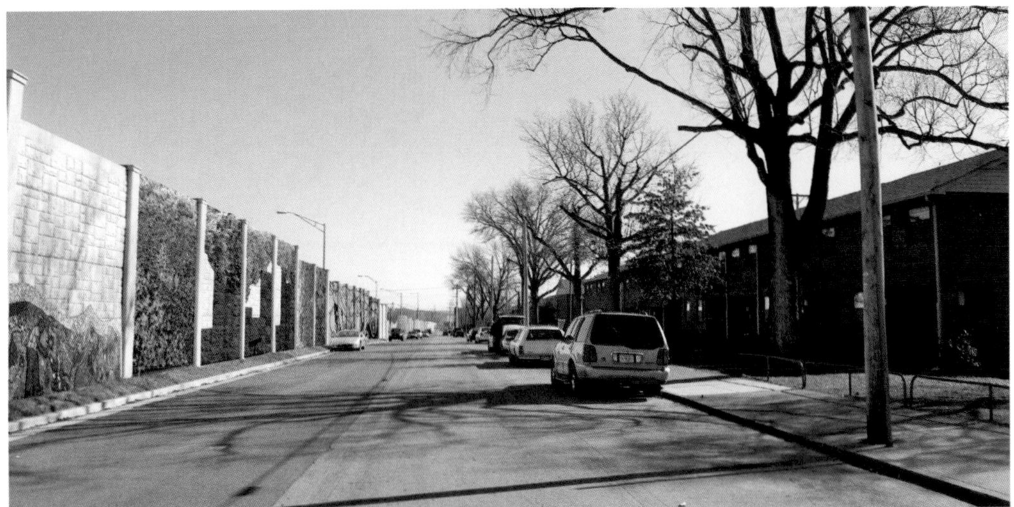

STRATEGY: *Install built and natural infrastructure to mitigate light, air, and noise pollution for residents living in close proximity to urban interstates. Owners and managers of outdoor venues in close proximity to urban housing should work with residents to develop a mutually acceptable plan for noise control consistent with Metro's "excessive noise" regulations (Ordinance No. BL2008-259).*

Conceptual design for "greening" an existing sound wall adjacent to the Sudekum apartments in South Nashville adorned with plantings and public art. Such walls mitigate freeway noise. Other buffers, such as dense plantings of evergreen trees, also remove pollution. *(Visualization, 2010: Ron Yearwood, NCDC)*

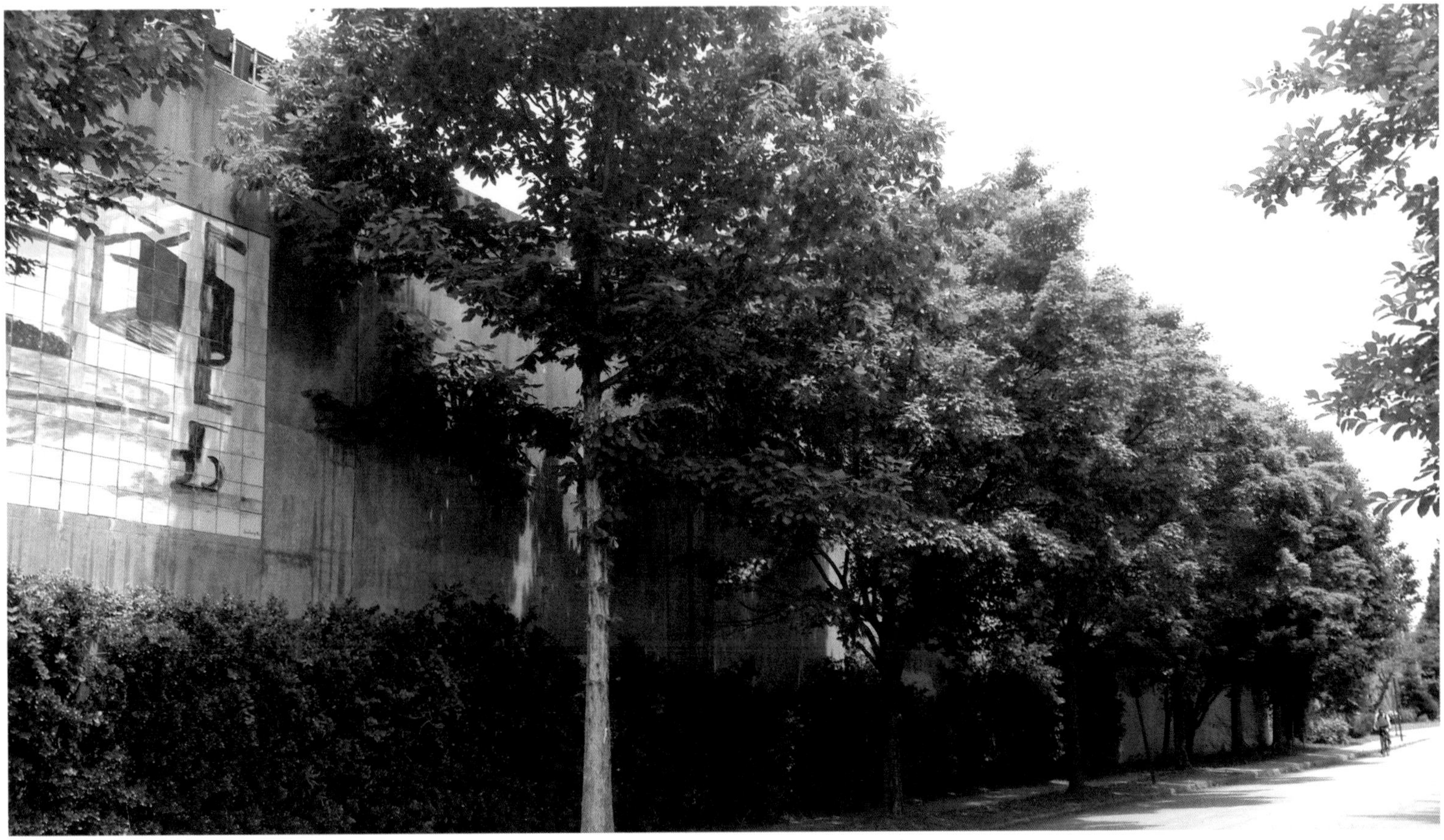

Sound wall and dense vegetation along the Husley Yard railroad corridor in Atlanta, Georgia, help protect nearby residents from noise and air pollution; the trees shade sidewalks during hot summers. *(2013)*

Bird's eye view of "Spaghetti Junction" in Northeast Nashville. The bloated interchange creates a daunting pedestrian barrier for residents of Sam Levy Homes—a 226-unit federal Hope VI public housing makeover—trying to access the businesses and public transit line on Main Street. Note also the vast amount of surface parking in the area, much of which is fully utilized only for Titans' football games. *(© 2012: Google)*

Right top: Plan for the roadway reconfiguration of "Spaghetti Junction" and 16 new urban blocks. *(Drawing, 2012: UTK College of Architecture and Design)*

Right lower: View of proposed redevelopment looking west from Main Street toward downtown Nashville. *(Rendering, 2012: Tyrone Bunyon, UTK College of Architecture and Design)*

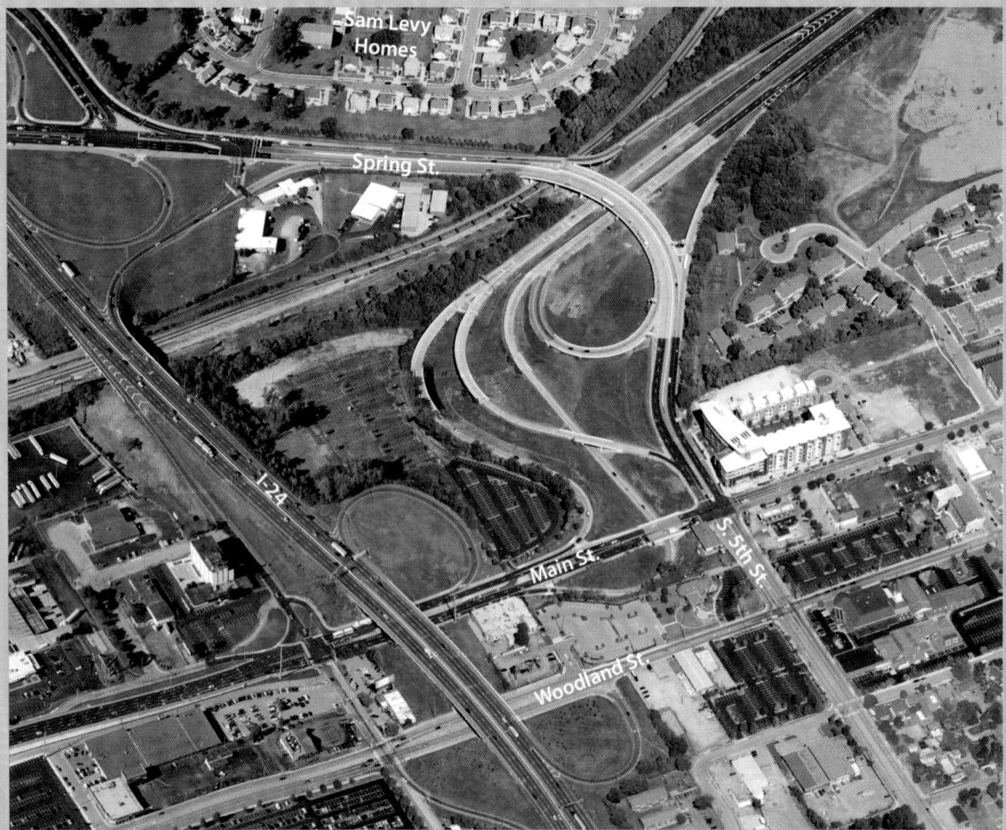

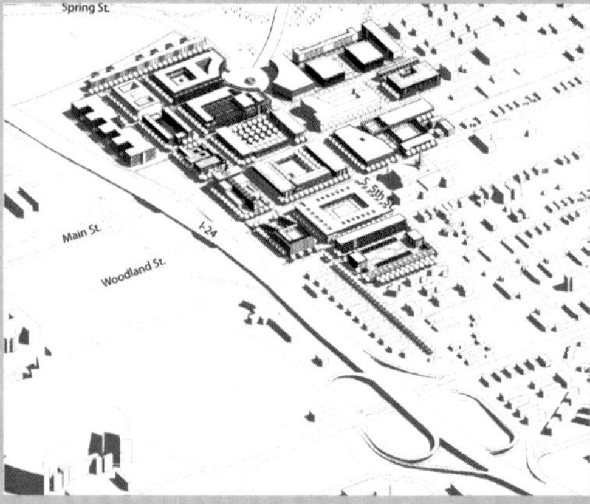

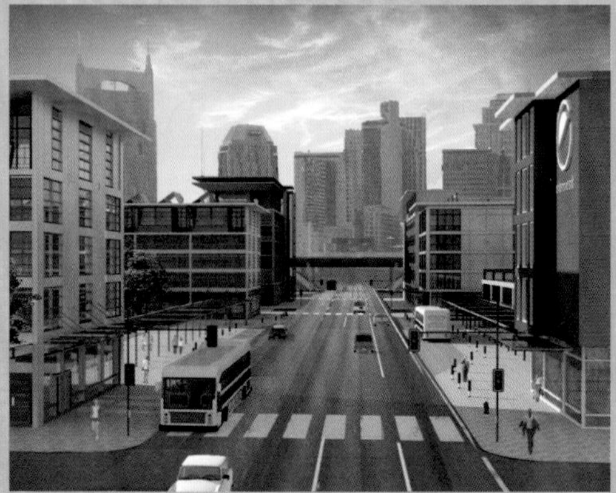

Spaghetti Junction Makeover

In response to the seeking-the-center trend in US metropolitan areas, with its resultant rise in property values, city officials and developers are pursuing opportunities offered by underutilized and economically underperforming parcels in urban areas. One obvious target is the land occupied by over-engineered and aging interstate cloverleaf ramps. Highway reconfiguration allows municipalities to create developable land, a limited commodity in the urban transect zone.

"Spaghetti Junction"—the phrase used in *The Plan of Nashville* to describe the convergence of Ellington Parkway, Spring Street, and I-24 in Northeast Nashville—sprawls over 95 acres just across the Cumberland River from the downtown core. Reestablishing a neighborhood street grid and designing more compact highway ramps would reapportion approximately 70 acres for private development. By comparison, the Gulch Master Plan encompasses approximately 60 acres and features over 4,500 residential units, 1.5 million square feet of office space and half a million square feet of retail and restaurants.

In 2012, University of Tennessee-Knoxville College of Architecture and Design professor T. K. Davis asked the students in his spring design studio to re-imagine the "Junction," following the precedent of the Gulch Master Plan and *The Plan of Nashville's* proposal for redevelopment of this site. Assuming the implementation of Nashville's East-West bus rapid transit, they designed a transit-oriented, mixed-use development with an emphasis on walkability. Sixteen urban blocks of mid-rise structures embrace the Fifth & Main building as a central component in an interconnected eastside neighborhood. Taking advantage of the site's natural gradations, the majority of parking is placed below street level.

The on/off ramp modifications in the students' schematic plan would alleviate the divisive impact of the highways, introduce high-performing development opportunities, create the potential for millions in new property tax dollars, and increase the density necessary to support public transit: all goals worthy of government investment.

—RON YEARWOOD
assistant director, NCDC

TRANSPORTATION

✓ Health-Promoting

Urban communities have a high level of transportation connectivity via a network of streets and sidewalks that serve automobiles, public transit, cyclists, and pedestrians. A street grid mitigates traffic congestion because vehicles can disperse through multiple routes to reach destinations. Bus service in the urban zone is usually more frequent due to the typically higher ridership levels.

✗ Health-Defeating

Traffic congestion on major roadways accessing downtown, especially near junctures with interstates, contributes to air pollution.

Because bus routes converge at downtown's Music City Central transit facility, riders traveling to destinations outside the core must often transfer, adding to their travel time. Such commuters may choose to drive, which lessens their physical activity and increases air pollution.

The limited number of dedicated bike paths within the city discourages cycling in urban areas, especially where there are high levels of traffic and congestion. Existing bike lanes are not buffered from vehicular traffic. Storm grates with vertical slots parallel to the curb—so-called "bike killers"—trap tires, send cyclists flying over the handlebars, and engender lawsuits against the city. Limited safety education for both cyclists and motorists contributes to dangerous conditions.

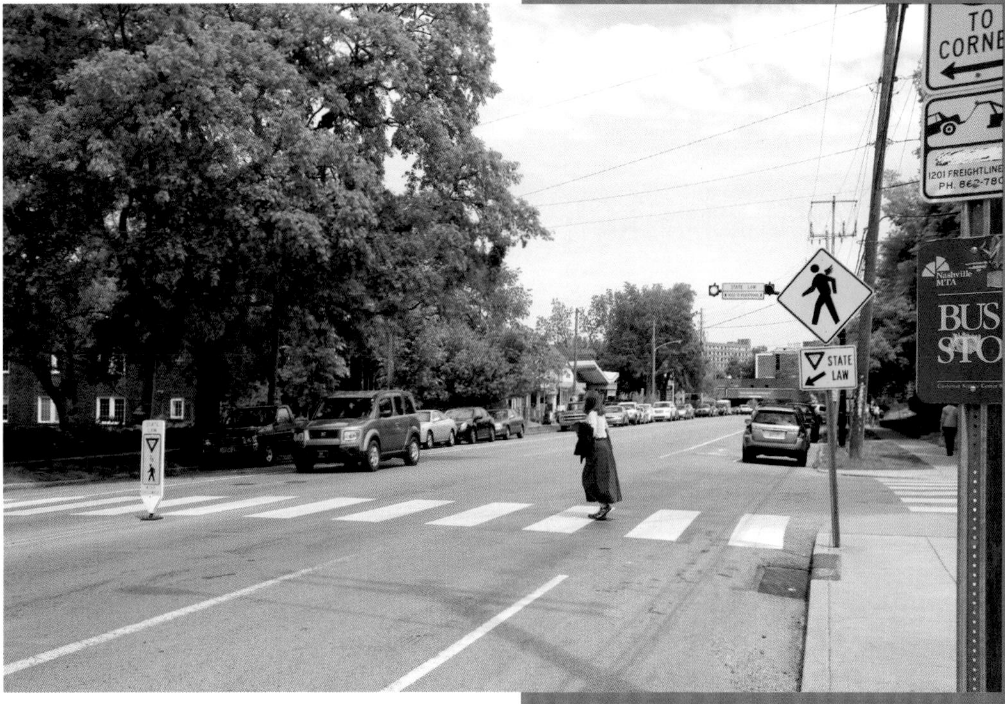

✓ Belmont Boulevard exhibits the multiple transportation options of what's called a complete street: sidewalks, bus stops, and dedicated bike lanes, as well as lanes for cars.[17] Note the enhanced pedestrian safety features, such as clearly marked crosswalks, planting strips to buffer sidewalks, and on-street parking that slows vehicular traffic. *(2013)*

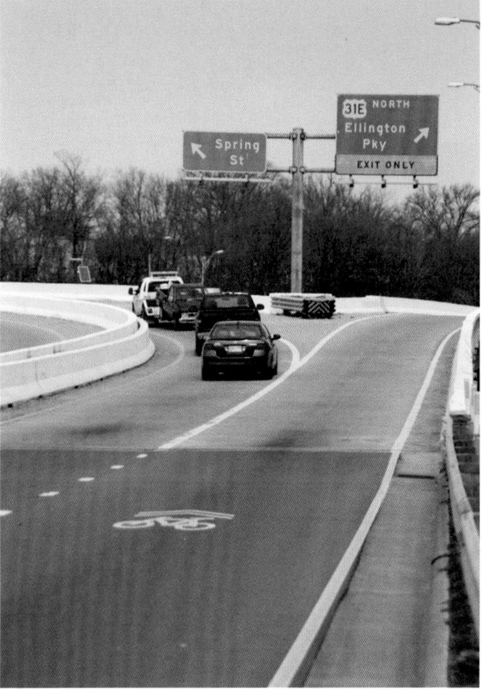

"Riding a bicycle should not require bravery. Yet, all too often, that is the perception among cyclists and non-cyclists alike."

Roger Geller, bicycle coordinator, Portland Bureau of Transportation

✗ Bike sharrow near Ellington Parkway misleads cyclists and motorists alike. Signage appears to direct bikes onto the parkway rather than toward Spring Street, exacerbating an already challenging cycling situation. *(2013)*

MTA's University Connector route serves TSU, Fisk, Meharry, Vanderbilt, Belmont, and Lipscomb, with connections to 11 different bus routes that radiate from the downtown transit hub. Note that a proposed extension would connect to Watkins College of Art, Design & Film. This route, introduced in 2012, was the first line connecting destinations that doesn't do so via the central hub *(Diagram over map, 2013: Eric Hoke, NCDC)*

Right top: The 28th/31st Avenue Connector just prior to its opening in 2012. This example of a complete street, which features Nashville's first protected bike lane, accommodates cars, public transit, cyclists, and pedestrians within a right of way that also includes sustainable landscaping and public art. *(2012)*

Right lower: Conceptual rendering of the Centennial Park stop on West End Avenue for a proposed BRT line that has yet to be implemented due to opposition by those concerned that the line's dedicated lane would increase auto congestion. *(Rendering, 2013: Transit Alliance of Middle Tennessee)*

STRATEGY: *Expand frequency of transit service in highly urban areas. Continue to implement more connector routes.*

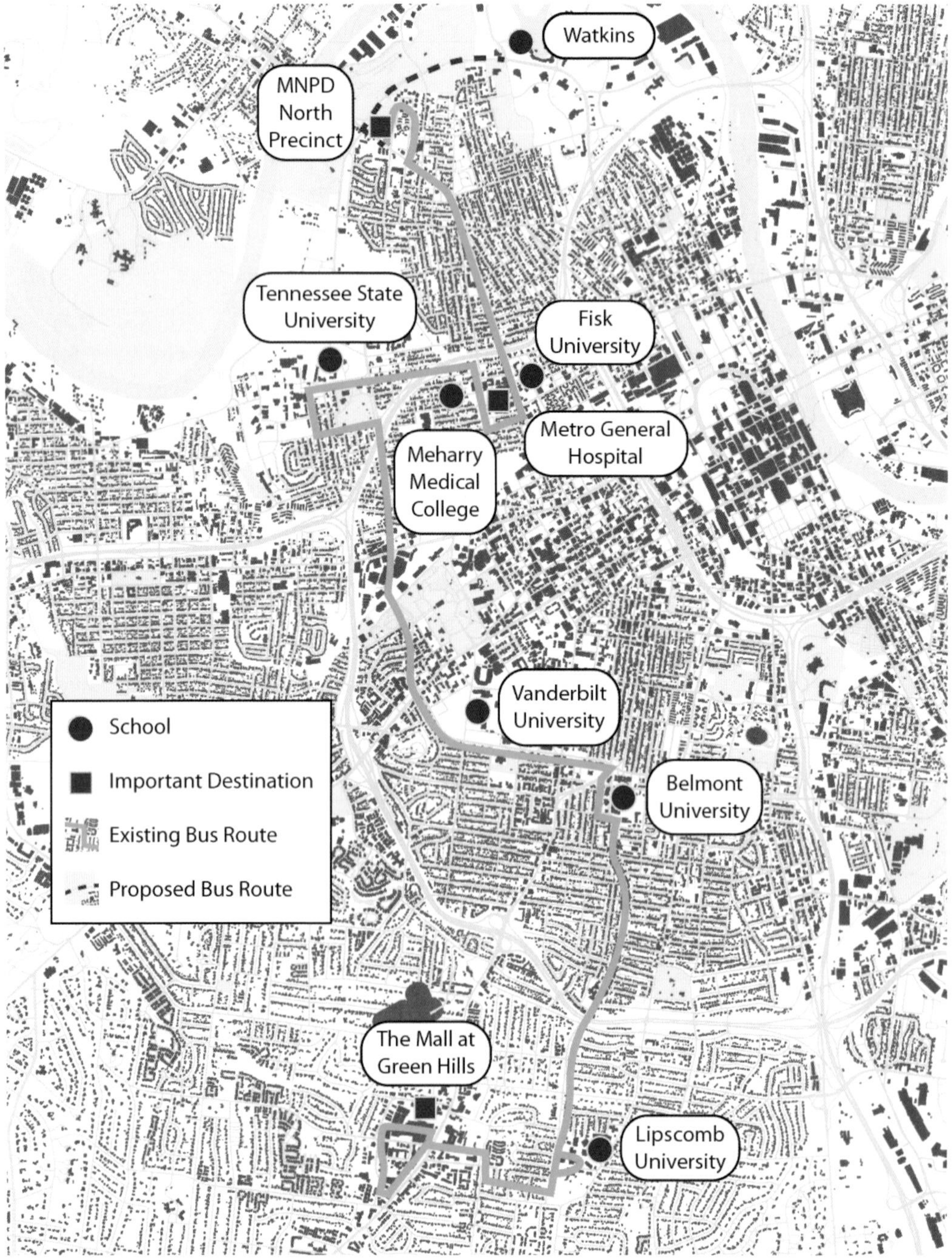

STRATEGY: *Enhance the multimodal transportation experience: public transit, automobiles, cycling, and walking.*

STRATEGY: *Implement Nashville's first dedicated lane bus rapid transit (BRT) line, the East-West Connector.*

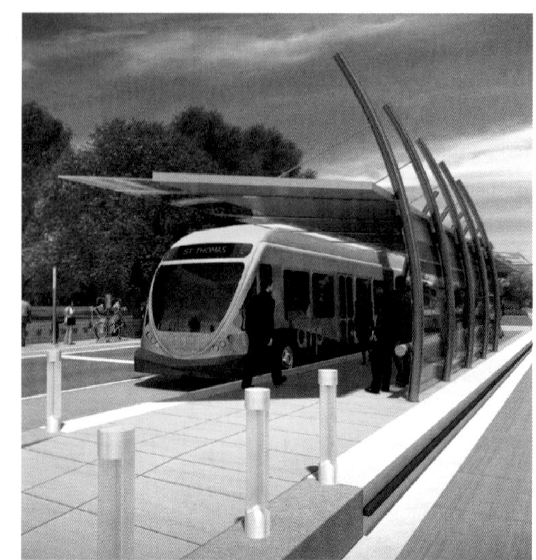

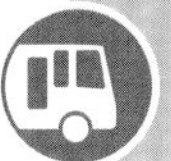

The East-West Connector

The Metro Transit Authority's 2009 Master Plan prioritized the Broadway-West End corridor to expand Bus Rapid Transit (BRT) services from Gallatin Road in East Nashville. "This corridor was selected," according to MTA, "because the route serves the densest segment of Nashville and Middle Tennessee. No other route connects as many critical economic elements including universities, hospitals, businesses, tourist and cultural attractions, entertainment venues, dense residential areas and centers of local, state, and federal government."[18]

In October of 2014, Mayor Karl Dean announced that he would no longer pursue federal funding for the project. What happened? The answer illustrates how practically and politically difficult it is—and will be—to retrofit for mass transit a transportation infrastructure designed for cars.

No one questions that congestion on Nashville's central East/West artery is bad—and certain to get worse. Thus it seemed logical to use this corridor for a transit line in its own dedicated lane to provide service faster than a single-occupancy vehicle and connect to the Gallatin BRT, which currently has the highest ridership in the system.

Such thinking, however, flies in the face of public transportation realities in Nashville: the South's long cultural linkage between transit ridership and low incomes (hence those who argued for a route on Charlotte Pike, immediately adjacent to African American neighborhoods); the fondness for the continuous turn-lanes on West End that provide access to venues with front-loaded parking; and the lack of recognition by older and wealthier residents that this plan focused on riders of the future: the millennials, who are eschewing drivers' licenses for ear buds and laptops on their public-vehicle commutes.

MTA is conducting public workshops to ascertain what Nashvillians want and will accept in public transportation. Stay tuned.

—CHRISTINE KREYLING

STRATEGY: *Increase the network of dedicated bike lanes. Implementation should be in the form of protected lanes that feature barriers physically separating cyclists from cars as much as possible. Such lanes are much safer than the traditional painted lines on pavement.*

A study of residents in Portland, Oregon, found that a majority—60 percent—want to ride their bikes, but are afraid a car will hit them.[19] With a goal of making Chicago the most bike-friendly city in the United States, city officials recently pledged to construct 100 miles of protected bike lanes by the year 2015.[20] After surviving a legal challenge by car-centric residents, the Prospect Park West protected bike lane in Brooklyn has reduced automotive speeding rates from 74 percent to 20 percent with crashes and injuries dropping by 63 percent. Travel time for motorists and congestion did not increase.[21]

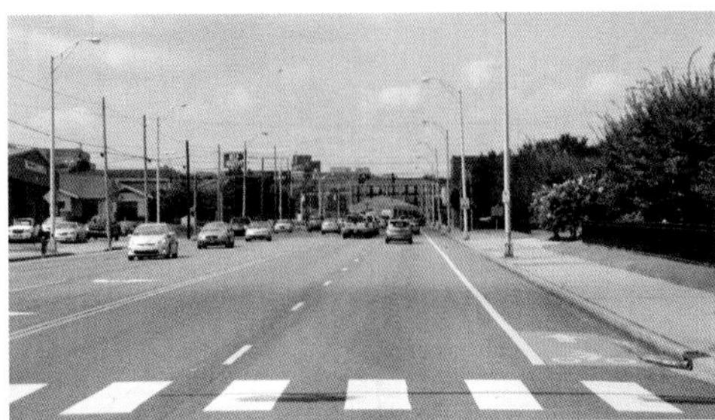

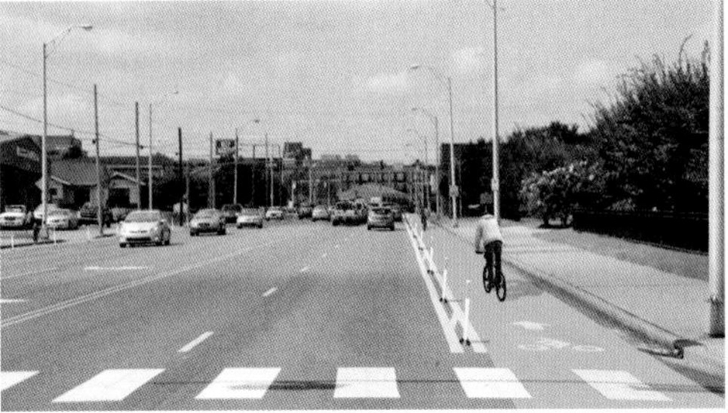

Far left: Existing cycling infrastructure on Charlotte Avenue. (2013)

Left: Conceptual illustration of Charlotte Avenue with dedicated bike rapid transit infrastructure, including protective bollards. A grade difference between bike lane and sidewalk would also increase safety for pedestrians. (Visualization, 2013: Eric Hoke, NCDC)

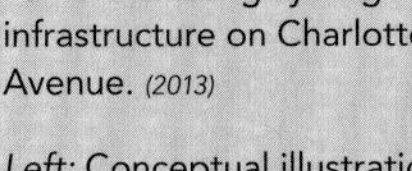

STRATEGY: *Expand the use of the B-cycle program, particularly in low income neighborhoods, to more commercial neighborhood centers in the urban zone, where residents might not have access to cars.*

This membership and fee-based bike-share program is designed to provide an alternative transportation option for business, shopping, and meal trips. Partner with business groups, multifamily residences, and universities in urban districts to install bike stations. (See Downtown transect zone chapter, p. 231 for further information on B-cycle.)

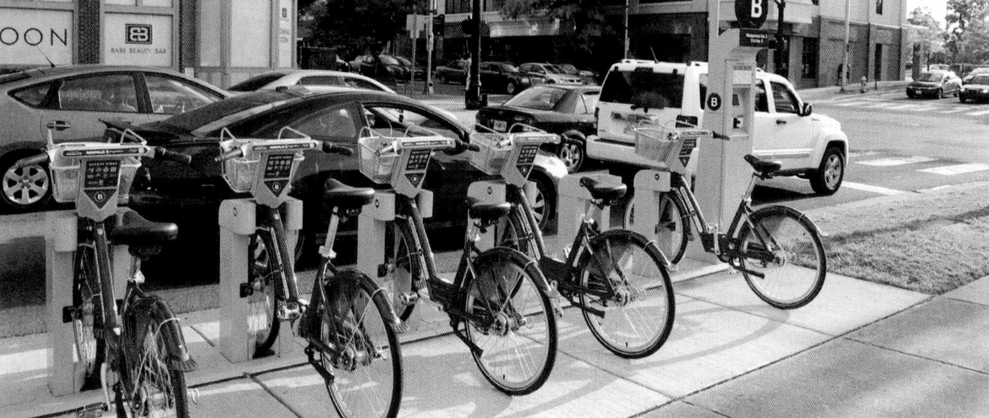

B-cycle station in Hillsboro Village. (2013: Nashville Downtown Partnership)

The plan to construct a greenway along I-440 is not new. The proposal was part of the original construction plans developed by the Tennessee Department of Transportation in 1980 but was never implemented. The proposed 3.6-mile greenway would connect Tennessee State University to Centennial Park, and then parallel I-440 all the way to the Tennessee State Fairgrounds and Trevecca University. *(Plan, 2013: Lose & Associates)*

Update: Mayor Dean's 2015/2016 budget allocates one million dollars to connect the 1.5 mile stretch between Hadley Park and Elmington Park. The city already owns the land, decreasing the cost of the project.

STRATEGY: *Implement the I-440 Greenway Plan as an alternative transportation corridor.*

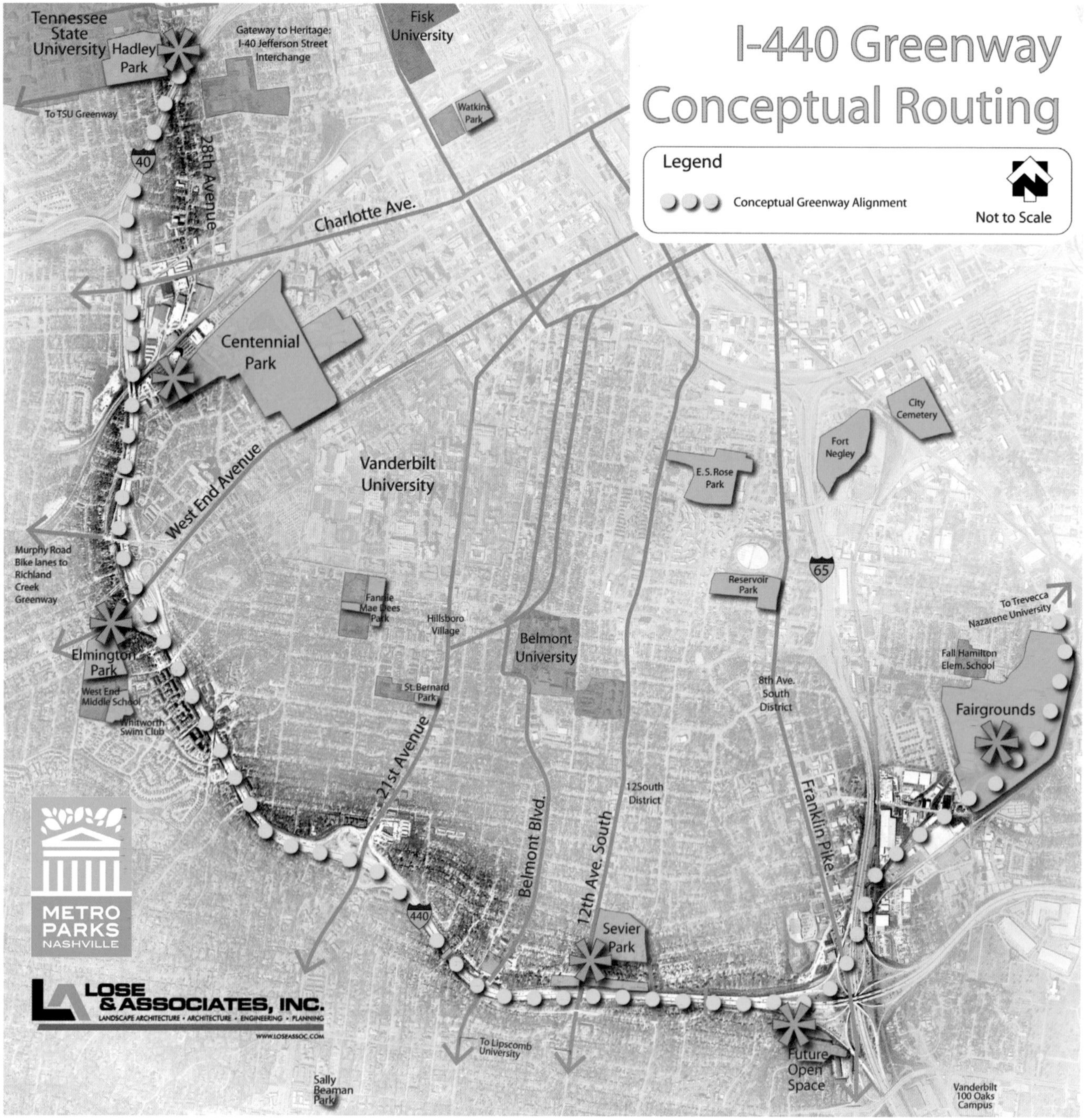

I-440 Greenway Conceptual Routing

Legend

Conceptual Greenway Alignment

Not to Scale

Tennessee State University
Hadley Park
Gateway to Heritage: I-40 Jefferson Street Interchange
Fisk University
Watkins Park
To TSU Greenway
28th Avenue
Charlotte Ave.
Centennial Park
West End Avenue
Vanderbilt University
Murphy Road Bike lanes to Richland Creek Greenway
Elmington Park
West End Middle School
Whitworth Swim Club
Fannie Mae Dees Park
Hillsboro Village
St. Bernard Park
21st Avenue
Belmont University
Belmont Blvd.
12th Ave. South
12South District
Sevier Park
To Lipscomb University
Sally Beaman Park
E.S. Rose Park
Reservoir Park
Fort Negley
City Cemetery
8th Ave. South District
Franklin Pike
Future Open Space
Vanderbilt 100 Oaks Campus
To Trevecca Nazarene University
Fall Hamilton Elem. School
Fairgrounds

METRO PARKS NASHVILLE

LOSE & ASSOCIATES, INC.
LANDSCAPE ARCHITECTURE • ARCHITECTURE • ENGINEERING • PLANNING
WWW.LOSEASSOC.COM

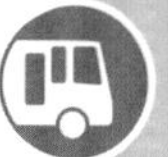

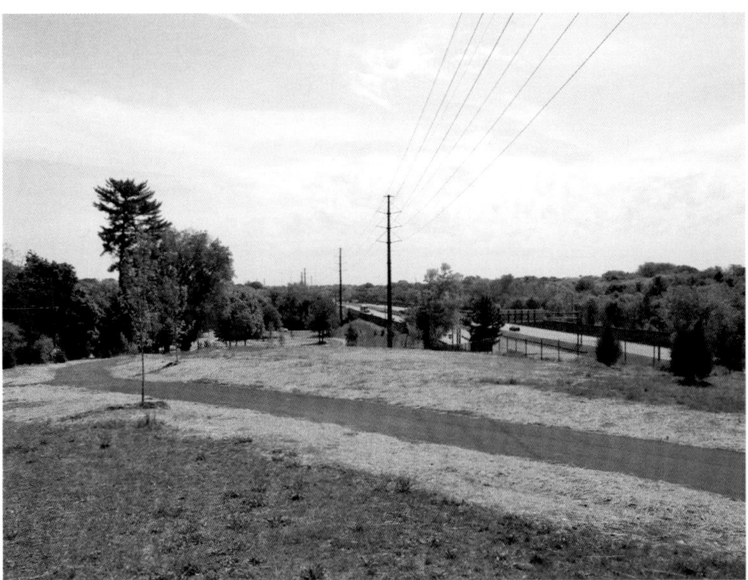

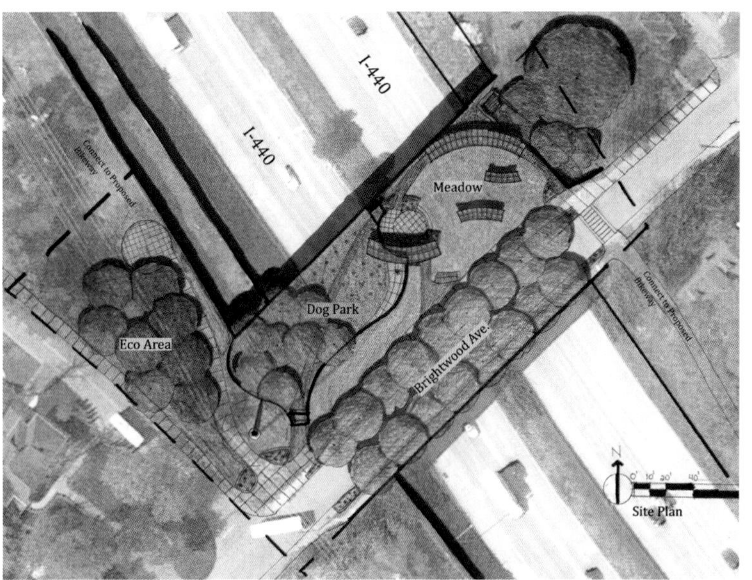

Left: New greenway adjacent to I-440 along Gale Lane from Granny White Pike to Lealand Lane is a step toward realizing the I-440 Greenway Plan. *(2013)*

Conceptual plan for transforming the greenspace on the existing bridge over I-440 along Brightwood Avenue into an active park space connecting two neighborhoods. *(Drawing, 2010: Brent Hunter, NCDC)*

STRATEGY: *Implement multimodal Sundays on prominent streets in Nashville to promote cycling, walking, and rollerblading and to build community interaction on a citywide scale.*

Ciclovía

Cities around the globe are developing innovative ways to create temporary civic spaces. "Ciclovía" (literally "bike path") began in Bogotá, Colombia, in 1976. Its intent was to create safe and fun environments for cyclists. Each Sunday, the city closed off portions of streets to all motorized traffic and welcomed pedestrians and cyclists. The temporary closure of roads to automobiles offered healthy recreation and social interaction activities.

San Francisco modeled its "Sunday Streets," which commenced in 2008, after Ciclovía. For ten Sundays out of the year, various streets around the city are closed to automobiles. In March of 2013, the city closed the entire length of its famous waterfront, Embarcadero. The streets were packed with cyclists and pedestrians encompassing all age groups. Activities and live music were dispersed along the three-mile route, including yoga classes, bluegrass string groups, impromptu dancing, street art, and pedal-car shows.

—RON YEARWOOD
assistant director, NCDC

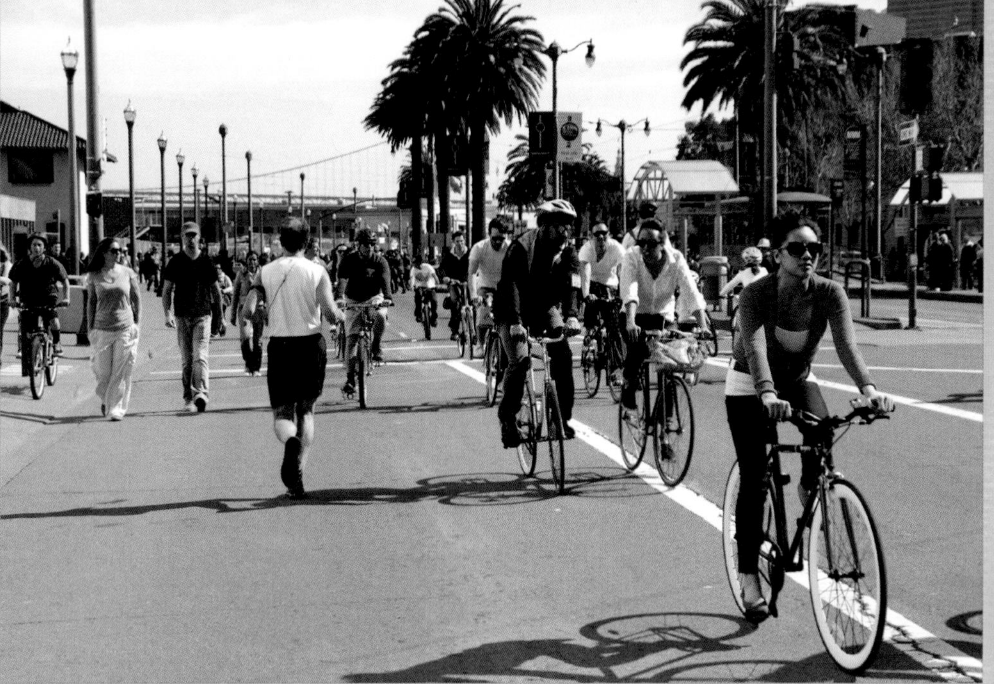

Sunday Streets along the Embarcadero in San Francisco. Note that the road closures do not disrupt the city's historic trolley line, which maintains its regular operation through the crowded street, emphasizing the symbiotic relationship between motorized transit, people, and bikes. *(2013)*

✗ Pre-improvements, Dickerson Pike was an environment hostile to pedestrians, cyclists, and transit riders. Note the continuous curb cuts, severely eroded sidewalk, inhospitable bus stop, and landscape dominated by utility poles and wires. *(2004)*

Streetscaping initiatives along the same section of Dickerson Pike restored sidewalks and added stamped crosswalks and bike sharrow. The lighting, however, remains car-centric. Note also the difference in pedestrian ambience between the portion of the sidewalk flanked by buildings and the sidewalk across the street with large curb cuts for "out front" parking. Urban redevelopment of these large parking lots will help complete the street's transformation to a truly walkable community. Although the use of painted and stamped asphalt crosswalks—an inexpensive way to replicate brick or other distinctive paving—emphasizes the walkway for both pedestrians and motorists, visibility erodes quickly without regular maintenance. *(2013)*

✓ Signage on Eastland Avenue in East Nashville alerts drivers to be cautious in this high traffic pedestrian area. Note the traffic calming feature of on-street parking and the planting strip flanking the sidewalk. The new commercial infill to the right is pulled up to the sidewalk in the manner of the traditional storefront to the left. *(2013)*

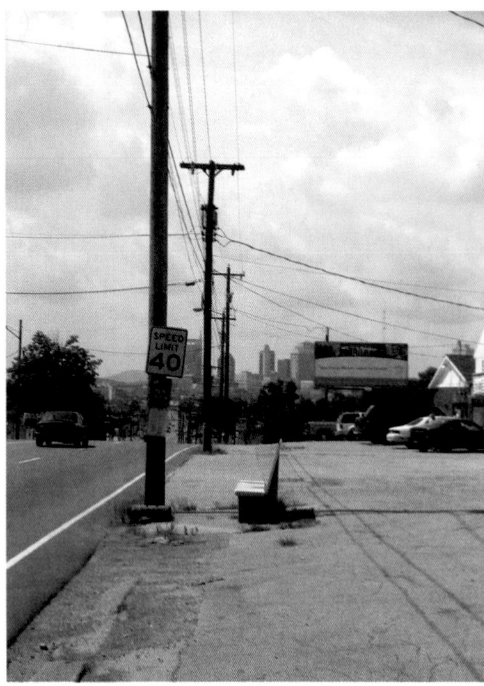

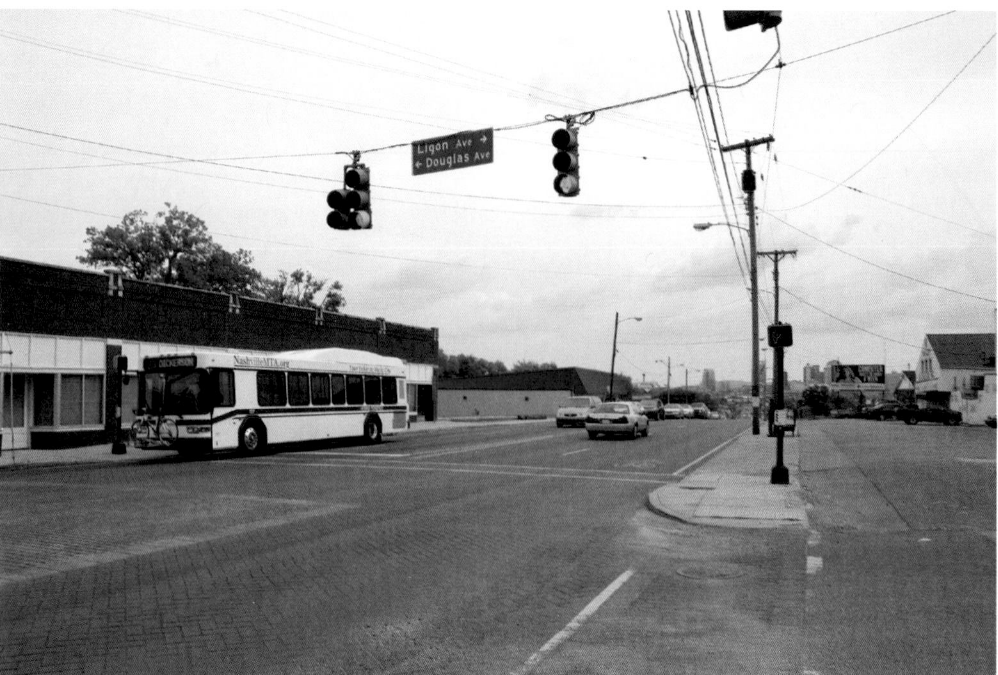

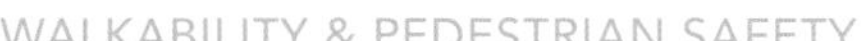

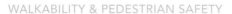

WALKABILITY & PEDESTRIAN SAFETY

✓ Health-Promoting

Sidewalks are abundant in urban areas; progress has been made toward the installation of pedestrian safety signage in some neighborhoods. Access to parks at both the neighborhood and regional scale through the greenway system provides urban residents with active transportation options as well as opportunities for exercise.

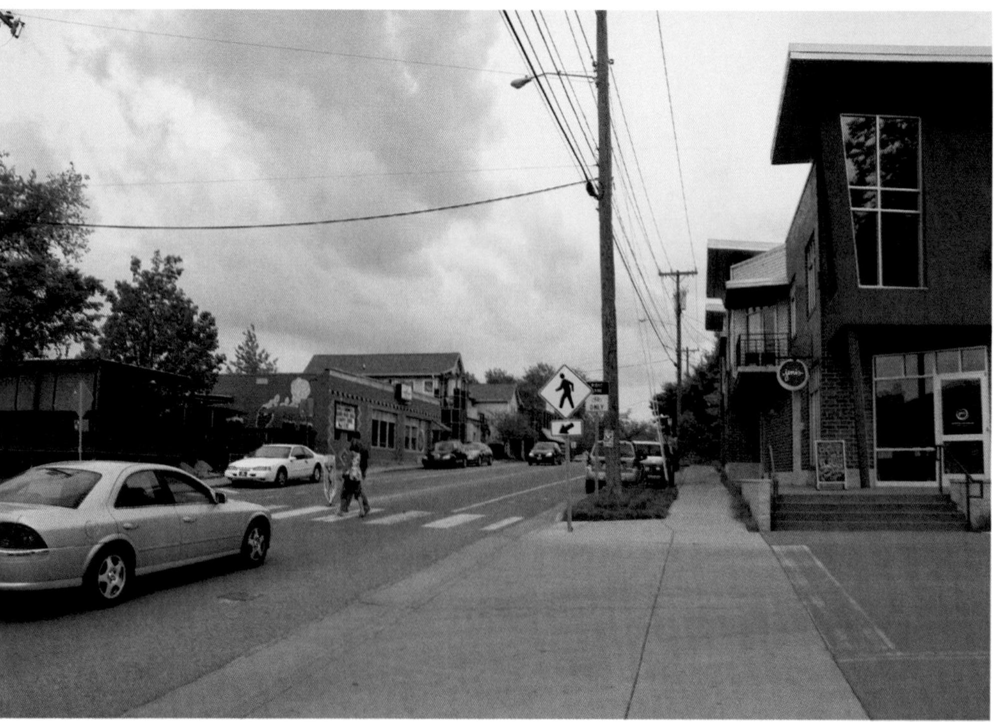

X Health-Defeating

While sidewalks are frequently present in the urban zone, some neighborhoods in the zone still lack them, and existing sidewalks may be poorly designed, too narrow, and exposed to vehicular traffic for safety.

Many urban areas also lack adequate pedestrian safety infrastructure: human-scale lighting, clearly marked crosswalks, and pedestrian signage.

Limited access highways and their interchanges present pedestrians in urban neighborhoods with challenging barriers to safety and connectivity. The noise and air pollution that characterize these highways also make walking unpleasant.

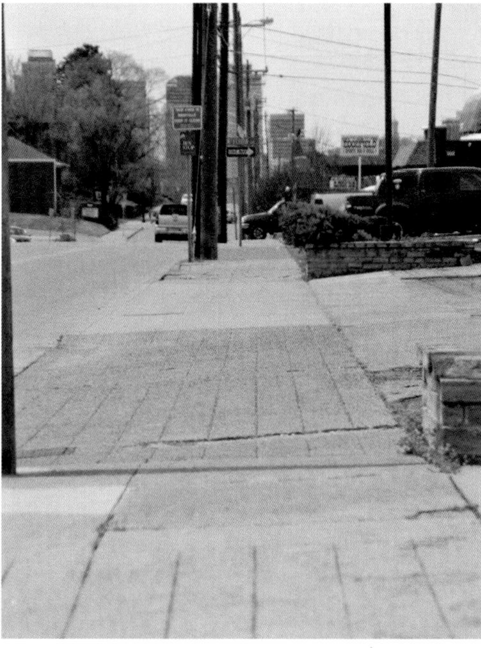

X Woodland Street in East Nashville just west of Five Points. Even in neighborhoods considered reliably walkable, excessive curb cuts bring pedestrians and vehicles into direct conflict. In the 1970s, Nashville's traffic engineers called for this section of Woodland Street to become four lanes with a 60-foot right-of-way. While this plan was fortunately never implemented, the suburban-style building setbacks, front-loaded parking, and curb cuts anticipating this change remain. *(2013)*

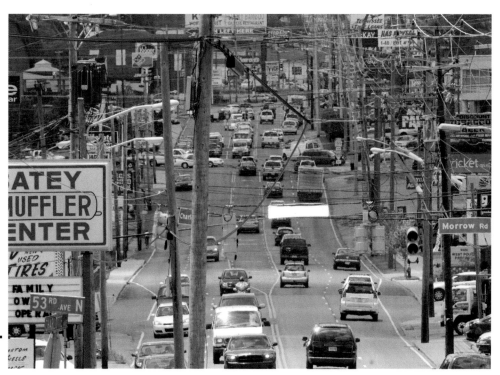

X This section of Charlotte Pike, which lies in the urban zone near the Nations neighborhood in West Nashville, visually defines "dysfunctional" for all transportation modes. Features that in particular test the pedestrian: the cacophony of auto-oriented signage, as well as sidewalks fragmented by curb cuts and utility poles. Note also the lone—some might say crazed—cyclist pedaling against the flow of car traffic. *(2012: Gary Layda)*

"Pedestrians should not be treated as second class citizens; actually, we are all pedestrians. Every trip begins and ends with walking, to places, to public transit, to the bike, or to the car. From the point of view of vulnerability the pedestrian is clearly on top. We need to make pedestrians the top priority in all cities, with emphasis on the children, the older adult, and the handicapped."

—Gil Penalosa, executive director, 8-80 Cities

A crosswalk signal at the Public Square that allows pedestrians to begin to cross the street before the light turns green for automobiles. Some signalized crosswalks in Nashville do not even operate for pedestrians unless they push a button for a "Walk" sign, reflecting a traffic engineering philosophy dedicated to moving cars. *(2013)*

STRATEGY: *Apply Metro's Complete Streets Policy to provide a network of sidewalks and bike lanes linking residential and commercial areas. It must be acknowledged, however, that the limited public rights-of-way in many traditional urban areas restrict full implementation of these policies, especially for infill projects. Planners and designers must often balance the need for greater building density with the desirability of wider sidewalks, bike lanes, and on-street parking. (For a fuller discussion, see "The Transect" chapter, "Making the Complete Street," p. 44.)*

STRATEGY: *Use traffic calming tactics in areas where pedestrians and automobiles intersect. Such tactics include crosswalks with pedestrian signage, as well as narrower lane widths, which decrease drivers' perceptions of their own safety and thus slow speeds. Another approach is the reduction in the number of permissible "right on red" automobile turnings at intersections with heavy auto traffic. While drivers are legally required to come to a complete stop before turning and must yield to pedestrians, many do not, and ticketing of violators by traffic police is minimal to non-existent. (See also the discussion in "Downtown Transect Zone," p. 232.)*

STRATEGY: *Introduce pedestrian-priority signalization for crosswalks throughout Nashville's urban areas.*

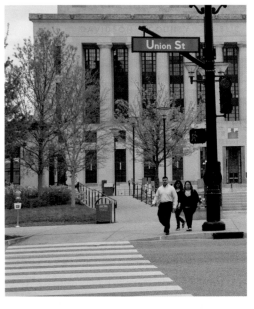

STRATEGY: *Mitigate the disruptive impact of interstate highways.* The Plan of Nashville *set forth a four-step plan for healing the scars created by interstates.*[22] *The steps range from making visual improvements to areas marred by these highways to actually removing highway segments and restoring the street grid.*

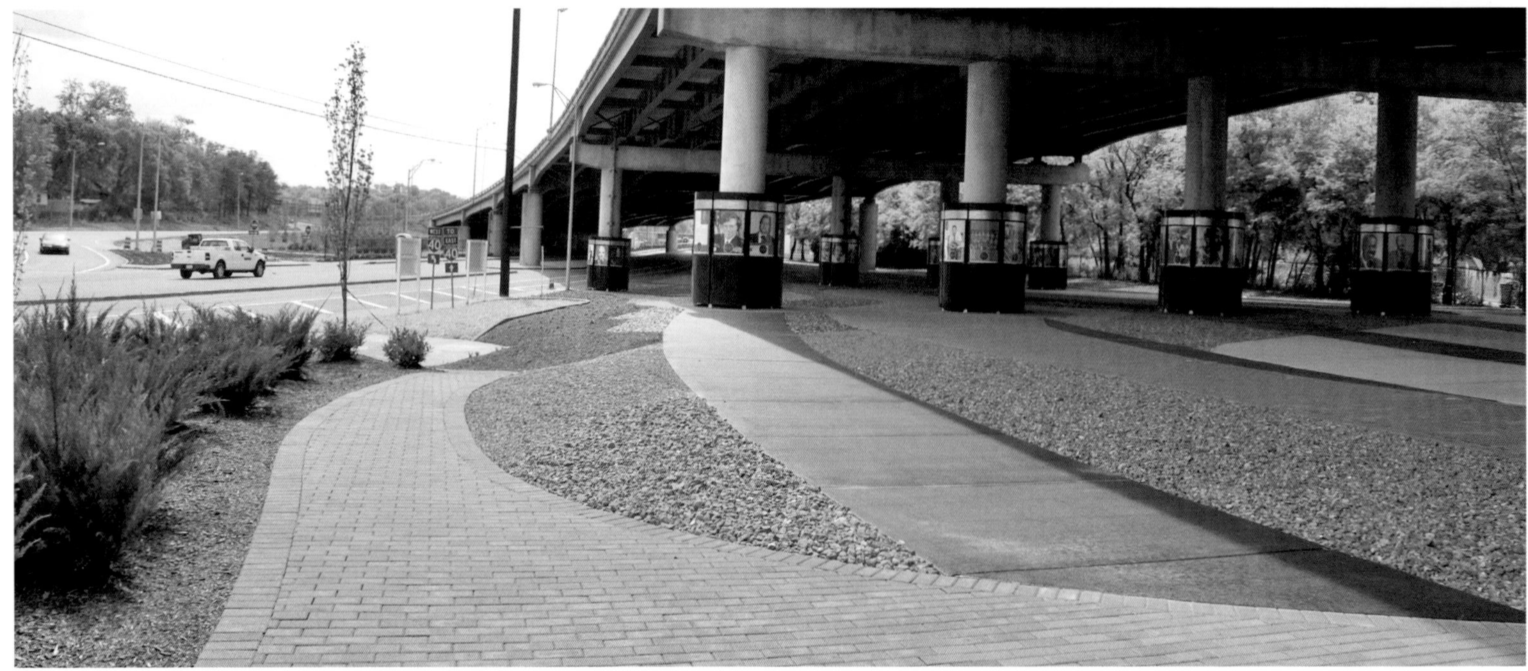

The Gateway to Heritage project on Jefferson Street is an example of step one of *The Plan of Nashville's* four-step program: cosmetic improvements. The project—which includes new landscaping, lighting, public art, and kiosks that tell the rich cultural history of the area—improves the quality of the street life below that had been so negatively affected by the construction of I-40. *(2013)*

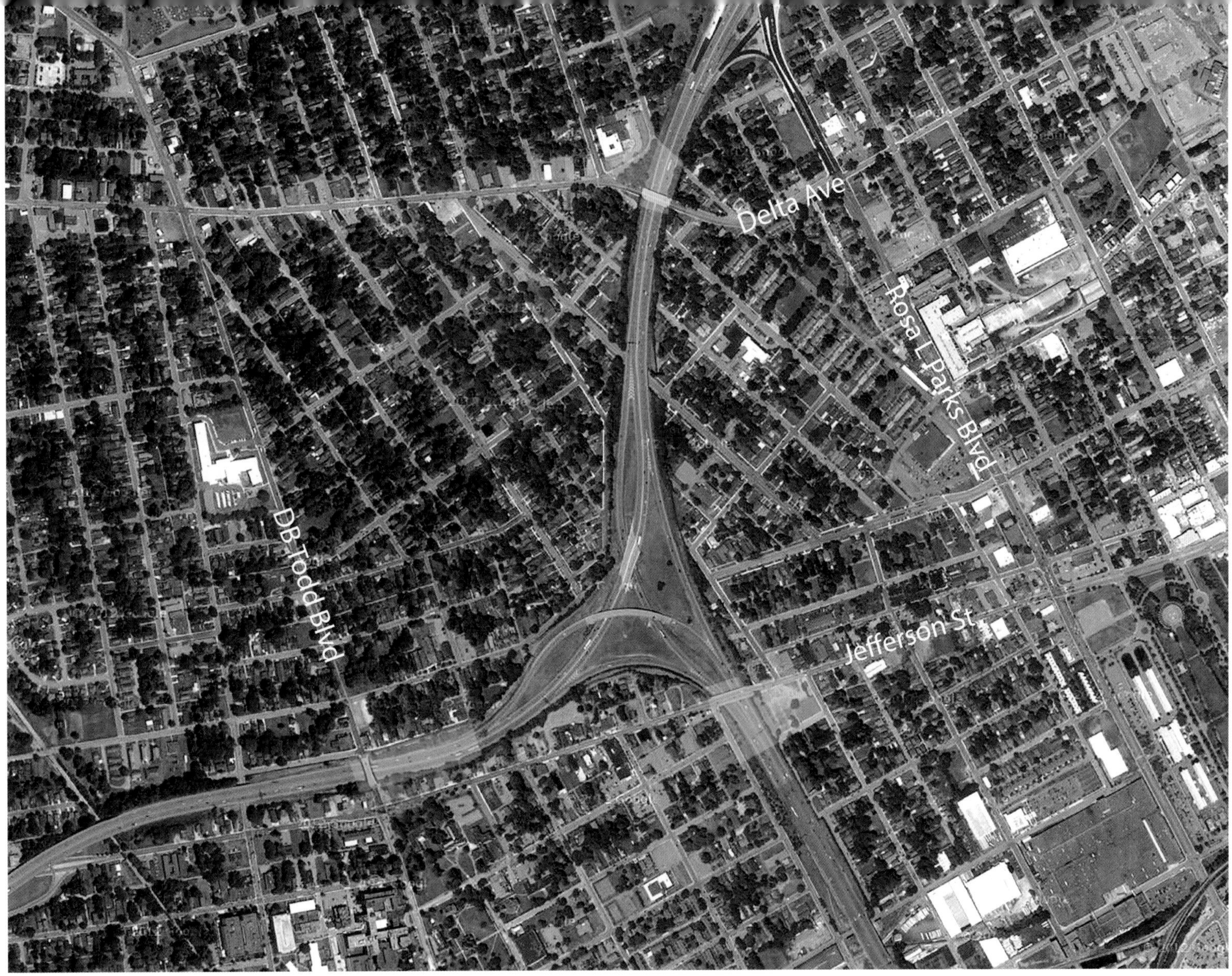

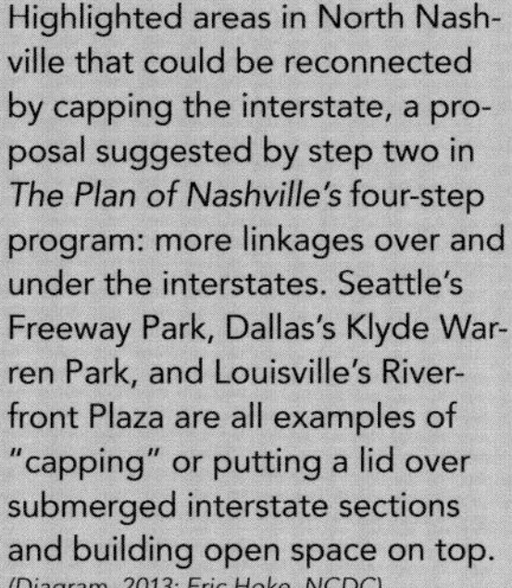

Highlighted areas in North Nashville that could be reconnected by capping the interstate, a proposal suggested by step two in *The Plan of Nashville's* four-step program: more linkages over and under the interstates. Seattle's Freeway Park, Dallas's Klyde Warren Park, and Louisville's Riverfront Plaza are all examples of "capping" or putting a lid over submerged interstate sections and building open space on top. *(Diagram, 2013: Eric Hoke, NCDC)*

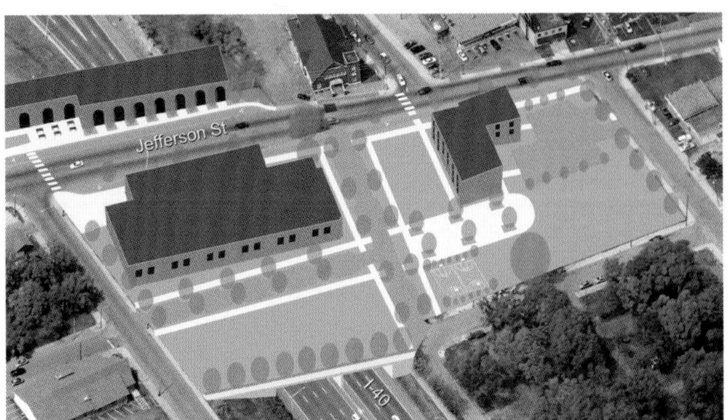

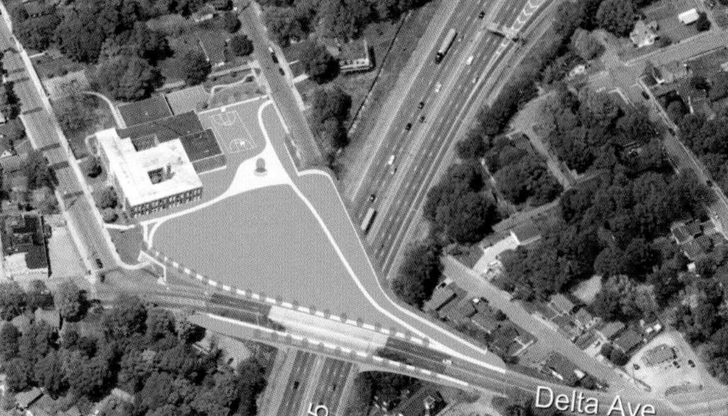

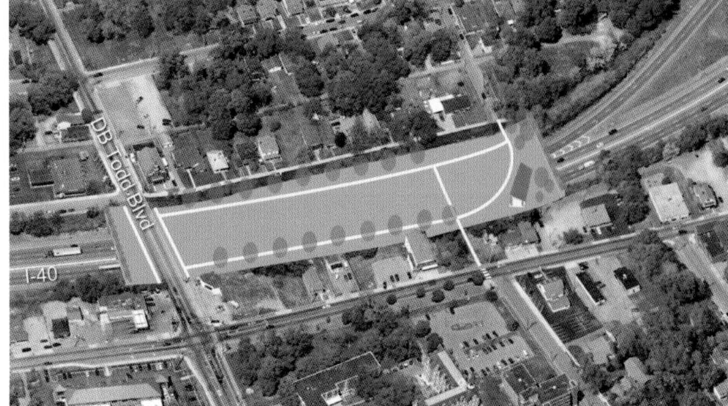

FOOD RESOURCES

✓ Health-Promoting

Increased numbers of pop-up farmers' markets, community gardens, and artisanal food shops, as well as stores and restaurants that feature locally grown and produced foodstuffs, have cropped up in Nashville's urban areas. The Healthy Corner Store Initiative, launched as a part of the Community Putting Prevention to Work (CPPW) federal grant to the Metro Health Department, has begun to address the availability of fresh produce in small convenience stores. Organizations such as Second Harvest, Nashville Food Project, and Nashville Mobile Market work to bring healthy food options, diet awareness, and cooking education to urban areas.

X Health-Defeating

Fresh produce is unavailable or can be difficult to locate in urban areas known as "food deserts." In place of healthy foods, these neighborhoods often feature a plethora of relatively cheap, calorie-dense (high fat and sugar) food options at fast food franchises, convenience stores, and gas stations. Residents in higher density multifamily housing may not have access to plots in which to grow their own food.

STRATEGY: *Make fresh, healthy food accessible for everyone.*

STRATEGY: *Connect people to food resources within their communities, with food deserts a particular target.*

STRATEGY: *Make the grocery store a building block in community planning.*

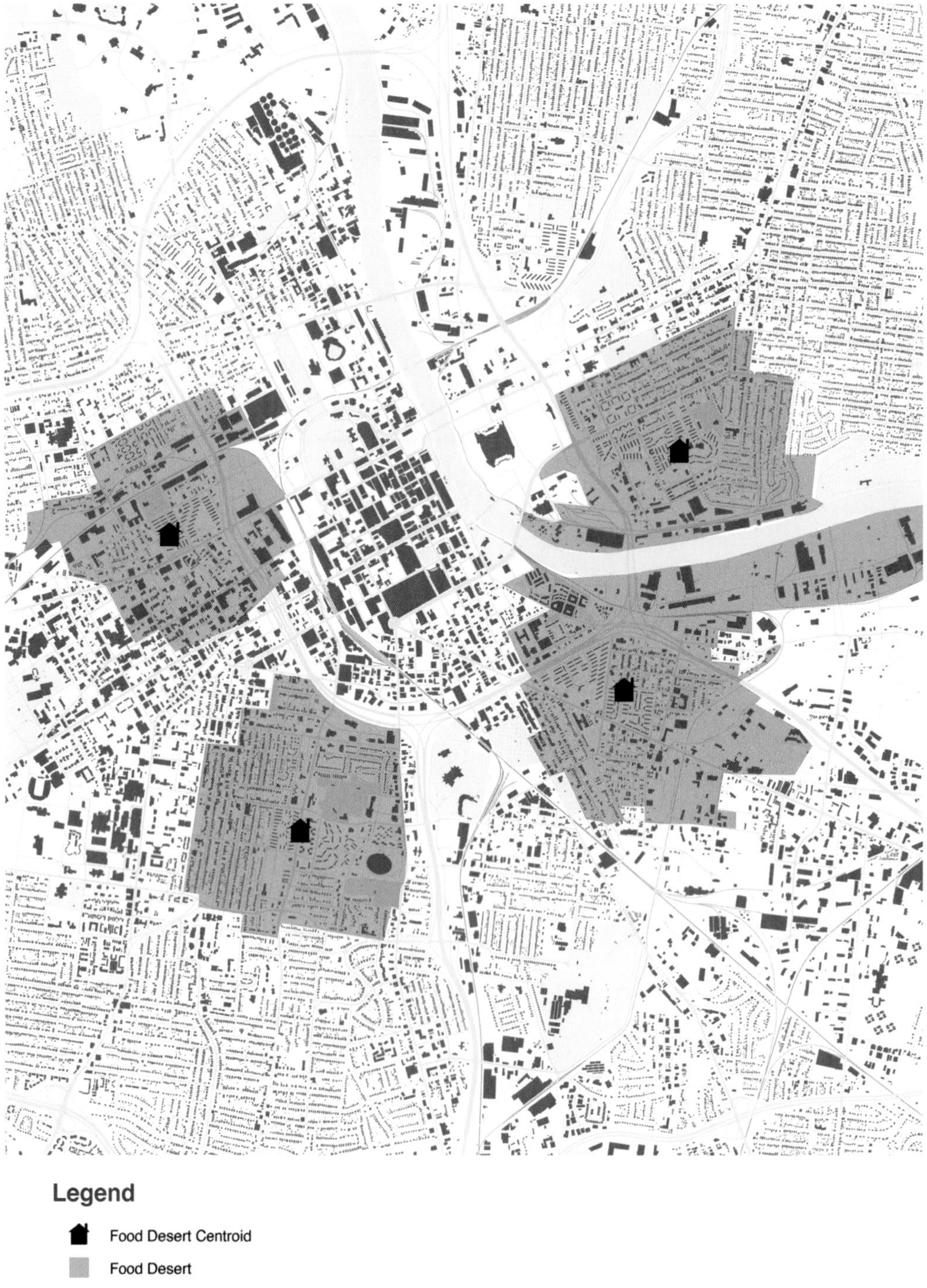

Legend

Food Desert Centroid

Food Desert

X Areas in Nashville's urban zone defined as food deserts by Tennessee State University urban geographer David Padgett. Food desert boundaries are based upon Census Block Groups selected within one mile of the center points (centroids) of inner-city communities having significantly high numbers of households without private automobiles. Data provided by 2009 American Community Survey (ACS) estimates and Metro Public Health Department. *(Based upon a 2013 map created by David A. Padgett, Tennessee State University. Diagram over map, 2016: Eric Hoke, NCDC)*

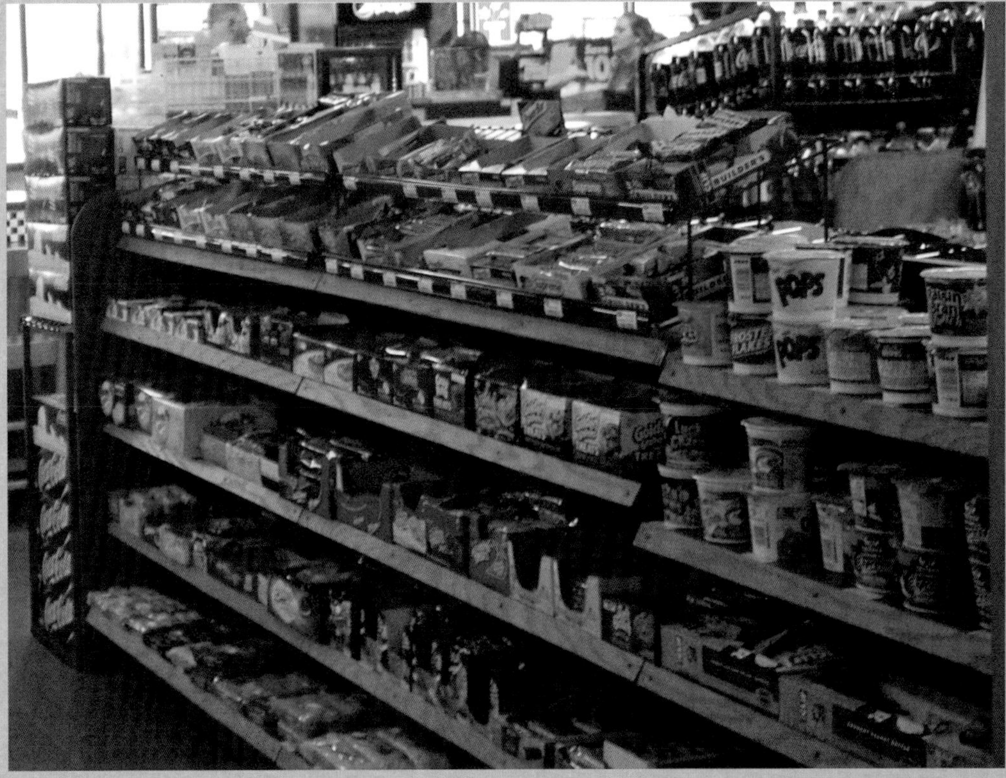

Typical items found front and center upon entering many convenience stores. *(2012)*

Grocery Rethink

It is an interesting but largely unremarked phenomenon that the dimensions of the American grocery store have expanded in rough sync with the national waistline. According to the Food Market Institute, the average size of United States supermarkets—note the "super"—was 18,000 square feet in the 1980s; by 2007 it was almost 50,000 square feet.[23] (By way of comparison, the main level of the grocery on the corner of 21st Avenue and Blair Boulevard, formerly Harris-Teeter, contains approximately 25,000 square feet.)

A minimum of 10,000 households is required to support a 50,000-square-foot store, according to authors Julie Campoli and Alex S. MacLean in *Visualizing Density*.[24] Catching this number of customers in most areas requires a wide net in terms of land area, meaning that the majority of patrons must drive. And finding sites in urban areas for the ever-bigger boxes is difficult and costly. The result has been that urban communities, especially those characterized by low-income residents, have sometimes become food deserts, where healthy, affordable food is difficult to obtain.

The model of the large supermarket was developed 50 years ago to serve families with children. This prototypical family drove a station wagon—later an SUV or minivan—to the market once a week and packed it with groceries. Changing demographics and shopping patterns, however, have made this model less valid for supermarket planning and development.

Households are shrinking in size— all those millennials and retiring baby boomers—while the number with two wage earners, who have less time for food prep, is increasing. Thus "the notable growth of deli sections in supermarkets, many of which now have seating sections and act as de facto restaurants," says Jason Scully in "Rethinking Grocery Stores."[25] Coffee bars are another new grocery amenity.

Scully notes a study showing that 23 percent of urban neighborhood residents in Seattle / King County walked to the grocery rather than drove by car, and only 7 percent of shoppers left with more than two bags. Another survey done in Houston found that 49 percent of shoppers went to the grocery at least twice a week. The increasing desire for fresh food leads to buying more frequently.

Locating smaller groceries within walking distance of a maximum number of households is a logical response to these trends. "When thinking about what constitutes a good neighborhood, [however], planners have yet to assign food and eating the same prominence as transportation, open space, and housing mix," Scully writes.

In "The Supermarket as a Neighborhood Building Block," authors Mark Hinshaw and Brian Vanneman urge planners to make grocery stores "cornerstones of great places to live."[26] They suggest that groceries in urban neighborhoods be located at or near the center of a neighborhood as an anchor of a community's main street. The store size can be determined by the amount of population within a half-mile walking distance. The walkable store will thus require fewer parking spaces and serve as a stimulus to other retail venues. As groceries become places to dine and socialize as well as shop, it's time that they take center stage in community planning.

—CHRISTINE KREYLING

Food on Wheels

The Nashville Mobile Market is a new take on an old practice: the itinerant vendors who once maneuvered horse drawn wagons, then small trucks, through urban communities, selling local produce, meats, breads, and other products to homemakers who'd wave them down from their porches and stoops.

While working at Shade Tree Clinic, a free clinic run by Vanderbilt students that he helped found, Vanderbilt University medical student Ravi Patel encountered low-income patients suffering from chronic conditions, such as hypertension and diabetes, related to a lack of healthy food in their diets. Ravi learned that, although they wanted to add fresh fruits and vegetables to their diets, they struggled to purchase them. These patients faced numerous obstacles to a healthy diet: a lack of grocery stores within walking distance, no cars of their own for travel elsewhere, and incomes insufficient to purchase costlier foodstuffs. They were essentially living in a state the World Health Organization defines as "food insecurity," experiencing physical, financial, and educational barriers to the availability and use of healthy foods. Recalling better days, the patients reminisced about the man who once sold fresh produce in their neighborhood from the back of a pick-up.

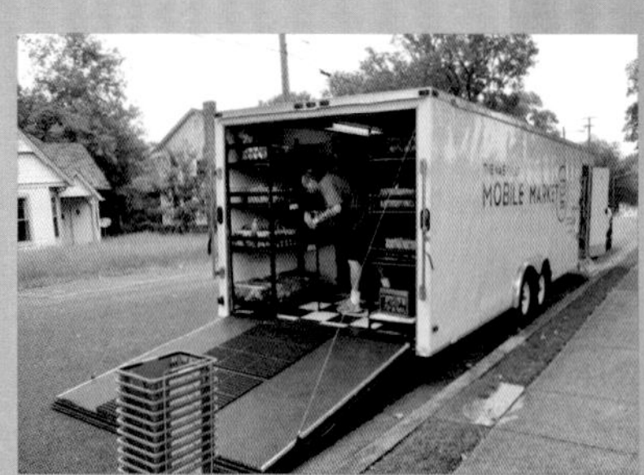

The Nashville Mobile Market on a street near the Vine Hill Apartments. *(2012: Nashville Mobile Food Market)*

Ravi decided to explore a new variation of this tradition of mobile food for people who are less so. By February of 2011, he had partnered with Organized Neighbors of Edgehill, Vanderbilt professors, and numerous Vanderbilt undergraduate and graduate students to bring the Nashville Mobile Market (NMM) into reality with a generous seed grant from the Frist Foundation. Two years of operation have built upon the principle that every neighborhood deserves access to healthy food at an affordable price.

The Mobile Market's updated model is a 28-foot trailer outfitted with shelving and refrigerators stocked with nutritious foods. We have expanded from three stops in the Edgehill community to 15 weekly stops in 12 locations across the city. That expansion, along with the community connections we have developed, has led to over $50,000 worth of healthy food purchases in Nashville's food insecure communities. The number of market transactions has increased by 50.2 percent in the last year alone.

Our experience has revealed food insecurity in Nashville as both pervasive and diverse, with myriad causes and complications impacting a variety of people. Initially, NMM saw its work as making healthy foods conveniently and affordably accessible in those communities without a good full-service grocery option. Other needs, however, have emerged.

Seniors without transportation or full mobility have difficulty reaching a store only several blocks away. Whole neighborhoods have become acculturated to consuming from fast food menus and convenience store freezers, stocking up on calories to stave off hunger and on processed goods to prevent spoilage. Lack of cooking and nutritional knowledge hinders healthy food purchasing, preparation, and consumption. In response, NMM has become a site of community-based learning on what to eat and how to cook it, supplemented by an educational series offered in conjunction with nonprofits and Metro Parks community centers.

NMM emerged from an intersection of academic, medical, and community concern. The program has remained focused on connecting Nashville's academic populations with its neighborhoods, functioning also as a learning lab for many, largely student, volunteer staff members. We respond to customer and neighbor feedback, aiming to be perceived not as a service provider but rather as a component of the community's life. In the end, lower prices, closer geographic availability of good food, nutrition education, and the development of trust among residents and volunteers will lead to healthier communities in Nashville.

—KELLEY-FRANCES FENELON
executive director, The Nashville Mobile Market

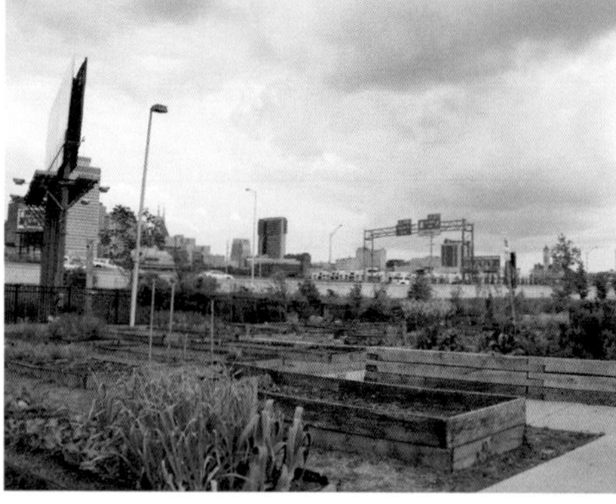

Top: "Farm in the City" at the J. Henry Hale Apartments on Charlotte Avenue offers community garden plots on a first-come, first-served basis for a low monthly fee. The garden also features a fruit orchard, tool shed, picnic shelter, compost bins, garden supplies, and water access. *(2013)*

STRATEGY: *Increase the availability of community gardening plots and farmers' markets in urban neighborhoods.*

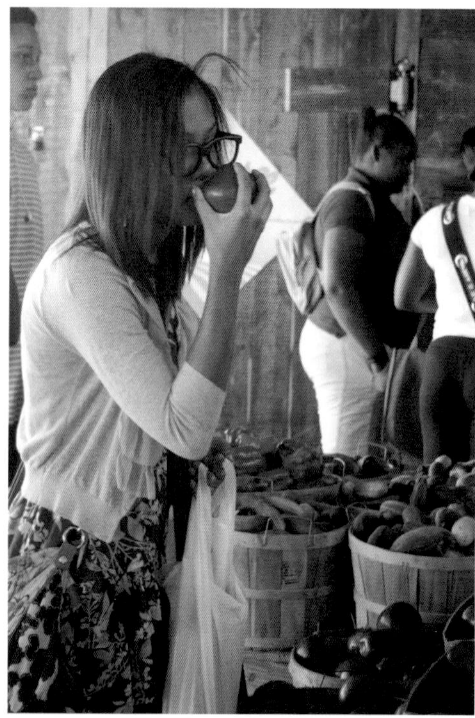

High school students get the feel of fresh local produce at the Nashville Farmers' Market as part of the Nashville Civic Design Center's *Design Your Neighborhood* program. *(2011: Jill Robinson, NCDC)*

STRATEGY: *Develop more opportunities for communities to learn how to grow and prepare food in healthier ways.*

The Plots Thicken

From vacant lots to schoolyards, community gardens are cropping up.

As the seeds of the local food movement take root in Nashville, urban farmers are repurposing the fallow lands of schoolyards, vacant lots, and industrial areas into fertile fields of sustainable agriculture. From Sylvan Park to Antioch, North Nashville to Edgehill, Nashvillians are staking out unexpected tracts of land on which to cultivate crops and nurture awareness of nature, nutrition, and the environment. Some urban gardens supply produce for people with limited access to healthy food, while others provide educational curricula or anchors for community-building efforts.

While the urban agriculture movement—and its feathered cousin, the urban chicken movement—has become popular in recent years, it used to be more underground. Metro codes did not explicitly support community gardens, so guerrilla growers, determined to cultivate land in the umbra of downtown, simply dug in. Conventional wisdom held that it was better to ask forgiveness than try to wrangle permission.

By 2009, urban farms were cropping up with such vigor and with so much support that council members from the urban districts drafted legislation that allowed community gardeners to come out of the shadows: to operate in full sunlight, so to speak. In July of that year, Mayor Karl Dean signed an ordinance that opened the door to community gardening projects such as The Farm in the City near the John Henry Hale Apartments on Jo Johnston Avenue, Perk Farm along Mill Creek in Southeast Nashville, and other unexpected pastoral patches within the urban core.

A partnership between Trevecca Nazarene University and Hands On Nashville, Perk Farm reclaimed vacant fields adjacent to an industrial plant to grow corn, cabbage, beans, broccoli, greens, peanuts, and basil. The crops harvested are used to create healthy meals for people living in food deserts nearby.

In the planting beds of the Chestnut Hill Community Garden on First Avenue South, neighbors came together to grow a diverse bounty of herbs and vegetables. For $10, gardeners can reserve their own irrigated garden plots. Strangers became neighbors as they shared complementary crops at potluck suppers in the garden.

At Wedgewood Urban Gardens near the Tennessee State Fairgrounds, the nonprofit Nashville Food Project took on responsibility for tending rows of okra, corn, cabbage, squash, and kale, as well as berry bushes and fruit trees that support the Project's hot meal delivery program. Tucked behind a busy thoroughfare, the rolling acre is home to a flock of chickens and two beehives. It has flourished as a community gathering space for movie nights and potluck events.

A look at the rapidly populating map of community gardens across Nashville shows a significant number of the projects on school campuses. At West End Middle School, for example, parents help tend the raised beds, teachers build curriculum around the garden, and students harvest herbs and vegetables to eat and even sell at a local produce shop. In 2012, the Nashville School Garden Coalition emerged to help educators integrate school gardens into their curricula and to pilot a garden-to-cafeteria program to increase the use of garden food in school lunches.

In conversations with community gardeners, one consistent theme emerges: for a community garden to succeed, there must be a committed individual or crew to shepherd the project through an entire growing season, from the early excitement of spring planting through the sweltering labors of summer maintenance.

"Nobody has any idea how much work is involved," says Nancy Stetten, a longtime volunteer who manages the colorful garden of vegetables and flowers at the front doors of Park Avenue Elementary in Sylvan Park. Over the years, as teachers have become more familiar with the garden project, they have invited Stetten and her co-volunteers into the school and led their students to the outdoor classroom. As more students and classes have participated in the school garden's

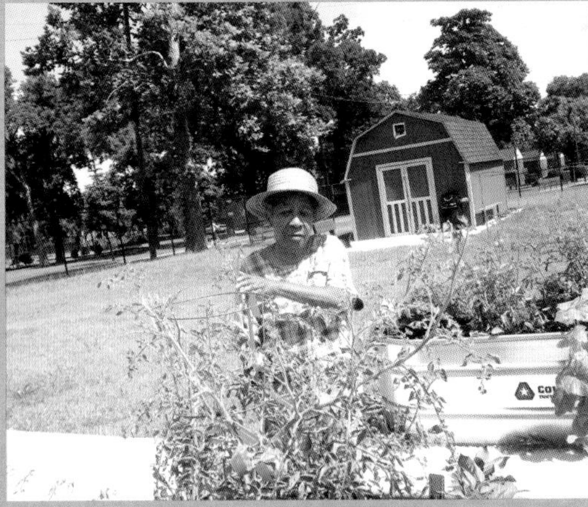

Garden harvest at the Edgehill Community Memorial Garden.
(2013: Alicia Smith, NCDC)

project-based learning, Stetten has applied for grants to buy equipment to accommodate them all. A former employee of the State Department of Education and a member of the Nashville School Garden Coalition, Stetten is exuberant about the opportunity to trade textbooks for hands-on learning tools such as seedpods, flowers, vegetables, and honeybees. With the help of towering sunflowers, she teaches students the basics of selective breeding. (Every fall, when she tells the class to pick one sunflower's seeds to save, they always choose the biggest one. "Aha! That's how they got big," she explains triumphantly.)

Using squash, beans, and corn—the so-called Three Sisters of the garden—Stetten introduces students to the symbiosis in which corn provides a climbing pole for beans, beans replenish soil with nitrogen, and squash vines suppress weeds; the triangular relationship provides longtime fertility for the soil. Pointing to a stand of corn growing by the front walk, Stetten describes an exercise she does with first-graders called "The Corn is as High as an Elephant's Eye," in which she introduces the basics of standard measurements. "We need standard measurements," she says with a twinkle in her eye and an infectious enthusiasm in her voice, "because you can't always get an elephant."

—CARRINGTON FOX
food writer, *Nashville Scene*

HOUSING

✓ Urban housing ranges from single-family dwellings to multi-unit residential buildings. Images clockwise from top left: 12 South, Gale Park, Cheatham Place, Fifth and Main. *(2013)*

✓ Health-Promoting

Housing stock in urban areas typically offers an assortment of types, sizes, prices, and options of renting or owning. This variety helps ensure diversity of residents and helps them age in place. Urban housing development has flourished in Nashville over the past decade and is being built at greater densities.

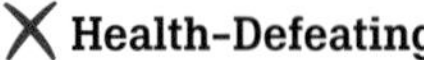

X Health-Defeating

The popularity of urban neighborhoods was evident in Metro Nashville's 2013 property tax reappraisal. Residential values have risen 14 percent since 2009 in the 37206 zip code of East Nashville, the highest increase in Davidson County.[27] While such escalations validate the urban quality of life, they can also have unintended negative consequences.

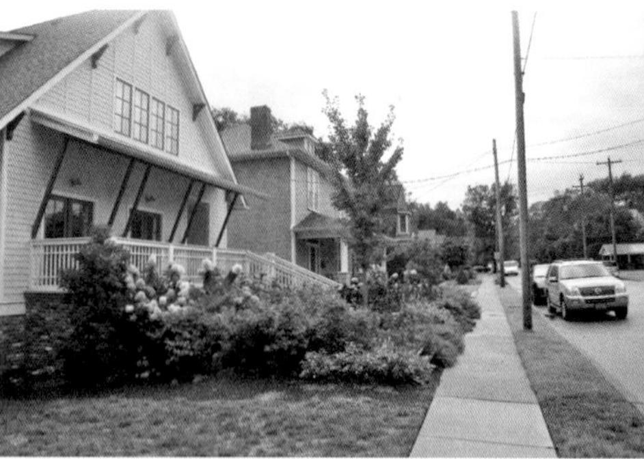

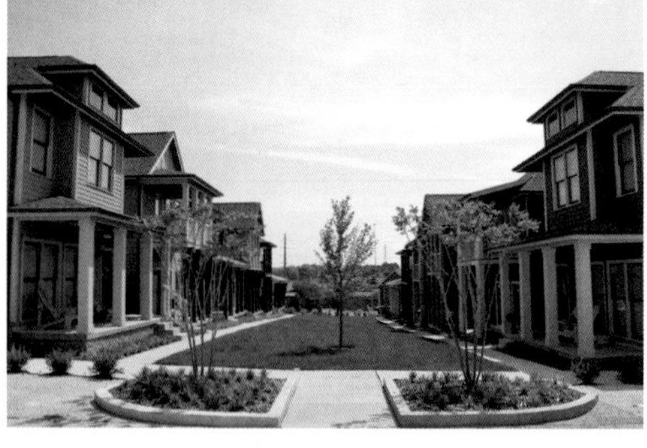

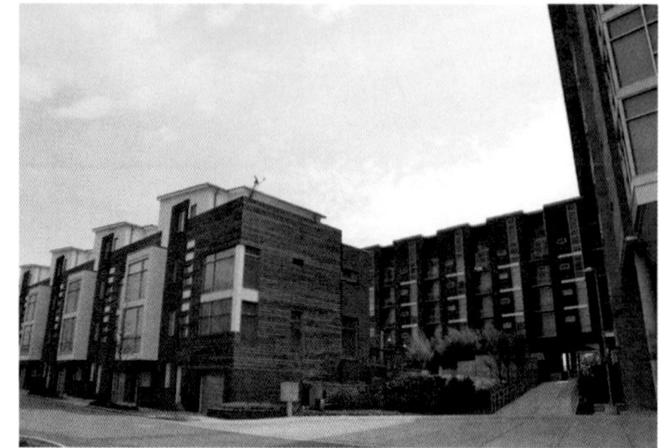

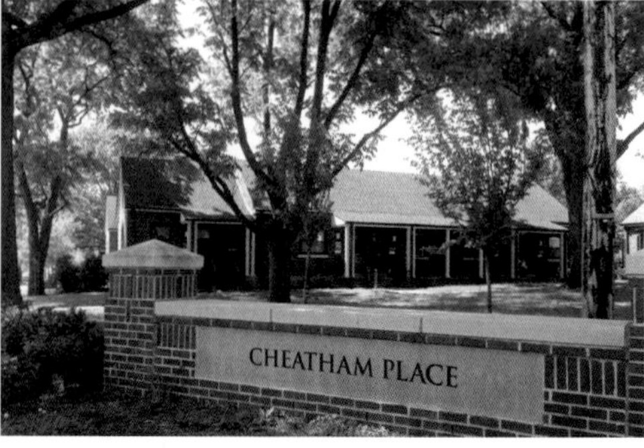

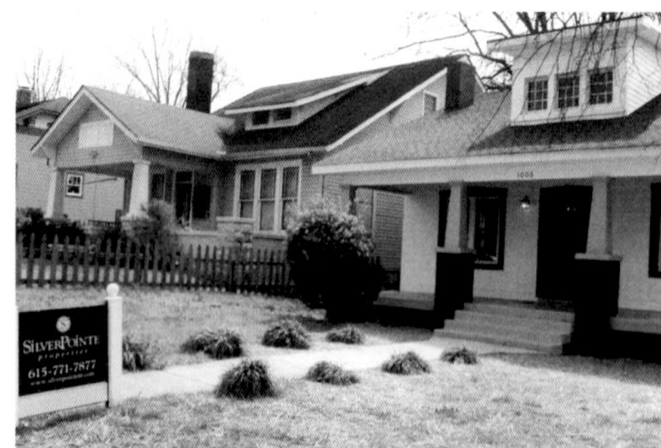

X West Eastland Avenue bungalow on the market. The renovation of historic urban homes helps stabilize and revitalize neighborhoods but subsequent increases in home prices, rental rates, and property taxes can force residents—many of them long term—out of the neighborhood. *(2013: Eric Hoke, NCDC)*

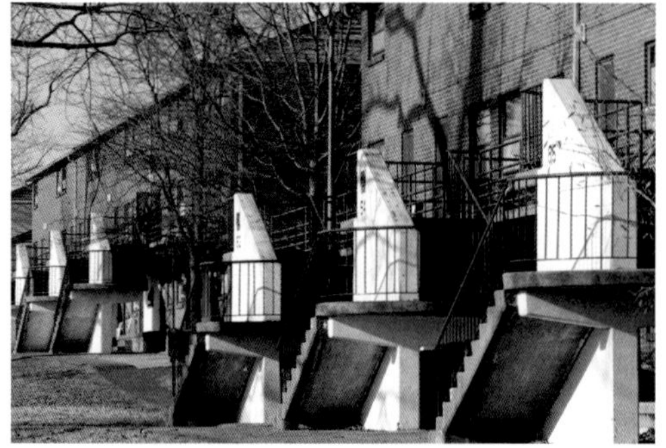

X View of Sudekum Homes public housing neighborhood from the pedestrian bridge over I-40. *(2011: Gary Layda)*

In addition to an upsurge in property taxes and rents, the increase in property values has also motivated developers and builders to tear down small houses and replace them with larger ones. These outcomes make urban neighborhoods less affordable, eroding socioeconomic diversity. Lower income residents compelled to relocate may find themselves in locations of less walkability, access to public transit, and healthy foods.

Bad urban design of public housing and federal policies regarding who would occupy it created isolated islands of concentrated poverty, racial imbalance, and crime. Originally intended to offer an alternative to slums for those suffering from the Great Depression, by the 1960s public housing had become warehouses for the permanently poor. In 1981 the federal government established preferences for those eligible for public housing that ensured residency by those with the lowest incomes. By 1996, when the preferences were abolished, the average income of residents had fallen from 33 percent of Nashville's median income to 17 percent.[28]

STRATEGY: *Build and preserve homes for everyone. Encourage affordable housing infill development within urban communities, especially on sites near public transit. Incentives for developers in other cities include density bonuses, as well as reduced permit and user fees. Charlotte, North Carolina, restricts its use of such strategies to census blocks with average home values above the city's median to keep low income housing from overwhelming neighborhoods that already have a lot of it.*

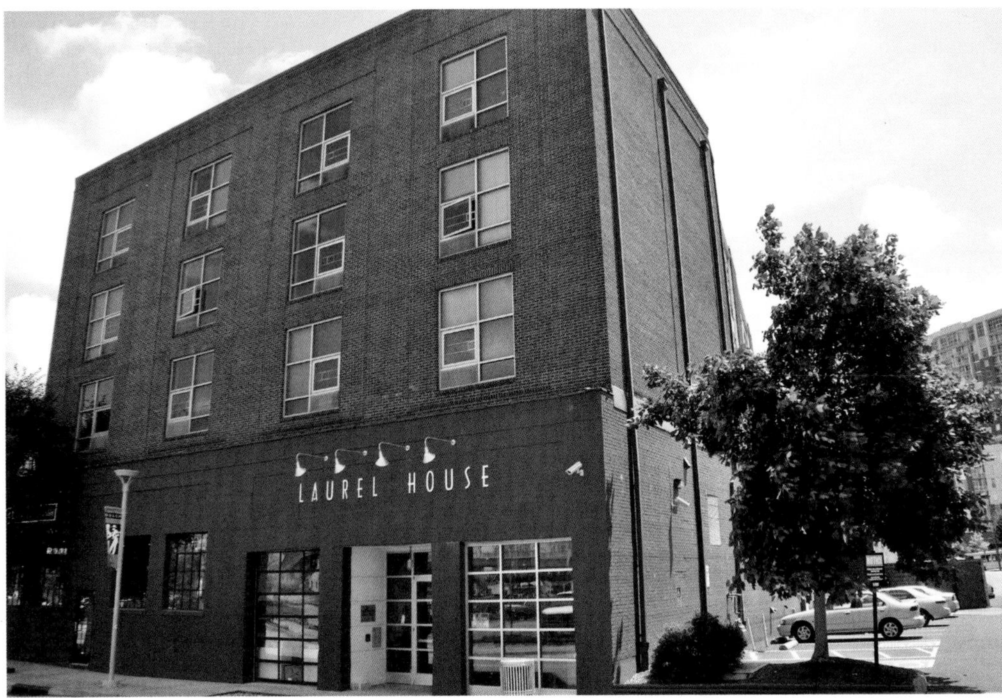

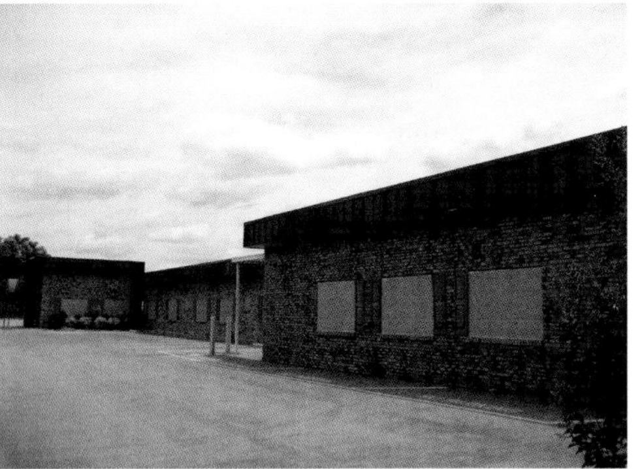

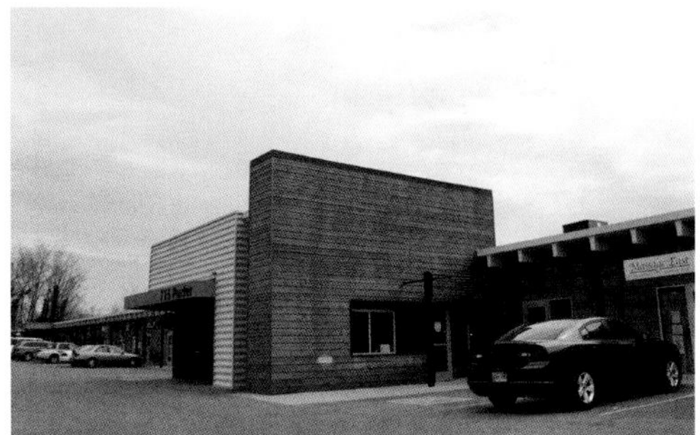

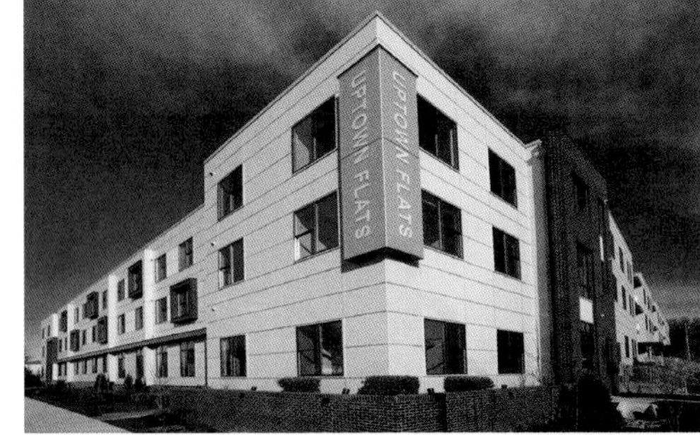

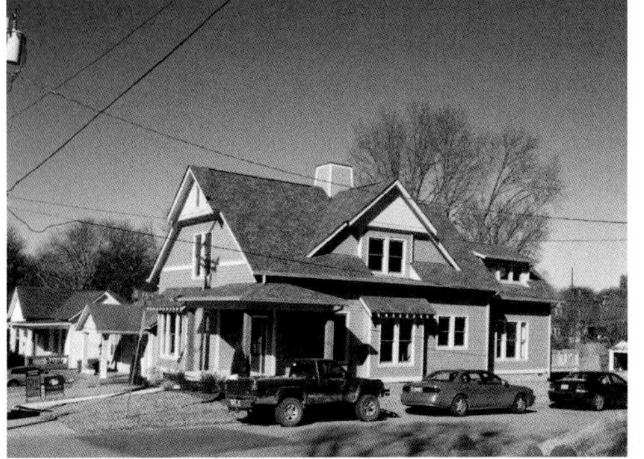

Far left: Laurel House, a 48-unit, mixed-use building in the Gulch, was developed in 2001 by The Housing Fund (THF), a private nonprofit, using federal low-income housing tax credits. In 2013 Metro established the Barnes Fund for Affordable Housing with $3 million in seed money from the city. These housing funds work in complementary fashion—THF offering loans, Barnes offering grants—to create new housing units and make existing housing more affordable, for people of low and moderate incomes. (See also "Housing for All," pages 50–51.) *(2013)*

Located at the corner of East Nashville's Eastland Avenue and Porter Road, this adaptive reuse of a former senior care facility damaged in the 1998 tornado offers 20 one-bedroom apartments designed for the hearing impaired. The property includes numerous green features, oversized windows, and designer finishes. In addition to housing, Porter East accommodates a preschool and a number of retail outlets.
Top right: **Before**
Next below: **After**
(2010: Urban Housing Solutions; 2013, NCDC)

Uptown Flats, a 72-unit community on Dickerson Road, provides affordable rental housing for Nashville's workforce. It is the first example of residential redevelopment along this commercial corridor. *(2013: Smith Gee Studio)*

New construction in the Lockeland Springs-East End conservation zoning district replaced a much smaller home. The traditional architectural style is compatible with the surrounding context, but the scale is not. *(2013)*

STRATEGY: *Preserve existing affordable housing stock by limiting teardowns of small single and multifamily houses.*

Their replacement by larger homes undermines neighborhood affordability and narrows housing options for single and senior households. To combat this problem, the Virginia state legislature, to use one example, has enabled cities, counties, and towns to establish housing rehabilitation zones that provide financial and regulatory incentives in designated areas.[29]

The rise in Nashville's land values, particularly in the urban zone, has made it profitable for developers to bulldoze small cottages built in the 1950s and 1960s. The site scraping is permissible even in historic and conservation zoning overlay districts when these structures are listed as "non-contributing" to the historic architectural character of the neighborhood.

At the time when these districts were surveyed by the Metro Historic Zoning Commission, preparatory to the application of preservation zoning overlays, most homes built after World War II were considered non-contributing. This practice followed federal guidelines that properties must be at least 50 years old to qualify for the National Register of Historic Places unless they have exceptional significance. Many of these cottages have now reached this age while retaining their original architectural integrity, however. A re-survey could put them in the "contributing" column and thus subject to demolition controls.

This new duplex in East Nashville lies in an area unprotected by preservation overlays. It is one of several new buildings on Boscobel Street completely incompatible with neighborhood scale or even basic principles of urban design—note the lack of a front door. The prominent placement of garage entrances on the front façade and the wide driveway are characteristic of suburban dwellings and hostile to the pedestrian character of the street. The design ignores the alley to the rear, which could have provided car storage access with minimal paving. The steep slope of the site coupled with all the concrete out front is a formula for stormwater runoff problems for the neighbors across the street. *(2013)*

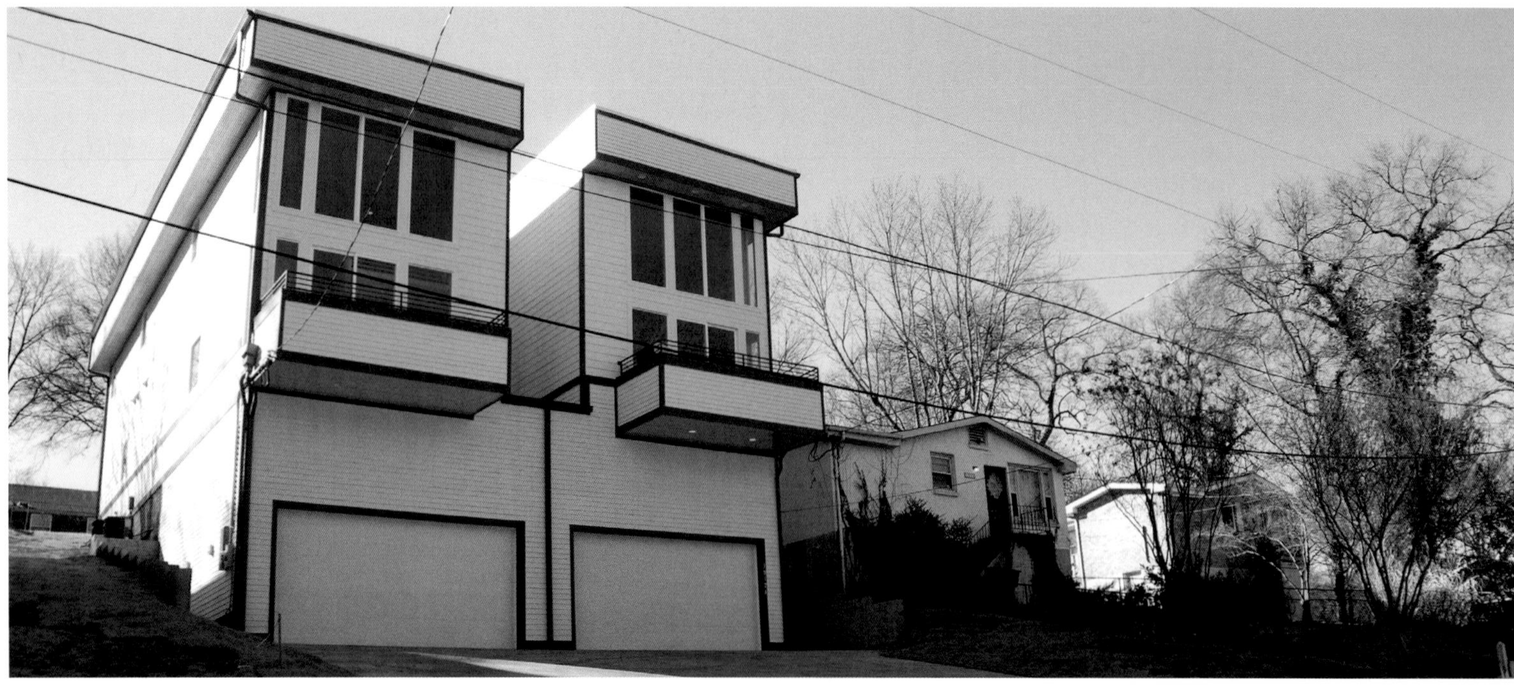

Home revitalization by the Habitat for Humanity's ReConstruct program. This Meridan Street home in East Nashville was built in 1890 and had a rich past, but had become neglected, then vacant. After damage by fire it was condemned by the city. The Metro Housing and Development Agency donated the house to Habitat for Humanity with the condition that the renovations follow the US Secretary of the Interior's *Standards for Rehabilitation.* Volunteers from local churches, government agencies, and preservation organizations like Historic Nashville assisted with Habitat's award-winning restoration and modernization.
Right: **Before**
Far right: **After**
(2010 Robbie Jones, Historic Nashville, Inc.)

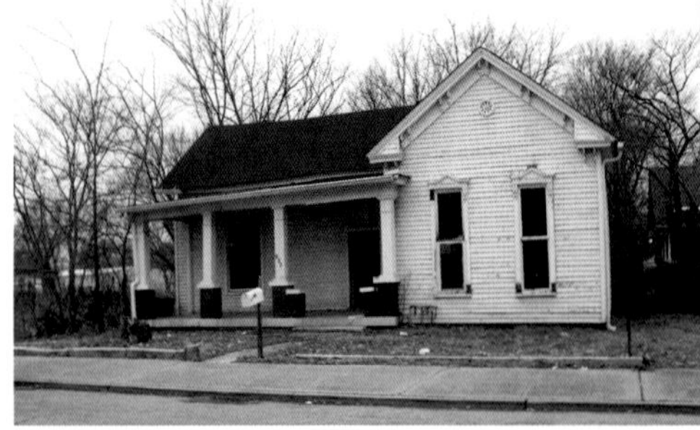

STRATEGY: *Emphasize the preservation of historic architectural character in the restoration or development of moderately priced housing stock, to help such buildings fit into the neighborhood context and not stand out as "affordable."*

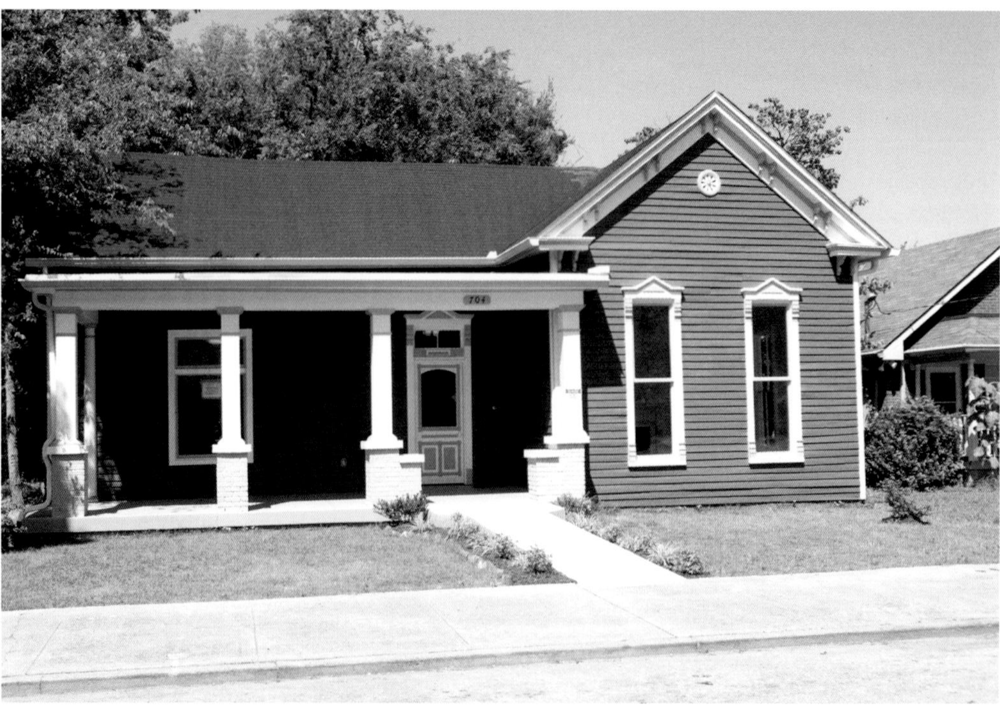

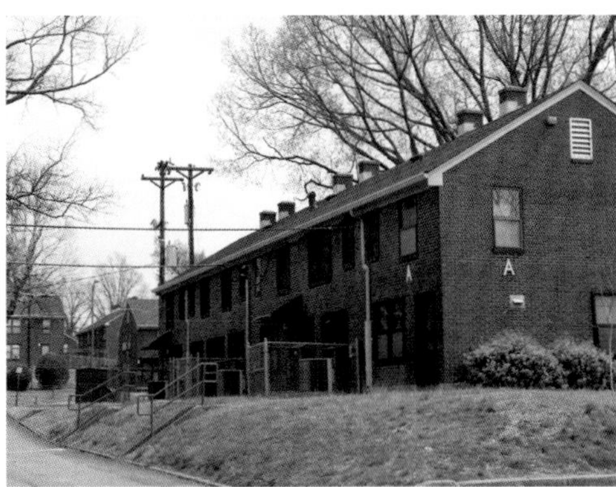

STRATEGY: *Redevelop or renovate public housing complexes to include a mix of uses and affordability levels. The variety in cost alleviates the concentration of poverty among residents that has been so detrimental to social stability in public housing. The mixture of uses should be planned to make daily needs a walkable proposition.*

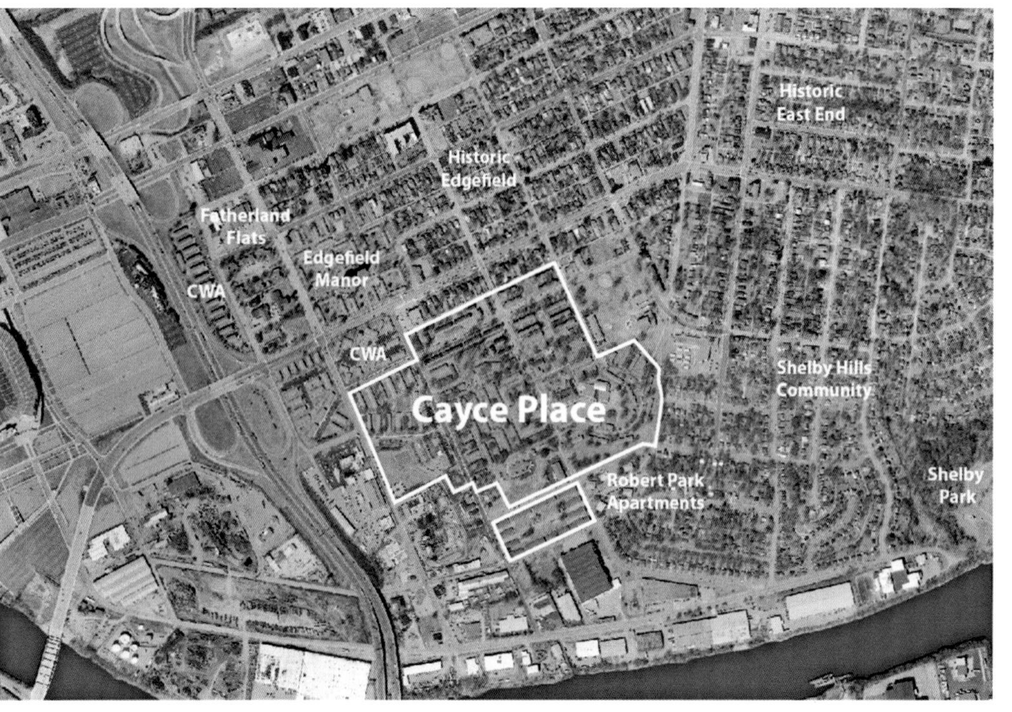

Cayce Place in East Nashville, the largest public housing complex in the city, contains 709 units occupied by 1,991 people. Completed in 1954, the aging development was designed in the typical government style of the times: superblocks of units perpendicular to the street—for surveillance of backyards—and a disconnected street system. Both design strategies were thought at the time to deter crime. *(2013)*

Existing aerial view of East Nashville shows Cayce Place's proximity to the Cumberland River and I-24. The CWA housing was acquired by the Metropolitan Development and Housing Agency in 2014, and will be redeveloped as a part of the new master plan for Cayce Place. *(2010: Metro Planning Department)*

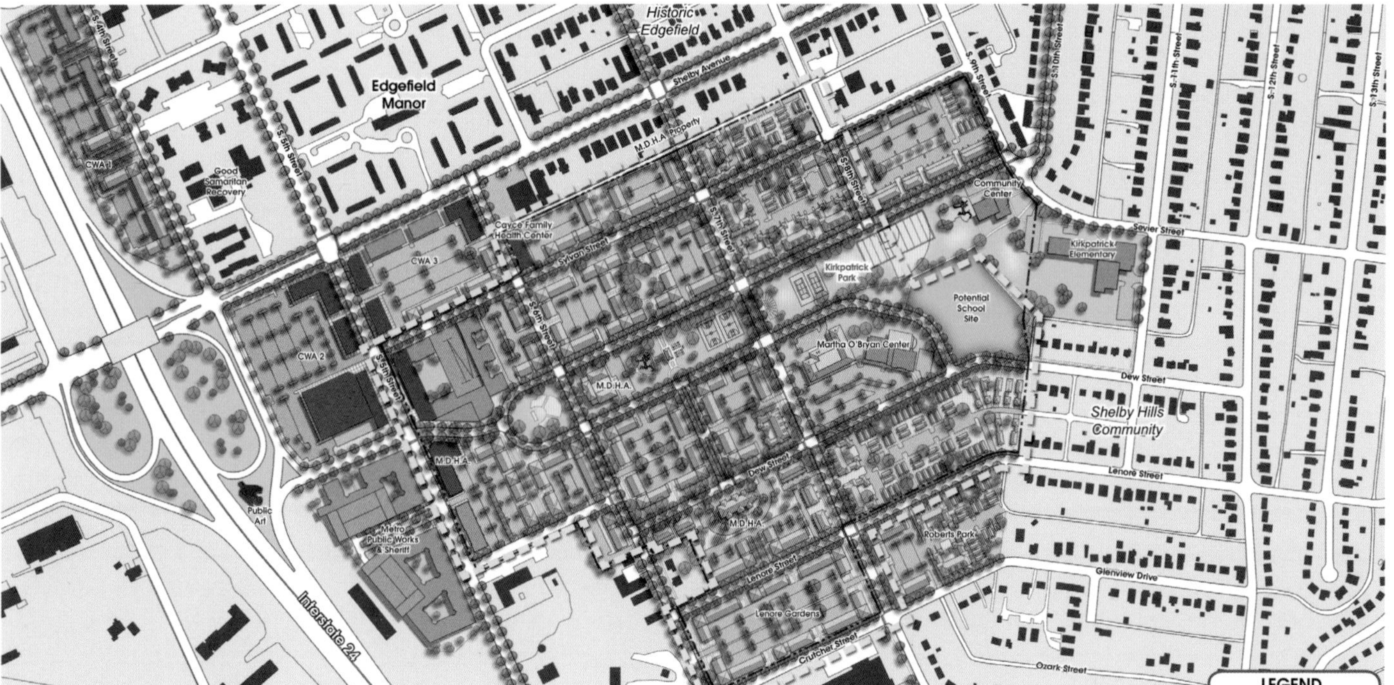

The vision for Cayce Place involved community meetings with residents and neighbors to consider opportunities for additional redevelopment, including connecting the neighborhoods of East Nashville to the river, the connection of Shelby Park to the East Bank greenway and downtown, and the redevelopment of East Bank industrial sites. Note the large central greenspace that serves as a defining feature of the plan. *(Plan, 2013: Metropolitan Development and Housing Agency)*

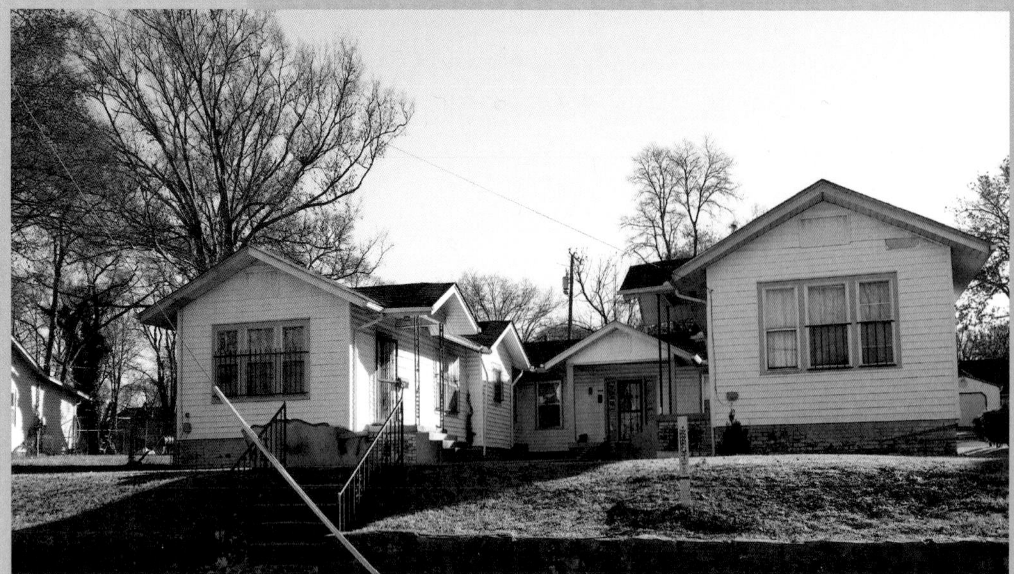

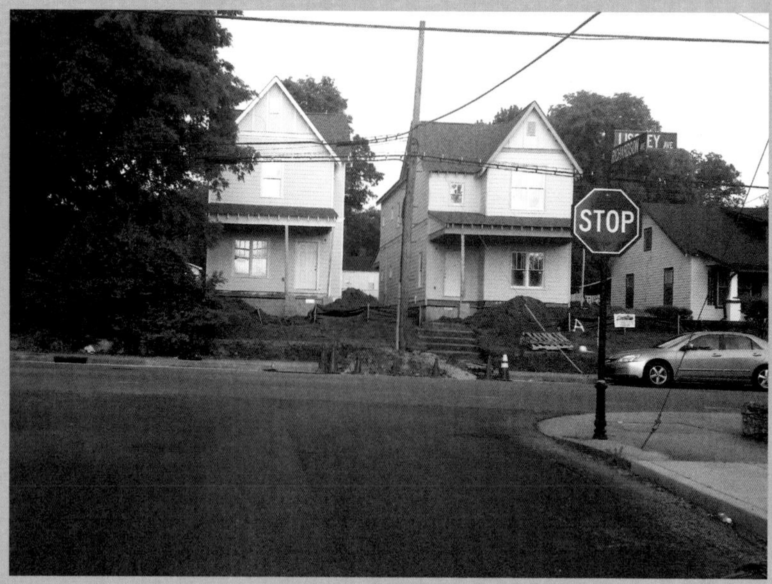

Affordable housing in Cleveland Park is routinely being demolished and replaced by larger, more expensive dwellings. *(2014: Sam McCullough)*

Cleveland Park: Displacement on Steroids

I have lived in Cleveland Park for 55 years. I can still walk through my neighborhood and recall the names and histories of most of the families who lived, and some who continue to live, in the old houses. But that is changing—rapidly.

Today my neighborhood is under siege by the forces of gentrification. Long-term residents like myself and many of my friends and neighbors are asking: How much longer will I be able to afford to live here, feel comfortable living here, will even recognize this place as home?

The Cleveland Park neighborhood lies north of Cleveland Street and takes its name from the park developed in 1963 that was part of the Nashville Housing Authority's urban renewal program in East Nashville. But the area called Northeast Nashville that contains Cleveland Park has a much older history.

The area's identity as an African American enclave began with the second contraband camp established by the federal troops in 1864. Without a bridge across the Cumberland—destroyed by retreating Confederates in 1862—the river was a barrier preventing thousands of fugitive slaves from reaching Nashville itself. "Because a major railroad ran through the community," writes historian Bobby Lovett, "the Union army used the contraband slaves there to build repair shops and warehouses on the eastern side of the river."[30] When Edgefield was incorporated as a separate city in 1868, the area north of the railroad tracks was called North Edgefield.[31]

Like many other first ring urban neighborhoods, Cleveland Park is located less than two miles from the center of downtown, between Ellington Parkway on the east and I-65 and Dickerson Pike on the west.[32] The construction of parkway and interstate in the 1960s created barriers that hemmed in the public housing project, first called Settle Court and later renamed Sam Levy Homes.These barriers created a series of dead-end streets—Lischey Avenue, Settle Court, and Foster Street—that became havens for the drug trade; the one-way-in-and-out pattern decreased pedestrian and vehicular traffic, removing watchful eyes from these streets.

Despite these depredations by government, Cleveland Park has been a middle-class, mostly black community and, for many, a desirable place to grow up. The diversity of income levels created a variety of housing options. Voucher-subsidized lodging through the Federal Section 8 program and low-income rentals were available to those needing the assistance. And home ownership was affordable to almost anyone who really wanted to posses his or her portion of the American dream.

That dream is now departing as fast as the long-time residents of Cleveland Park. We are losing the historic character of our neighborhood—the houses that we could afford and that we loved. Our homes are being replaced by oversized boxes: too big for our lots and our incomes. The average income for current residents is less than $32,000/year.[33] Yet new infill houses can easily cost from $300,000 to over $450,000. Older homes are being flipped for prices triple what rehabbers paid for them. Rental housing rates are upscale: $1,500 to $2,400 a month. The result is that many have been displaced from housing they had rented for 10

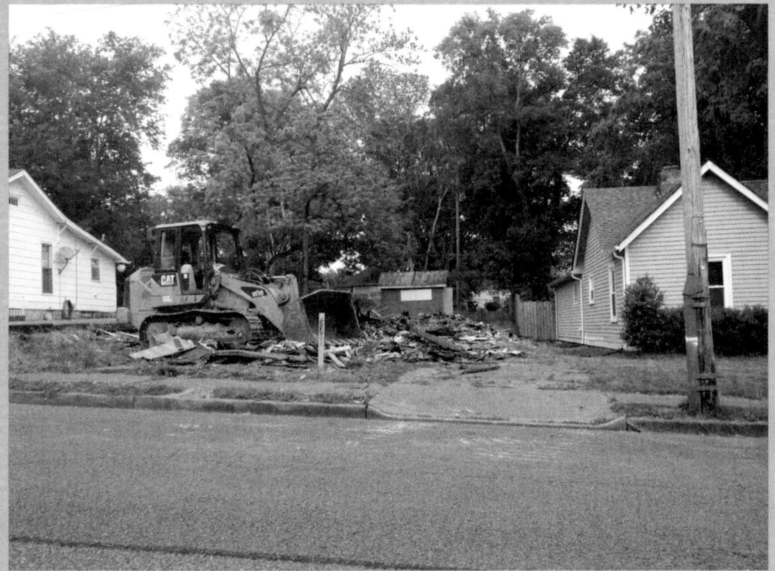

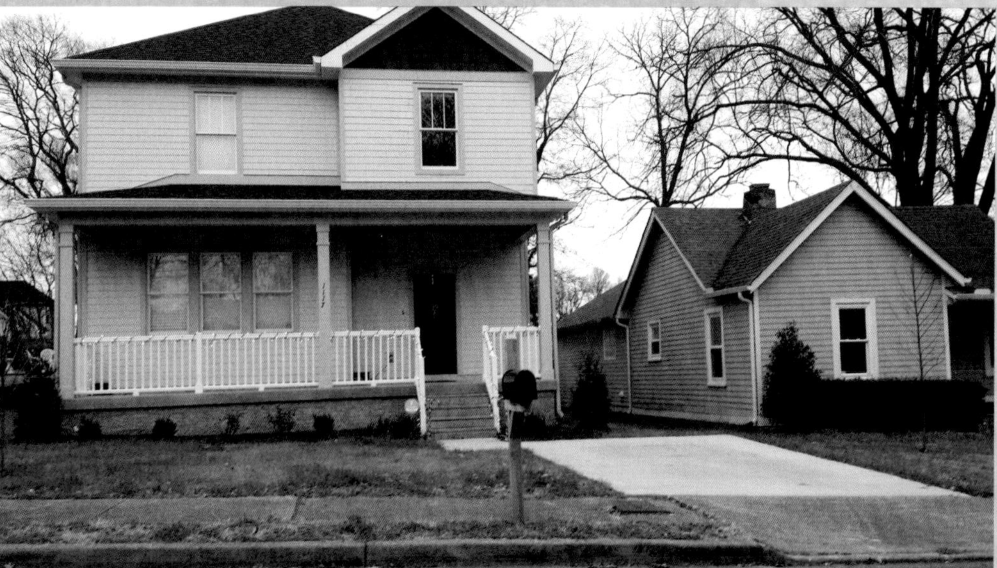

or 15 years—and they can't afford new quarters in the neighborhood.

Cleveland Park was once a close neighborhood. But it is turning into a place I don't know with new residents I don't know. Long-time inhabitants such as myself fear that, as property taxes go up, older residents and families will go out.

For about 25 years or so, during the 1970s, 1980s, and early 1990s, Cleveland Park had its fair share of crime: drug dealing on the streets and shootings that produced a high murder rate. Residents who had been here for years got tired of being captive in their homes. We came together and formed the Cleveland Park Neighborhood Association at a community meeting in 2003 to turn things around. New residents who arrived during the bad years came willing to work and with a mindset that old and new were in it together. We all watched out for each other. We labored to create a new reality and reputation for Cleveland Park. Apparently it worked because everyone is interested in our neighborhood now.

This is a familiar story all across Nashville: East Nashville, West Nashville's Nations, North Nashville's Salem Town, and South Nashville's Chestnut Hill. Long-term residents joined with the so-called urban pioneers and invested decades lobbying government officials, elected representatives, police, and codes enforcement—you name 'em—to bring back an urban neighborhood that had been eroded by government neglect and policies such as urban renewal. The success of their efforts is now illustrated by steeply rising property values.

This is good if you want to sell your house. It's not so good if you want to stay, due to the equally steep rise in property taxes. And if you want to buy or must rent—and have an income with fixed limits—you're out of luck.

One former resident wanted to come back and purchase the old family home when it came on the market. She qualified for a mortgage for an amount some percentage over what the seller had paid for it. But the asking price was out of her range, and she forever lost the opportunity to return to the family home.

The insensitivities of the recent crop of new residents are also an issue. They move to Cleveland Park because they say they want to feel the vibes of an urban neighborhood. But then the newcomers complain to Metro Codes about the properties of residents with limited means, generally elderly, who apparently don't live up to their standards. The neophytes rarely speak to their neighbors. They do not seem to understand the values or the workings of a true community.

Change is underway and can't be stopped. But the changes need to include old and new, white and black. The lawmakers should stand by the side of the residents and hold developers accountable for retaining diversity and a mix of affordability. That is what makes a real community.

—SAM MCCULLOUGH
founder and president emeritus of the
Cleveland Park Neighborhood Association

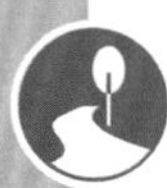

Urban parks range in scale and function from large regional parks to small community pocket spaces. Shelby Park in East Nashville (top), East End Methodist park on Holly Street (middle), Monroe Street playground in North Nashville (lower). *(2013)*

Private greenspace in the urban zone varies in size from an intimate backyard in Germantown (top) to a large shared courtyard at 5th and Main (lower). *(2012: Brian Phelps and Chris Whitis; 2012: Teresa Blackburn)*

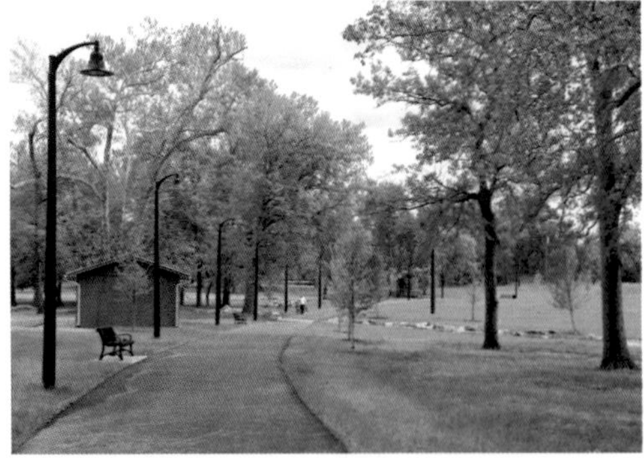

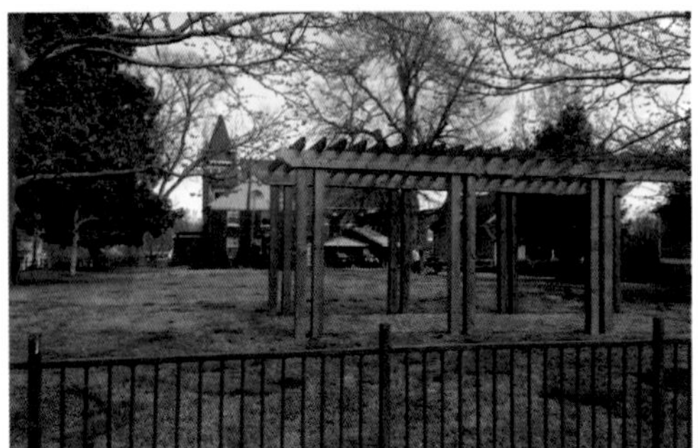

PARKS AND OPEN SPACE

Health-Promoting

A wide variety of park sizes and recreation amenities can be found in urban neighborhoods: pocket parks, regional parks and greenways, community centers, sports fields, and community gardens.

GreenBikes, a Metro program that began in 2010, offers free use of touring bicycles, helmets, and locks at eight community centers throughout the city, as well as at the Shelby Bottoms Nature Center and the Music City Star Riverfront Station. The locations are directly linked to 94 miles of greenways and 133 miles of on-road bike lanes and shared-use bike routes. Bikes may be checked out at one station and returned to any other during operating hours. Riders may obtain a free membership online or at bike stations with a proof of identity and current address.

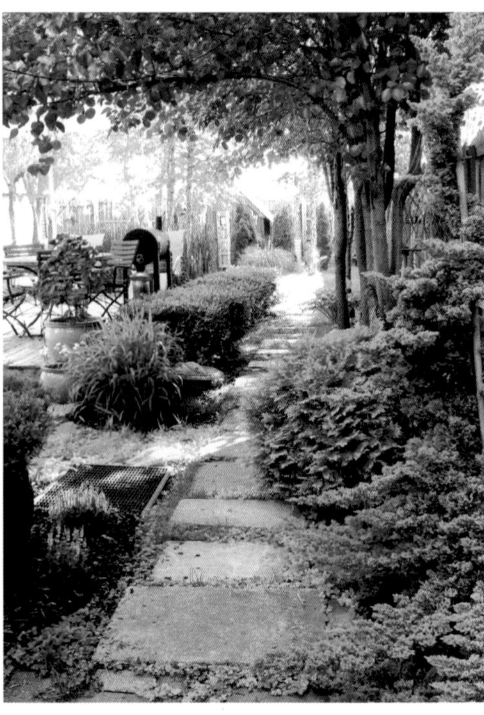

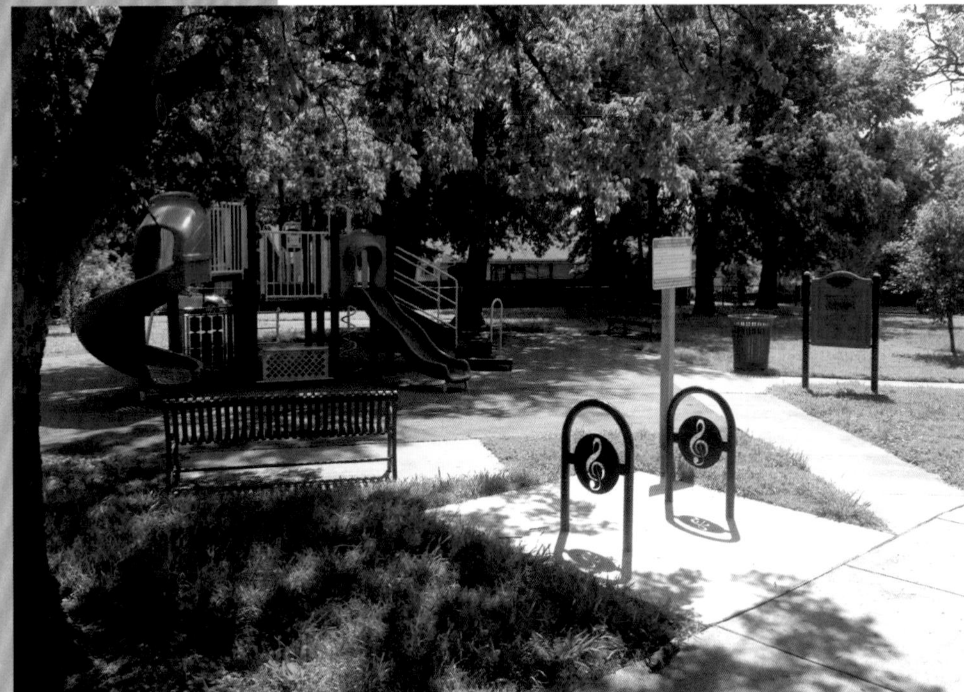

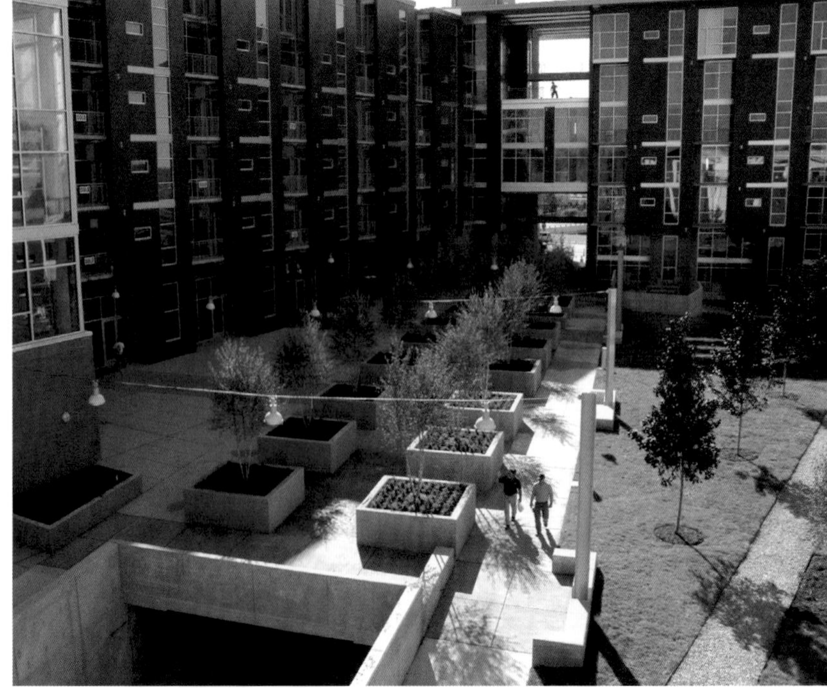

✗ Health-Defeating

There is insufficient tree coverage in many urban neighborhoods, which has a negative impact on health.[34] Trees remove pollutants from the air; release fresh oxygen; absorb stormwater and reduce flooding; cool air temperatures, reducing energy costs and countering the heat island effect; and provide shade for walkers.

Urban trees, however, require significant maintenance to grow and prosper. Irrigation and regular upkeep are necessary for urban trees to survive to maturity. Cuts in the budgets of the Public Works and Parks Departments have limited the city's ability to grow its tree canopy. Lacking a concerted effort by private property owners and developers of new infill to plant trees to shade the public rights-of-way, canopy coverage will continue to decrease.

STRATEGY: *Target tree planting initiatives, both public and private, in urban communities that have insufficient tree canopy coverage.*

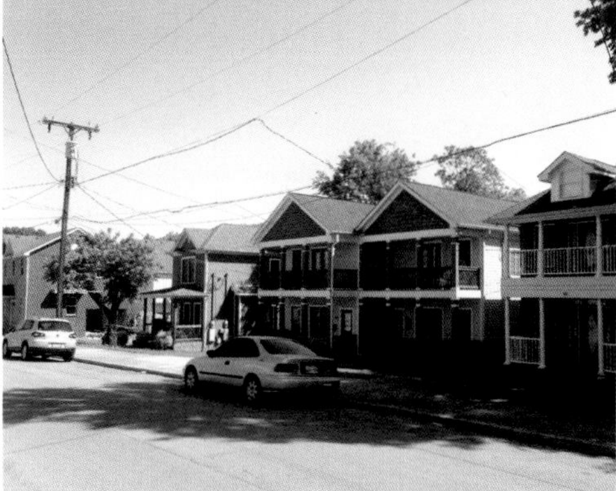

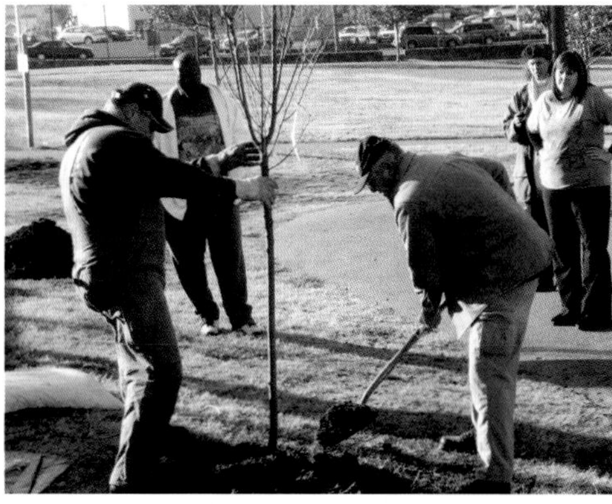

Left: New development within the urban transect zone has the potential to include more street tree plantings, like this section of Sixth Avenue North in Salemtown, which currently lacks front yard trees or a planting strip in the public right-of-way. Note also the presence of overhead utilities, which limit tree plantings to smaller ornamentals rather than large shade trees. Relocating utility lines to alleys would allow more trees out front. (2013)

Right: Volunteers plant trees in targeted neighborhoods across the city at the annual Releafing Day, begun by the Nashville Tree Foundation in 2002. (2012: Cumberland River Compact)

STRATEGY: *Increase environmental education. Include consideration of the total ecosystem in urban policy and planning to create natural ways to reduce the negative impact of buildings and runoff.*

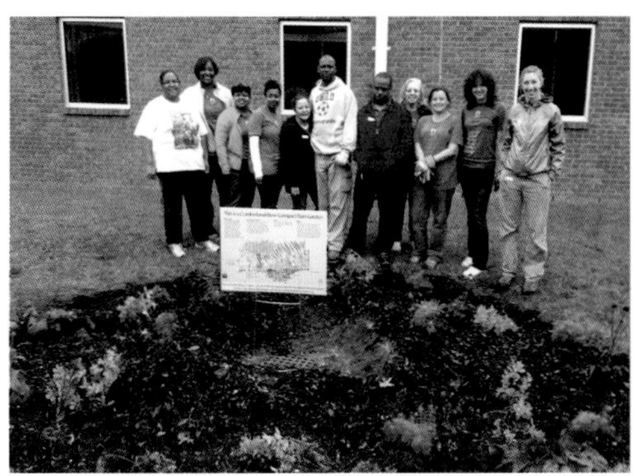

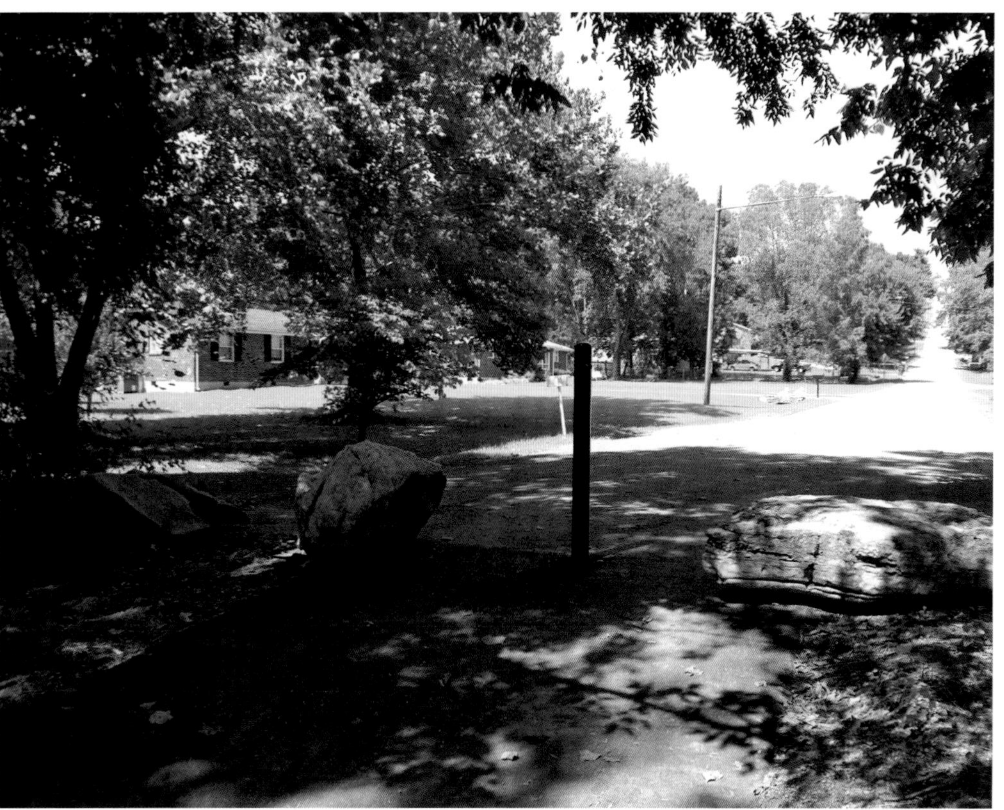

Left: Rain garden built at Charlotte Park Elementary School in West Nashville. Metro Water Services and the Cumberland River Compact established a five-year partnership beginning in 2009 to build 300 rain gardens, plant trees, and teach people about water quality issues and other sustainability issues. (2012, Cumberland River Compact)

Right: A new trail-head funded by Metro Parks Department with a matching grant from the Tennessee Department of Environment and Conservation connects the Riverside neighborhood to the Shelby Bottoms Greenway. (2013)

CASE STUDIES

CHESTNUT HILL AND GERMANTOWN

The urban transect zone is defined by its form: an integrated mixture of housing within walking distance of neighborhood-scaled commerce and open space, laid out along a well-connected street system, with side-walks, bikeways, and transit lines providing multiple transportation options. This is the "complete urban community."[35] The character of urban neighborhoods, however, may vary widely in their cultural, socioeconomic, and ethnic backgrounds as well as in the degree that they achieve "completeness." The following case studies of Chestnut Hill and Germantown illustrate how these distinctions may require specific strategies to improve the health of residents.

Chestnut Hill (formerly Cameron Trimble) and Germantown are neighborhoods of approximately the same size, situated on the south and north sides of the downtown core, respectively. Both are historic communities severely impacted by federal urban renewal policies as well as interstate construction, which led to their deterioration as residential neighborhoods.

The federal census tracts in which Chestnut Hill and Germantown lie encompass more territory than the neighborhoods themselves. But the data for these tracts can reveal the differences between the two.

The census tract that includes Chestnut Hill also includes the large public housing complexes of Napier Place and Sudekum Apartments. The Chestnut Hill census tract, therefore, has a higher poverty rate—74 percent—with more people dependent on public transit and carpooling than the Germantown census tract, which contains the older and smaller public housing of Cheatham Place. The large number of children residing in Napier and Sudekum also mean that the population of the Chestnut Hill tract is younger.

The census tract in which Germantown is located also includes Salemtown, Hope Gardens, and Buena Vista. The median value of housing in the Germantown census tract is $193,800, higher than the metro Nashville median of $145,521. Even so, 41 percent of the tract's population is below the poverty level, illustrating one of the contradictions of gentrifying urban neighborhoods.[36]

Definition of Family / Non-family

Family = Contains at least two people related by birth, marriage, or adoption. Family households are of two types:

- **Married** = When a married couple is considered the householder
- **Other** = When a single man or woman is considered the householder and lives with other family

Non-family = This may be one person living in a household or multiple people who are not related to each other.

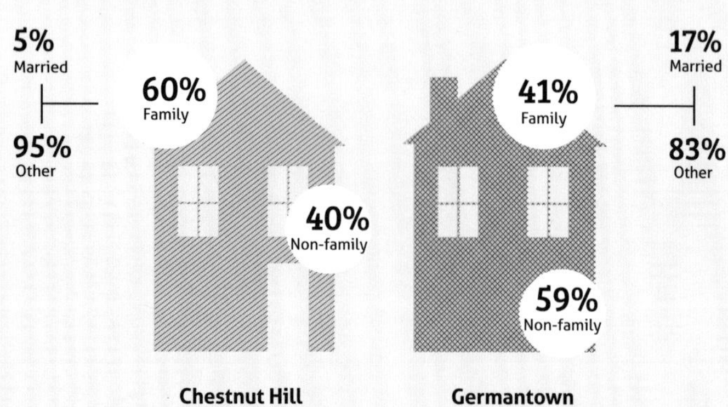

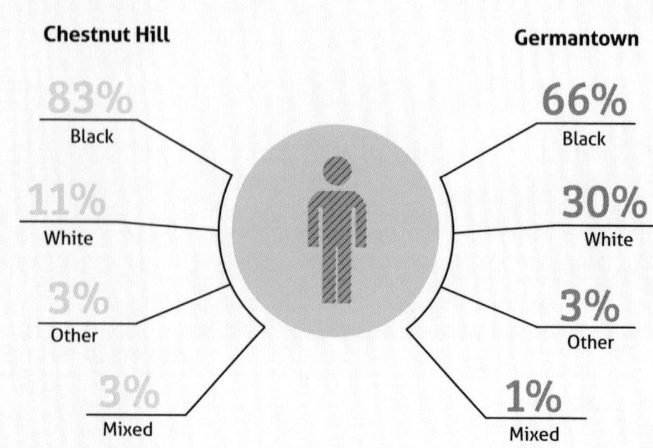

Information graphics, 2013: Ashley Nicole Johnson

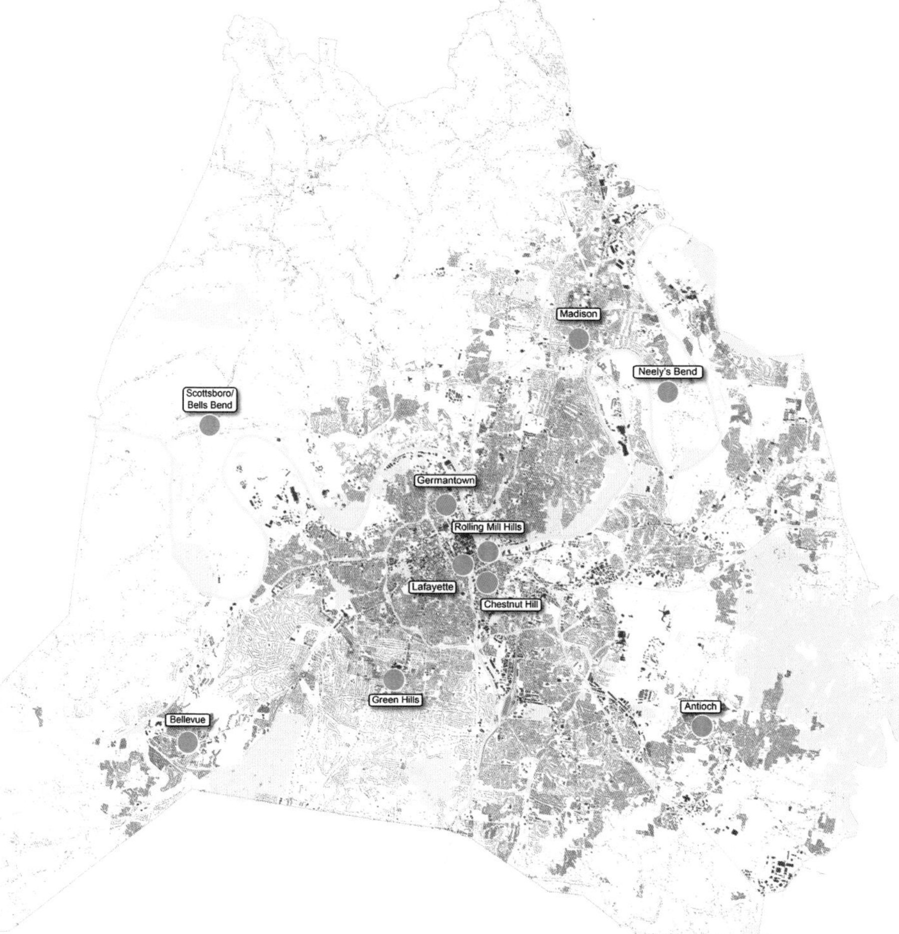

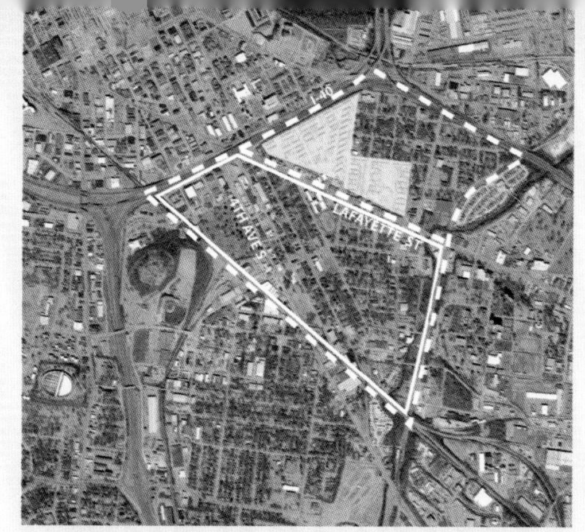

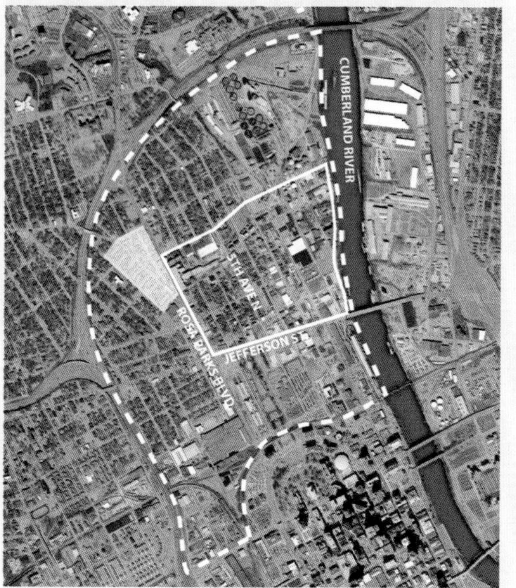

Map of case study neighborhoods with Chestnut Hill and Germantown marked in blue. *(Diagram over Map, 2013: Eric Hoke, NCDC)*

Top: Aerial of Chestnut Hill, outlined in white, with dotted line indicating the census tract in which the neighborhood lies and nearby public housing—Napier Place / Sudekum Apartments—in shaded area. Note the proximity of public housing to I-40, an indication of the close planning ties between low-income housing and the interstates—and the double whammy these developments had on existing neighborhoods. *(2010: Metro Planning Department)*

Lower: Aerial of Germantown, outlined in white, with dotted line indicating the census tract in which the neighborhood lies and nearby public housing—Cheatham Place—in shaded area. *(2010: Metro Planning Department)*

Income

Chestnut Hill

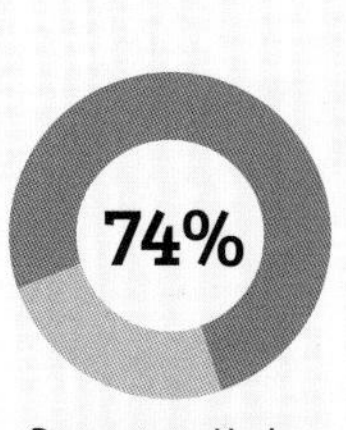

Percentage Under Poverty Level

$11,509
Median Income

Germantown

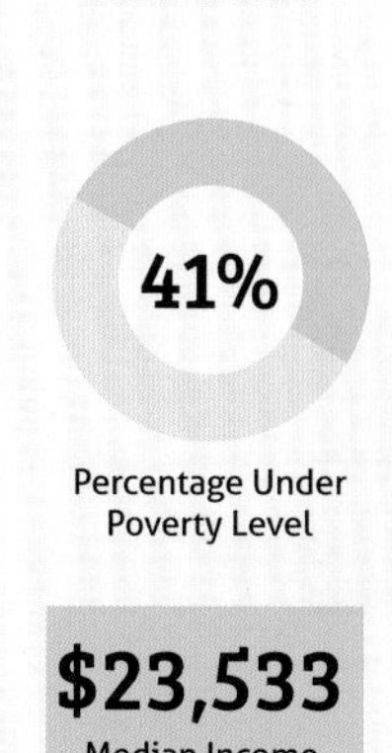

Percentage Under Poverty Level

$23,533
Median Income

Age Demographic

Chestnut Hill

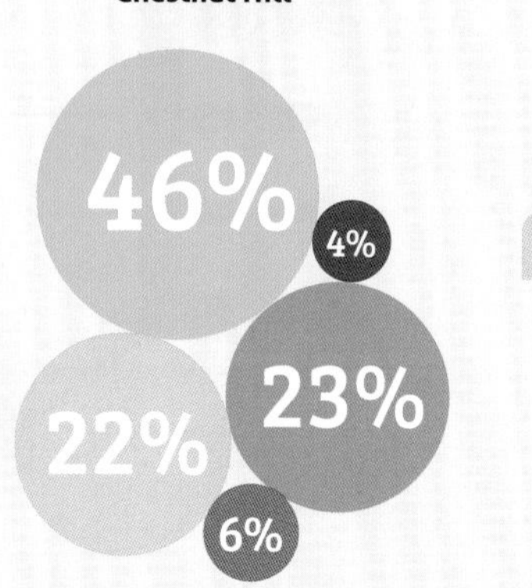

Germantown

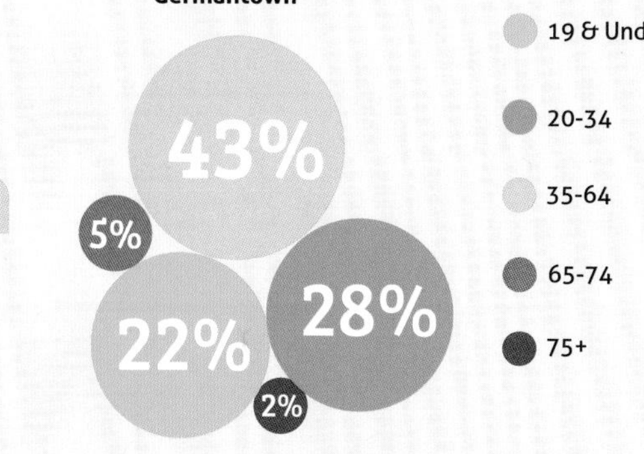

Demographic data from the US Census Department's 2010 American Community Survey (5 year estimates). At the time of research for this publication, the 2010 dataset was the most current data available. For the case studies, neighborhood boundaries were identified and data was then collected from the census tracts that best corresponded to those geographic boundaries.

Aging in the Place We Call Home

When my husband and I bought a house in East Nashville in 1985, we were in our 30s. We didn't consider what life there—or life anywhere—would be like in our 60s and 70s, much less 80s. We were just budget constrained and liked old houses. And we had, except for a regrettable two-year stint in "Bulldog Estates"—the suburban-style faculty-housing ghetto of Mississippi State University—always lived in neighborhoods where we could walk to bus, stores, and park.

During house hunting, we briefly flirted with a 1960s ranch in Hillwood. I liked the mid-century modern aesthetic. My husband pointed out that the location would be a radical departure from life as we'd known it. The lot was two acres, we didn't even own a lawnmower, we had only one car, the neighborhood had no sidewalks, the bus line was hiking not walking distance, and the closest retail was big box heaven. Enough said.

So we purchased a rambling, Victorian fixer-upper two blocks from Five Points. The reaction by many of my husband's colleagues at Vanderbilt University was that we'd gone to the dark side. They suggested that this course of action would result in our being held up at gunpoint, slain in our bed, and—most importantly—no one on the faculty would come to our house for parties.

A lot of sweat equity, neighborhood activism, and one tornado later, we have aged in place, having hosted a number of parties at which Vanderbilt faculty, staff, and students were prominent among the attendees. And we intend to dwell in East End until we are certifiably demented, when we probably won't know, or care, where we are.

Of course, we're now in our 60s and it seems advisable that we downsize sooner rather than later from our nine rooms of high maintenance. Condos are out because we have too many pets for shared walls and mini-yards. But we should be able to find something nearby that's easier and cheaper to keep up, if the teardown specialists will be good enough to leave some of the small stuff standing.

Our determination to stay in the Near East is in part due to the fact that we have aged in a place where life is possible when one can no longer drive. We can walk or bike to groceries, hardware store, bank, library, post office, BRT line—downtown takes 15 minutes—recreation center, park, greenway, and a variety of nice restaurants. Of equal significance is that we are part of a community that we have helped to build and grow, with longtime friends who've hoed the row beside us. We want to enjoy the fruits of our labors.

—CHRISTINE KREYLING

STRATEGY: *Create communities that enable aging in place, defined by the Centers for Disease Control and Prevention as "the ability to live in one's own home and community safely, independently, and comfortably, regardless of age, income, or ability level."*[37]

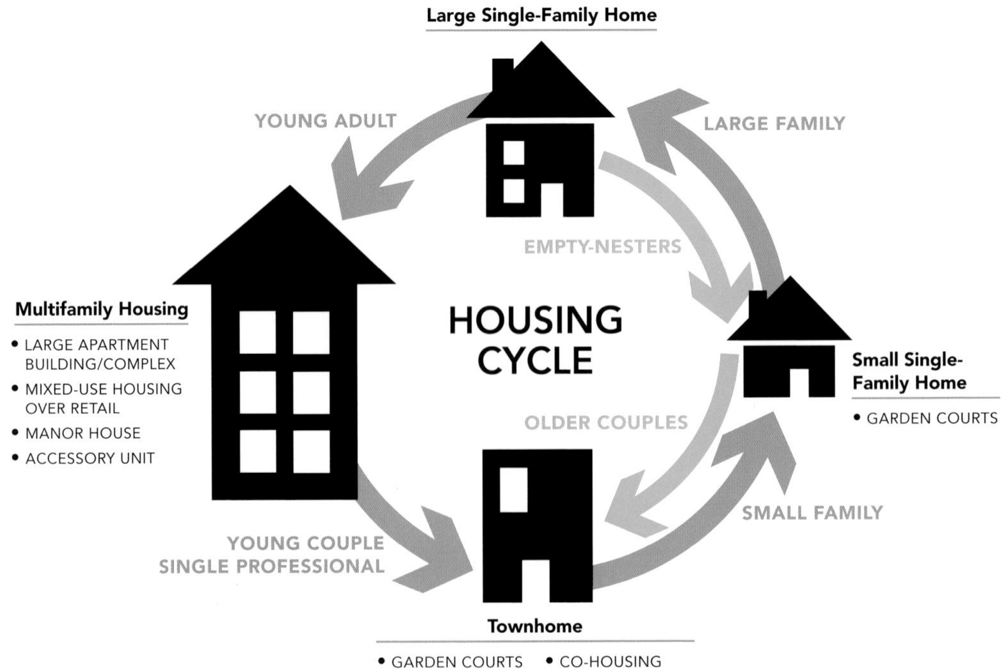

The different housing types potentially experienced across one's lifetime. This image is an update to a graphic that appeared in the Cumberland Region Tomorrow's *Quality Growth Toolbox*, 2007. *(Diagram, 2013: Deborah Brewington, Vanderbilt University Creative Services)*

CHESTNUT HILL

Formerly called Cameron Trimble, and before that Trimble Bottom, Chestnut Hill has a rich African American heritage.[38] After the Union occupation of Nashville in 1862, the federal forces established three so-called contraband camps to house fugitive slaves who had fled to the city for protection and were considered the contraband of war. One of the camps was near the site of Fort Negley because the army employed the slaves in its construction. The fort became part of the largest fortification of a city outside of Washington, DC, and "the most important Civil War structure for which Negro artisans and laborers contributed their talents," according to historian Bobby Lovett.[39]

After the war, some of the emancipated blacks settled nearby, just south of Murfreesboro Pike and a mile from the fort, on land sold to the freedmen by Republican John Trimble. The area became known as Trimble Bottom because of its low-lying position along Brown's Creek.

Central Tennessee College in 1894, looking south toward Chestnut Street. This site is now occupied by Cameron School. The school was named for Henry Alvin Cameron, an African American science teacher and community leader who enlisted during WWI at the age of 45 and died in battle. *(1893: Metro Nashville Archives)*

In 1867 Central Tennessee College, founded by northern Methodists for the education of the freedmen, opened on Maple Street, now First Avenue South. The college established the Meharry Medical Department in 1875. This was the first facility in the South to train black doctors. With more than four million freed black people in the region, the need was critical. Central Tennessee changed its name to Walden University in 1900, regrouped as a junior college in 1922, and closed completely in 1929. The Meharry program split from the university in 1917, winning its own charter as Meharry Medical College.

The medical school's students, doctors, and nurses took up residence on Trimble Bottom's western hills, with less affluent blacks occupying the flood prone and unhealthy bottomlands. Meharry was a dominant force in Cameron Trimble until the college moved to North Nashville in 1931. Meharry professors and staff followed. The neighborhood became dominated by the working class.

In 1913, Chestnut Street Park opened on Third Avenue South and Chestnut Street. A year later it was renamed Louise and Rebecca Dudley Park in memory of two daughters of Park Commissioner Robert Dudley, who died when the family car was hit by a train. At this time there was only one city-owned park open to African Americans: Hadley Park in north Nashville, which was founded in 1912. Seven years earlier Preston Taylor had established his Greenwood Park for blacks on property he owned at the southwest corner of Lebanon Road and Spence Lane.

The existing Tennessee State Fairgrounds was once home to the 125-acre Cumberland Park, which began hosting horse races in 1891 during a time when Tennessee rivaled Kentucky as the center of Thoroughbred breeding and racing. The fairgrounds, which opened in 1906, were connected to downtown via a trolley line that terminated farther south at the Radnor rail yards.

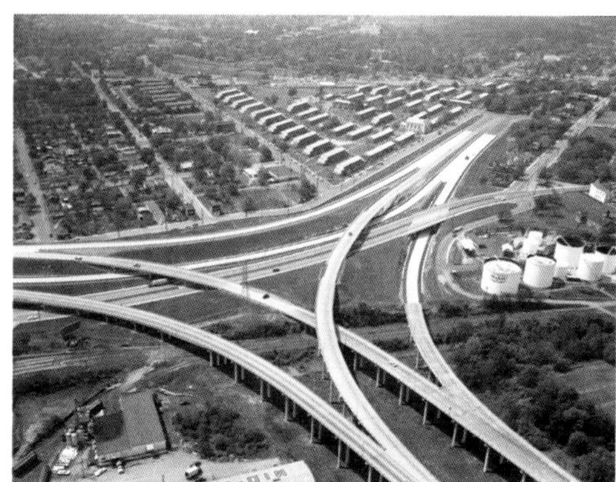

The construction of I-40 in the 1960s cut off Cameron Trimble from Rutledge Hill and downtown, creating a physical and psychological barrier. The two roadways running underneath the new interstate, Second and Fourth Avenues, became fast-moving one-way streets. This further altered the character of the once pedestrian-friendly neighborhood. Note the superblocks of Sudekum public housing in the top right of the photograph. *(1965: Tennessee State Library and Archives)*

Top left: Cameron Middle School (on the left) is easily accessed by the Chestnut Hill community's sidewalks. *(2013)*

Top right: Nashville's first example of shared equity housing was built by the Nashville-based nonprofit The Housing Fund on Third Avenue South. Called "Our House," the program enables home ownership for people whose incomes and expenses make it impossible for them to save for a down payment or qualify for a mortgage loan for repairs. The shared equity program provides substantial down payment assistance—up to 25 percent of the purchase price—as a zero interest, due-on-resale loan. In return, the buyer shares a portion of the appreciation in the value of the home at the time of resale with The Housing Fund. The Fund leaves its equity in the house for the next income-eligible purchaser, thus preserving affordability over successive generations of homeowners. *(2013)*

Duplex infill housing on Second Avenue South was built on formerly vacant lots by David Pritchard, long-time Chestnut Hill resident turned developer. Note the traditional urban form of the building, with front porches and parking out back. *(2013)*

The Federal Housing Act of 1937 provided local housing agencies with funding for slum clearance and new public housing developments. The slums were bleak, unsafe, and unhealthy, without access to city water and sewer lines. Infant mortality, tuberculosis, homicide, and truancy rates were considerably higher than in the rest of Nashville.

Cameron Trimble, along with many other inner city neighborhoods, received large-scale public housing blocks. The federal programs vastly improved infrastructure in these neighborhoods, but the housing developments were ill conceived. J. C. Napier Homes was constructed in South Nashville in 1941 and Tony Sudekum Homes in 1953. The complexes replaced blocks of so-called blighted single family homes with barracks-style housing and gradually devolved into areas of concentrated poverty and crime. Today, Sudekum has 443 apartments and Napier Place has 378.[40]

In 1997, residents created the Trimble Action Group (TAG) to give the community a voice. TAG fought zoning changes detrimental to residents, completed neighborhood audits on topics such as codes violations to gain the attention of city government, and helped the Metro Planning Department and the Nashville Civic Design Center develop a neighborhood plan for the future. TAG also partnered with the Metro Development and Housing Agency to plan the use of federal community development block grants (CDBG) earmarked for the area that were received from 2001 to 2003.[41] A walking track was installed at Dudley Park, custom signage went up around the neighborhood, benches were placed at bus stops, health and safety improvements were completed for homes owned by income-eligible individuals, lots were acquired for new home construction, and improvements made to the community garden. TAG continues to advocate for redevelopment, preserving existing housing, and encouraging single-family homes to be built on vacant lots.[42]

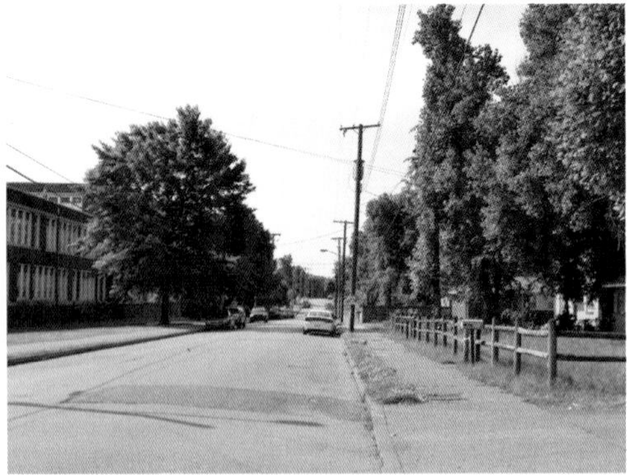

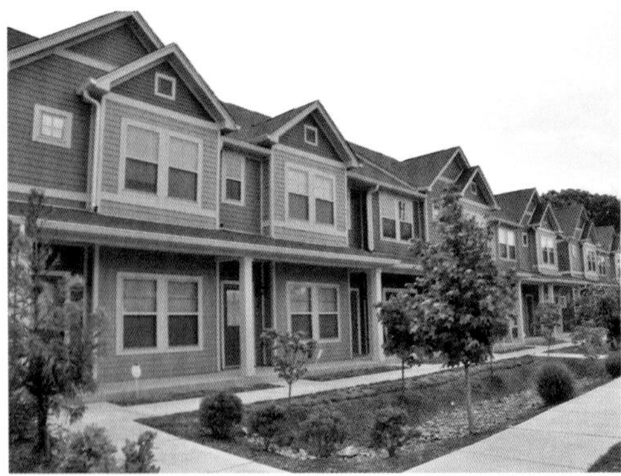

In 2005, residents renamed the neighborhood Chestnut Hill in the hope that the rebranding would aid renewal efforts. The economic downturn stalled redevelopment until recently, however. Significant transformation is now evident, with the aid of both private and public funding, including an $8 million federal stimulus grant. The federal grant supported the construction or renovation of more than 126 apartments and townhomes within Chestnut Hill. Other projects include new mixed-use development with 10 residences and 2,000 square feet of retail space.

Sensitivity to pricing out long-time residents has been at the forefront of the planning process for the community as it strives to maintain affordability while improving living conditions for residents.

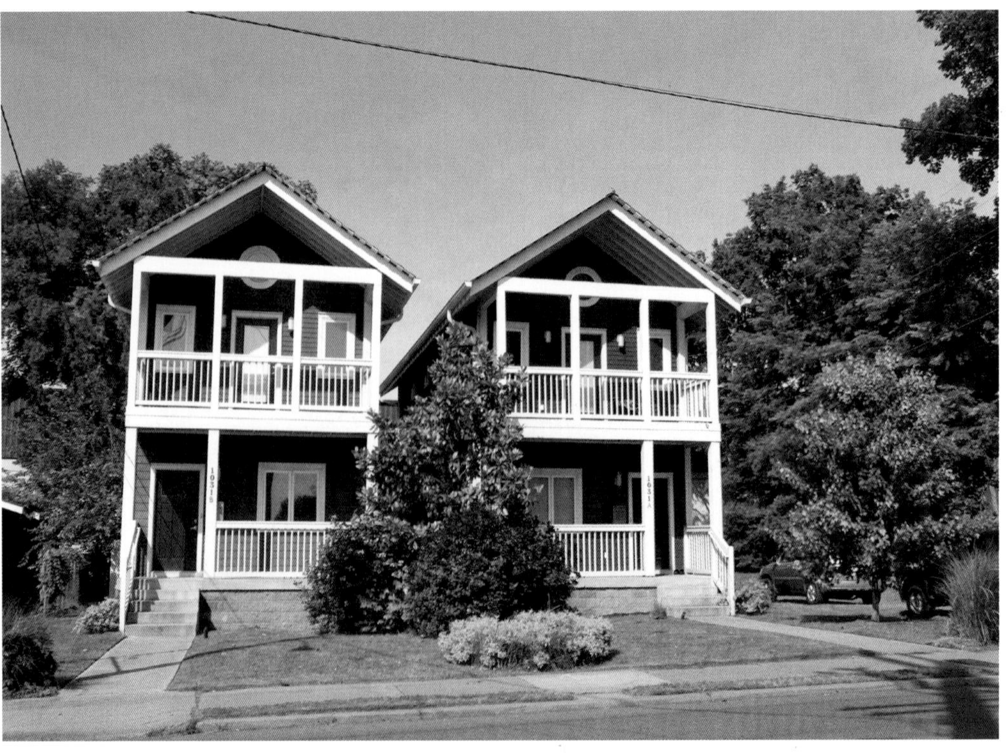

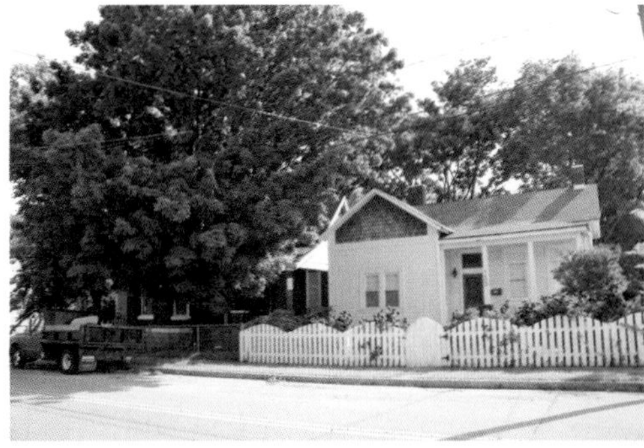

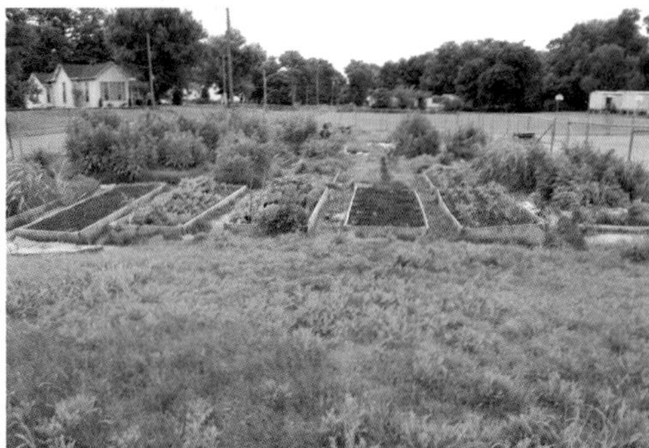

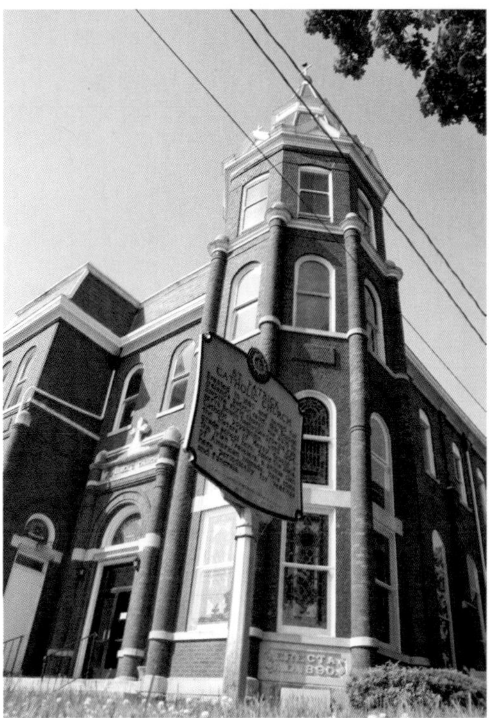

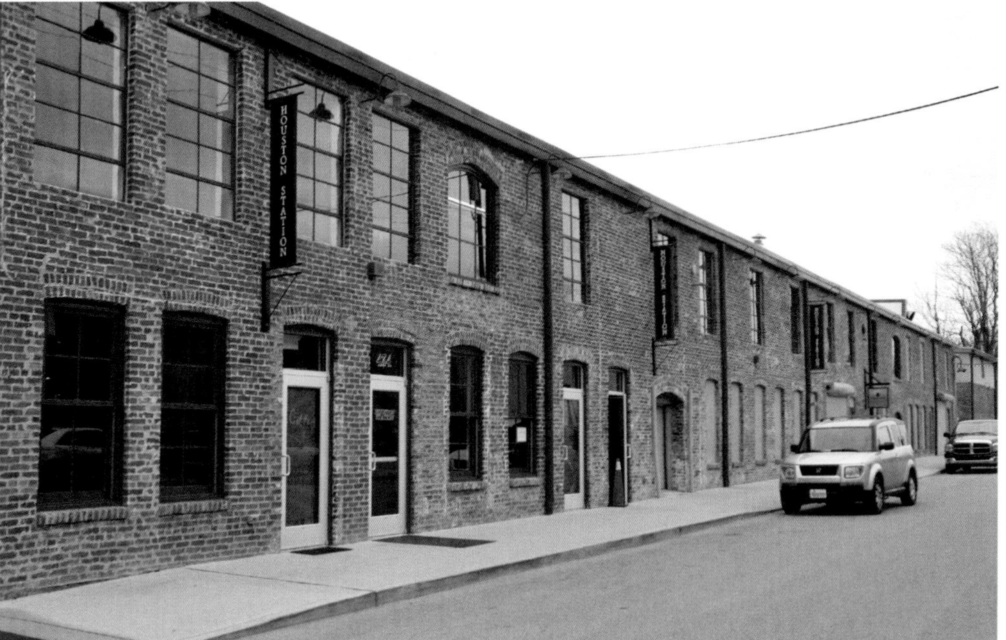

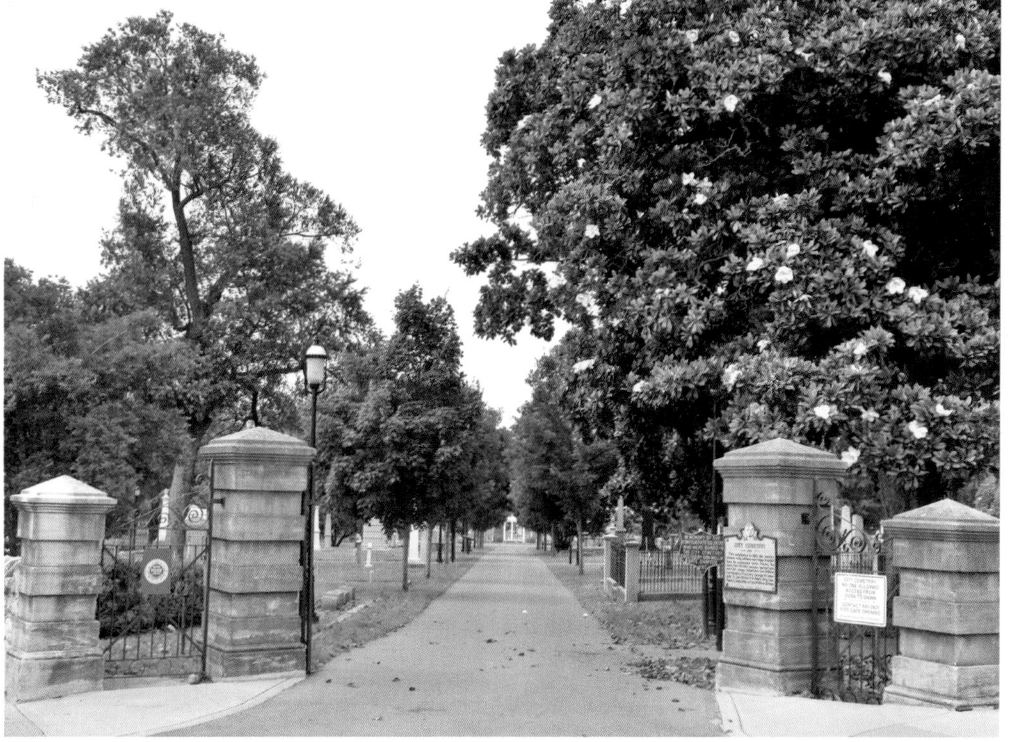

Far left, top: A large portion of Chestnut Hill's housing stock is made up of small, older structures. (2013)

Far left, center: Community garden located on the grounds of the Johnson School at the corner of Chestnut Street and First Avenue. Such gardens make underutilized school property productive for the whole neighborhood. (2013)

Far left, lower: St. Patrick's Catholic Church has been a prominent architectural feature and community anchor within Chestnut Hill since the 19th century. (2013)

Left, top: Houston Station is an adaptive reuse of a 19th- and early 20th-century manufacturing complex located just south of Chestnut Street on Houston Street that once served as the home of the May Hosiery Mill and the American Syrup Company. These warehouses stood largely vacant from the 1970s through the 1990s. Their restoration and conversion to quarters for events and businesses related to art and music offers an example for recycling the many formerly industrial properties that still exist in the neighborhood. (2013)

Left, lower: The City Cemetery, which opened on January 1, 1822, and is the oldest continuously operated public burying ground in Nashville, was listed on the National Register of Historic Places in 1972. Its 28 tree-shaded acres offer a pleasant place to walk and present a history of the city in microcosm, with tombstones designed by William Strickland and the final resting places of city founders James and Charlotte Robertson, Revolutionary War soldiers, four Confederate generals, the man who named the American flag "Old Glory," 15 mayors of Nashville, and two of the original Fisk Jubilee singers. (2013)

View of Second Avenue at the intersection with Lafayette Street, looking north. This intersection is particularly problematic for pedestrian crossings. *(2013)*

Center: Existing view of Chestnut Street and Third Avenue South with four lanes for vehicles and massive utility infrastructure. Note, however, the new townhomes and retail spaces developed by the nonprofit Urban Housing Solutions (on the right). *(2013)*

Far right: Proposed view of Chestnut Street with road diet and streetscaping improvements. The plan includes new features such as on-street parking, pedestrian-scaled lighting, crosswalks and new landscaping. *(Visualization, 2013: Eric Hoke, NCDC)*

Right: Concept for a segment of the Brown's Creek Greenway corridor through Chestnut Hill and beyond. *(Diagram over aerial, 2013: Eric Hoke, NCDC)*

Far right, center and lower: Existing conditions on Creek Street, which lies alongside Brown's Creek in Chestnut Hill, and vision of proposed new greenway. *(Visualization, 2013: Eric Hoke, NCDC)*

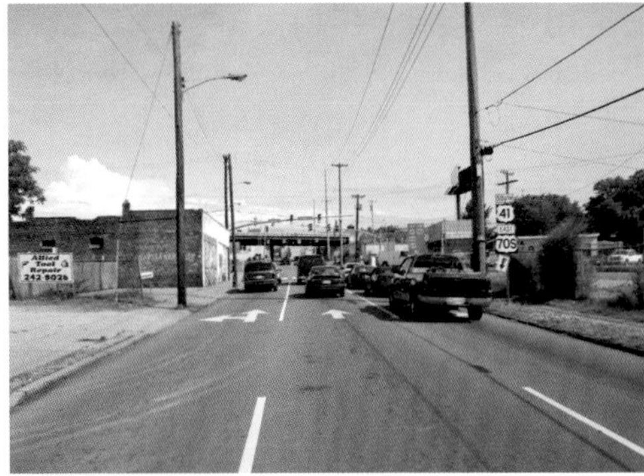

STRATEGY: *Develop a plan for traffic calming on Second and Fourth Avenues South to enable a more pedestrian-friendly environment.*

The reordering of traffic engineering priorities is a major need of Chestnut Hill in order to to increase walkability for residents and demote the emphasis on vehicular through traffic. To feed traffic to and from the interstate, largely composed of commuters to downtown, Second and Fourth Avenues were transformed into one-way pairs of three lanes each. The result for Chestnut Hill was two corridors of high-speed traffic hurtling through the neighborhood, a condition antithetical to walking, cycling, and urban living in general. As long as the interstate exists, however, the cars and trucks heading to and from the interchanges must be considered in any traffic plan for the area.

One way to slow vehicular speeds would be to convert Second and Fourth Avenues to two-way traffic. The impact on interstate access must be studied to ascertain if this is workable, however. Narrowing the lanes is another traffic calming device to be considered.

What is certain is that in the past, the living conditions and pedestrian safety of Chestnut Hill were sacrificed for the sake of through traffic and the downtown commuter. A reordering of this priority to bring parity to the two conflicting needs would yield a different traffic pattern.

STRATEGY: *Perform a road diet on Chestnut Street with on-street parking, buried utility lines, landscaping, and new lighting to create a pedestrian-friendly "Main Street" for the neighborhood.*

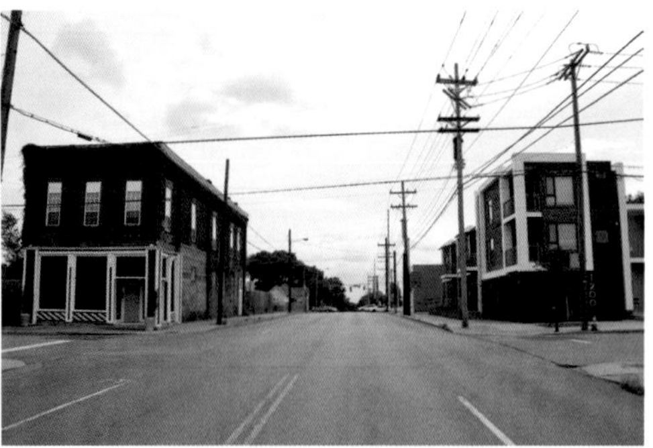

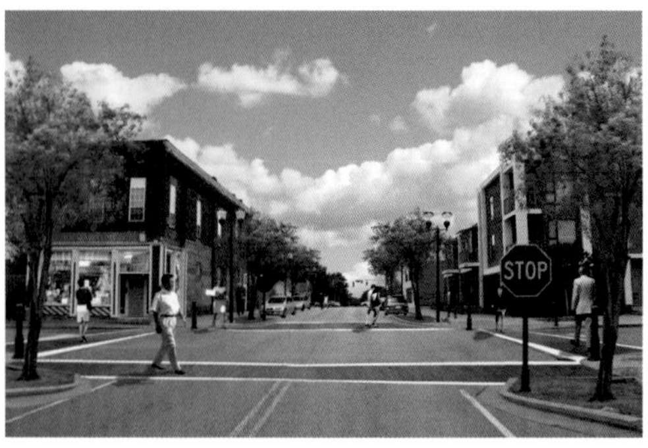

STRATEGY: *Develop a greenway along Brown's Creek to connect the Cumberland River to the park proposed for the floodplain at the Tennessee State Fairgrounds. Install community gardens within the creek's bottomland as it passes through Chestnut Hill.*

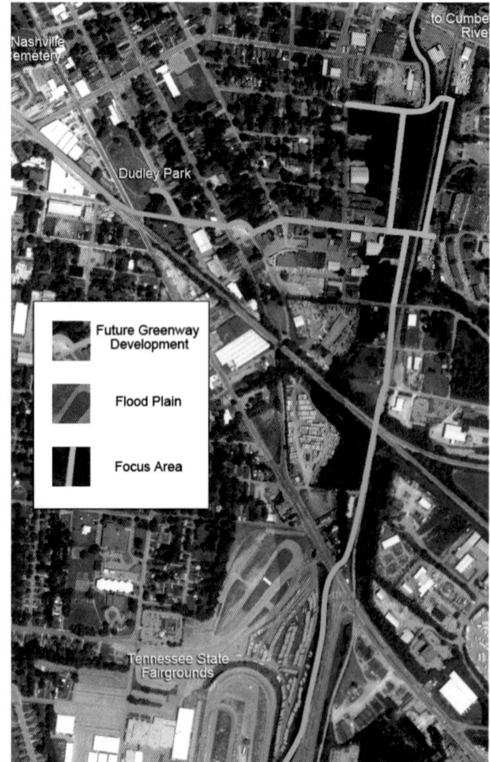

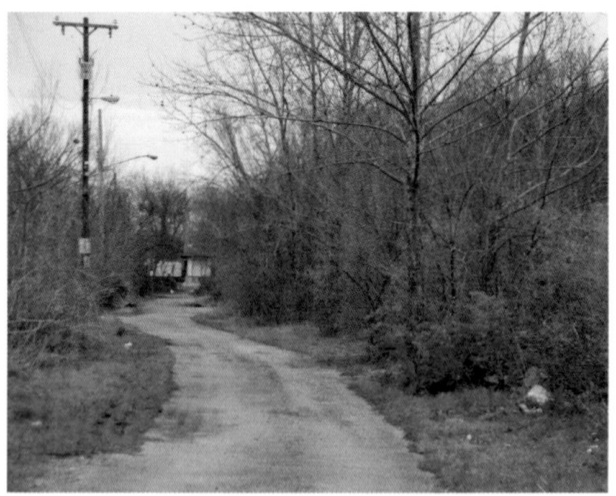

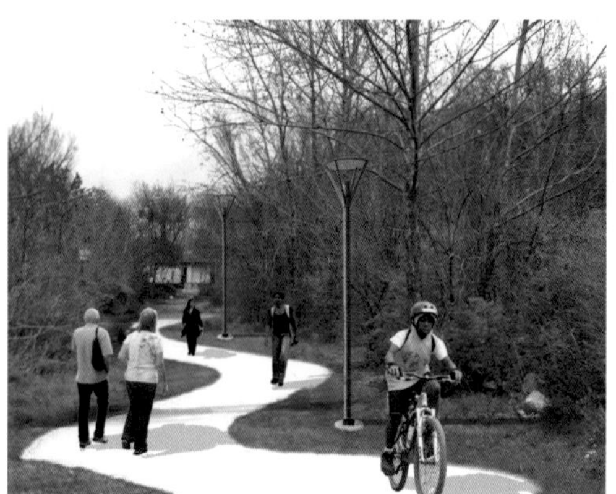

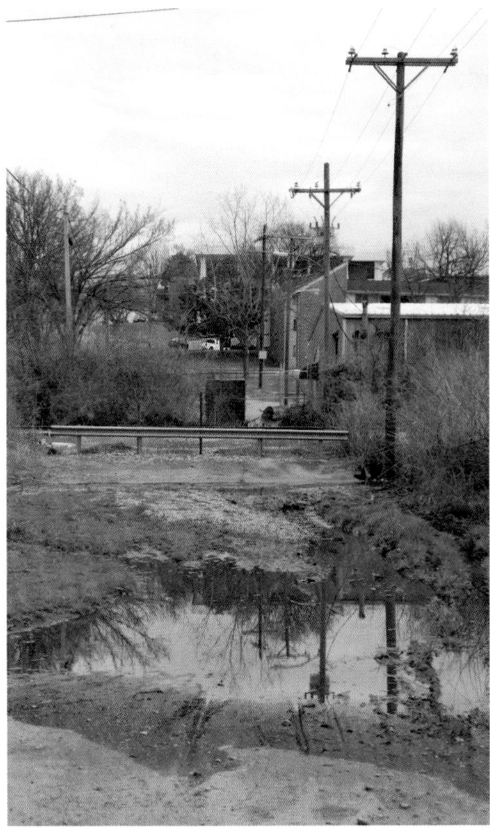

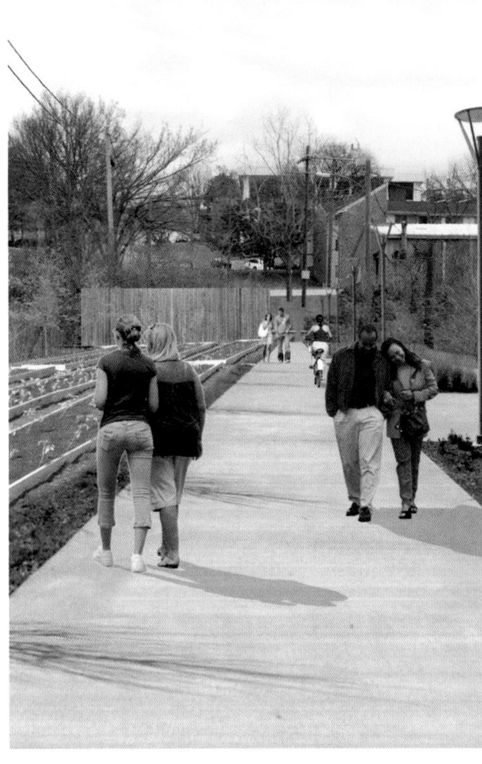

Far left: Hart Street is currently fractured by fencing and a vehicle barrier. *(2013)*

Left: A proposal for new pedestrian connections to Trevecca with community gardens and greenway. *(Visualization, 2013: Eric Hoke, NCDC)*

STRATEGY: *Connect the Chestnut Hill neighborhood to Trevecca Nazarene University across Brown's Creek via Hart Street.*

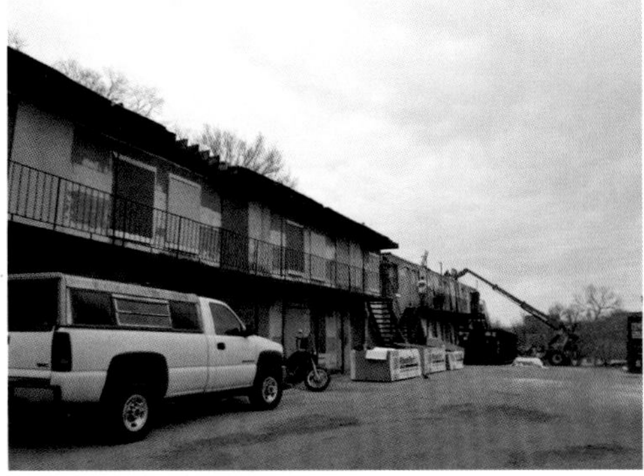

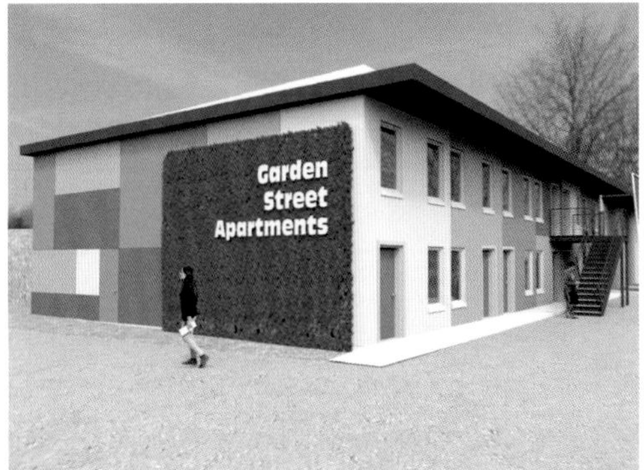

A dilapidated apartment complex along Garden Street under redevelopment by nonprofits Castanea and Urban Housing Solutions to provide sustainable affordable housing options in Chestnut Hill. *(2013; Rendering, 2013: Urban Housing Solutions)*

STRATEGY: *Continue infill development on vacant lots that incorporates mixed income housing as well as retail and business spaces. Rehab or redevelop neglected and condemned properties.*

GERMANTOWN

Even before there was a Nashville, the area that now includes Germantown was well-trafficked.[43] The pattern of hoofprints and then footprints was imprinted on the land due to the salt lick and sulphur spring that lay just east of what is now the Bicentennial Mall. Lick and spring attracted animals who, in turn, attracted the Native Americans who hunted them, followed later by French trappers and traders.

In the late 18th century, David McGavock acquired 640 acres in present-day Germantown, a portion of the 2,240 acres he would eventually acquire through purchases and inheritance.[44] The McGavocks gradually sold off parcels of land for farming. In the 1830s and 1840s agriculture gave way to residential development, largely occupied by Germans. Prominent among these immigrants were the Buddekes (groceries and whiskey), Neuhoffs (meat packers), Gersts (brewers), and architect Adolphus Heiman. In 1865 Germantown was incorporated into Nashville proper.

Many of the new residents set up shop as butchers, an occupation they brought with them from the Fatherland, using backyard sheds as slaughterhouses. This cottage industry earned the area the nickname Butchertown. Beginning in the latter decades of the 19th century, cotton mills arrived, diversifying the local economy. Germantown reached its industrial peak in the years immediately before World War I, with meat packing and textile manufacturing as the predominant employment opportunities.

The development of refrigeration in the early 20th century brought meat from outside suppliers to Nashville, creating competition for the locals. To stay in business, the butcheries consolidated and expanded into large meat packing houses that eroded the residential character of the neighborhood. During World War I, anti-German sentiment swept the nation and people of German ancestry

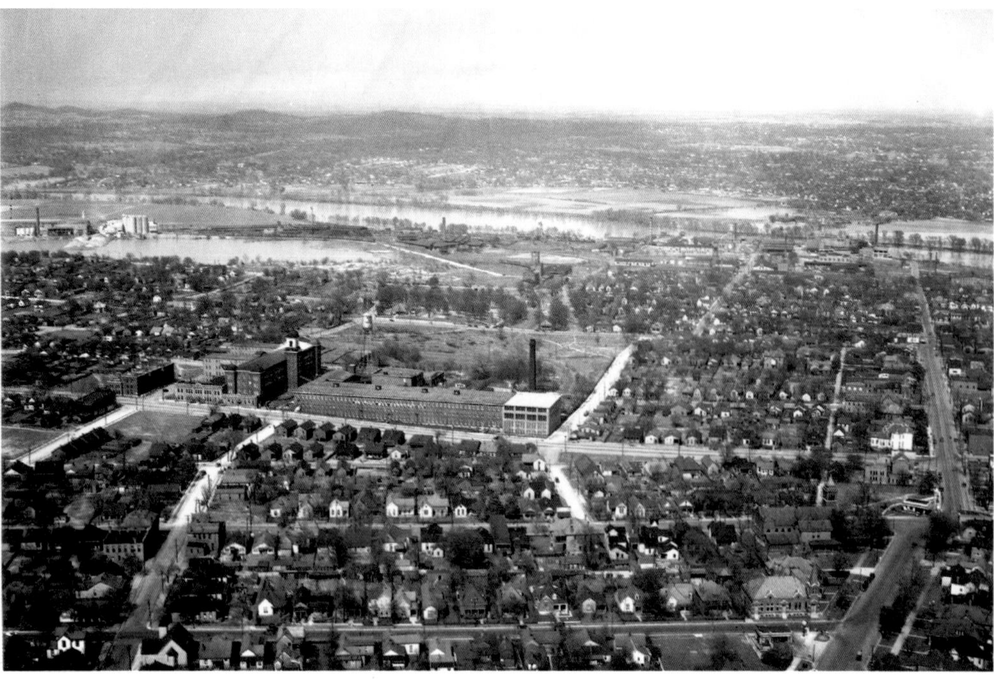

Aerial view of Germantown in 1934. The Werthan Bag Mill on Eighth Avenue is located in the middle of the image and the Neuhoff complex on the west bank of the Cumberland River is in the upper right. Many of the homes in the foreground were subsequently torn down to build Cheatham Place public housing. *(1934: Walter Williams, Jr. Collection, Metro Nashville Archives)*

were viewed with suspicion and hostility. Nashville churches catering to this population ceased conducting services in German, and German language newspapers switched to English. Residents of German background began to disperse throughout the city in an attempt to assimilate into the larger population.

Germantown's once well-maintained and stately homes were subdivided into apartments and rented or turned into boarding houses. The area was zoned industrial and historic homes were replaced by warehouses, machine shops, and other heavy commercial and industrial uses.

In the 1950s, urban renewal efforts utilizing federal funds cleared slum housing around Capitol Hill, pushing its residents northward. I-40 sliced through North Nashville in the 1960s, sundering the connectivity between Germantown and its surrounding neighborhoods.

It wasn't until the 1970s, when interest in historic preservation and urban living emerged across the United States, that revitalization commenced in Germantown. A small group of pioneers purchased neglected homes to prevent their demolition and bought up vacant property that they later sold to developers interested in rebuilding the community. Prostitution and drug dealing were routine problems, but residents remained determined to make a new neighborhood on the old foundations.

In 1979, Germantown was listed as a district on the National Register of Historic Places. The application described Germantown as "one of the most architecturally and socially heterogeneous neighborhoods in Nashville," noting that there is a significant concentration of Victorian architecture, as well as Italianate, Queen Anne, Eastlake, and "shotgun."[45] The city began a series of public infrastructure improvements and funded opportunities designed to make the neighborhood more attractive to investment, including brick sidewalks, pedestrian lighting, and low-interest loans for historic home restoration. Zero-interest loans were also made available to businesses and restaurants willing to locate in Germantown.

In 1989, Governor Ned Ray McWherter unveiled plans for the 19-acre Bicentennial

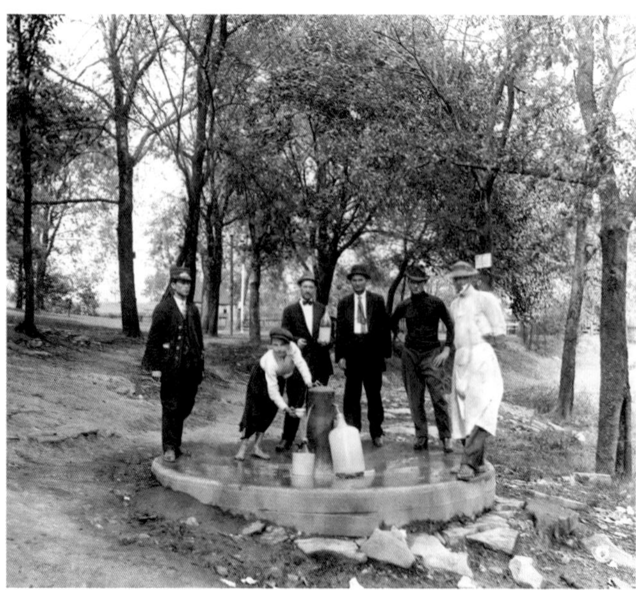

Right, center: Nashvillians collecting sulfur water from the spring in Morgan Park. *(Date unknown: Metro Parks Department)*

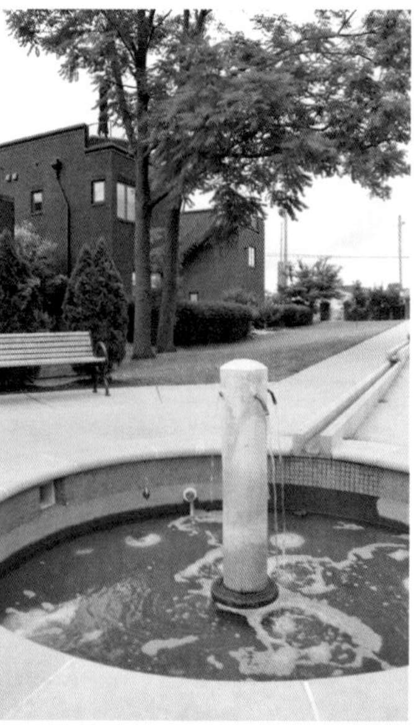

Far right: The well in Morgan Park, now capped and replaced with a decorative, non-drinking fountain. The park, which was once the city's botanical garden but had decayed before its recent renovation, now features a link to the city's greenway network. *(2013)*

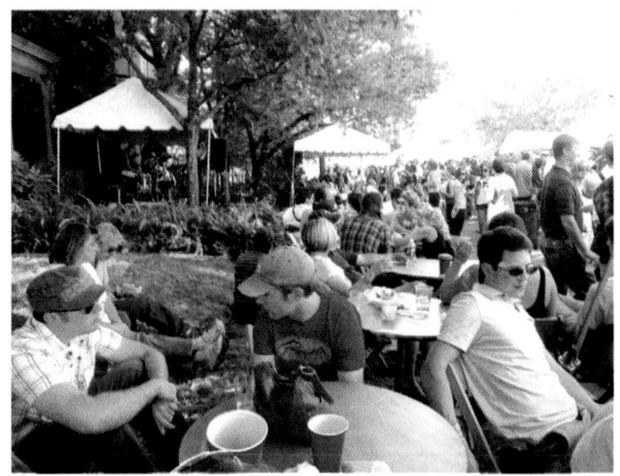

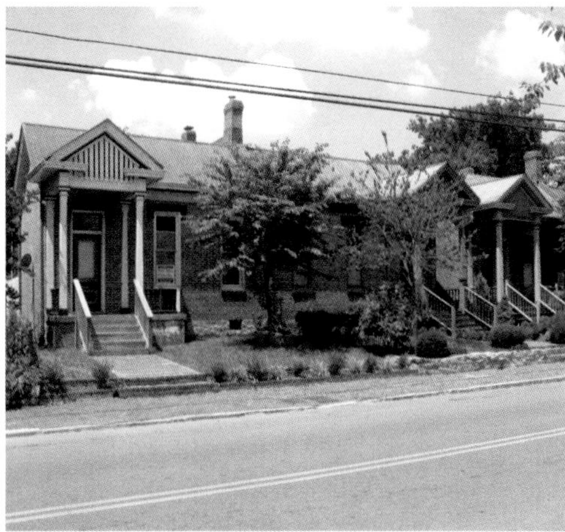

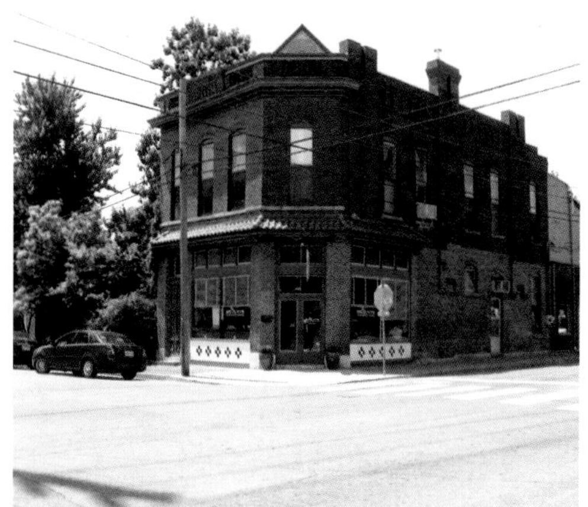

Mall, to be located on blocks of light industry and the old farmers' market immediately south of Germantown. The market was relocated to new quarters on Eighth Avenue South (now Rosa Parks Boulevard). As a part of the plan, the Metro

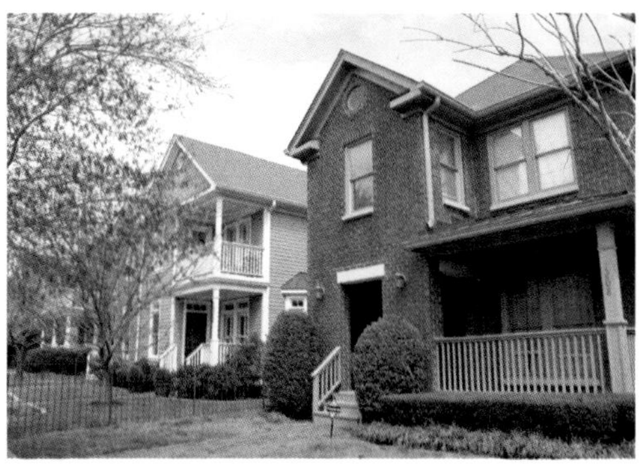

Development and Housing Agency (MDHA) created the Phillips-Jackson redevelopment district for Germantown in 1993. New projects were held to stringent design guidelines and land-use requirements. Tax increment financing (TIF) supported a new grocery store and pharmacy and helped finance larger-scale residential developments that otherwise would not have been realized. In 1998 Germantown went from an industrial to a mixed-use zoning designation.

Residential infill projects have consisted primarily of single-family homes on vacant lots and condo developments on larger vacant parcels. Rehabs include the Werthan Mills buildings, which have been converted to loft condominiums.

In the past few years, industrial and large commercial property owners, as they relocate outside Germantown, have also sold property to developers. Within the 18-square-block area,[46] a number of mixed-use developments, with office and retail space on the ground floor and condos above, have been added to the landscape. Health care technology and web marketing companies are moving into the neighborhood.[47] As one of the few residential areas within walking distance of downtown that has retained its historic charm, Germantown remains poised for further attention.

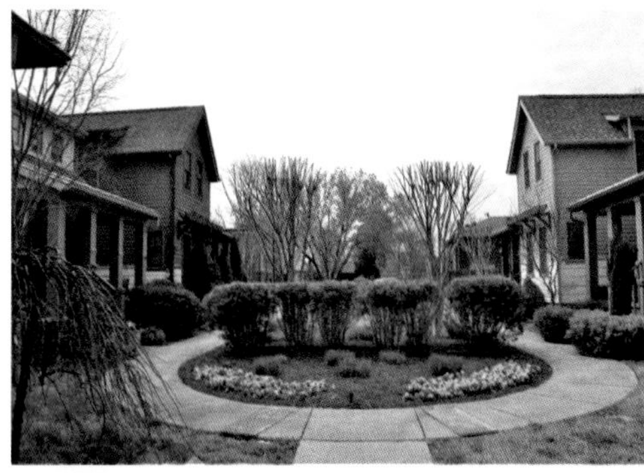

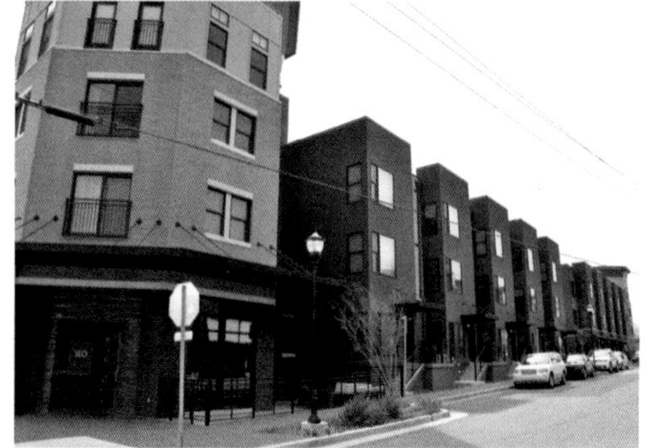

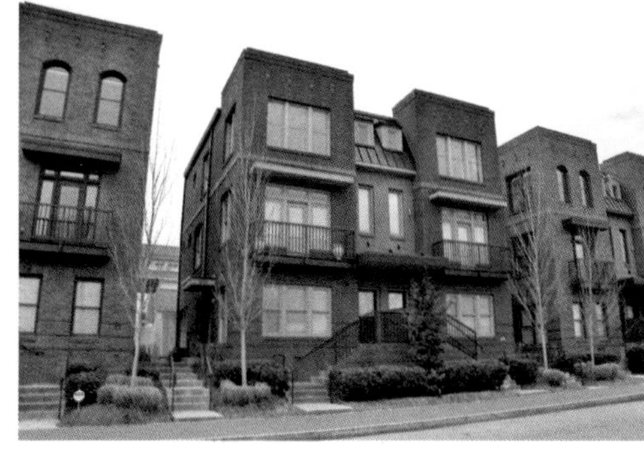

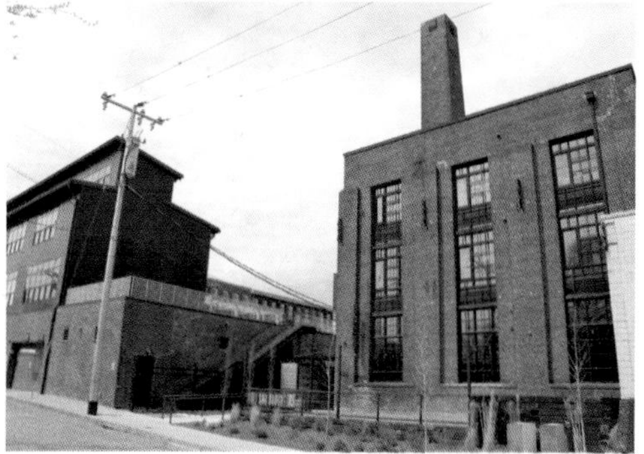

Far left, top: Germantown activists created Oktoberfest in1980, celebrating the food, music, and dance of the neighborhood's German heritage. The neighborhood festival, one of the largest in the city, attracts more than 70,000 people each October. The streets become pedestrian-only and feature a 5K run, street vendors, artists, music, and, of course, beer. *(2012: Teresa Blackburn)*

Center left, top: Restored row houses on Fifth Avenue North in Germantown. *(2010)*

Left, top: The Mad Platter restaurant at Monroe Street and Sixth Avenue North. Historic commercial structures throughout Germantown have been transformed into restaurants, shops, and offices. *(2010)*

Far left: Residential infill by Germantown Partners on Fifth Avenue North (1997). The site had once been slated for an auto emissions testing center. MDHA sold the land to the developers for a minimal price, but the developers needed zoning variances to permit narrower lot widths than the city's subdivision policies then required. The new single-family homes were the first in decades in the neighborhood. Urban infill was a new concept in the city, and the success of the project proved that there was an interest in urban living. *(2013)*

The 21st century has seen a wide variety of housing types constructed in Germantown. Examples include (clockwise) single-family courtyard housing, apartments, adaptive re-use lofts, and row houses. *(2013)*

The Station Lofts at Cheatham Place is affordable housing in a dense residential building located at the edge of Germantown on Jefferson Street. *(2013)*

STRATEGY: *Keep Germantown affordable.*

Unlike Chestnut Hill, Germantown does not lack the basic built-environment factors of the prototypical healthy urban community. The neighborhood has access to healthy food via a large grocery and Nashville's central farmers' market. Germantown also has sidewalks, a neighborhood-scale public park, public transit service, and a link to the greenway system.

The risk for Germantown is its becoming an upscale enclave surrounded by poorer neighborhoods. Its increasing lack of affordability is a warning to every urban neighborhood where revitalization efforts are underway.

Thus, the key strategy for Germantown is the incorporation of affordable housing in future residential development.

STRATEGY: *Capitalize on Germantown's proximity to downtown by extending eastward the pattern of mixed-use infill development on vacant and underdeveloped lots. This would create a more continuous urban fabric all the way to the Cumberland River, engaging the Neuhoff complex as part of the neighborhood.*

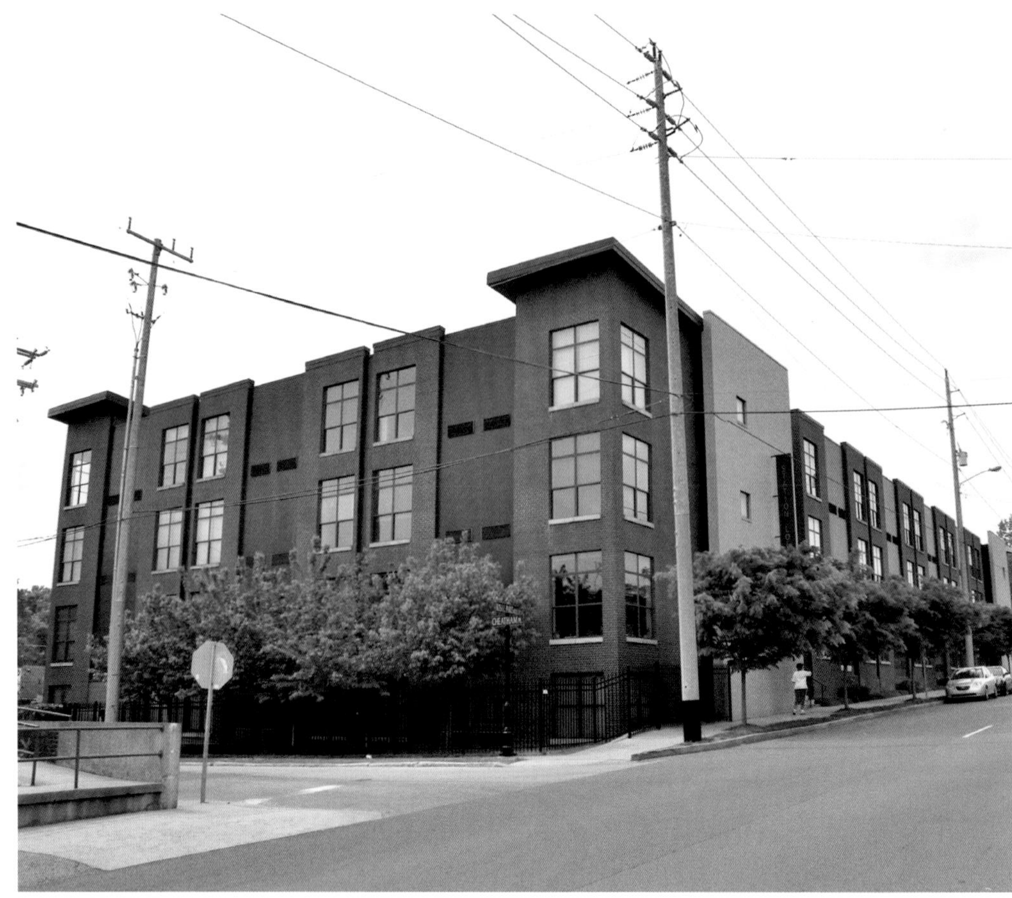

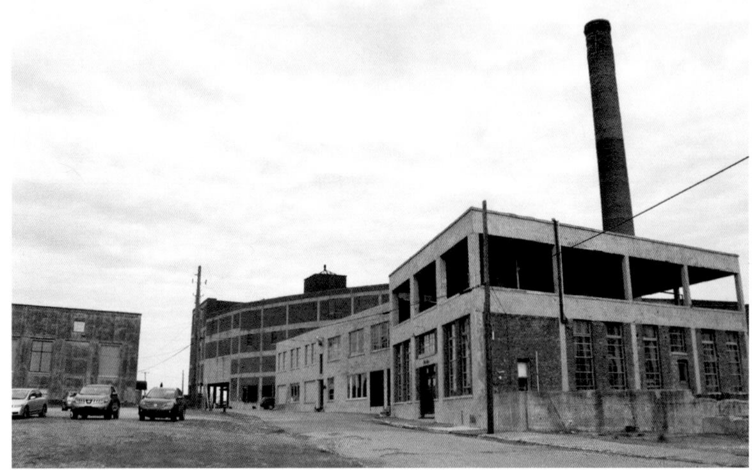

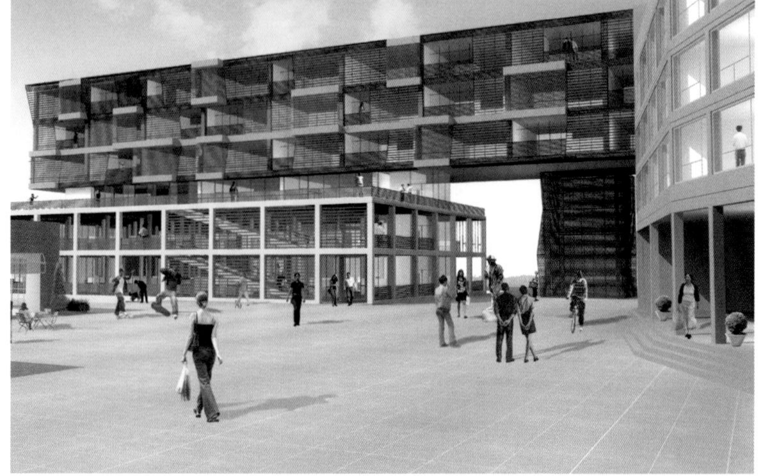

Right: The Neuhoff meat packing plant, built in 1906 and situated along the Cumberland River, closed in 1977 and stood vacant for over two decades. The McRedmond family, the current owners, commissioned from SHoP Architects of New York a master plan for redevelopment whose vision is for a mixed-use complex with an arts focus. The complex now houses the Nashville Jazz Workshop and artisan boot-maker Peter Nappi, and regularly hosts programs devoted to the arts and design. *(2013)*

Far right: The former animal holding pen at Neuhoff is re-imagined as a mix of uses below new housing, topped by a green roof. *(Rendering, 2007: SHoP Architects)*

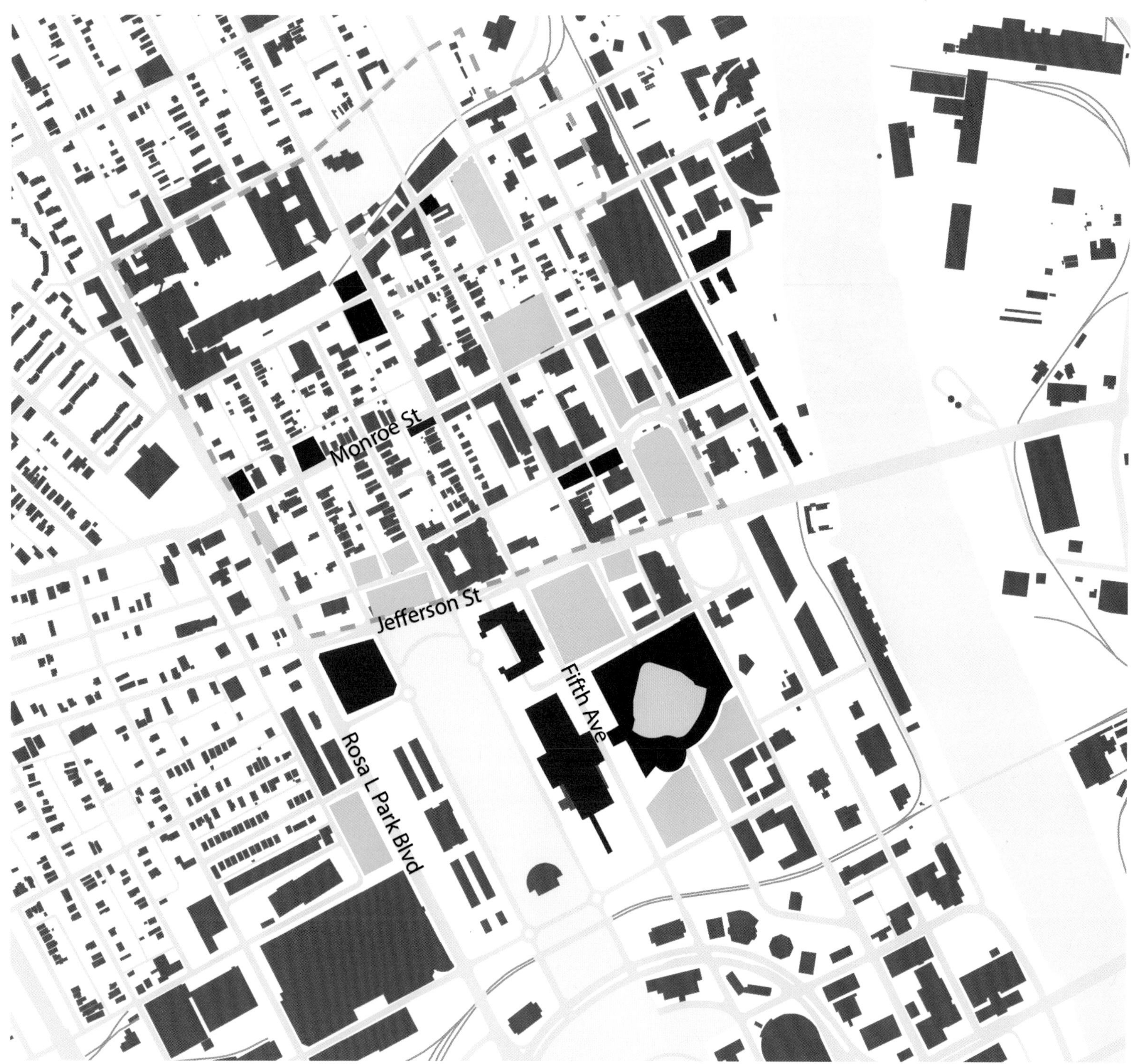

Intense infill development in the relatively compact 18 block Historic Germantown neighborhood. Dark blue represents recently completed projects; light blue are projects under construction; red are planned. *(Diagram over map, 2015: Eric Hoke, NCDC)*

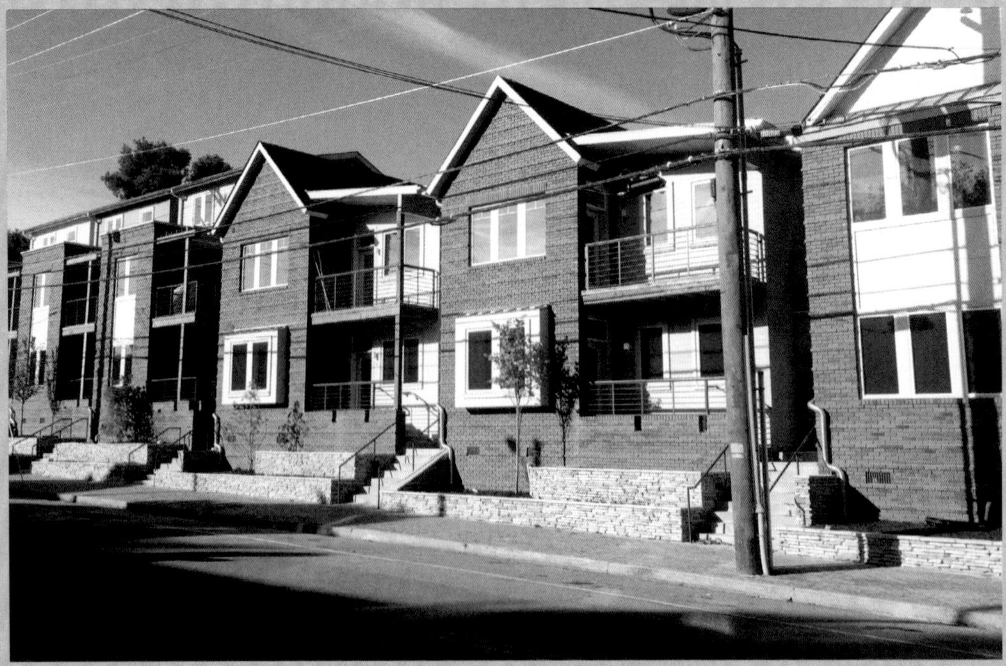

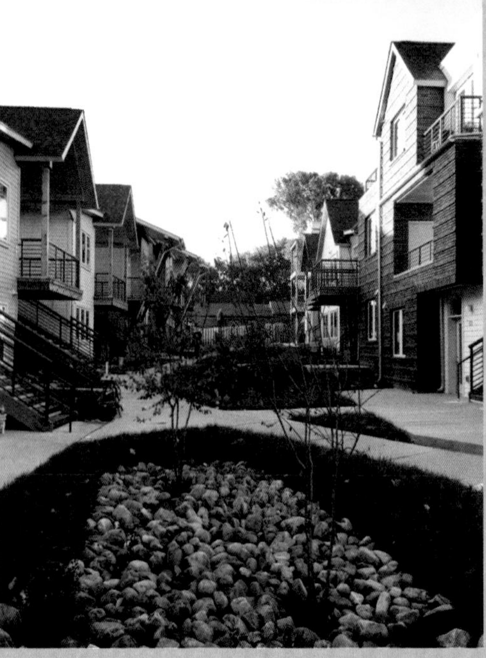

Cohousing at the intersection of 5th Avenue and Taylor Street in Germantown. *(2015: Gary Gaston, NCDC)*

Cohousing for Nashville

Cohousing is an exercise in collaboration. Residents actively participate in both the design and operation of their community.

Private homes in a cohousing development contain all the features of conventional homes, though they are often much more compact. Residents have access to extensive common facilities: open space, courtyards, community gardens, playground, and a common house where residents may choose to share cooking responsibilities and dine together as a group.[48] Weekly chores, such as yard work, are also shared among the residents. Cohousing thus provides a lifestyle with many amenities at an affordable price.

The ideal makeup of cohousing residents is multigenerational. Retired seniors may play the part of caregiver for residents with children, while younger residents can provide assistance with errands to those who need it, creating social cohesion resembling that of an extended family.

The decision-making process for a cohousing community is not hierarchical. Residents own individual units and may buy and sell them as they please, but the members of the community run the homeowners' association. Consensus among all residents is used to solve problems and make decisions. Everyone is encouraged to take part in whatever capacity they can best serve.

In an effort to promote the concept of cohousing in Nashville, the Civic Design Center hosted Cohousing Week in September 2010, which consisted of a panel discussion among enthusiasts, a lecture by a cohousing designer from Atlanta, and a public workshop that explored concepts for four potential sites around Davidson County.[49] One of the sites, located in Germantown, broke ground in September 2013 and became Nashville's first cohousing development when completed in 2015.

Most cohousing projects do start with a "burning soul," someone who has the passion to begin the process of forming a cohousing community. In Nashville, that person is Diana Sullivan, who has served as the principal promoter for Nashville's first cohousing development and spent the last several years cultivating relationships with people who want to live in this type of community.

The plan for Germantown cohousing includes 25 condos with a common house on almost an acre of property. The site is within walking distance of grocery stores, coffee shops, restaurants, the farmers' market, and two parks, as well as being bikeable to downtown. The site plan includes edible landscaping with fruit trees and planter beds for growing vegetables. A rain garden system runs through the center of the site to catch rainwater, creating a stream that eliminates the need for an underground retention system. The project is one of the first to feature Metro Stormwater Division's low-impact development (LID) guidelines.[50]

—GARY GASTON
executive director, NCDC

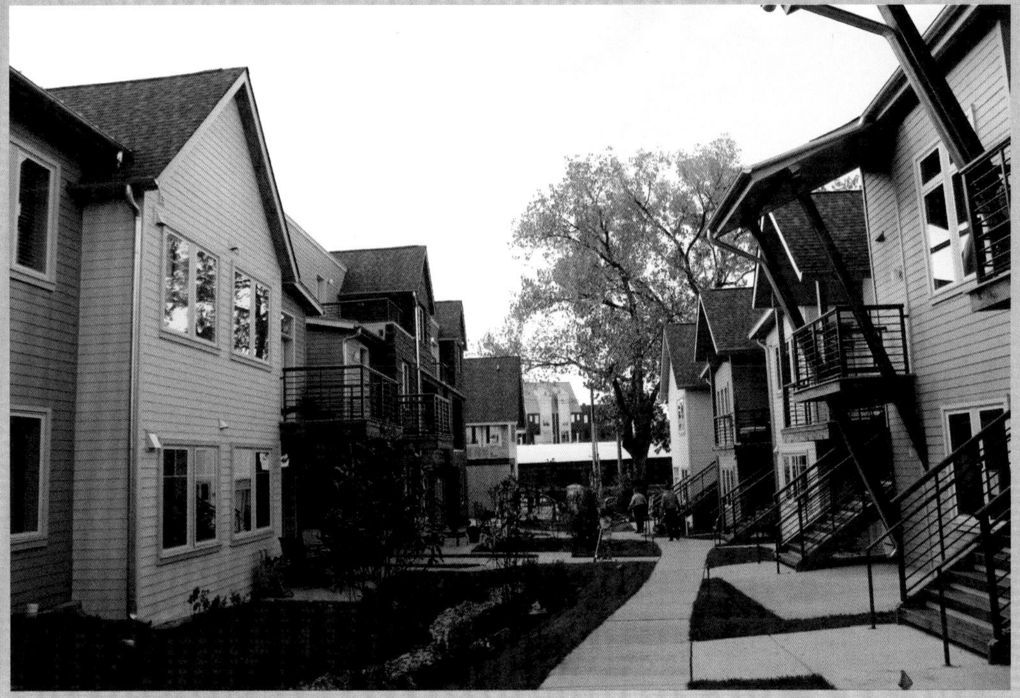

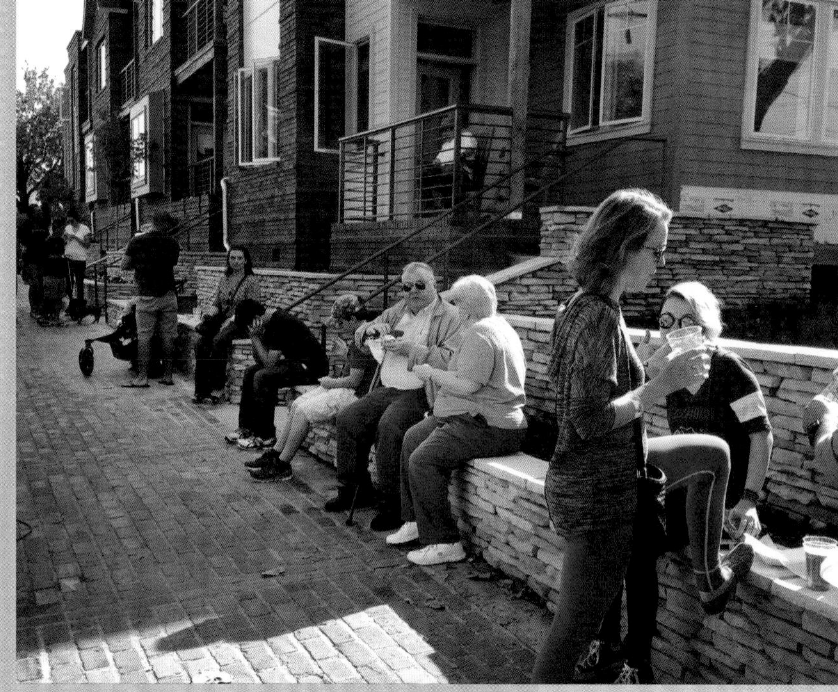

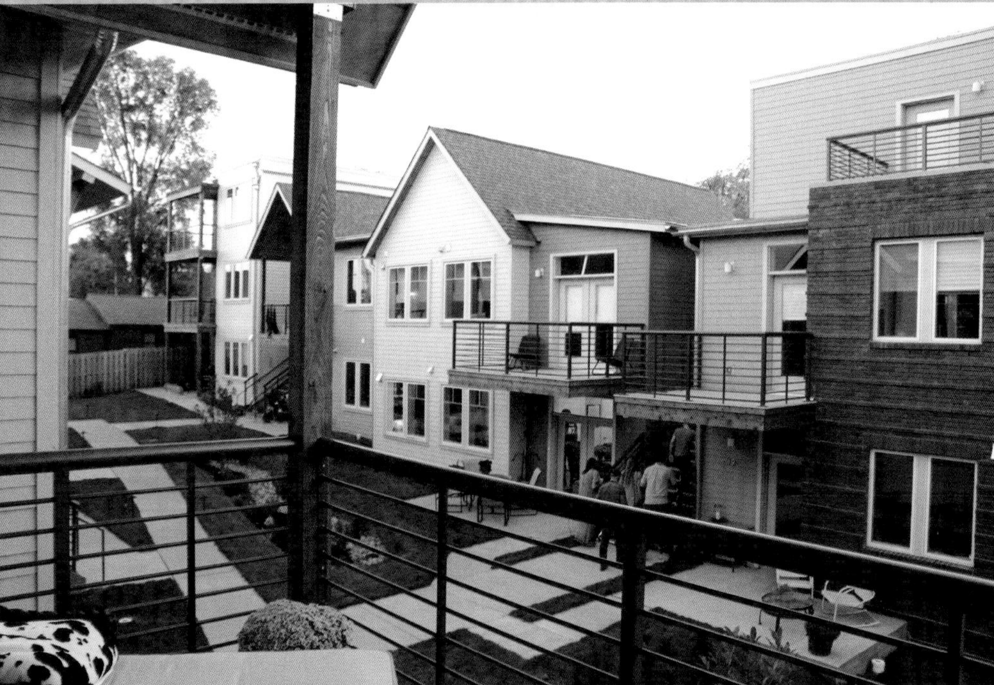

"It's a simple and basic idea to be intentional about the community in which I live, to share resources, to share time, to be supported and to support."

Patrick Nitch, Germantown Cohousing resident (2015)

Above: The exterior stone retaining wall along Fifth Avenue North was designed to be a feature that helps engage with neighbors. This intention was fulfilled shortly after the cohousing opened during a community festival. *(2015: Chris Corby)*

Cohousing courtyard design encourages interaction among residents through balconies, wide patios, and large windows in the rear-facing kitchens that front onto walkways. Note in the top left photo the presence of two large, mature cottonwood trees that were saved and incorporated as a landscape feature. *(2015)*

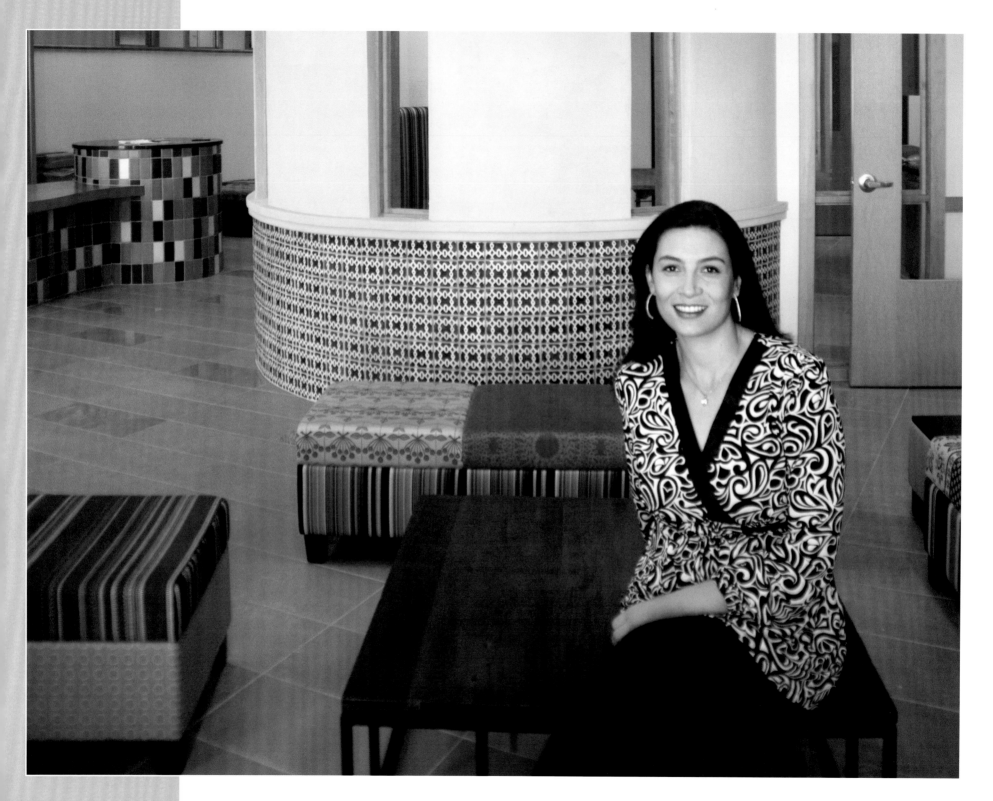

MARTHA SILVA

"I am not from the United States, and the multicultural environment in Antioch made me feel comfortable," says **Martha Silva,** 35, who moved to Middle Tennessee five years ago and is the director of economic integration at Casa Azafran Community Center.

Silva finds in southeast Nashville the excitement of a shopping and business destination, access to public transit as well as to I-65 and I-24, housing that is still affordable, and a population of immigrants from around the world.

"You can find Kurdish people, Middle Eastern people, a lot of Asian people, and Hispanic," Silva says. "Immigration has been seen heavily in Nashville for just the last 15 to 20 years, so this is still a young community. We haven't built that separation between us that you find in New York or Washington or Boston. We are all living together. We are all new in town."

Though Silva's employer, Conexión Américas, was created to serve the Latino community, Casa Azafrán, the organization's new community center on Nolensville Pike, houses 10 nonprofits within its brightly painted 28,000 square feet that provide all immigrants with affordable health care, free financial advice, and a series of English and computer classes. Event and gallery space is used for entertainment, arts, and dance. A community kitchen is available to food entrepreneurs, serving as a commissary for food trucks as well as a laboratory, catering hub, and classroom. "There is no community center like this in the whole city, so it's not just for this area, it's for Nashville," Silva says.

People can easily find fresh foods, including items from their native homelands, in stores serviced by public transport. "We have the big box stores we all know that offer fresh food, plus the little markets that are the small businesses of the immigrants," Silva explains. "They offer a huge variety of fresh food of their own plus food that Americans will feel familiar with." A formal farmers' market began in 2013 in Antioch, meeting weekly during growing season. And one enterprising Egyptian man peddles fruits and vegetables on Nolensville Pike from 8 a.m. to 6 p.m. "He himself is a little, little farmer's market," she says.

Southeast Nashville's rapid ascension as a hub for newly arrived immigrants has thrown into high relief the area's lack of long-range transportation planning. Murfreesboro and Nolensville Pikes are the main arterials. With the increasing popularity of the commercial district and all of the new residential neighborhoods that feed into these pikes, the roadways have become heavily congested.

"Traffic is really affecting the area right now," Silva says. "It can easily take me 35, 40 minutes on Nolensville Pike during the peak morning and afternoon hours to get from home to downtown and the same coming back. When developers build those brand new, pretty subdivisions, they don't think about access to them." Silva also worries that if there is another flood and people have to evacuate, for many there is only one way out. "This is my biggest complaint about the area: the primary means of access is Nolensville Pike and it's absolutely not enough."

Some residents use sidewalks and public transportation. But Silva says few walk along Bell Road near the Global Mall at the Crossings (formerly Hickory Hollow Mall). Silva laments the lack of pedestrian safety and accommodations for cyclists, who can be spotted riding on the intermittent sidewalks that do exist.

While energizing, living in this bustling center has some disadvantages. "There is a lot of visual contamination because there are a lot of signs, a lot of advertising," Silva says. Some of the businesses are less than desirable as well. "I would like to shut down some of the businesses that don't promote the financial stability of the community. There are a lot of check-cashing places; you see a new one every day. The operators are targeting low-income people that live check by check, and they take advantage of them."

Parks and greenspace are also scarce. According to Silva, "Coleman Park, [at the busy intersection of Thompson Lane and Nolensville Pike], is the only park that is well used. There are little parks like Antioch Park on Blue Hole Road, but they are too tiny, not like a community park where you can really do something." Residents frequently go to the parks in nearby Smyrna.

Silva recently moved with her growing family to the Lenox Village neighborhood because she liked the new homes and the walking trails, but staying close to work was important. "The markets, the commercial buildings, the variety of cultures, I like all that," she says.

"My beautiful daughter Sofia was born in June 2013. I am very proud to be the mother of a true Nashvillian. I can't wait to buy her first pink cowboy boots."

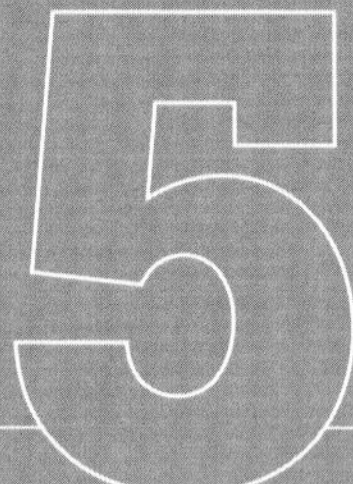

STRATEGIES

Transform underdeveloped centers into "Complete Centers" that function as mixed-use areas with access to all the basic needs for living, working, and recreation.

Establish public transit hubs in centers to anchor circulator routes in surrounding neighborhoods.

Create safe pedestrian and bicycle connections to centers from surrounding residential areas.

Ensure a wide variety of healthy food options in centers.

Establish a range of housing types and sizes within centers to ensure a wide variety of households and affordability.

Incorporate new public spaces and parks into centers, including areas for both active and passive recreation that are accessible to the entire community.

THE CENTER TRANSECT ZONE

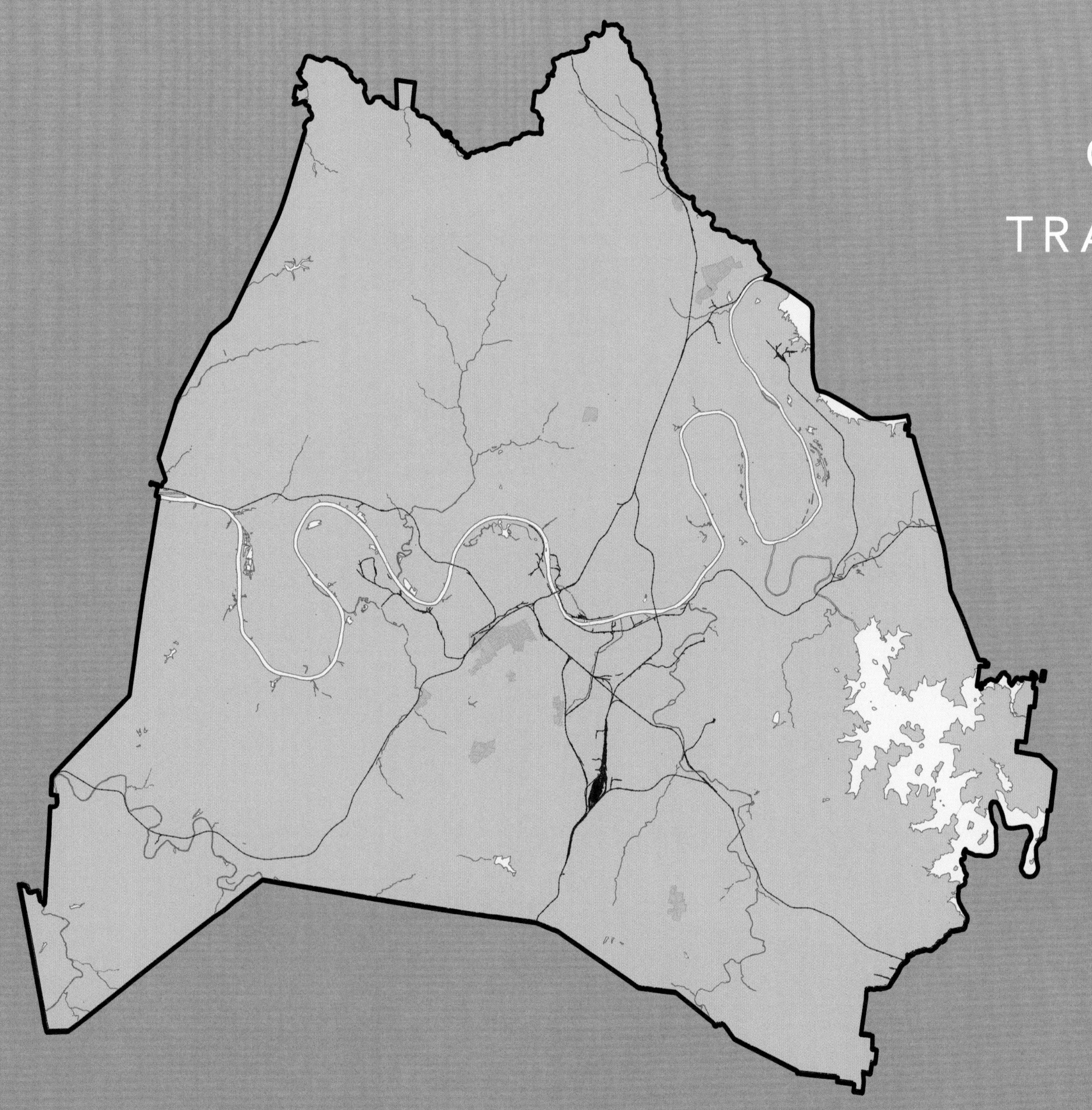

Davidson County, highlighting the areas identified by Metro's Planning Department as having the potential to evolve into true or complete centers. Centers can be distinguished by scale of catchment area (i.e., whether they serve several communities, Davidson County, or the Middle Tennessee region as a whole).

(Map, 2014: Metro Planning Department)

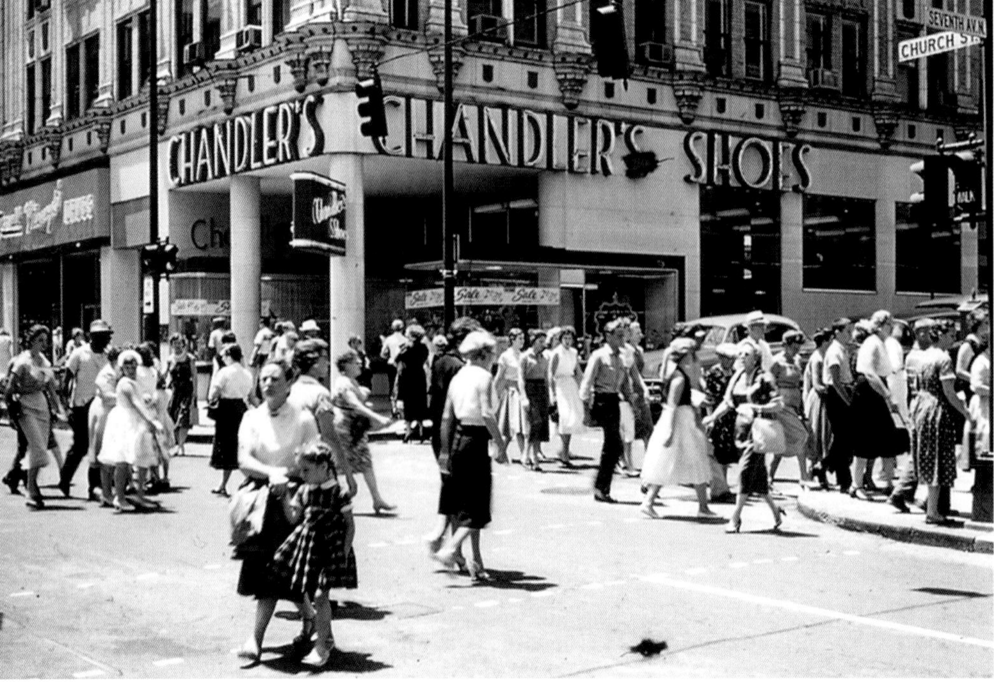

Shoppers at the corner of Church Street and Seventh Avenue in downtown Nashville when Church Street was still the retail center for the region. People rode the bus or drove to downtown and then walked between their various destinations. *(ca. 1950s: Metro Nashville Archives)*

THE EVOLVING CENTER

The centralized marketplace has functioned as the essential space for commerce and civic transactions since humans first began to structure urban communities. In describing the ancient cities of Mesopotamia and Egypt, urban historian Lewis Mumford stresses the nature of the market as an *urban* institution whose function was the "procurement, storage and distribution" of goods. Its permanence in the life of the city was dependent on reliable mass transport, originally via waterway, and a population large enough to provide merchants with a good living and sufficient urban workshops to produce goods for general sale.[1]

In the United States, the modern version of the marketplace is still dependent on mass transport. But that transport system is global and involves a network of trucks, railroads, air freight, and huge container ships. In addition, the marketplace itself now includes a virtual component. The physical marketplace has become much less urbanized and is spread out along major commercial corridors.

The shift away from downtown as the central marketplace to suburban strips and shopping centers scattered throughout an entire region began with the rise of the automobile as the vehicle for personal transportation. As discussed more extensively in the Suburban chapter, cars enabled Americans to live farther from an urbanized core. Individualized transportation brought numerous amenities to locations within closer driving distances to suburban homes, but these amenities were laid out for access by private automobile.

The development of big-box grocery stores, department stores and smaller retail specialty

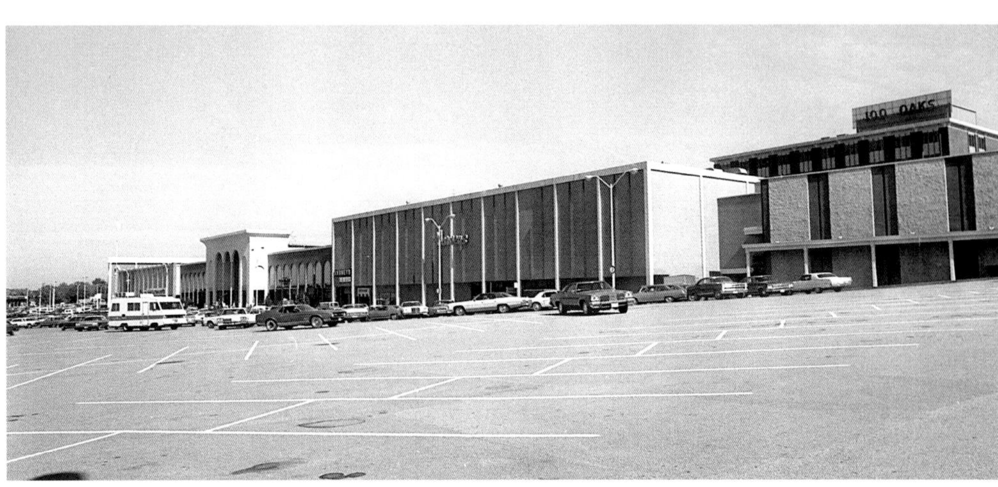

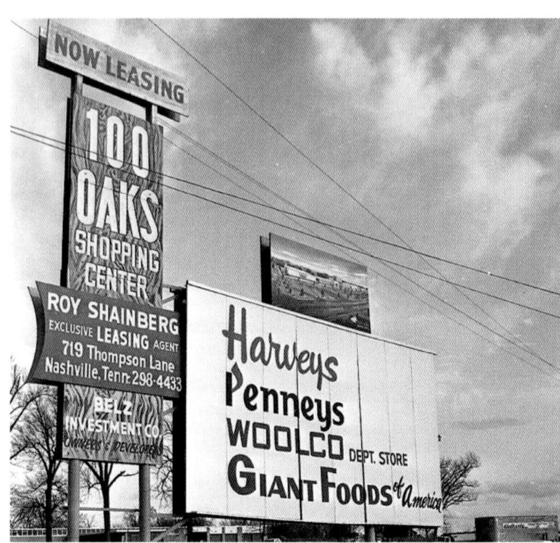

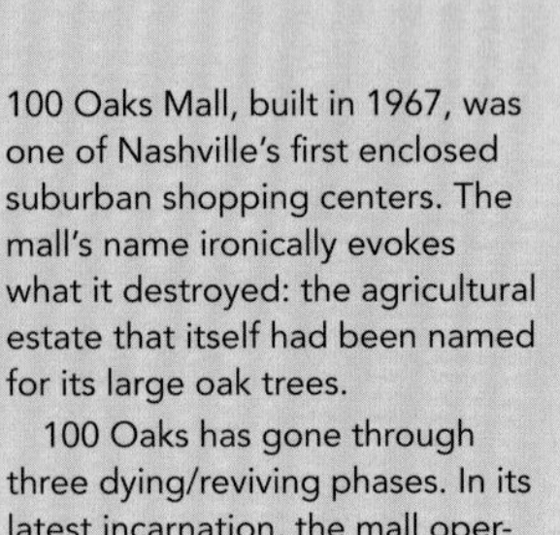

100 Oaks Mall, built in 1967, was one of Nashville's first enclosed suburban shopping centers. The mall's name ironically evokes what it destroyed: the agricultural estate that itself had been named for its large oak trees.

100 Oaks has gone through three dying/reviving phases. In its latest incarnation, the mall operates as a shopping center on the ground level, with offices and clinics for the Vanderbilt University Medical Center on its second. *(ca. 1967: Metro Nashville Archives)*

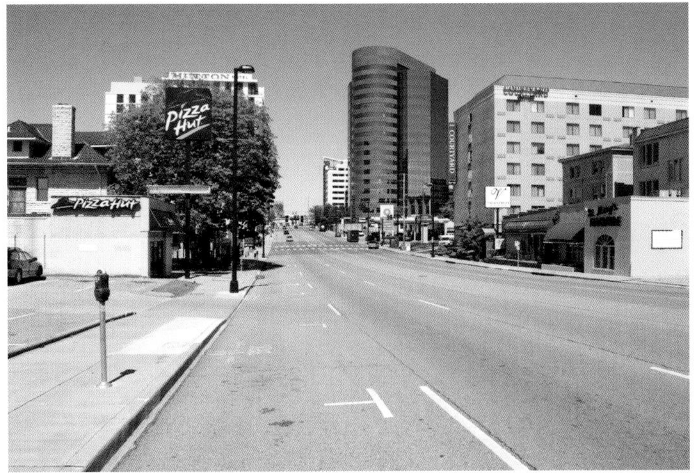

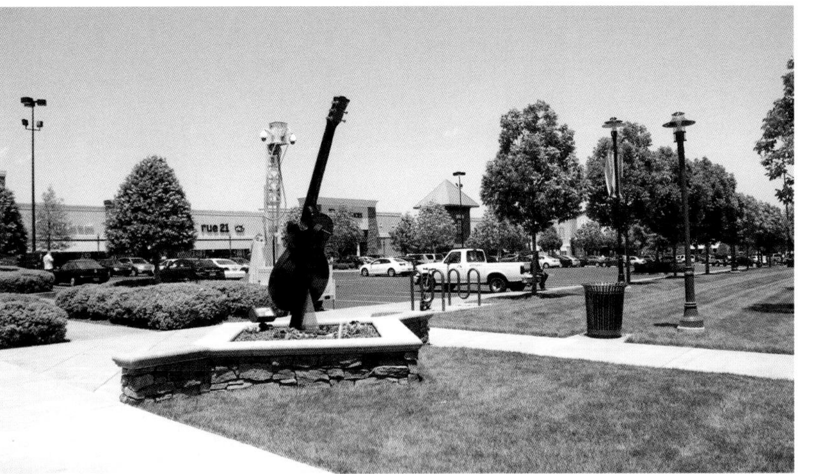

Left: Midtown's wide range of uses and densities, its location along West End Avenue—the city's busiest commercial corridor—the connectivity of its street network, and the increasing presence of residential units make the area a prime candidate for evolution into a true center. But the presence of suburban-style venues, such as drive-thru fast food shops and numerous curb cuts in the sidewalk network, indicate that midtown still has some evolving to do. *(2013)*

Right: The Nashville West Shopping Center incorporates a public park space and includes sidewalks, bike racks, and art, but it is still auto-centric in its design. *(2014)*

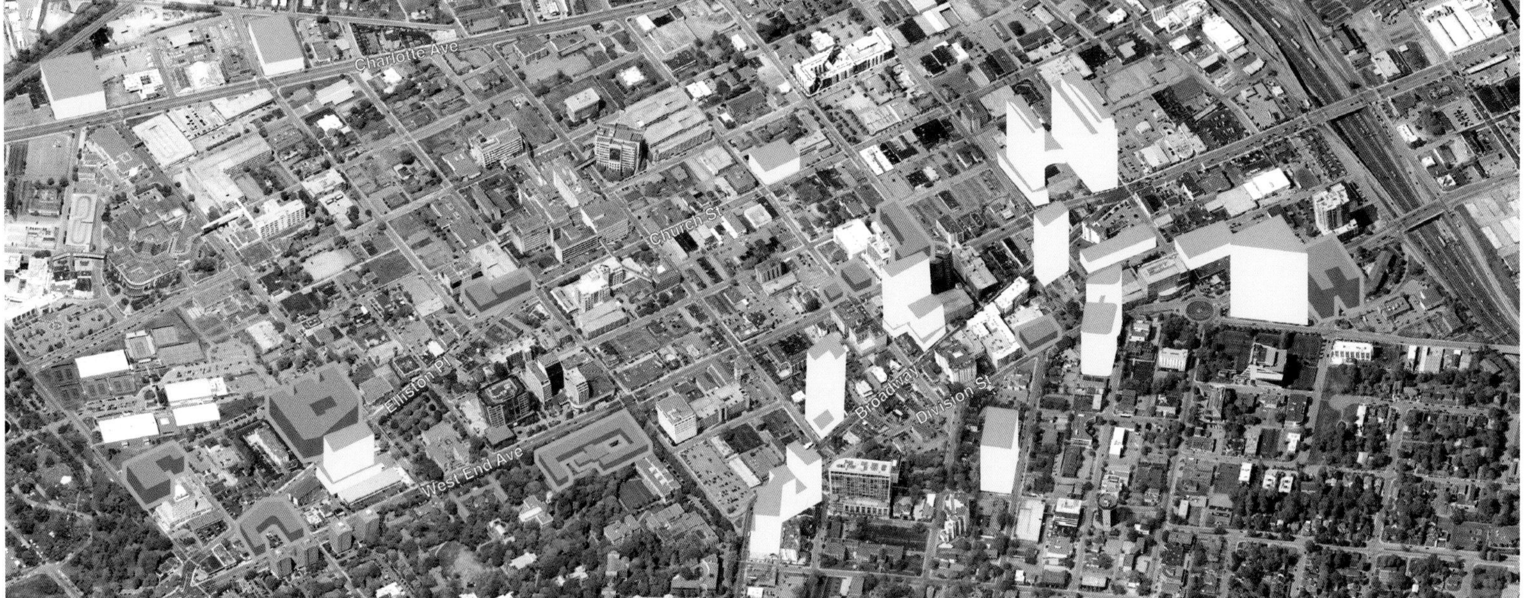

Midtown Nashville as a true mixed-use center with proposed and potential development highlighted in orange. Recently completed projects are shown in gray, outlined in orange. *(Photo simulation, 2015: Eric Hoke, NCDC)*

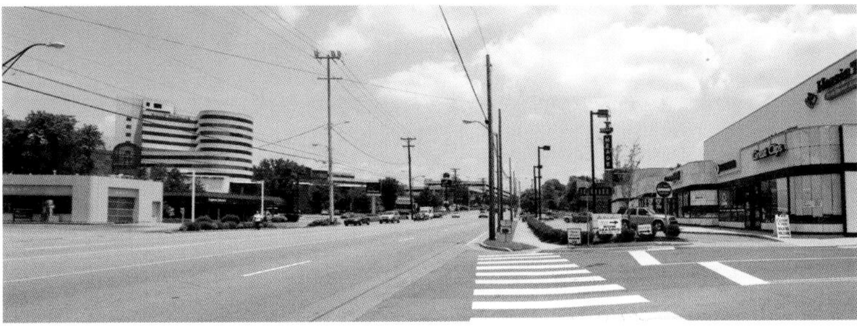

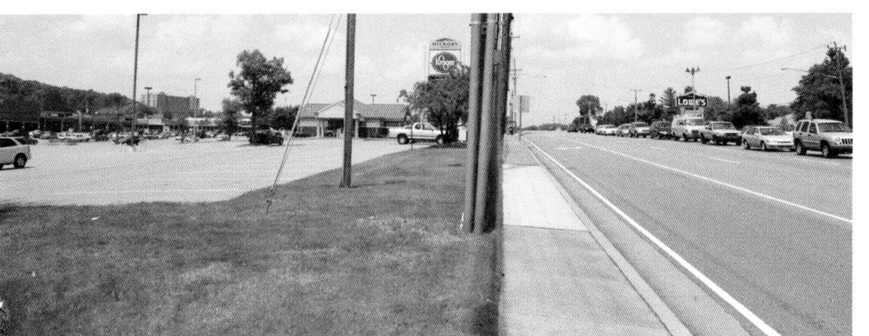

Left: Shopping centers in the Belle Meade area line both sides of Harding Road. Some pedestrian improvements, such as sidewalks and landscaping, have occurred, but connectivity is still intermittent and the car still dominates the shopping experience. *(2013)*

Right: The intersection of Nolensville Road and Old Hickory Boulevard is typical of Nashville's commercial intersections: wide roads and narrow sidewalks with little pedestrian protection from vehicular traffic. *(2011)*

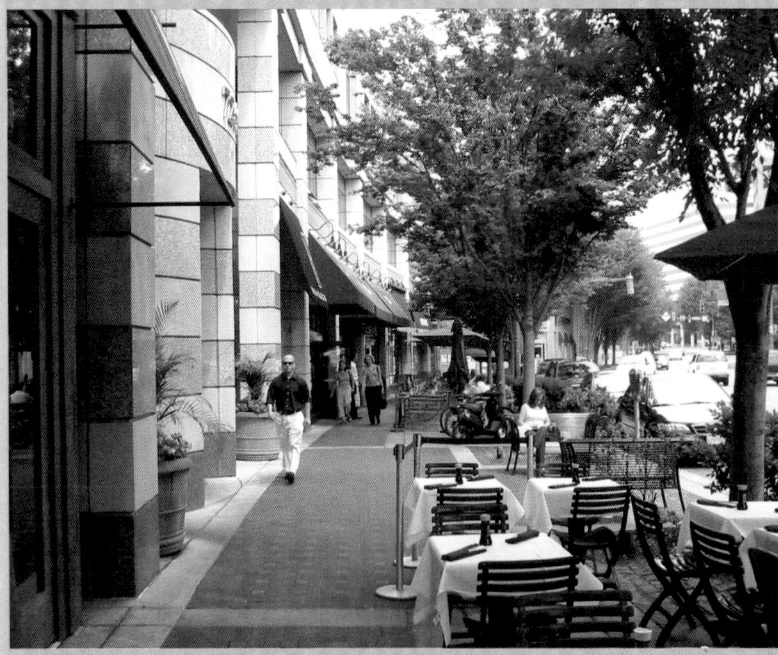

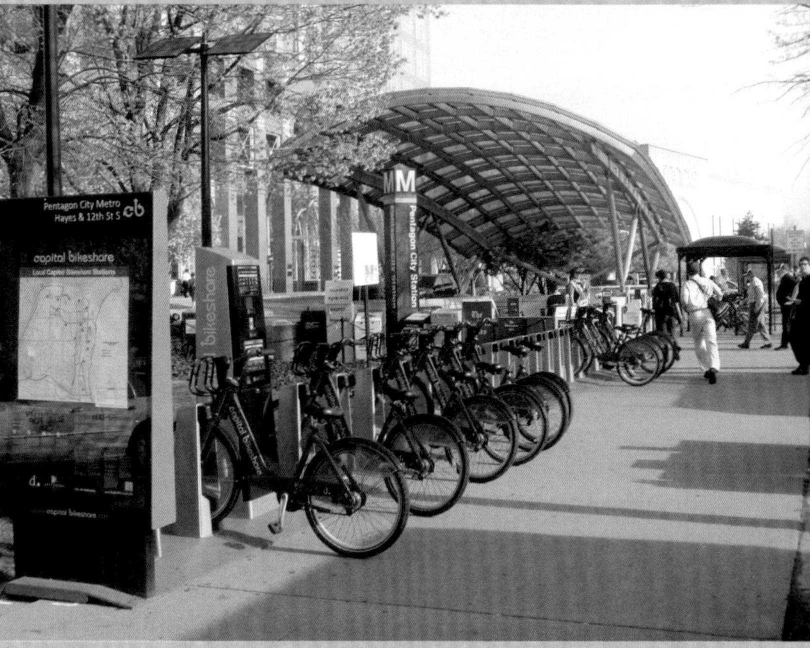

Characteristics of the true center in Arlington, VA: residential integrated into the land-use mix, mid-rise-minimum buildings, good access to public transit, wide sidewalks with landscaping and/or on-street parking to buffer pedestrians, and central open space. In Nashville's suburban areas such features occur, if they occur at all, in fragmentary fashion. *(2008: Brian Phelps and Chris Whitis)*

THE TRUE CENTER

Public transit service is the key enabler of the center as a complete community. Without mass transit that is easy to use and provides high frequency of service, the characteristics of the true center—continuous urban fabric, with an integrated mixture of land uses, presented in a walkable format—are not possible. That's because too much space must be dedicated to the movement and storage of cars.

This is the lesson taught by Arlington, Virginia, and the Pearl district of Portland, Oregon.

World War II brought boom times to Arlington, as people who poured into Washington, DC, to work for the federal government sought housing in nearby communities. By the 1960s, suburbanization had eroded the old commercial center of Clarendon in Arlington County, which lacked a generous supply of parking for the cars that were now the transportation mode of choice. Many shoppers migrated farther out to new retail centers in new suburbs. Some of Arlington's government officials began to push for new highways, widened roads, and more surface parking.

Regional transportation planners countered with a vision for rapid transit that became the Washington Metro system, with two lines for Arlington. The Orange Line was laid along the commercial corridor between Rosslyn and Ballston that included Clarendon. To support the new mass transit line, plans were made for an increase in the density of commercial and residential land uses near the line despite the fears of nearby residents about the impact on neighborhood character. Today Arlington is a vibrant urban center and a model for the transformation of suburbia.[2]

During the first half of the 20th century, Portland's Pearl District, located along the Willamette River, prospered as the industrial and warehouse quarter of the city. As transportation patterns shifted from river and rail to trucks, highways, and air, the area became marginalized. In the 1970s Governor Tom McCall created a task force to develop a new vision for the district; the task force recommended replacing the old Harbor Drive Highway with a public waterfront park.

A streetcar system was developed to serve new residents, who had converted old warehouses into loft living, and the workers at small businesses incubating in the "Pearl." Revitalization of the district has played a key role in Portland's growth management, whose goal is to absorb new populations and businesses without contributing to sprawl.[3]

— CHRISTINE KREYLING and
JOE MAYES, research fellow, NCDC

shops, restaurants, medical offices, and a variety of commercial and office services within close proximity to residential subdivisions is the defining characteristic of suburban sprawl. The low-rise profile of this development has utilized thousands of acres of land. The drive-and-park infrastructure that characterizes low-density suburban development patterns obstructs alternative transportation modes, particularly walking, and thus inhibits exercise as part of the daily routine as well as social interaction.

The question today is how to enable large suburban commercial areas to evolve into true centers. The Metro Planning Department defines the center transect zone as "where multiple neighborhoods and communities meet." Ideally they would "feature a mixture of housing convenient to commercial, employment, and recreational land uses, and provide multiple modes of transportation with sidewalk and bikeways or multi-use paths and facilities for mass transit."[4]

Nashville currently lacks centers that function as complete communities.

The Planning Department has initiated policies to help transform these commercial areas into more mixed-use community hubs. These include zoning changes along commercial corridors to allow high-density mixed uses, including residential, which was previously prohibited.[5] In particular, the addition of what is called the Specific Plan District to the zoning menu enables developers to plan integrated mixed-use projects for specific parcels, streamlining the development process by eliminating the need for a more general zoning change, which usually results in costly delays.[6]

CENTER ZONE BASICS

For planning purposes, center transect zones exhibit the following characteristics:

Centers in Nashville (Existing)

- **Multiple uses and functions—including commercial, office, and retail—accommodated on a more intense scale than all but the downtown transect zone**
- **Land uses often segregated**
- **Extensive commercial and retail with little residential integrated into the mix**
- **Underutilized high-density development zoning**
- **Significantly larger buildings, in terms of footprint, than those typically found in the surrounding community**
- **Automobile-oriented infrastructure**
- **Significant amounts of surface parking**
- **Food access typically dominated by large grocery stores, fast food, and chain restaurants oriented to patrons arriving by car (except in Midtown)**
- **Positioned on major thoroughfares served by public transportation**
- **Few to no open spaces or parks**

Centers in Nashville (Ideal)

- **Multiple uses and functions—including commercial, office, and retail—accommodated on a more intense scale than other transect zones**
- **Intensely developed as complete communities with an integrated mixture of land uses, including residential**
- **Buildings oriented toward transportation corridors and other prominent streets**
- **Active, pedestrian-friendly streets**
- **Multimodal transportation access**
- **Big-box groceries and restaurants well oriented to pedestrian customers, with smaller markets and locally owned restaurants integrated into the mix**
- **Open spaces in the form of pocket parks, plazas, and roof gardens**

According to the 2010 US Census Bureau statistics, the center transect zone in Davidson County has an estimated population of 4,249 residents and contains 3,262 acres, less than one percent of the county's land area.[7] Centers represent the second smallest transect zone in area, after the downtown zone.

Many of Nashville's commercial areas are oversupplied with retail space at the expense of other land uses. Along the arterials, there is more commercial zoning than can be fully and efficiently utilized. The low scale of much suburban commercial development and the vast acreage of surface parking present significant opportunities for diversification through reinvestment and redevelopment.

Creation of a wide range of housing choices and mixed-use developments in the center zone, along with increased access to multimodal transportation choices,[8] can accommodate the estimated 200,000 new residents (100,000 new residential units) Nashville-Davidson County expects over the next 20 years.[9] According to Arthur Nelson, an expert on public finance, economic development, and metropolitan development patterns, Nashville will build an estimated 1.2 billion square feet of new nonresidential space between 2013 and 2040, with an approximate value of $250 billion. Nelson estimates that all of Nashville's predicted growth and expansion needs can be accommodated within the existing commercial nodes and along the commercial corridors across the city.[10]

SHAPING HEALTH IN THE CENTER TRANSECT ZONE

NEIGHBORHOOD DESIGN AND DEVELOPMENT

The goal is to develop centers that connect to surrounding communities via sidewalks, bikeways, and mass transit; encourage higher levels of physical and social activity; feature safe streets for pedestrians; and decrease automobile congestion. New development should provide facilities that accommodate transit shelters and street crosswalks, improving transit experience and safety.

STRATEGY: *Infill vacant lots and redesign underutilized sites to transform current centers into truly mixed-use nodes.*

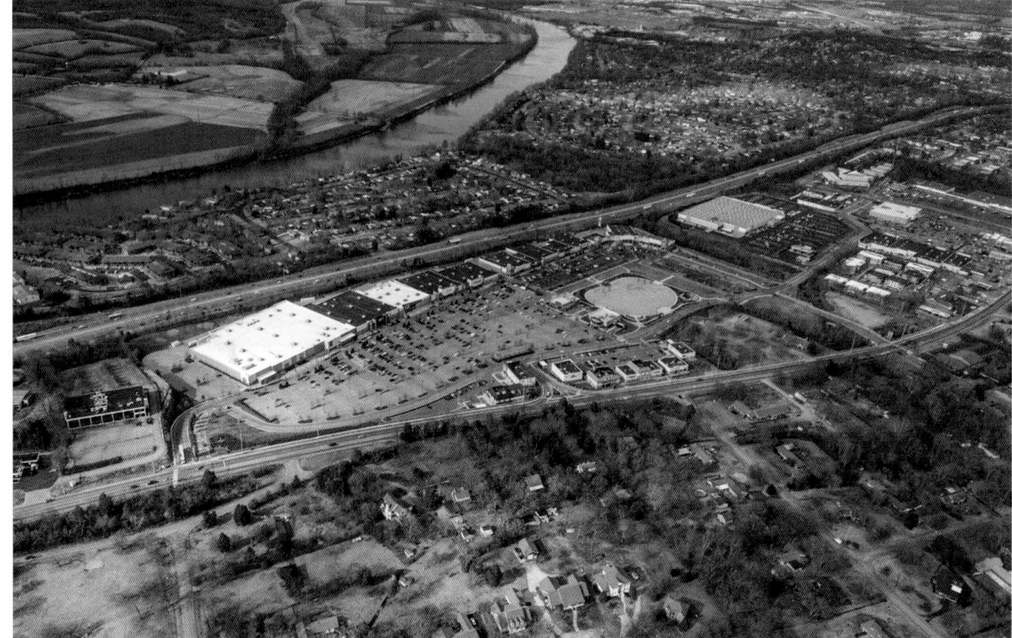

Aerial view of Nashville West, one of the city's newest shopping centers. Note the disconnect from surrounding residential areas; the rural farmland across the river is Bells Bend. *(2013: Gary Layda)*

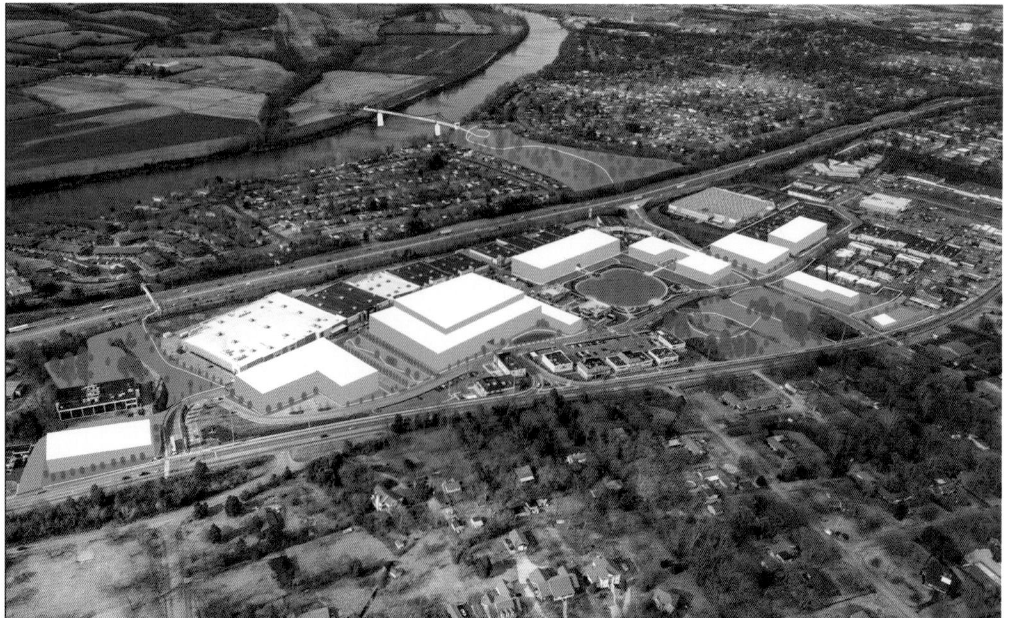

Nashville West reimagined as a complete neighborhood with infill uses taking up large expanses of existing surface parking lots. Car storage is in parking structures wrapped by ground-level retail, and topped by upper-level office and residential spaces. Note the pedestrian bridge connection to the natural areas and park of Bells Bend across the Cumberland River. *(Visualization, 2014: Eric Hoke, NCDC)*

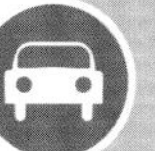

TRANSPORTATION

STRATEGY: *Increase public transit options within centers by providing circulator routes that connect to surrounding neighborhoods.*

STRATEGY: *Provide increased bicycle infrastructure to and within centers to accommodate short trips from surrounding residential communities. Include bicycle racks close to shops, restaurants, and grocery stores.*

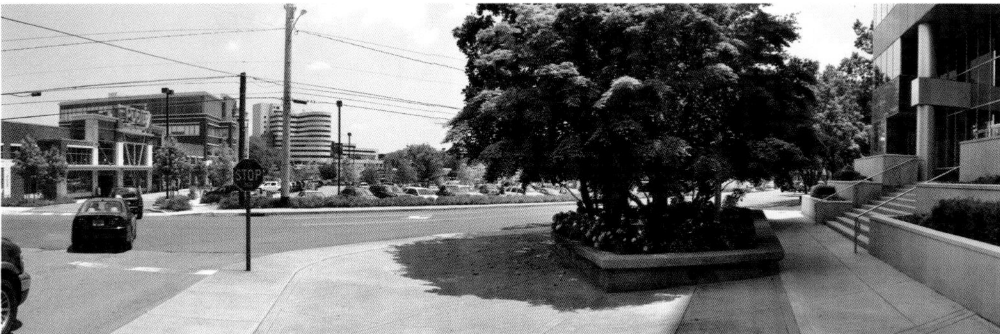

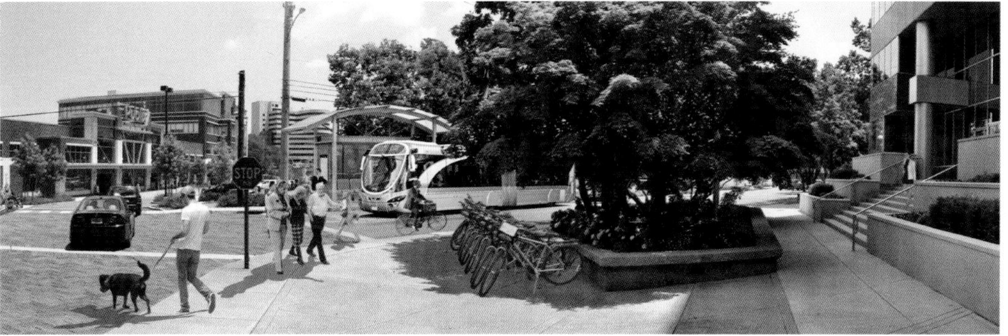

Before/after: Transportation mini-hub in the Belle Meade neighborhood near the White Bridge Road and Harding Pike intersection would accommodate rapid transit service, a bus circulator route, and bike station. The location is also near a trailhead for a Metro Parks greenway. (Visualization, 2013: Ron Yearwood, NCDC)

WALKABILITY AND PEDESTRIAN SAFETY

Because of the car-centric design of buildings and infrastructure, centers tend to be inhospitable to pedestrians. Vehicular proximity, noise, and exhaust on often narrow and fragmentary sidewalks discourage walking, just as the large amount of easily available parking adjacent to the road encourages driving.

STRATEGY: *Create safe pedestrian connections—from surrounding residential areas as well as within centers—through a reduction in curb cuts, design of buildings that front streets, and parking located behind the buildings to reduce pedestrian and automobile conflict.*

STRATEGY: *Develop parking shared by venues in the form of garages to enable patrons to walk between shops.*

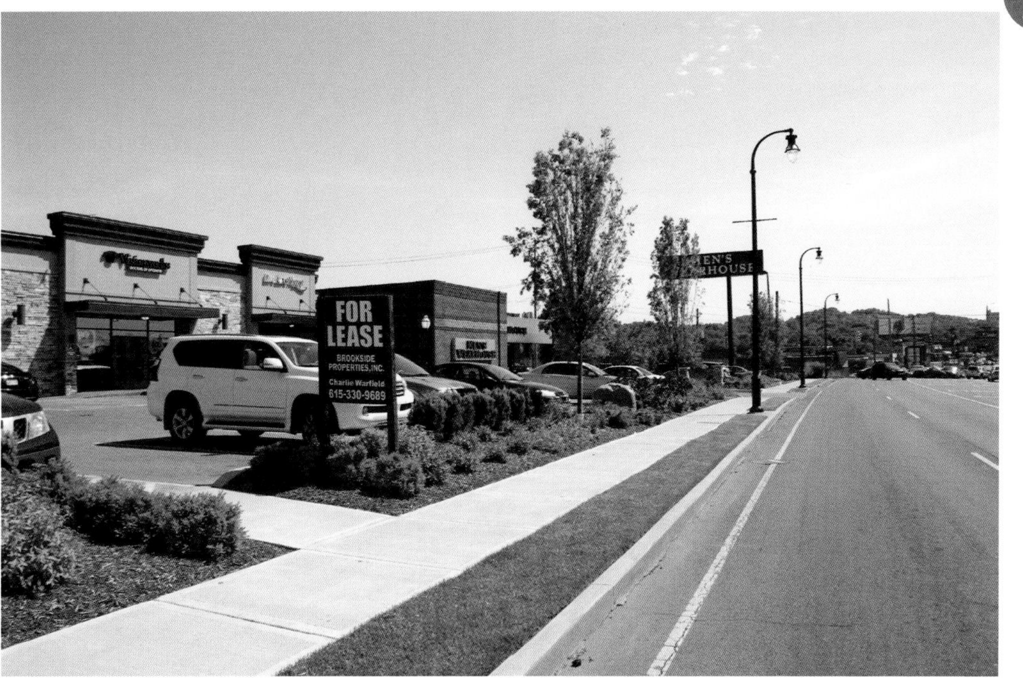

Recent pedestrian improvements along Hillsboro Road in Green Hills incorporate new sidewalks and a planting strip that separates pedestrians from automobile traffic. The out front parking, however, requires curb cuts and inhibits street-level interest for walkers. (2014)

FOOD RESOURCES

Centers are typically well served by grocery stores. An abundance of fast-food emporiums in centers, many with drive-thru options, enable easy consumption of high-calorie, low-nutrition foods, however.

STRATEGY: *Develop infrastructure to support, and orient buildings to emphasize, pedestrian-accessed restaurants rather than drive-through dining. Outdoor dining patios enhance street life, which makes for a better pedestrian experience.*

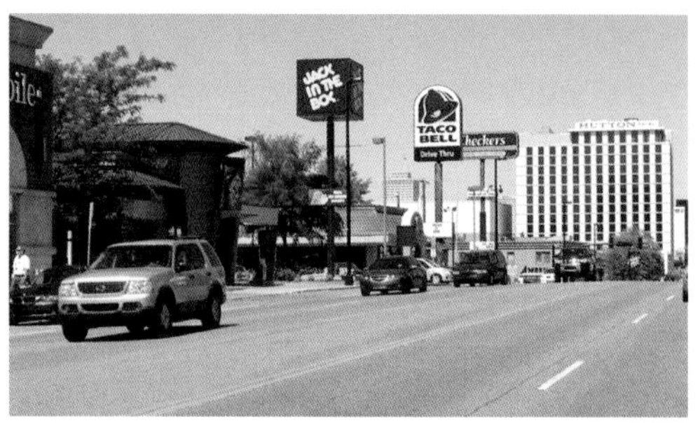

This cluster of fast food restaurants on West End Avenue in Midtown enables people to consume high-calorie, low-nutrition food with ease. The curb cuts such venues require are dangerous for pedestrians. *(2015)*

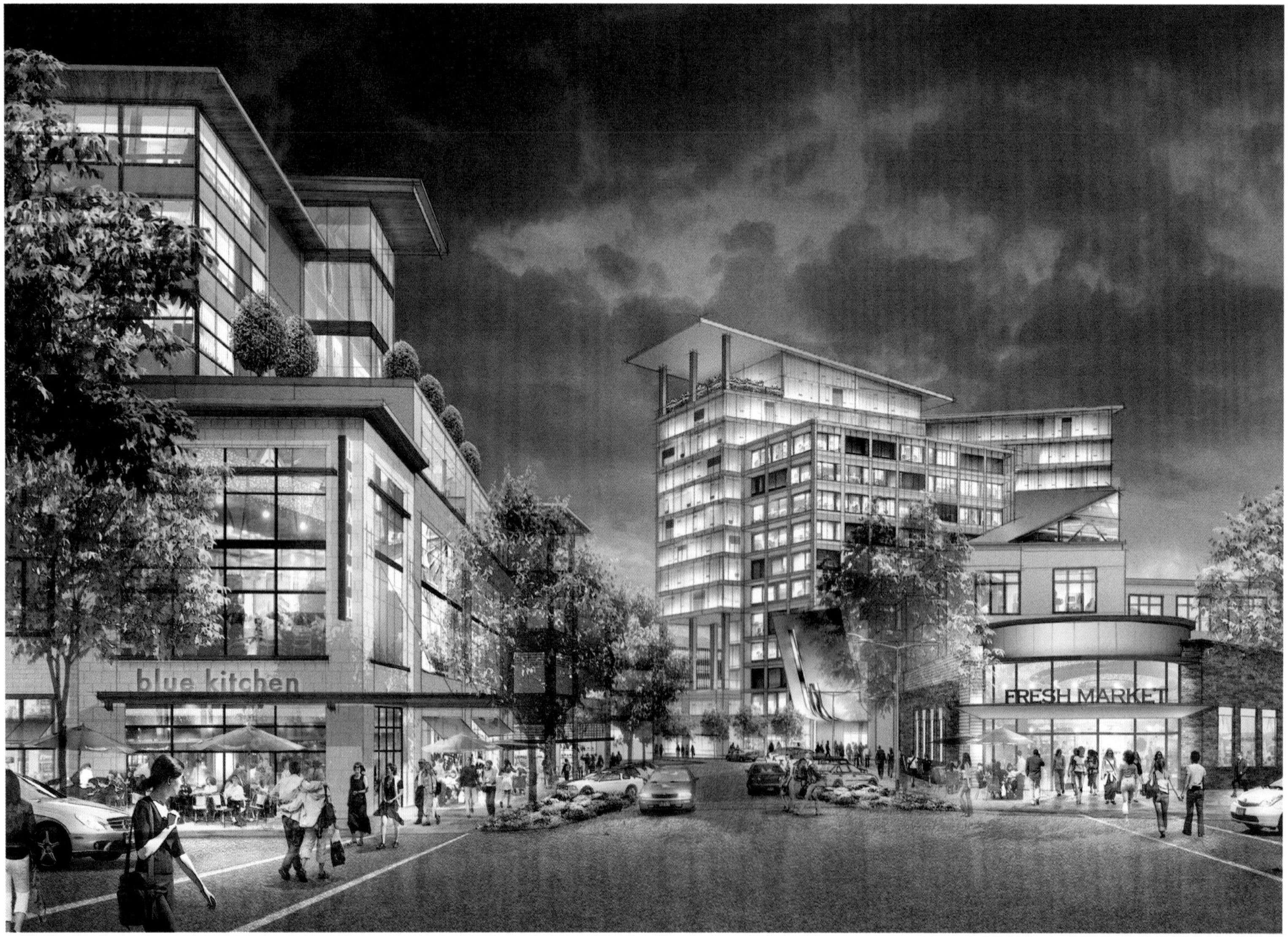

Master planned development called oneC1TY, located on Charlotte Avenue at 31st Avenue, features high-density development, mass transit accommodations, residential units, ample open spaces, numerous restaurants with outdoor dining areas, and a grocery store. *(Rendering, 2011: oneC1TY)*

HOUSING

STRATEGY: *Increase housing within centers to enable residents to access commercial spaces without driving.*

STRATEGY: *Include a diversity of sizes and levels of affordability for housing in centers so that retail and restaurant workers can reside locally, thus reducing vehicular demand and congestion.*

PARKS AND OPEN SPACE

Most centers lack parks and open space, except for that dedicated to car storage. Existing pocket parks and plazas are often small and uncomfortable due to the high volume of surrounding vehicular traffic.

STRATEGY: *Provide a wide variety of open spaces and parks within centers for recreation and passive contemplation: pocket parks, open plazas, rooftop gardens, and open space amenities including water play features, amphitheaters, and patio seating.*

Dog parks offer opportunities for social interaction for people as well as canines. Linear greenways can link various areas within a center as well as to surrounding neighborhoods.

STRATEGY: *Mitigate noise and air pollution with landscaping.*

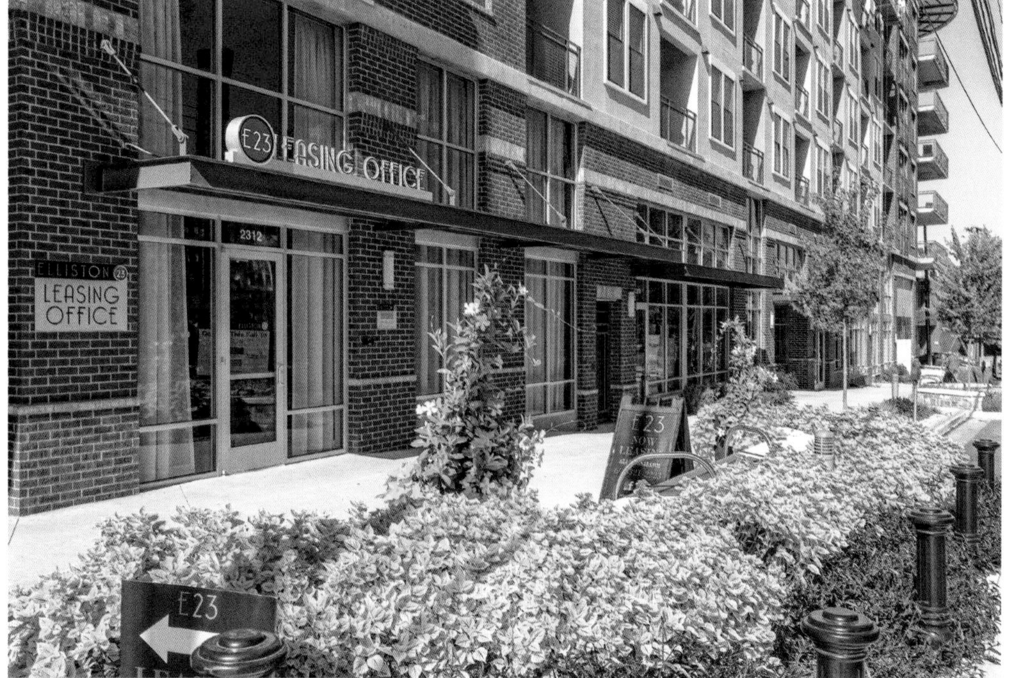

New residential building in the Midtown neighborhood features 331 units and seven retail spaces on the ground level. The project was built on a portion of the former Father Ryan High School campus that had lain vacant since the school's demolition in 1995. *(2015: Zach Rolen, Southern Land Company)*

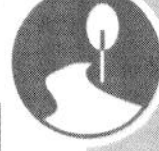

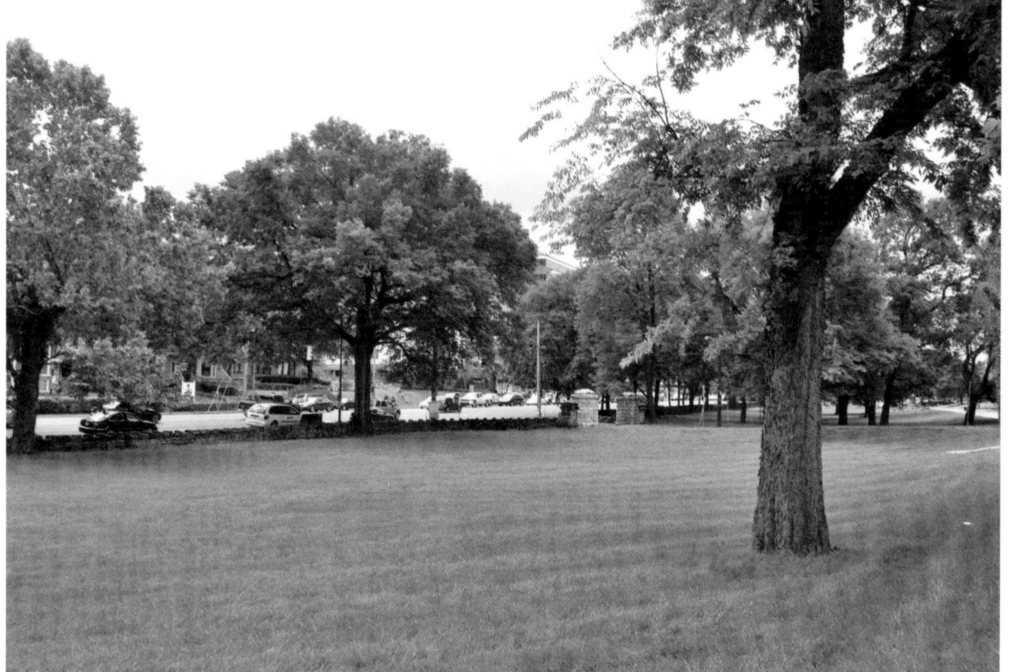

Large linear green space along West End Avenue provides shaded informal open area for neighboring residents and is screened from the intense traffic by large trees and an historic stone wall. *(2010)*

CASE STUDIES

ANTIOCH AND GREEN HILLS

Considered from a distance, Antioch and Green Hills have much in common. They share accelerated growth and development fueled by proximity to large shopping malls developed for regional appeal. Both are located along historic pikes that are now major arterials and feature auto-centric design. Both are also currently facing planning decisions regarding development patterns that could determine their futures as true centers. But there the similarities end.

Antioch is a largely working-class community that is home to many of Nashville's recent immigrants. Green Hills is home to Davidson County's wealthier citizens and has some of its most expensive real estate, whether as cause or result.

The recession of 2008 and the opening of newer retail centers that competed for shoppers hit Antioch's Hickory Hollow Mall hard. The closing of retail anchor stores in 2010

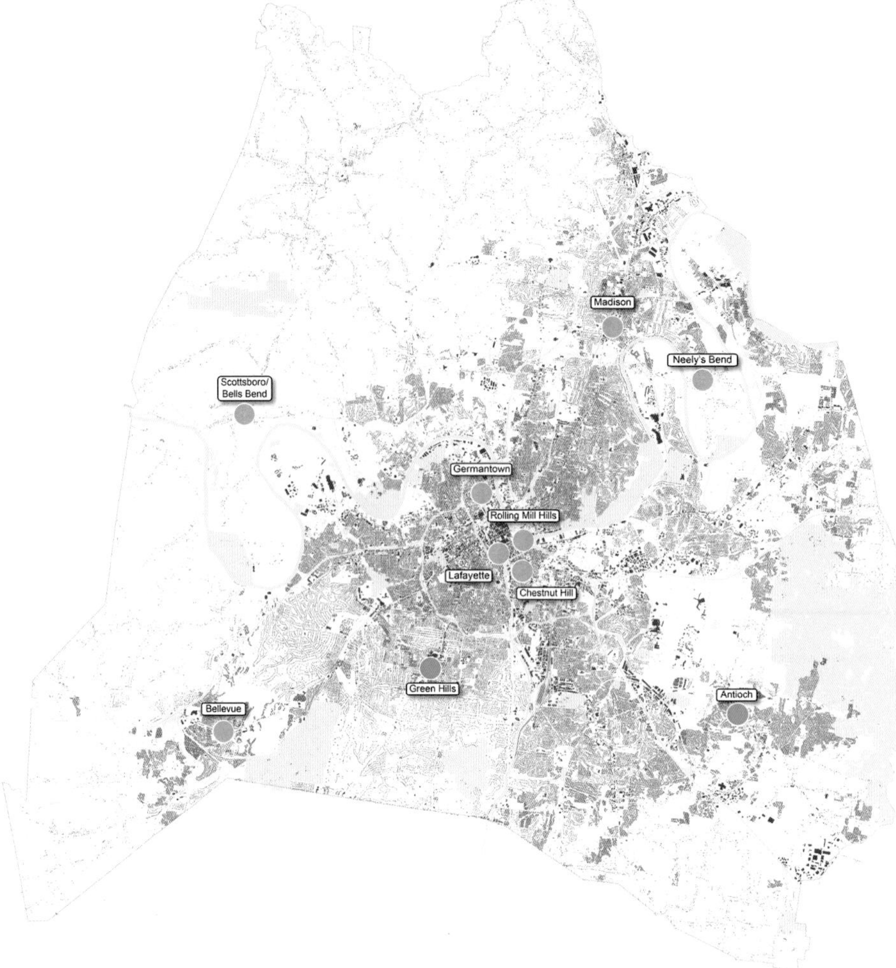

Map of case study neighborhoods with Antioch and Green Hills marked in blue. *(Diagram over Map, 2013: Eric Hoke, NCDC)*

Definition of Family / Non-family

Family = Contains at least two people related by birth, marriage, or adoption. Family households are of two types:

- **Married** = When a married couple is considered the householder
- **Other** = When a single man or woman is considered the householder and lives with other family

Non-family = This may be one person living in a household or multiple people who are not related to each other.

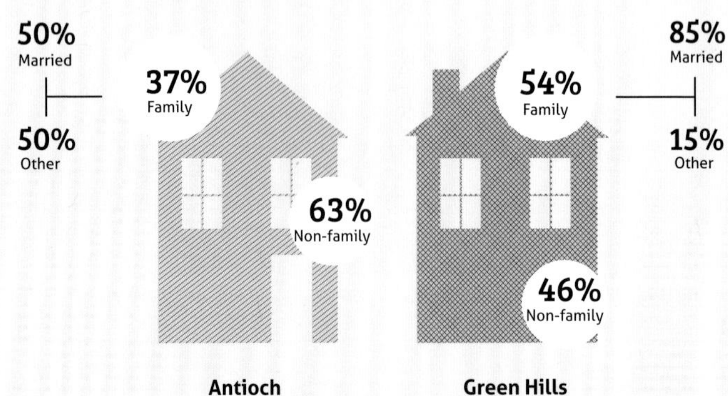

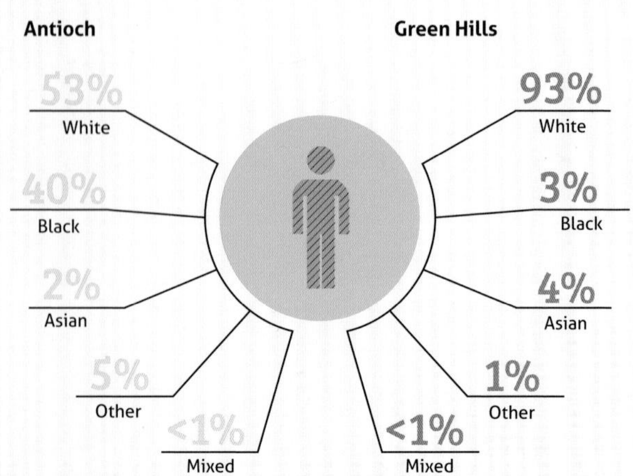

Information graphics, 2013: Ashley Nicole Johnson

signaled the decline of the area. The mall closed in 2012. The area was officially declassified as a center by the Metro Planning Department because it lacked the amenities that draw regional shoppers.

Green Hills, on the other hand, is flourishing. High-end department stores, mid-size shops, and boutiques abound in the expanding mall and surrounding developments. Residents fearful of increased traffic congestion and the transformation of existing community character view skeptically new higher density projects planned to meet future growth projections.

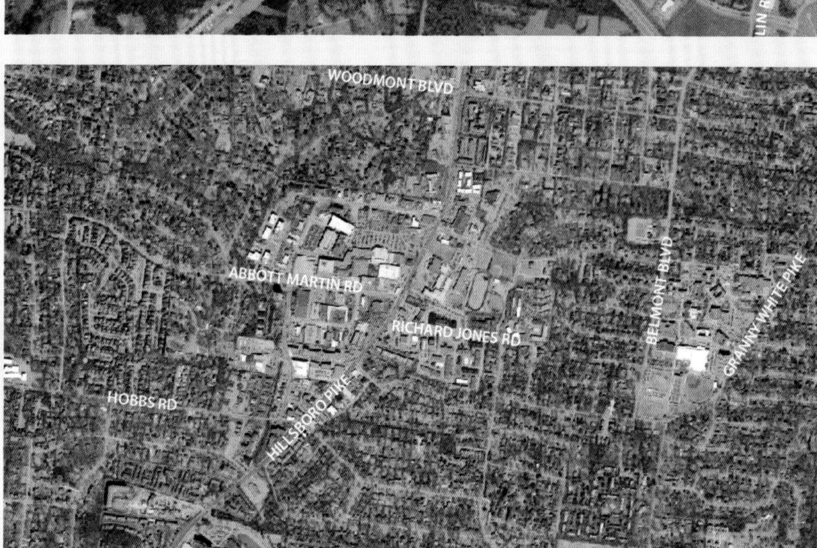

Aerial images of Antioch *(top)* and Green Hills *(bottom)*. Note how much more coarsely grained and disconnected is Antioch's newer street network than that in Green Hills. (2010: Metro Planning Department)

Income

Antioch

20%

Percentage Under Poverty Level

$39,282
Median Income

Green Hills

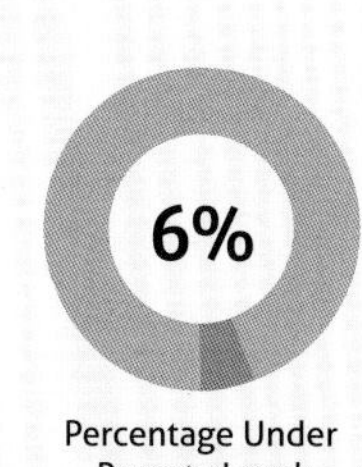

Percentage Under Poverty Level

$79,143
Median Income

Age Demographic

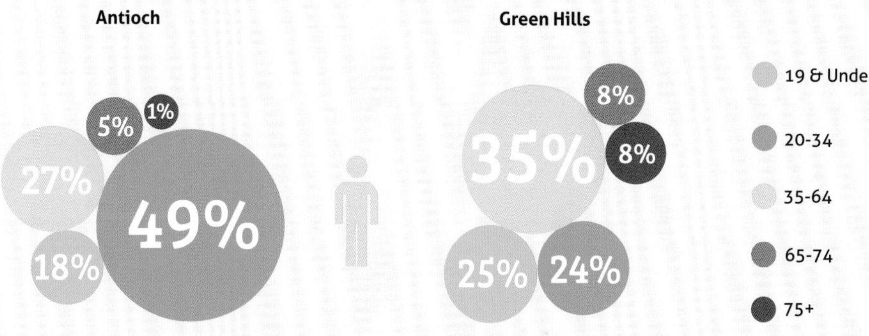

Demographic data from the US Census Department's 2010 American Community Survey (5 year estimates). At the time of research for this publication, the 2010 dataset was the most current data available. For the case studies, neighborhood boundaries were identified and data was then collected from the census tracts that best corresponded to those geographic boundaries.

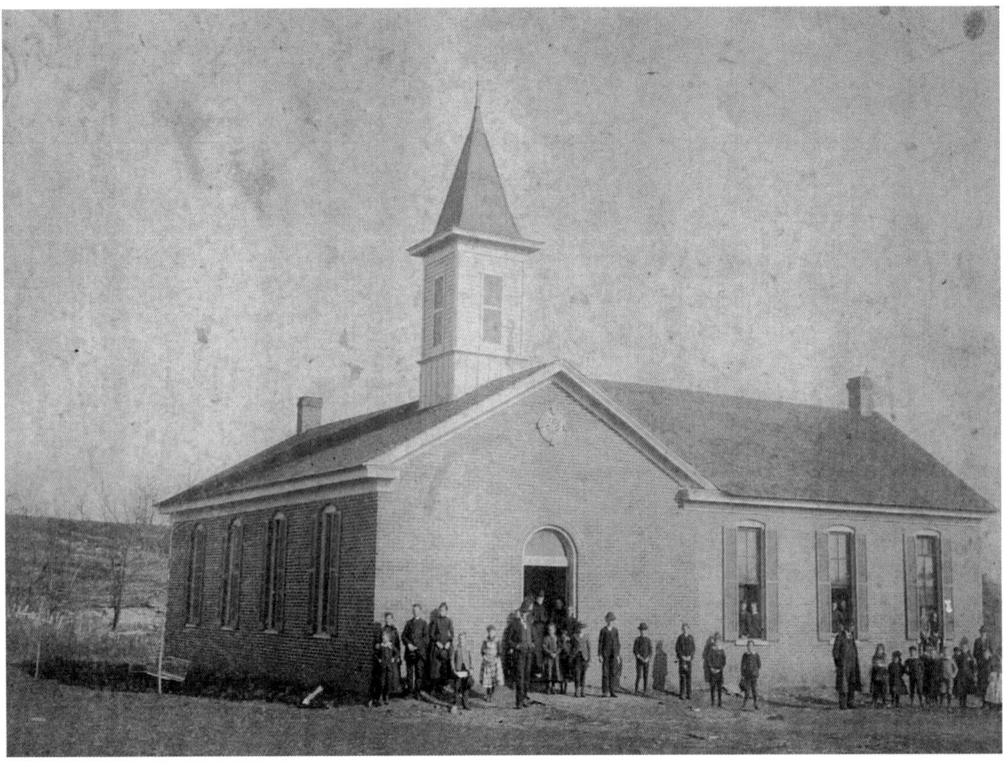

Antioch area church.
(ca. 1910: Metro Nashville Archives)

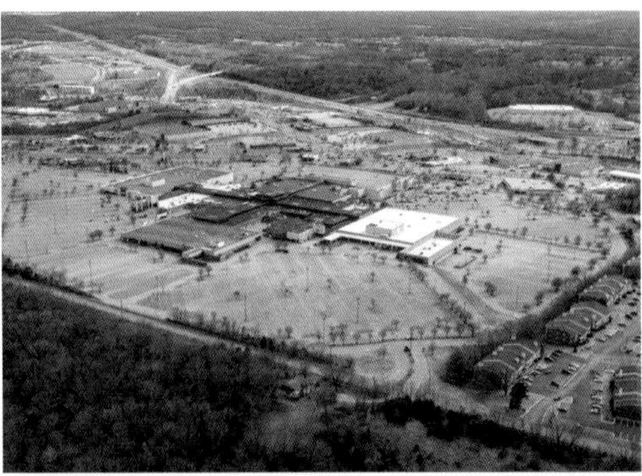

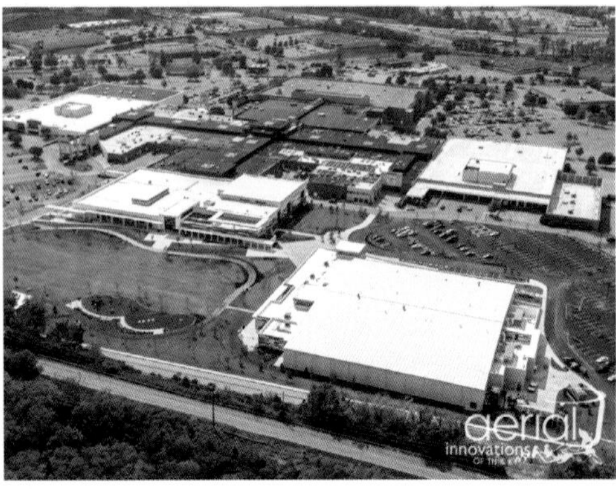

Right: Aerial views of the former Hickory Hollow Mall area from 2013 and 2014 show a stark contrast in the amount of redevelopment that has taken place in a relatively short time span. *(2013: Gary Layda; 2014: Aerial Innovations)*

ANTIOCH

The ancient city of Antioch, which lay on the Orontes River in what is now Turkey, was once the residence of half-a-million people and rivaled Egypt's Alexandria as the chief city of the Near East. But it is the city's Biblical associations as a center of Hellenistic Judaism and early Christianity that have made the name Antioch popular in the United States for educational institutions, churches, and towns.

Nashville's Antioch began at what is now the convergence of Antioch Pike, Hickory Hollow Parkway, Blue Hole Road, and Mt. View Road, and was originally little more than a cluster of houses and farms along Mill Creek.[11]

Around 1810 a small group of residents in the area began organizing what they called the First Baptist congregation. In 1820 a property owner by the name of Charles Hays donated land beside Mill Creek to be used for a church building to serve as the center of the small community.[12] Hays called it Antioch Baptist Church. The village has been known as Antioch ever since.[13]

Most of Antioch's early inhabitants were farmers who travelled to Nashville via the Mill Creek Valley Pike, completed in the 1840s. In 1851 the community got a railroad stop. The railroad allowed easier access to downtown Nashville—the trip by road could take half a day—and was vital to Antioch's growth.[14] By making it possible for workers in the city to live in Antioch, the railroad enabled the scattered settlement to coalesce into an actual town.[15] By the 1880s the village included a post office, a few stores, and a railroad depot at which four trains stopped.[16] With the arrival of the automobile, however, the train became less and less important, until the line was primarily used only for mail delivery. The depot was ultimately demolished.[17]

Having never formally incorporated as a town, in the years following World War II Antioch became a suburb for workers commuting to and from Nashville whose distinction from the larger city was largely its postal address.[18] The village center was obliterated by suburban-style development.

From the 1960s to the 1980s, Antioch's population grew 16-fold.[19] In 1978 came the opening of the Hickory Hollow Mall. The mall and the affordability of Antioch's housing drew new residents. In 1991, however, the Cool Springs Galleria opened in nearby Williamson County, drawing away a significant number of Hickory Hollow's customers.

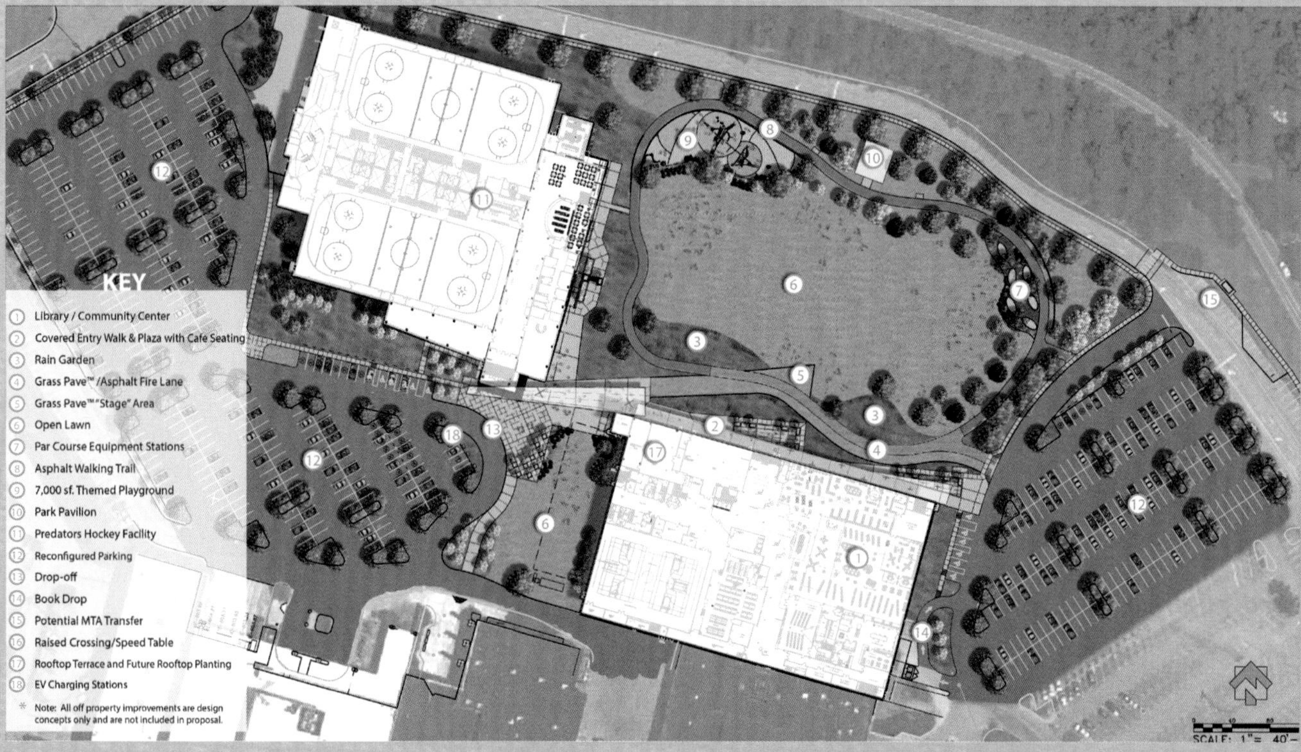

Site plan for the Commons at the Crossings at the former location of the Hickory Hollow Mall. *(Plan, 2014: Metro Parks Department)*

In early 2013 the Metropolitan Government of Nashville & Davidson County conducted a qualifications-based competition to convert a shuttered suburban retail mall into the Commons at the Crossings to feature the new Southeast Regional Community Center and park as well as a branch public library.

New programming for the facility includes a 60,000-square-foot LEED Silver building containing the new branch library and community center. The state-of-the-art library features designated children and youth areas, computer workstations, and a community room and café. The community center includes a gymnasium with fitness areas, an elevated walking track, and green roof with a terrace. As part of the project, a new 3.5-acre park replaced an asphalt parking lot. The park has a quarter-mile walking trail with six fitness stations along the eight-foot-wide path.

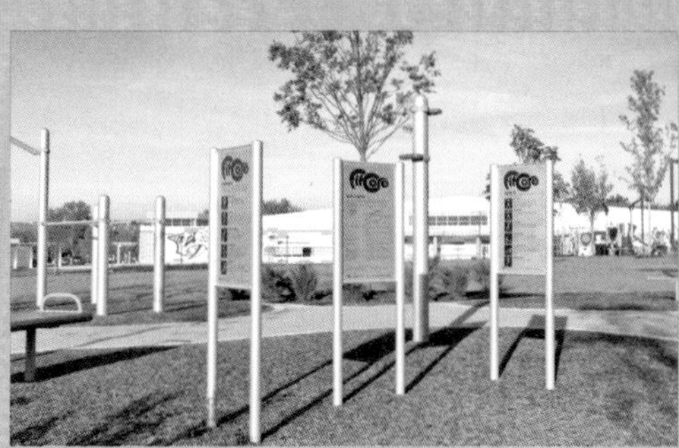

The new Southeast Community Park features six fitness stations (par course), a commitment by the city to active, health-oriented design. *(2014: Lose & Associates, Inc.)*

The Southeast Davidson Ice Center includes two ice rinks for recreational skating, hockey leagues, and figure skating. The building also houses staff offices, a skate rental center, a pro-shop with equipment repair center, a video training room, and a concession facility. The facility manager of the Ice Center will be the Nashville Predators, Nashville's National Hockey League team.

This redevelopment project incorporates several sustainable features that were part of Metro's program requirements:

- rain gardens and bioswales to reduce runoff from the site;
- ample windows and skylights to allow natural light to flow into the building;
- geothermal heating and cooling system to reduce energy cost;
- electric car charging stations to encourage reduction of greenhouse gas emissions;
- bicycle racks to promote alternative transportation access to the site, and access to mass transit to reduce parking requirements;
- native plants for environmental benefits and reduction of irrigation requirements;
- recycling program throughout the complex.

This investment by Metro government is a catalyst to make the former Hickory Hollow Mall a vibrant contributor to the quality of life in the Antioch community.

—CHRIS CAMP, president, Lose & Associates, Inc.

Changing demographics in the surrounding area—large increases in minority and low-income families—and the decline of brick and mortar retail due to the advent of online shopping further stressed the mall.[20]

When the recession hit in 2008, Hickory Hollow's anchor stores began to close. With the loss of Macy's, Sears, JCPenney, and Best Buy, shoppers had fewer reasons to visit. Responding to vacancies and crime problems, mall officials sent tenants their "final vacate" notices in June of 2012.[21]

Efforts by government and local individuals to revitalize the area have produced hopes for a comeback. In 2012 Nashville State Community College opened a satellite campus in the former Dillard's department store, which complements Metro's Academy at Hickory Hollow in providing education resources to the area.[22] In late 2012 Metro bought the space vacated by JCPenney and began turning it into what is called The Commons at the Crossing, with public spaces including a library, a regional community center, and a park, complete with public art. The following summer Metro announced a public/private partnership to purchase additional mall space and build an ice rink to serve as a practice facility for the National Hockey League Predators and for use by the community when not needed by the team.[23]

The city's investment led to the purchase of the rest of the mall by a local investment team, Global Mall Partnership. In 2013 they opened the Global Mall at the Crossings, marketing to the area's ethnic diversity.[24] The space continues to struggle, however.

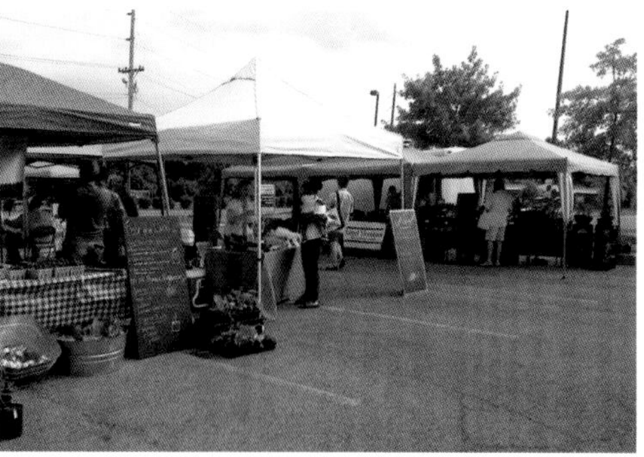

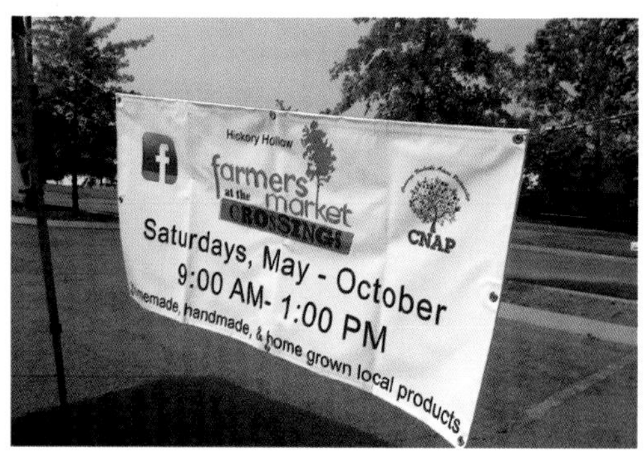
Hickory Hollow
farmers market at the CROSSINGS
CNAP
Saturdays, May - October
9:00 AM- 1:00 PM
handmade, & home grown local products

The farmers' market at the Crossings commenced in 2013 in the Lakeshore Christian Church parking lot at the intersection of Bell Road and Bell Forge Lane in Antioch. *(2014: Molly Martin)*

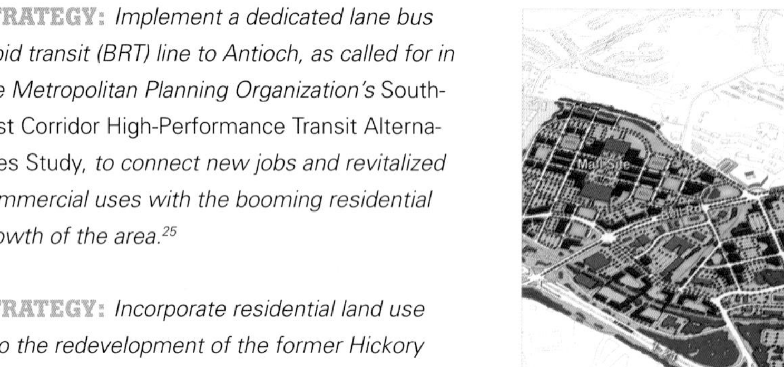

STRATEGY: *Implement a dedicated lane bus rapid transit (BRT) line to Antioch, as called for in the Metropolitan Planning Organization's* Southeast Corridor High-Performance Transit Alternatives Study, *to connect new jobs and revitalized commercial uses with the booming residential growth of the area.*[25]

STRATEGY: *Incorporate residential land use into the redevelopment of the former Hickory Hollow Mall.*

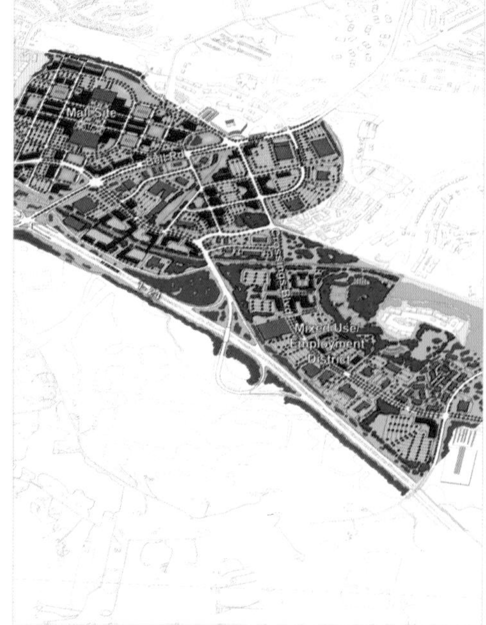

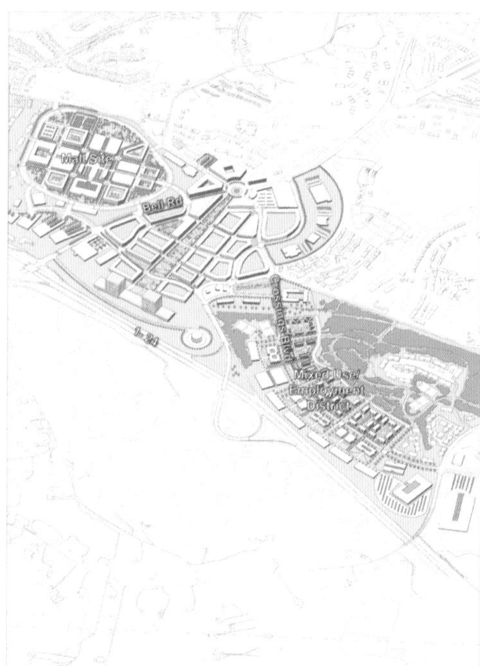

Left: Metro Planning's concept plan for the redevelopment of the Hickory Hollow Mall site features a grid of streets with sidewalks and an integrated mixture of land uses. *(Plan, 2012: Metro Planning Department)*

Right: Concept plan by University of Tennessee architecture students includes a similar mixture of uses, but has a denser development pattern and is more transit focused than that of the Metro Planning Department. *(Plan, 2013, University of Tennessee College of Architecture and Design)*

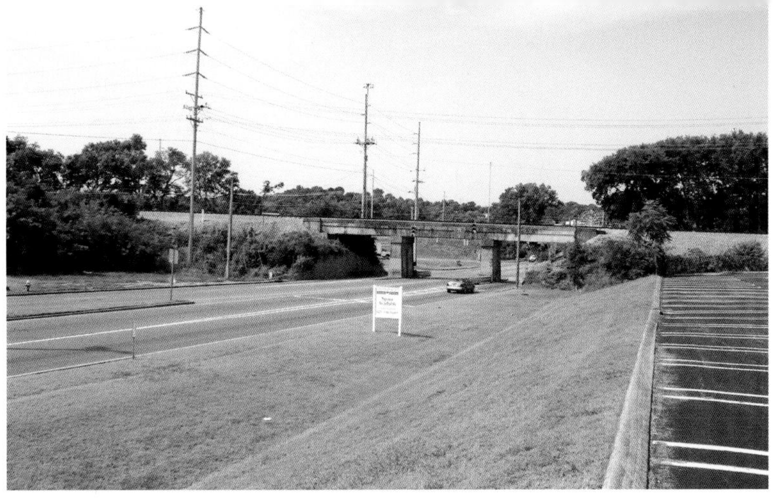

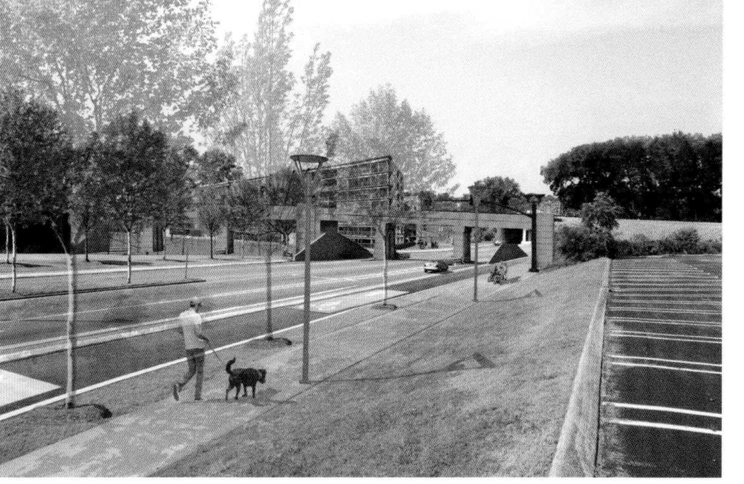

Pedestrian improvements at the Bell Road and CSX Railroad crossing would improve safety for those walking, biking, and taking public transit. *(2013; Visualization, 2013: Ron Yearwood, NCDC)*

STRATEGY: *Implement pedestrian and bicycle improvements in Antioch, focusing on connections between surrounding residential neighborhoods and retail shopping areas, utilizing greenways, sidewalks, and bike lanes.*

STRATEGY: *Implement a greenway loop in Antioch that connects existing and future park space with neighborhoods, offices, and shops.*

STRATEGY: *Implement a new regional park to the south of I-24 in the Antioch community, as identified in* NashvilleNext.[26]

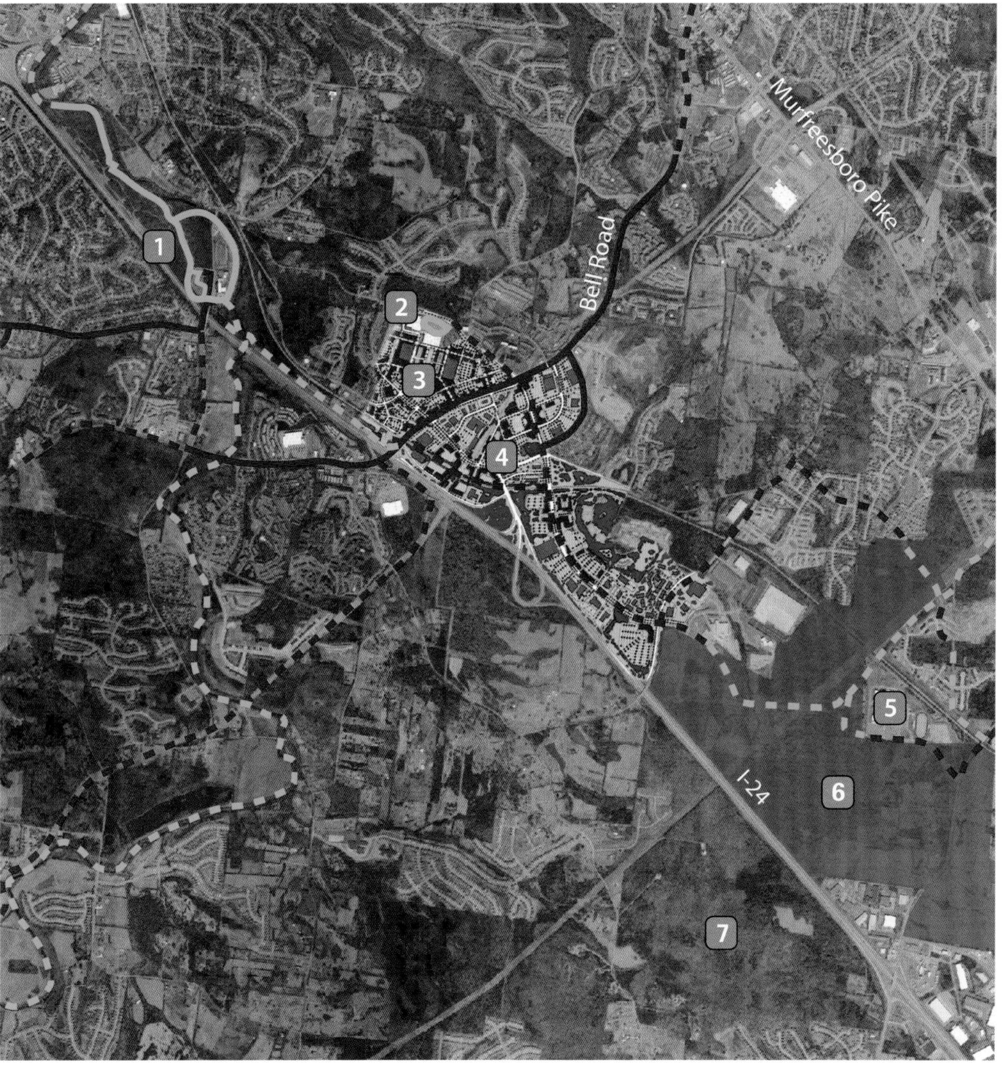

Existing and potential greenways and bikeways in Antioch to connect the community. Solid green lines represent existing greenways; dashed green represent potential ones. Solid red lines represent existing bike lanes; dashed red, potential ones. Update: in 2015 Metro Parks, with assistance from the Joe C. Davis Foundation and the Conservation Fund, announced the acquisition of 591 acres to form the new Southeast Park. *(Diagram over aerial, 2015: Ron Yearwood, NCDC)*

1 Antioch Park
2 Community Center, Library, Park
3 Global Mall at the Crossings
4 Crossings Event Center
5 Cane Ridge High School
6 Southeast Park
7 Proposed park expansion

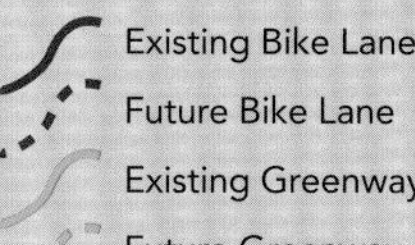

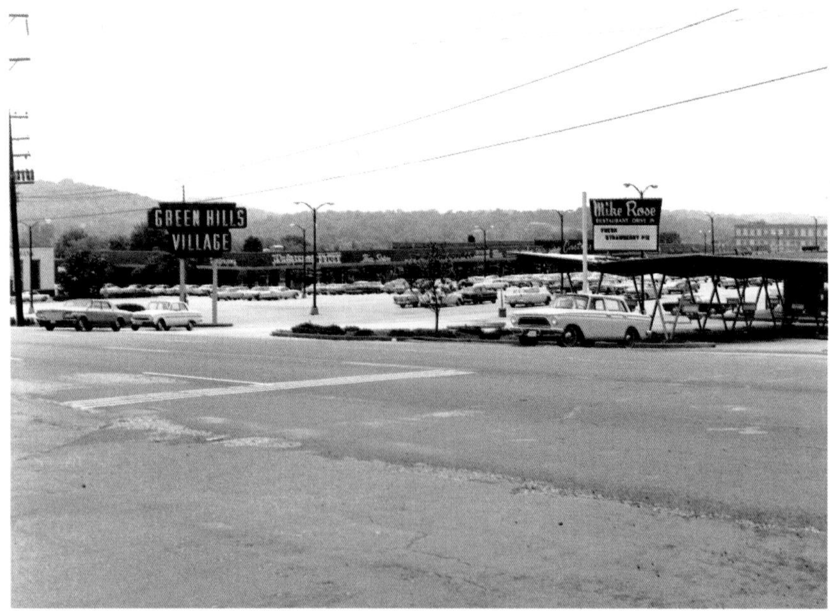

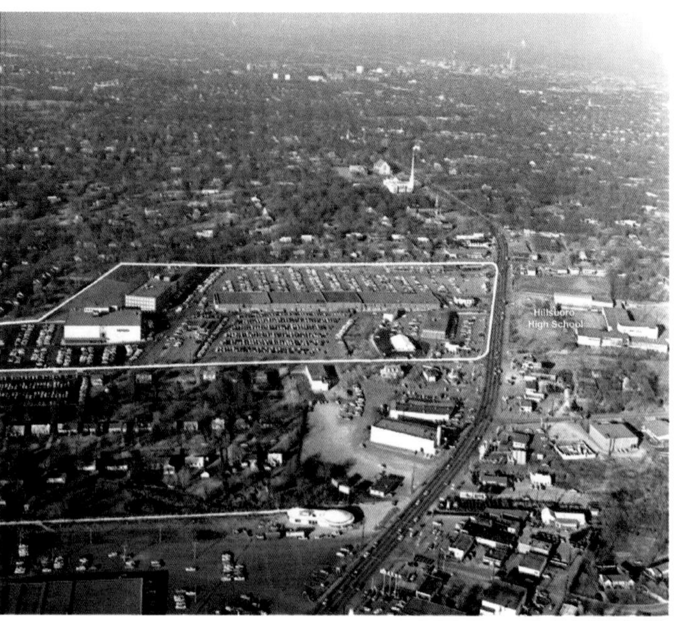

Left: Green Hills Village Shopping Center.

Right: View looking north to Green Hills Village. Note the residential neighborhoods adjacent to the shopping center's large surface parking lots.

The residential boom of Green Hills led to the development of a $2.5 million strip-style shopping center, Green Hills Village, which opened in 1953. Originally home to just 25 stores, the shopping center has gone through several phases of expansion and today is known as the Mall at Green Hills, home to over 80 retail shops. What was once a neighborhood commercial center is now a regional shopping destination.[27] *(ca. 1950s: Metro Nashville Archives)*

GREEN HILLS

The Green Hills neighborhood isn't particularly hilly by Nashville standards, nor as green as it was in the days before suburbia hit with its full impact after World War II, when commerce burgeoned on the stretch of Hillsboro Pike (US Highway 431) between Crestmoor and Hobbs roads, and large stretches of earth and Sugartree Creek were paved over. But the residential streets are still leafy and the 37215 zip code is one of the most prized in Metro Nashville.

Green Hills was never separately incorporated and thus lacks formal boundaries. Residents typically define their neighborhood as lying just south of I-440 to the east and west of the major arterial, Hillsboro Pike, running to Harding Place on the south. Real estate agents, who prize the Green Hills label, often use a broader definition.

Originally outside the reach of streetcars or urbanized infrastructure, Green Hills was a largely rural community of farms and private estates until well into the 20th century.[28] The area's undeveloped nature is indicated by the fact that it was home to the Nashville Golf and Country Club in the early 20th century and subsequently to Nashville's first airfield, Hampton Field. The landing strip lay in a pasture on the E. L. Hampton farm, between what is now Golf Club Lane and Woodmont Boulevard, and operated between 1917 and 1921.

In 1930 the population of the entire 7th Civil District of Davidson County (which included Green Hills and most of South Nashville) was only 6,254 and had neither post office, library, nor school.[29] A drive down Hillsboro Pike, then a tree-lined country lane, was recommended as a scenic escape from the hustle and bustle of city life.[30] When Hillsboro High School first opened its doors in 1939, only 164 students enrolled, taught by seven faculty, with twelve graduates in the first class.[31]

By 1950 all had changed. With the popularization of the automobile, Green Hills rapidly developed as a residential neighborhood for middle- and upper-class families. Between 1940 and 1950 the area was the fastest growing in Davidson County.[32] Soon the majority of the large farms and estates were subdivided for single-family homes or, occasionally, duplexes. Lots were large due to the use of septic systems for sewage disposal until their replacement with sewers.

Green Hills Village–turned–Mall at Green Hills has spawned other commercial development along Hillsboro Pike. The pattern has been largely in strip-shop format, with parking out front. Some strips are in a U-configuration, with parking shared among the shops in the U. Larger stores feature their own car storage, often fenced off to keep customers of other stores from poaching spaces. Logically enough this blueprint has produced a

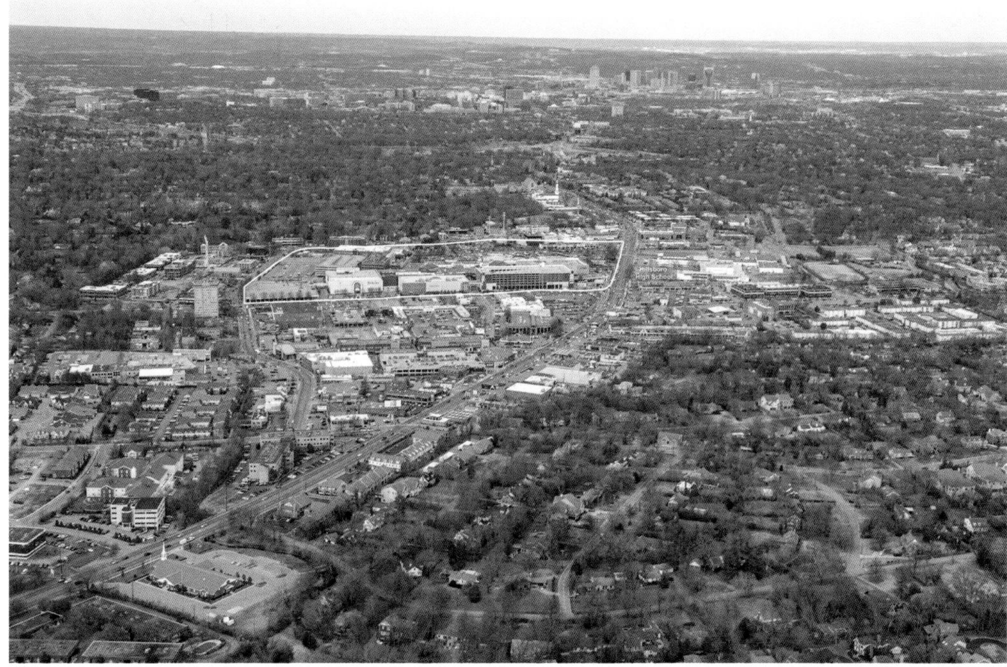

View looking north to the Mall at Green Hills. The tall, white-steepled church visible in both photographs is the Woodmont Christian Church, designed by architect Edwin Keeble, who also designed the current Hillsboro High School. *(2013: Gary Layda)*

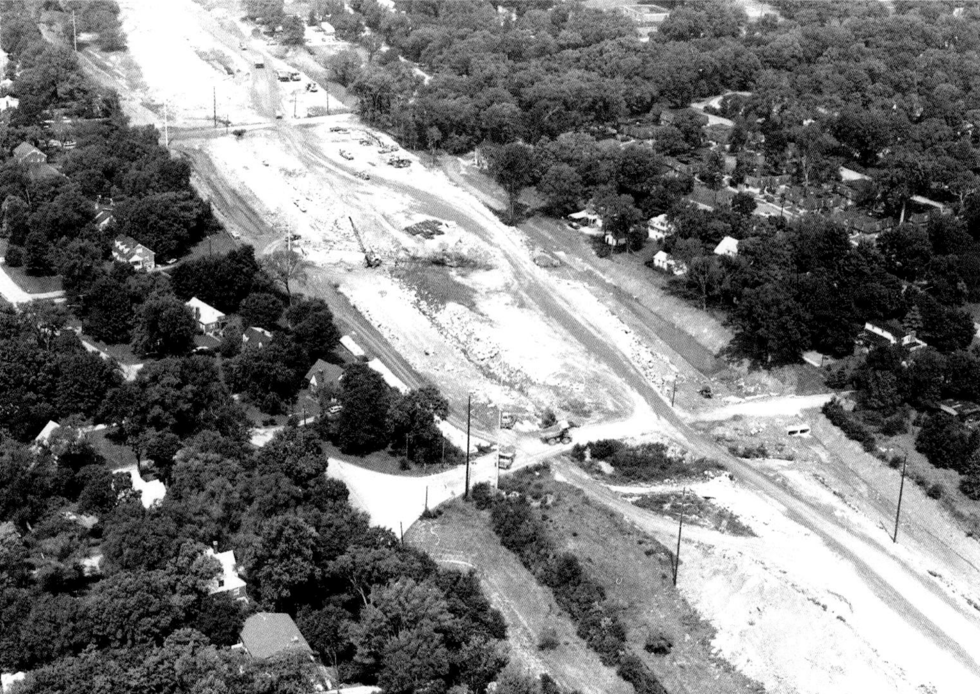

I-440 under construction. *(1983: Courtesy of Tennessee Department of Transportation)*

general lack of pedestrian connectivity.[33] As congestion has increased on Hillsboro Pike, wily consumers seek "back door" routes to all the commerce, increasing car traffic on the two-lane collector streets that are primarily residential in land use—but feed into the commercial area—to the general distress of residents on those streets.

The original orientation as a market center for the adjacent suburbs is evidenced by the infrastructure problems, which will be difficult to solve. Unlike other malls in Nashville, Green Hills Village was not developed in conjunction with an interstate interchange and associated wide ingress and egress roads. Such roads have rights-of-way that can be reworked to accommodate sidewalks, bike lanes, and transit-dedicated lanes. The four travel lanes of Hillsboro Pike, with an additional turn lane commencing some distance south of I-440, do not have this capacity.

The closest interstate, I-440, was constructed in the mid-1980s, long after the commercial development patterns were established. The beltway, promoted as a roadway to relieve traffic pressure on collector streets, particularly Woodmont Boulevard, has largely failed in this purpose. As a limited-access highway, I-440 disrupted the network of neighborhood streets, concentrating vehicular traffic on the major arterial of Hillsboro Pike. In addition, streets feeding onto Hillsboro Pike along the commercial section often fail to align at the crossing point, requiring separate signals. The result is an irrational concentration of cars, shops, parking lots, signage—and consistent congestion.

Residential forms in Green Hills have evolved as well. The neighborhood's first apartment buildings began showing up fewer than 10 years after the completion of the original mall.[34] Despite residents' concerns about increased traffic congestion and the erosion of residential character, the rapid pace of development has continued to the present day.[35]

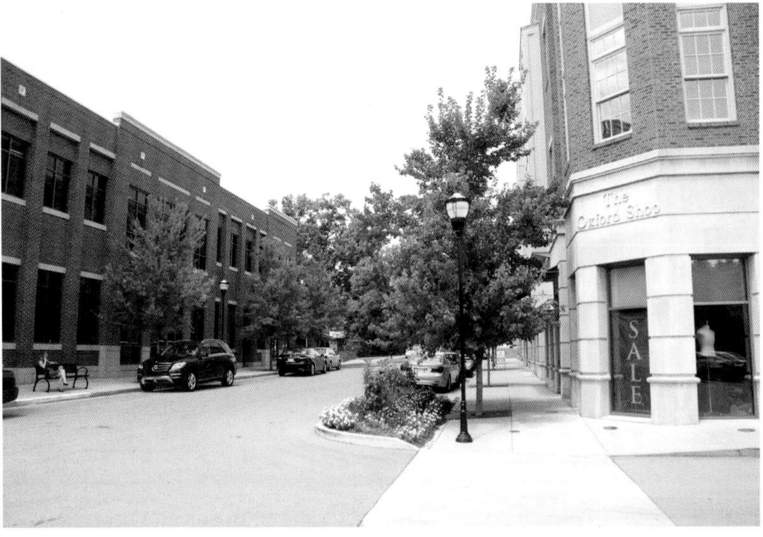

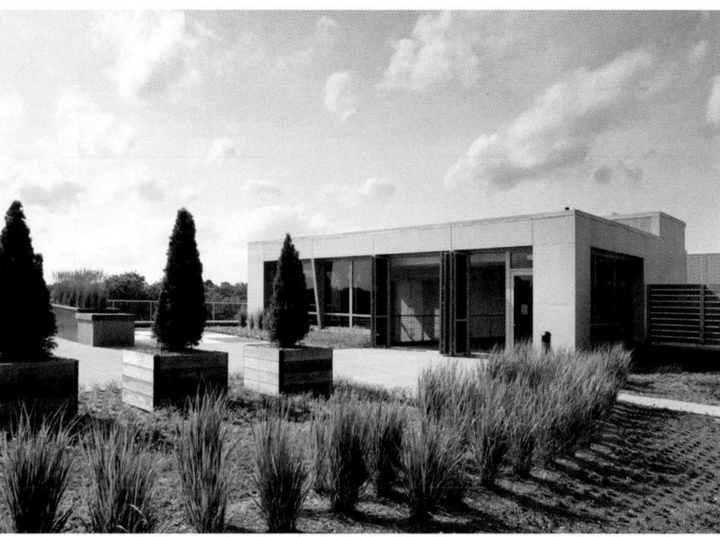

Bedford Commons, designed by Hastings Architecture Associates, was created in Green Hills in the first decade of the 21st century after numerous meetings among planning officials, designers, developers, and community groups to create a mixed-use plan for shopping, office, and residential venues in a walkable design. *(2012)*

Green roof in Bedford Commons provides an open space amenity for the tenants, while slowing rainwater runoff. *(2009: © Jim Roof Creative, Inc.)*

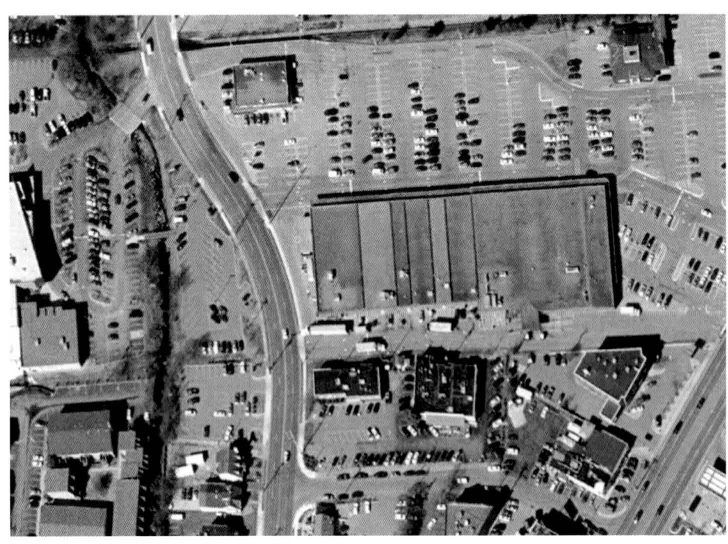

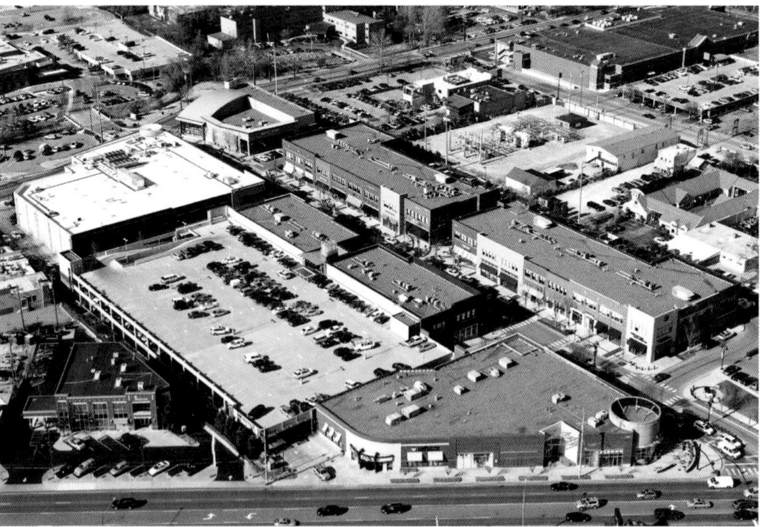

H. G. Hill Realty tore down its Green Hills strip mall and opened the Hill Center in 2007. The transformation of the Hill's grocery site, with its acres of surface parking, into the Hill Center in Green Hills is a good example of transforming suburban development patterns into a more walkable enclave. Note the densification of the site as well as the structured and on-street parking in the redevelopment. Long-term plans include adding a residential component, which would make the center fully mixed use. *(Aerial image, 2002: © Google; 2012: Aerial Innovations)*

In 2003 residents joined with Metro planners to try to prepare for new development. The creation of the *Green Hills Urban Design Overlay* (UDO) standard guidelines and the Bedford Avenue UDO call for an integrated mix of land uses, pedestrian-friendly streetscapes, and the addition of open space.[36] The UDOs, though voluntary, have been used by developers to create mixed-use, walkable projects, such as Bedford Commons and the Hill Center.

These more urban development forms, however, are fragmentary. The general built environment in Green Hills still does not encourage a healthy, active lifestyle. But public sentiment is shifting away from the car-centric format. A 2012 Livability Project for Green Hills, created by the Nashville Civic Design Center in collaboration with resident and community stakeholders, suggests building a greenway around the core of Green Hills, improvements in sidewalk connectivity, and creating a community-focused public space by making use of Hillsboro High School's green lawn as a neighborhood commons.[37]

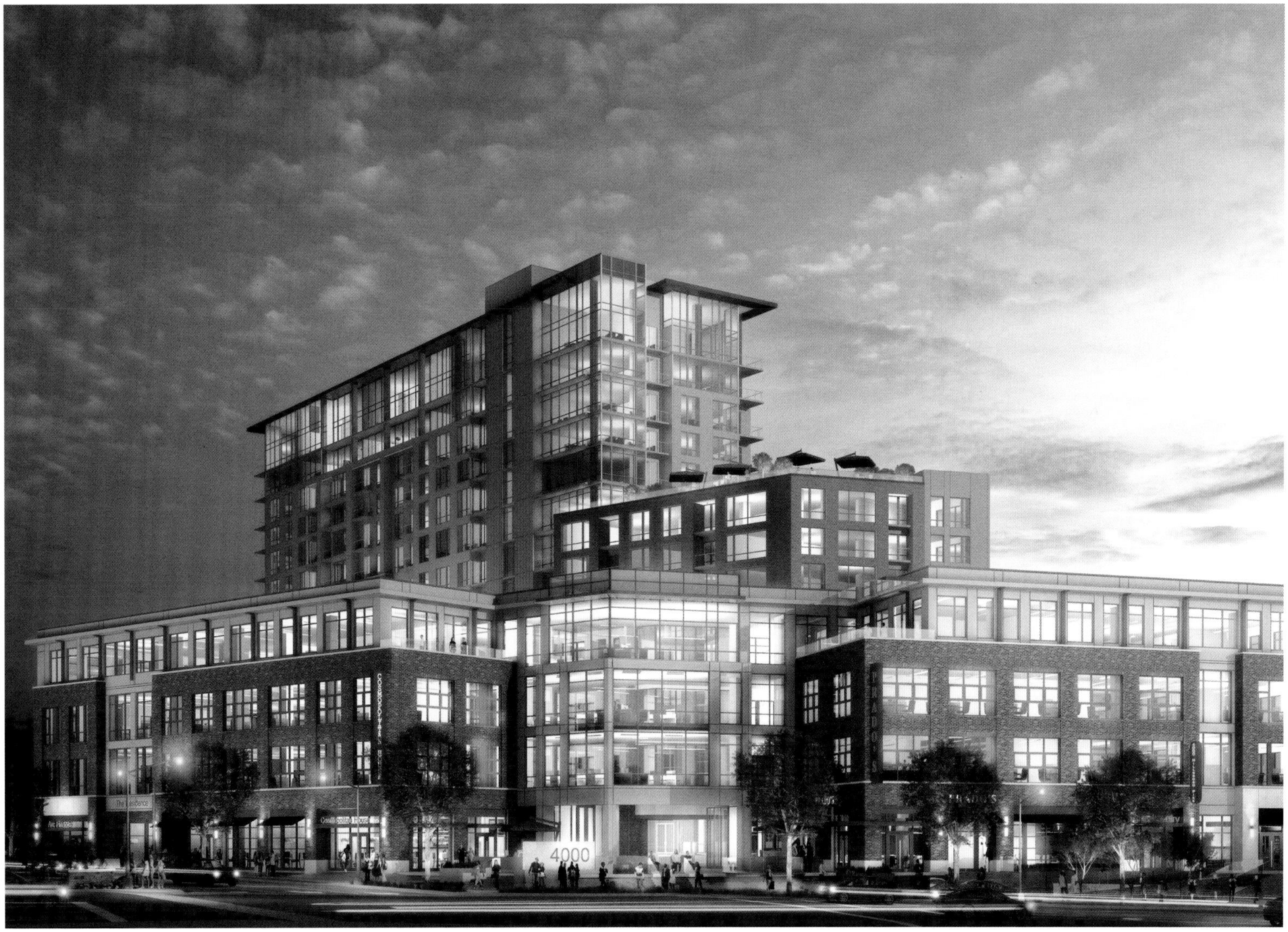

STRATEGY: *Increase density of mixed-use development with a strong residential component along Hillsboro Pike to place residents within walking distance of shops and create a larger ridership pool for public transit, meanwhile protecting existing neighborhoods served by local streets. While this development is necessary to transform the Green Hills commercial area into a true center, the transition period will be challenging due to the limited capacity of existing roadways.*

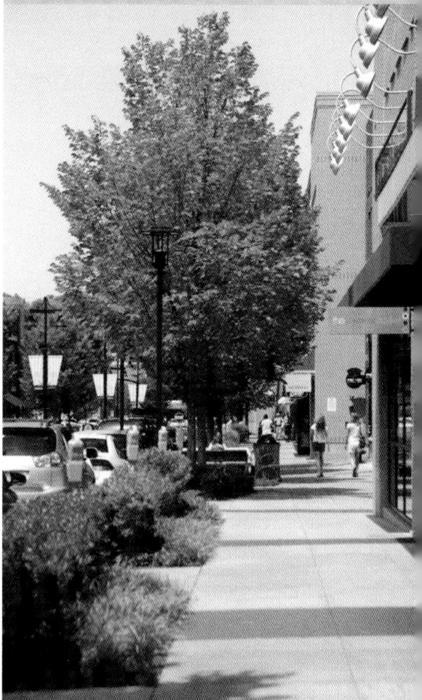

Above: The Hill Center's "Main Street," with trees, frequent pedestrian crosswalks, and sidewalk entrances. Shoppers park in a hidden parking garage and stroll down sidewalks filled with more than two dozen specialty shops, restaurants, and the anchor, a Whole Foods grocery store. *(2013)*

Southern Land Company's 18-story tower, known as 4000 Hillsboro, now under construction at the intersection of Hillsboro Pike and Richard Jones Road. The project features a mixture of residential, retail, and offices, as well as structured parking and pedestrian-oriented street infrastructure. The controversial development was initially proposed to be 22 stories and generated two lawsuits by the Green Hills Neighborhood Association that reflect neighborhood opposition to its density—85,500 square feet of commercial space and 301 residential units—and height. *(Rendering, 2014: Southern Land Company)*

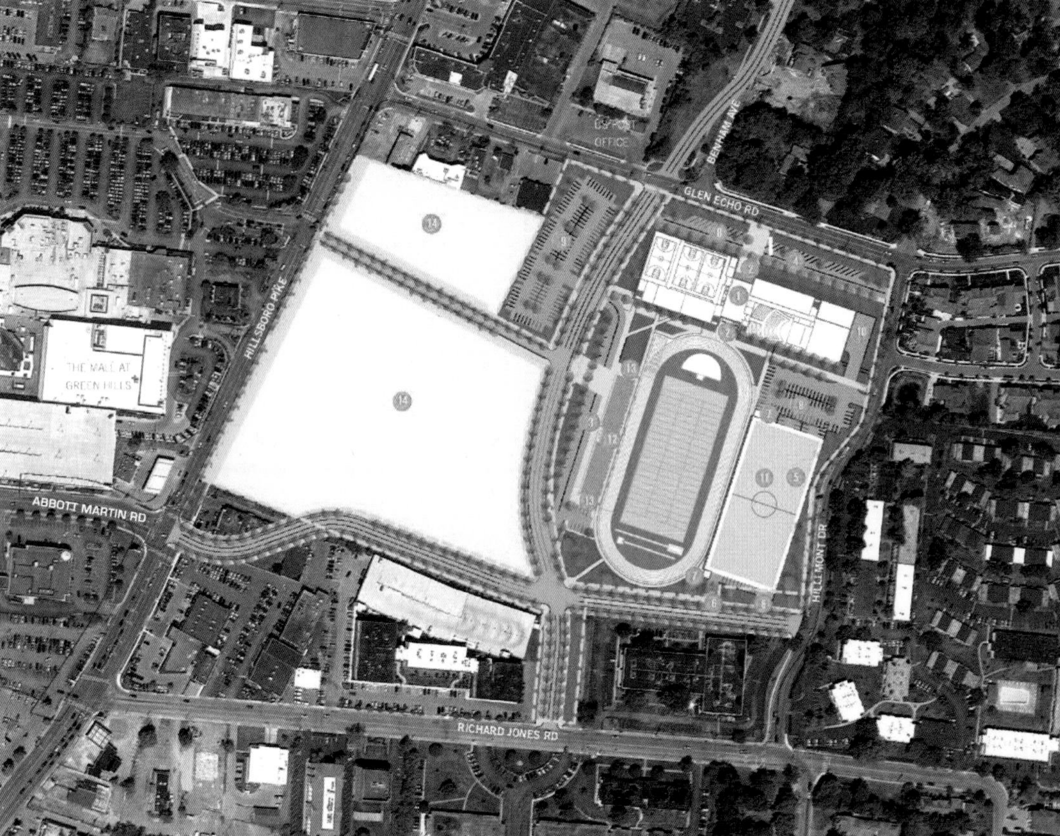

1. PROPOSED SCHOOL
2. MAIN ENTRY
3. BUS DROP-OFF
4. PARENT/STUDENT DROP-OFF
5. STRUCTURED PARKING BELOW
6. VEHICULAR ENTRANCE
7. PEDESTRIAN TOWERS
8. VISITOR PARKING
9. STAFF PARKING
10. SERVICE / LOADING
11. MULTI-PURPOSE FIELD
12. STADIUM
13. STADIUM ENTRY
14. FUTURE DEVELOPMENT

A proposal for rebuilding Hillsboro High School. The site plan includes new roads to connect and extend Abbott Martin Road and Bellham Avenue through the site, increasing much-needed street connectivity.

But there are negative aspects to the plan. The proposed sale for new private development of the property fronting on Hillsboro Pike would eradicate the current lawn at this location, eliminating the possibility of its use as public open space. And the plan requires the demolition of the existing school, one of Nashville's prime examples of mid-century modern architecture designed by Edwin Keeble. *(Plan, 2015: Perkins + Will)*

STRATEGY: *Realign the disjointed cross streets to help improve connectivity and reduce traffic congestion. Note: this will require trades of land with private owners.*

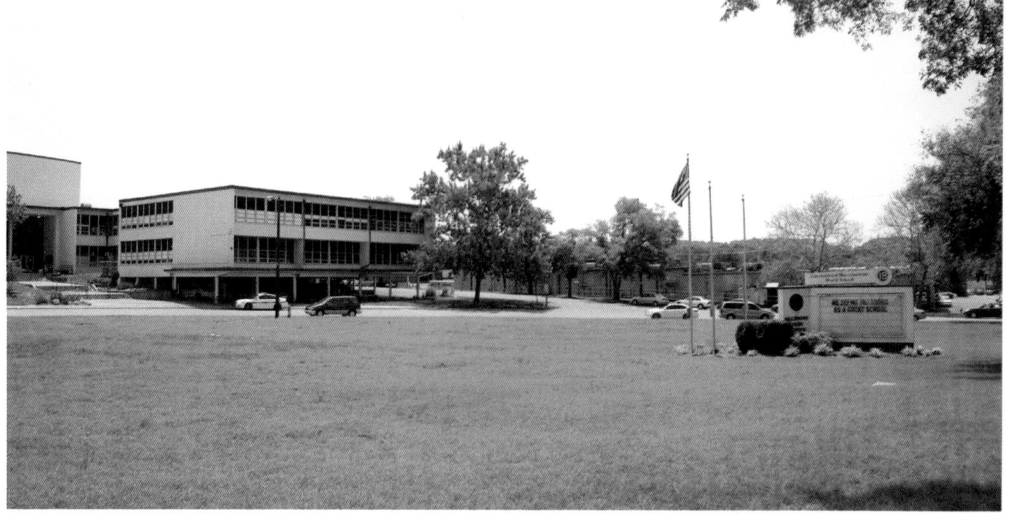

The current Hillsboro High School is fronted by a large lawn. If the proposed site plan is fully implemented, it should incorporate new civic park space to be shared by the school and the community at large. *(2015?)*

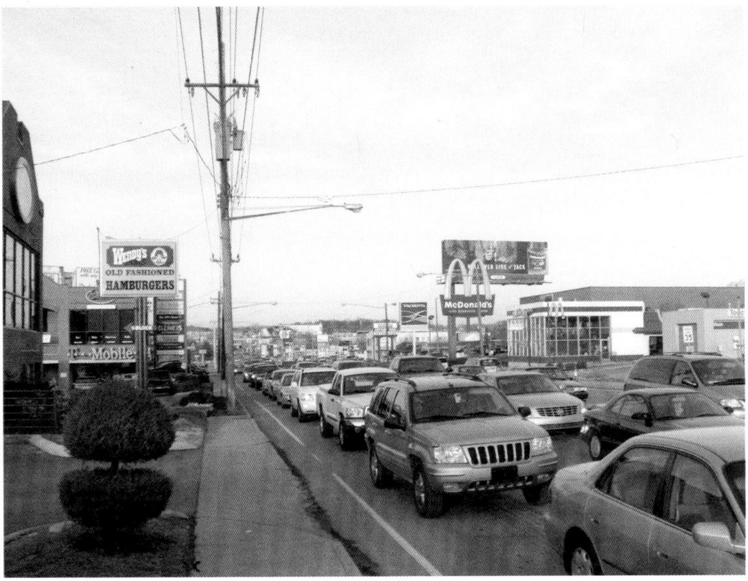

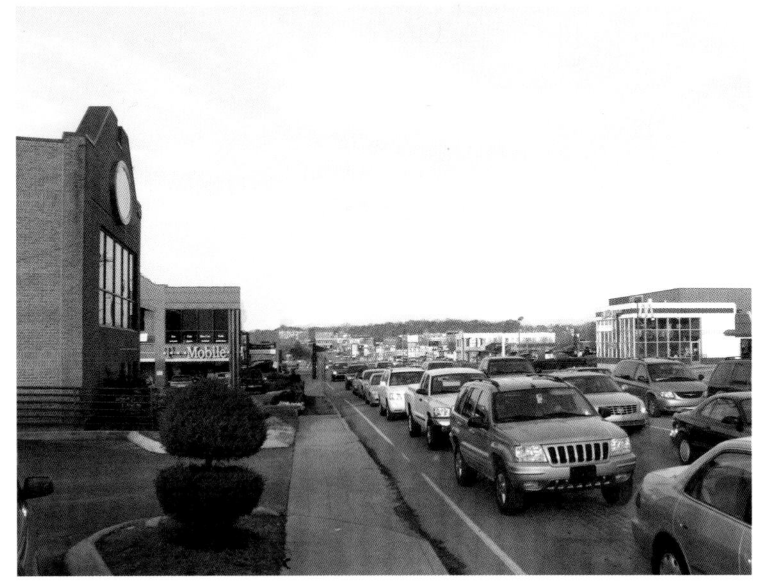

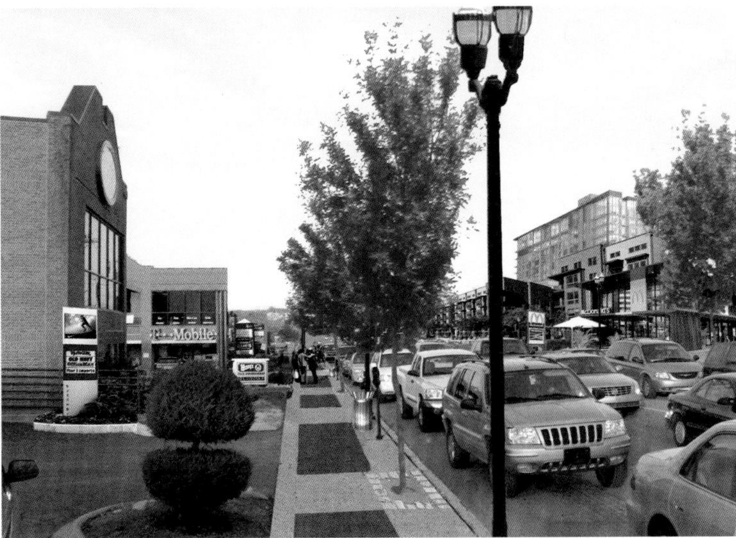

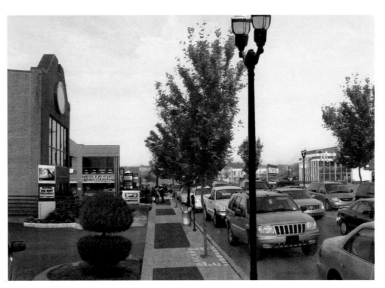

Phases of transformation proposed for Hillsboro Pike.

Clockwise from left: Existing condition; removal of signage; implementation of streetscaping; and new higher density infill development. *(Visualizations, 2005 and 2014: Parvathi Nampoothri and Eric Hoke, NCDC)*

STRATEGY: *Redesign the streetscape of Hillsboro Road through Green Hills to incorporate more pedestrian-friendly design.*

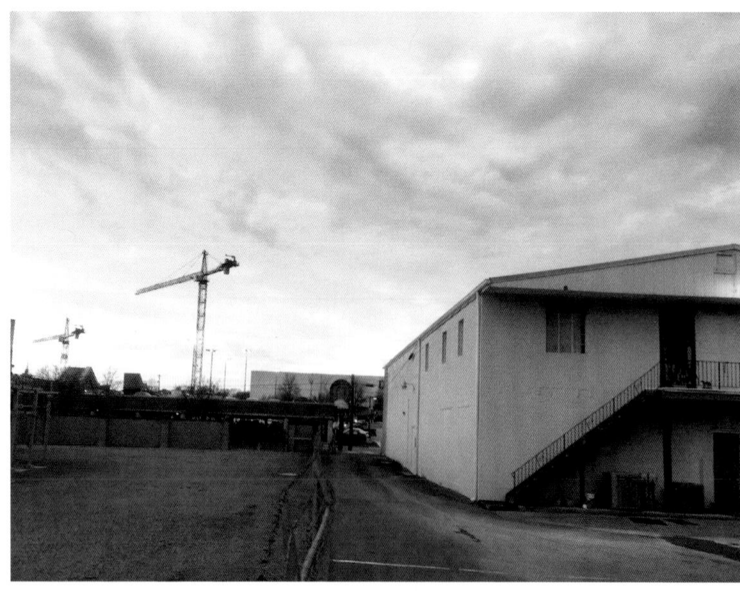

Stark existing conditions of potential pedestrian connection between the Hill Center and Bandywood Drive, with the Mall at Green Hills in the distance. *(2015)*

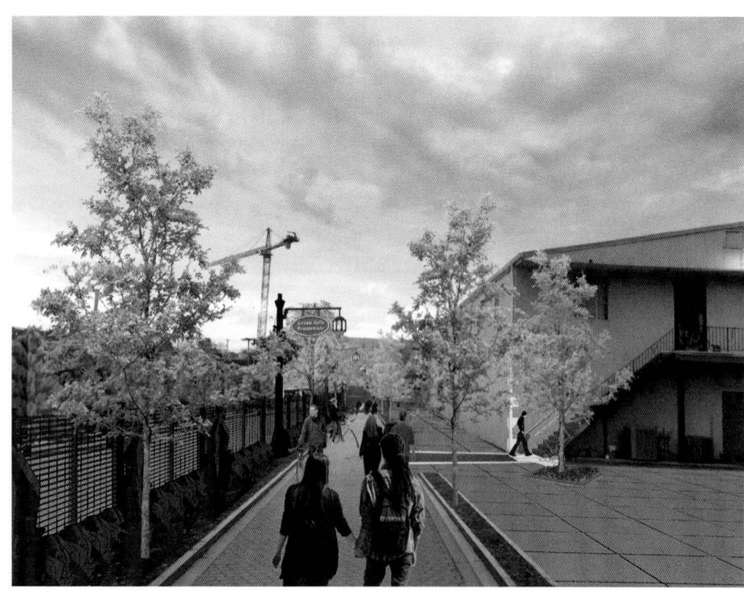

Same connection with pedestrian upgrades as proposed in the Green Hills Area Transportation Plan. *(Visualization, 2015: Eric Hoke, NCDC)*

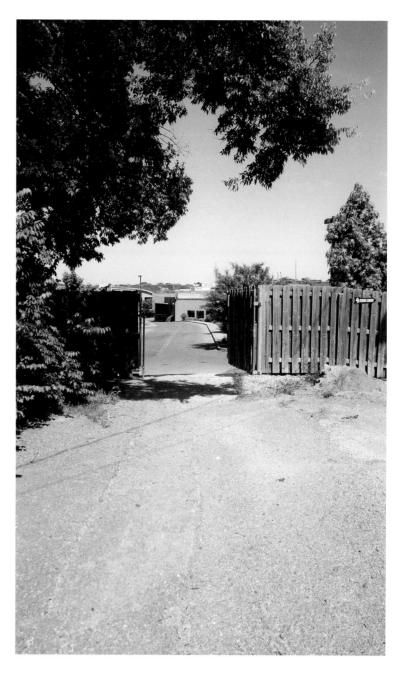

Right: Potential pedestrian and bicycle pathways to connect residential neighborhood in Green Hills to the community YMCA and numerous shops. Currently, a gate at the end of Warfield Lane obstructs access. *(2014)*

STRATEGY: *Develop a system of connected pedestrian and bicycle pathways between retail and residential areas to encourage accessibility by means other than the automobile.*

STRATEGY: *Create a green-belt loop around Green Hills incorporating pedestrian and bicycle routes among neighborhoods and commercial areas, offering safe recreational options.*

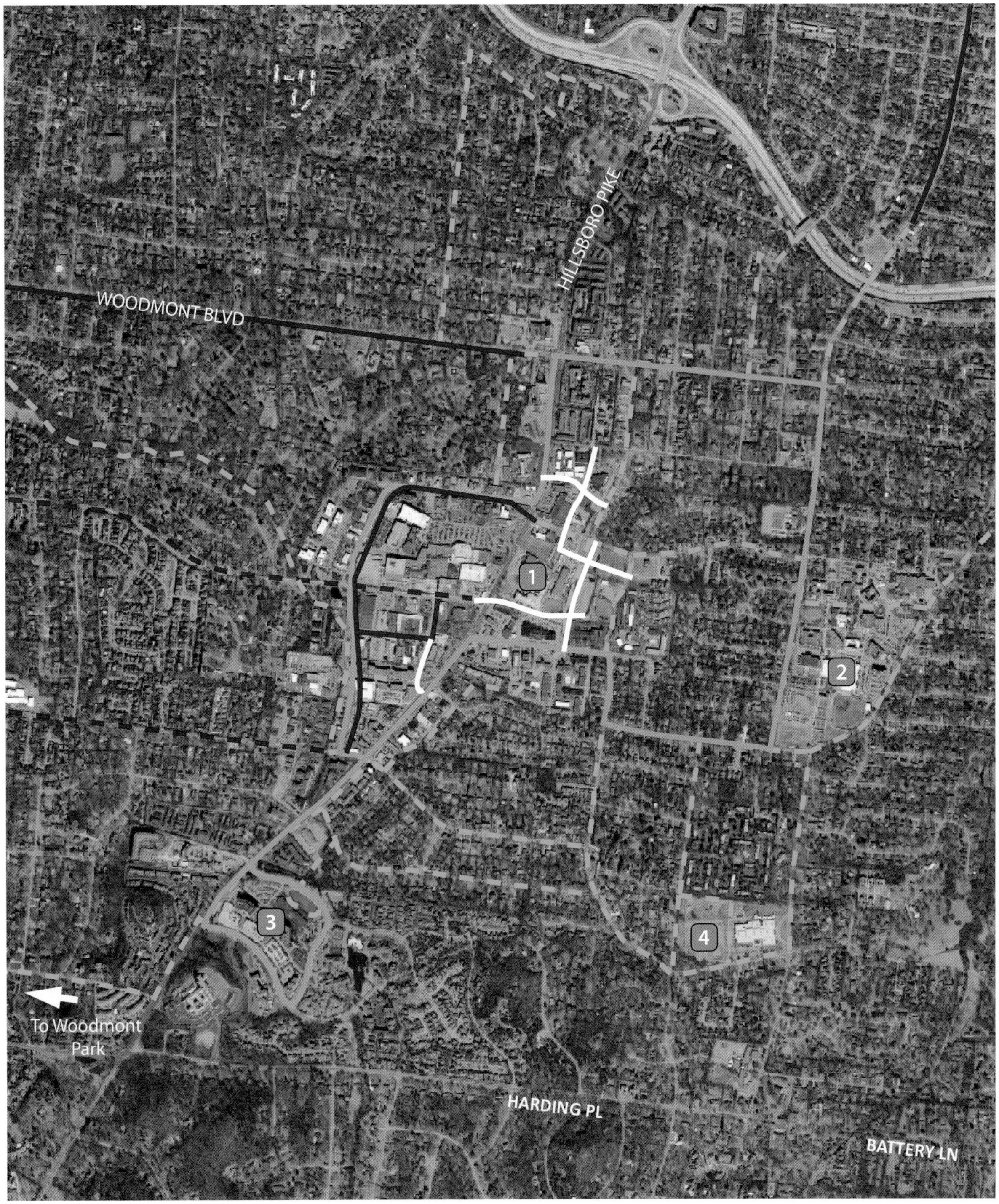

Existing and potential greenways and bikeways in Green Hills can serve to connect the community. Dashed green lines represent potential greenways. Solid red lines represent existing bike lanes; dashed red, potential ones. Solid white represents future roadway connections. Note the lack of existing greenways in the area. *(Diagram over aerial, 2015: Eric Hoke, NCDC)*

1 Hillsboro High School
2 Lipscomb University
3 Park and Ride
4 Green Hills Park

Existing Bike Lane
Future Bike Lane
Transit Circulator
Future Multi-Use Path
Future Road

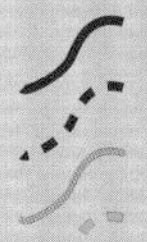

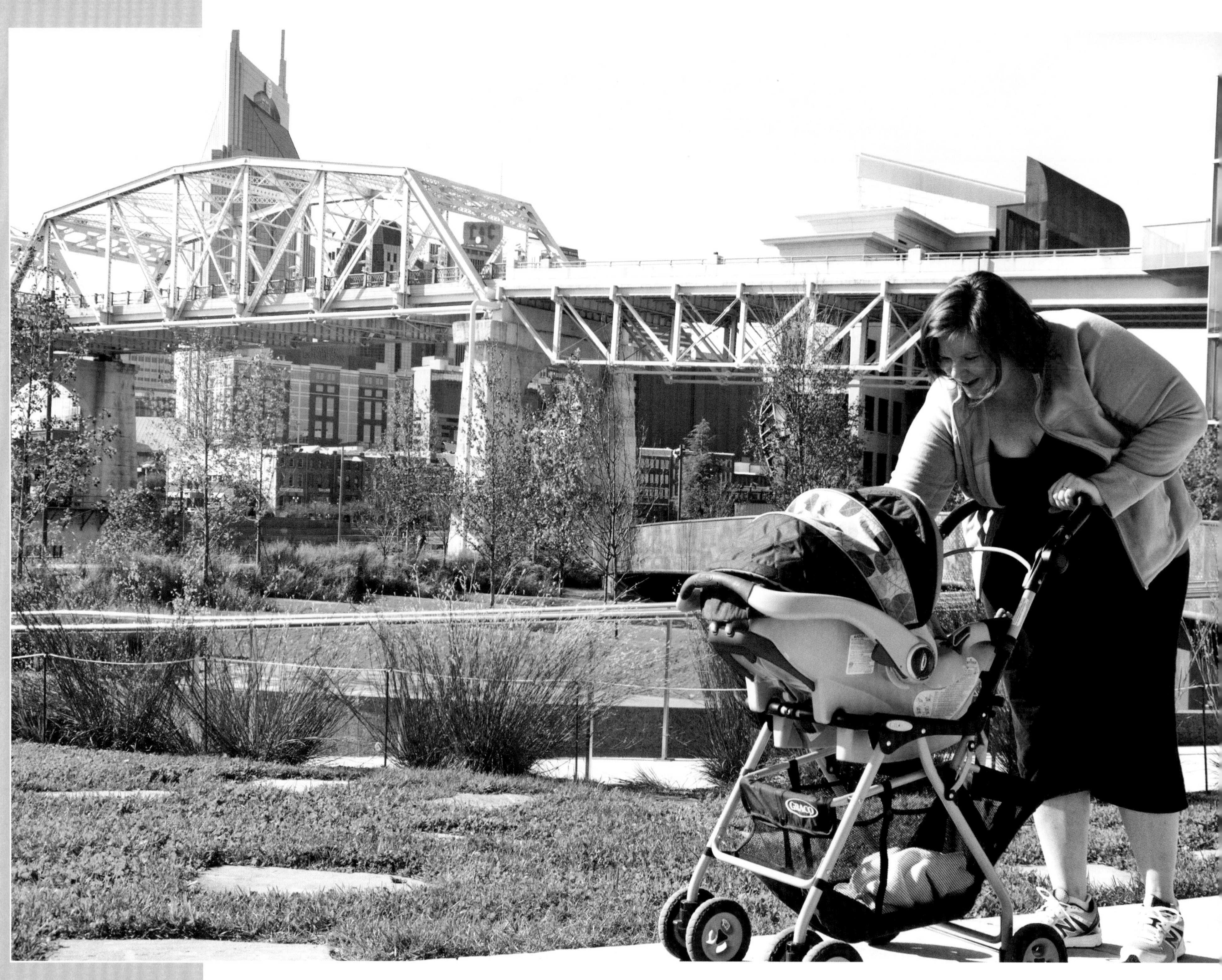
GRACO

CLAIRE CLAYTOR

City living, especially for children, is an anomaly to many Nashvillians. "We've been stopped a lot by people asking us, 'You live downtown with this little baby?'" says **Claire Claytor,** 30, an intern architect with Gresham Smith and Partners. "Yes!" she answers. "People do it all over the country, all over the world."

Claytor liked the idea of walking from home to work and to Riverfront Park, but it was her husband who really wanted to experience urban life. "Tim grew up in a rural area and he wanted to live in the thick of things, be surrounded by people in constantly changing environments," she says. "He likes to take a lawn chair out and sit on Second Avenue in the summer and just watch people walk by."

The couple and their kids, Leo and Ruth, live in the Quarters, a warehouse on Second Avenue converted to lofts for rent in 1986 that became condos in 2005. Claytor says there are tradeoffs to living in a 1,000-square-foot space on the fourth floor. "You can't buy a giant vat of peanut butter, just a little jar. But we don't mow a yard, we get to share beautiful public spaces and see the city evolve, instead of living on a cul-de-sac."

Claytor sees commuting by foot as a great perk. "Walking to work is wonderful," she says. "It's a great transition from the rush of getting ready and then arriving at work and needing to focus. Just that little bit of walk is great. When I lived in Mt. Juliet I commuted to downtown. I've never smoked a cigarette in my life, but I would get to work and think, 'Man, I need a cigarette.' I'd be in a foul mood, stressed on interstate traffic, which is no way to start the day. How do people do this every day for years and years?"

Transportation downtown, however, can also be challenging. Pushing a stroller has highlighted lapses in handicapped access. And when Claytor does have to take the car, it's a hassle. "Leaving downtown to do major grocery shopping is difficult," she says. "We park across the street, in the Commerce Street garage, so we have to load up children and gear and then get to the car to go off campus."

The Music City Circuit offers free service in the downtown area, and Claytor can often be seen on the bright green, clean-diesel-hybrid bus, heading to the Farmers' Market or the Gulch. "If downtown isn't going to have some of the amenities that are in East Nashville or farther west, I would love the ability to hop on public transit to get to them. To spend an hour reading or playing with our kid and not be behind the wheel so much would be awesome."

Claytor is a big fan of the new Cumberland Park, which flanks the river on the East Bank and opened in 2012. "The first time I went over there I actually cried. I thought, 'Wow! This is what we've been wanting,'" she says. "It's awesome to see people flock to that park from other parts of Nashville. I didn't expect people to come downtown to go to a park."

Claytor has a long wish list for the downtown core. She would like more pocket parks, a larger grocery store, and a place to buy basic clothing items. Another craving: healthy food stores and dining options that would appeal to residents and tourists alike, such as a Turnip Truck, which currently has stores in East Nashville and the Gulch. Retrofit part of the old Convention Center into a downtown movie theater. And open up storefronts on First Avenue, so that you can shop and stroll along the river.

Add to the list safer, more direct routes for getting around by bike. "I don't see us ever taking our kids bicycling except on a greenway—it's just dangerous," Claytor says. "A lot of cyclists and drivers don't know the actual rules of the road and tend to get very angry at one another. We've had a couple of near run-ins when biking downtown. Lots of honking, drivers telling us to get on the sidewalk, which is illegal!" In addition, bicycle lanes are often inadequate. "They just magically disappear and you've got to veer back into traffic. Some of the lanes are fairly treacherous with potholes and cracks," she says.

Claytor hopes for new development that will include some larger units for families. "Given the right opportunity, more people would enjoy downtown living. And if the people come, then the businesses and the amenities will come."

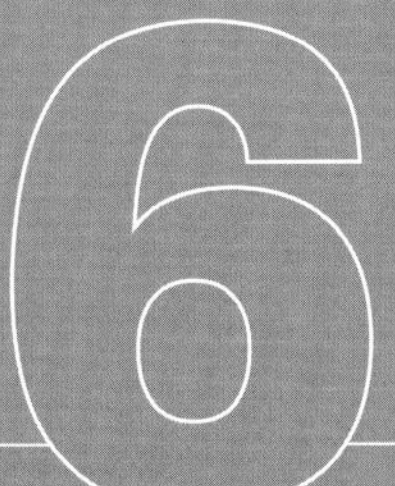

STRATEGIES

Focus on making downtown a complete neighborhood, with more residences and the necessities for daily life.

Infill vacant lots, surface parking lots, and empty upper floors of existing buildings.

Increase the frequency and hours of operation of public transit service.

Enhance cycling safety for commuters and residents, and create a network of protected bike routes through downtown.

Improve the pedestrian experience by upgrading the streetscape with more trees, benches, and public restrooms.

Limit pedestrian/vehicular conflict by giving crosswalk priority to pedestrians over automobiles and limiting vehicular right turns on red lights.

Enhance mobility for wheelchairs and strollers.

Develop a mid-size, full-service grocery store in the downtown core that features fresh produce and healthy take-out at prices reasonable for all shoppers.

Increase healthy food options in the concessions of publicly owned venues.

Increase housing diversity in terms of affordability and household types.

Create new open spaces, parks, and recreational uses in the core, and activate existing underutilized spaces.

THE DOWNTOWN TRANSECT ZONE

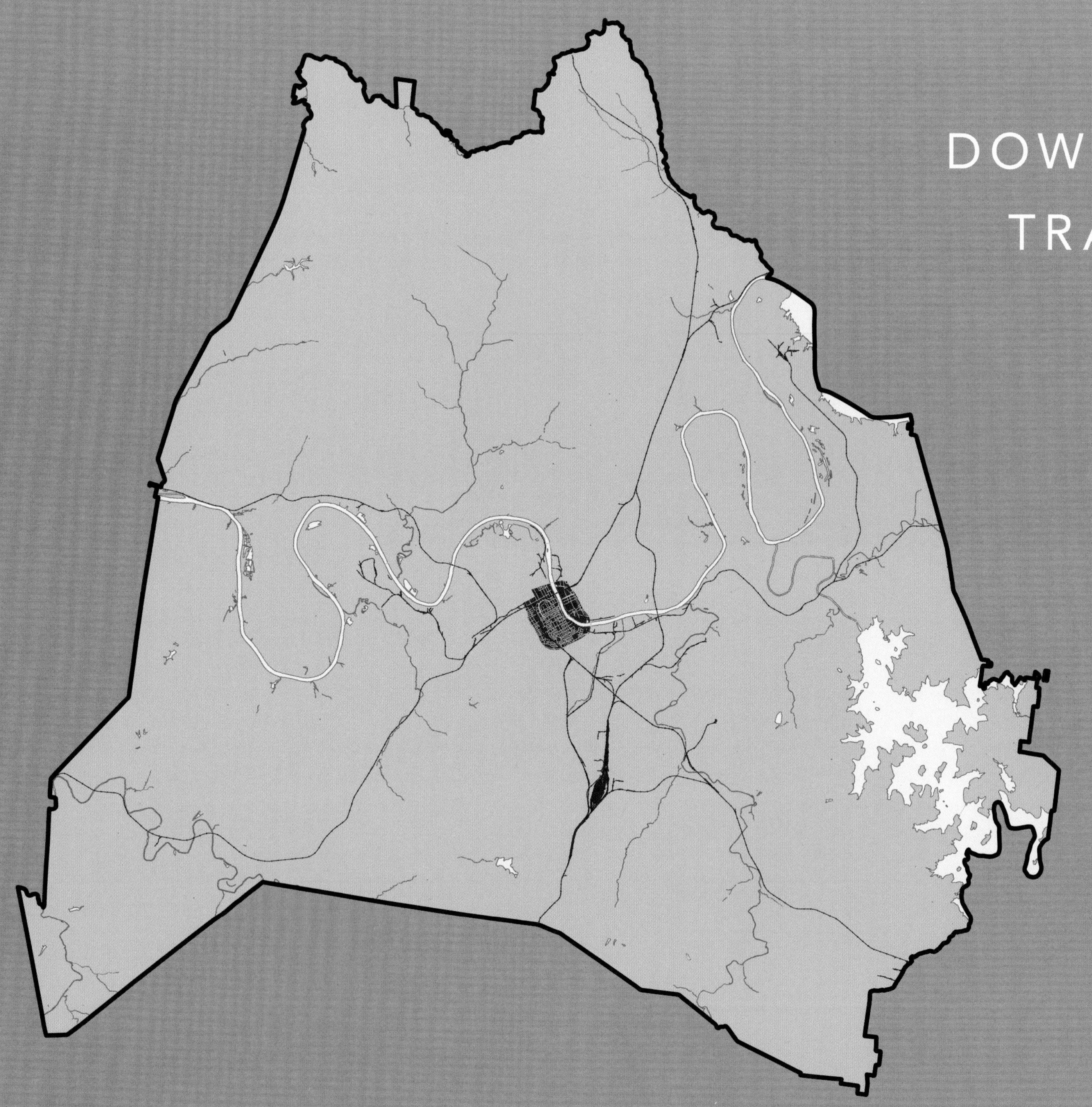

Davidson County, highlighting all areas in the downtown transect zone, also called the "core." The boundary defining this zone is the I-40, I-65, and I-24 interstate loop that encircles the western, southern, and eastern portions of downtown, including the East Bank of the Cumberland River. Jefferson Street is the boundary to the north. (Map, 2014: Metro Planning Department)

DOWNTOWN

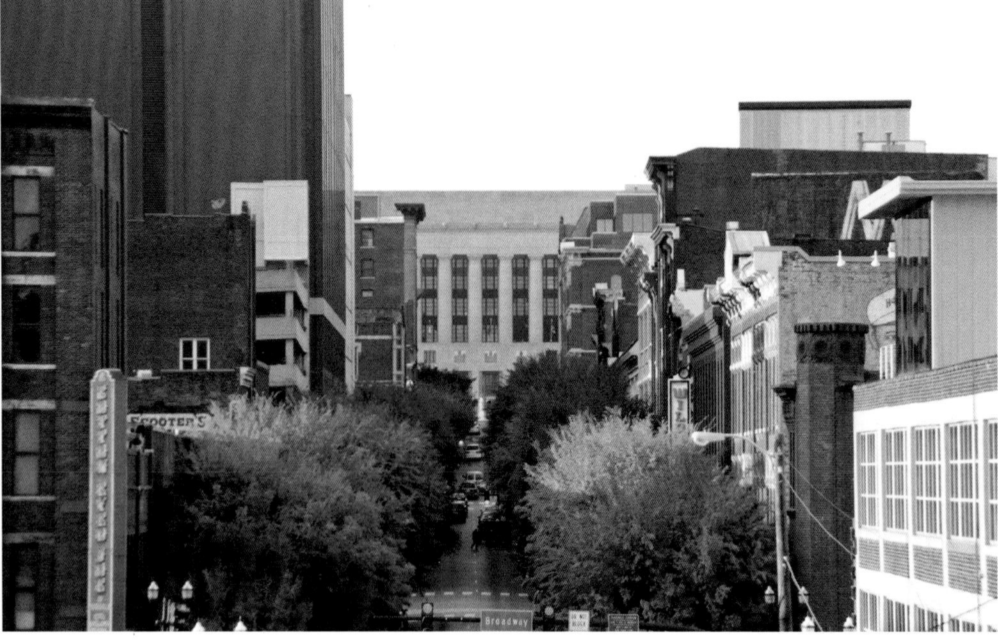

When it was Market Street, Second Avenue was the hub of Cumberland River trade. Now the street is part of The DISTRICT, the heart of Nashville's entertainment quarter. *(2013)*

CITY LIVING

Looking north from Broadway up Second Avenue, we see commerce crowned by government. The Victorian warehouses that line the avenue are evidence of Nashville's reason for being. The city began life as a Cumberland River port, distributing animal pelts, timber, and the products of agriculture to the region and beyond. The Courthouse and its public square are evidence of something else again. After the bustle of capitalism, the eye comes to rest on the civic place that binds enterprising individuals into a community.

Downtown Nashville is the binding agent of the region, an area encompassing 10 counties and over 1.8 million people.[1] Since the 18th century turned into the 19th, all of Middle Tennessee's major roadways—in traffic engineering lingo, "arterials"—have led to the central city. That's where people who lived and worked in the region wanted and needed to go to sell and buy, to meet and greet. But arteries are dependent on a healthy beating heart. Despite the loss of commerce and residents to suburbia, Nashville's core is still home to the highest concentration of government and private business offices, cultural and tourist amenities, all located in a relatively compact area of just under 1,600 acres.

We tend to define downtown visually by its buildings: State Capitol and Metro Courthouse, historic churches and honky tonks, symphony hall and skyscrapers, arena and convention center. But it is the transportation infrastructure—Cumberland River, streets and pikes, railroads, interstate highways—that has shaped the central city for better and worse.

The first permanent settlers, from North Carolina, staked their claim to Middle Tennessee land by building a fort along the west bluff of the Cumberland River in 1780.[2] They called the place Nashborough, changed to Nashville after the

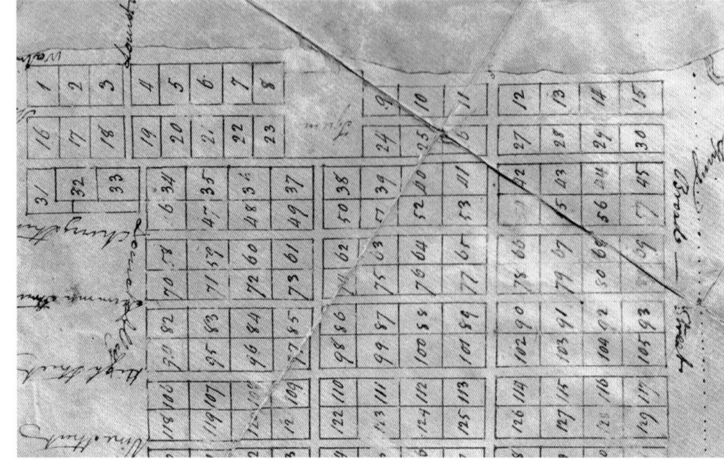

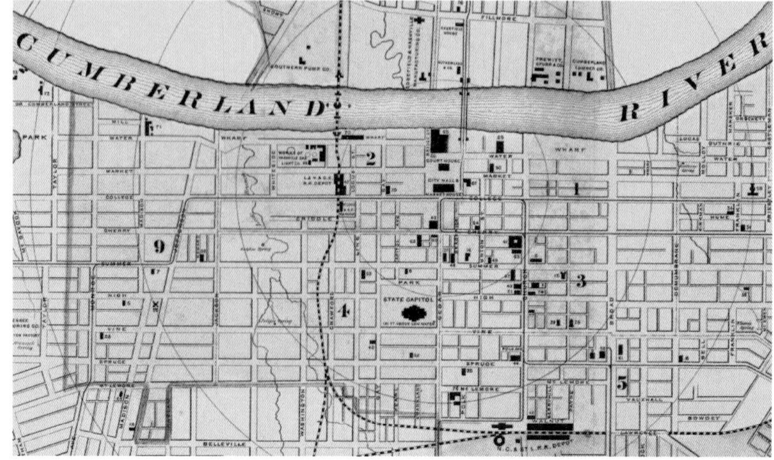

Left: Map after the original plat by Molloy; copy made for John Overton. Note the perfect grid of streets, which were laid out without regard to changes in topography. This regularity would be modified as lots were subdivided and developed. *(Map, 1789: The Tennessee Historical Society, Tennessee State Library and Archives)*

Right: Mid-19th-century map of Nashville. Note the irregularities in street widths and connectivity, as well as lot sizes. Molloy's checkerboard had adjusted to commercial reality. *(Map,1860s: United States Army, Military Division of the Mississippi. The Library of Congress)*

Revolutionary War to remove the stain of England. In Nashville's early years what would later be called downtown was the only thing that qualified as "town" at all. The history of the city as a whole, therefore, and that of the core are more or less interchangeable during this period.

In 1784, surveyor Thomas Molloy platted the nucleus of the downtown we know today along the Cumberland: a town of one-acre lots with a four-acre public square on the high point of the bluff. Broad Street defined the southern edge and terminated at what would become the city wharf. Nashville's commercial transportation centered on the wharf until the railroads gained ascendancy in the 1860s. Thus most of the historic pikes, bringing farmers and their products to market, led to what became Broadway.

The first locomotive arrived in Nashville via boat in 1850. By 1861 five railroad lines serviced the city, which had to accommodate the infrastructure. The tracks were laid in ravines and lowlands unsuited to other development, such as in what is now known as the Gulch. During the Union occupation of Nashville in the Civil War, when the railroads flourished with government subsidies, the tracks became a rough loop around the core. When the interstates superseded railroads 100 years later, the roadbeds followed the same downtown loop.

After the Civil War, its central location made Nashville a trade hub between the Midwest and the deeper South. The city evolved into a center for wholesale groceries, manufacturing, and banking. The business district expanded into formerly residential areas, raising property values. The factories, stockyards, and warehouses clustered around the transportation infrastructure needed to do business, primarily the railroads. The Cumberland River was the main pathway for lumber, with most of the mills located on the East Bank.

Industry increased air pollution. Those families who could afford the costs for land and

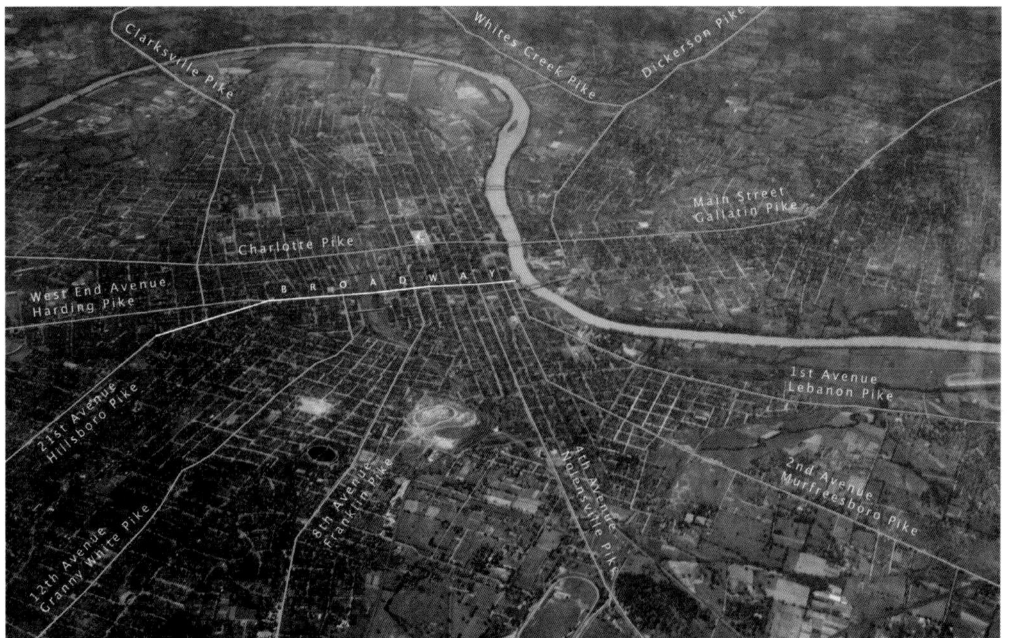

Historic pikes (highlighted) terminating in downtown Nashville. These roads were laid over the footpaths by which bison and other animals threaded through the hills to reach the salt lick north of downtown, near today's Bicentennial Mall. When incorporated into the city's street system, the pikes supplied an unpredictability and irregularity to the pattern of the core. *(1934: Metro Planning Department; diagram, 2004: NCDC)*

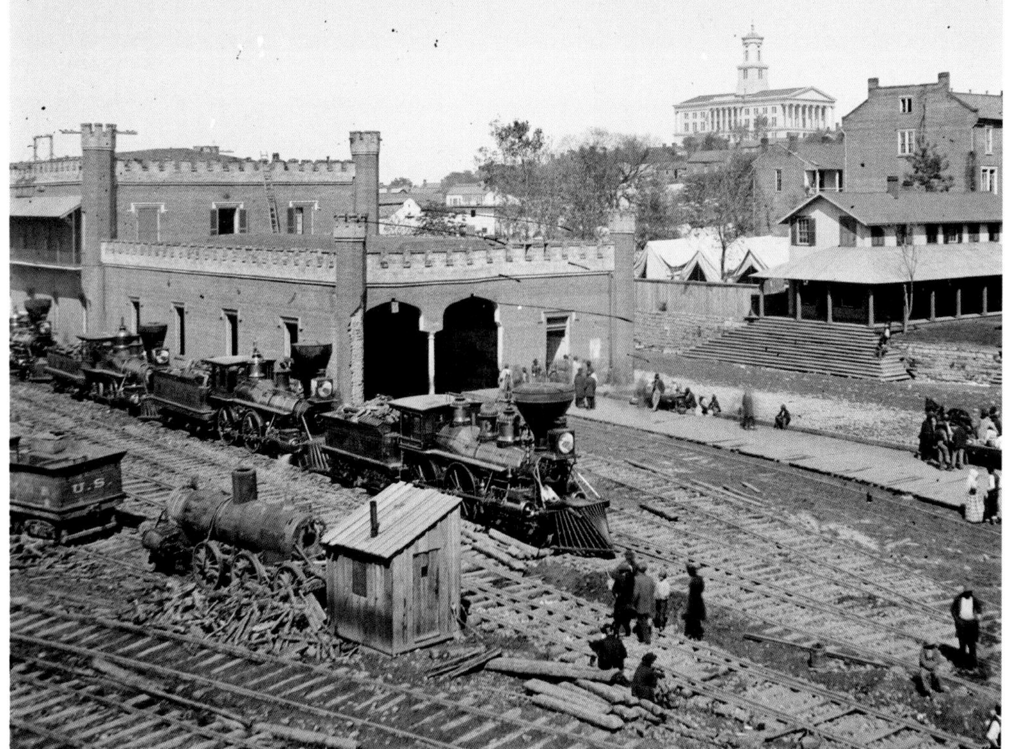

The selection of Nashville as Tennessee's capital in 1843 led to the development of Cedar Knob for the Capitol building, seen here in the background. Until the advent of skyscrapers, the Capitol defined the Nashville skyline. In the foreground, the crenellated Nashville & Chattanooga depot, which stood in the Gulch north of the current location of Union Station. *(1864: Library of Congress)*

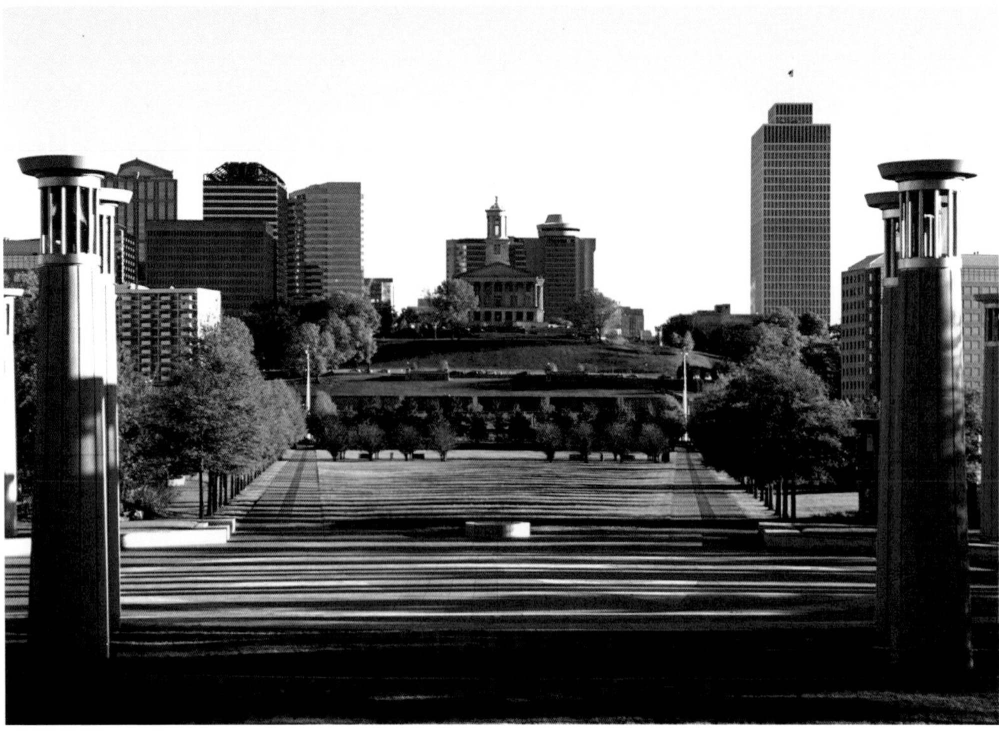

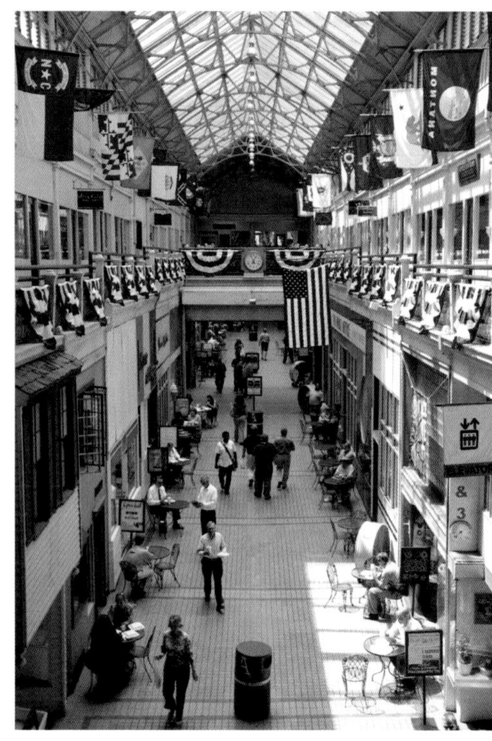

Left: Nashville's Bicentennial Mall, designed by Tuck-Hinton Architects, was the first significant greenspace in downtown. The Mall opened in 1996, ironically in the same area that the editor of a local newspaper had unsuccessfully proposed for the city's first park in 1856. *(2010: Gary Layda)*

Right: The Arcade, which opened in 1903, is a pedestrian-only connection between Fourth and Fifth Avenues. Such arcades were common in the 19th century and increased the value of mid-block land by giving such property more store frontage. Nashville's example, one of the few surviving in this country, shelters two tiers of offices and shops. Today it is an especially popular lunch destination. (2013)

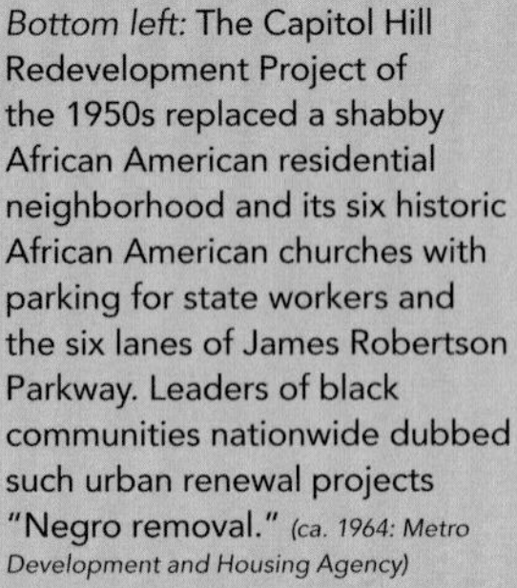

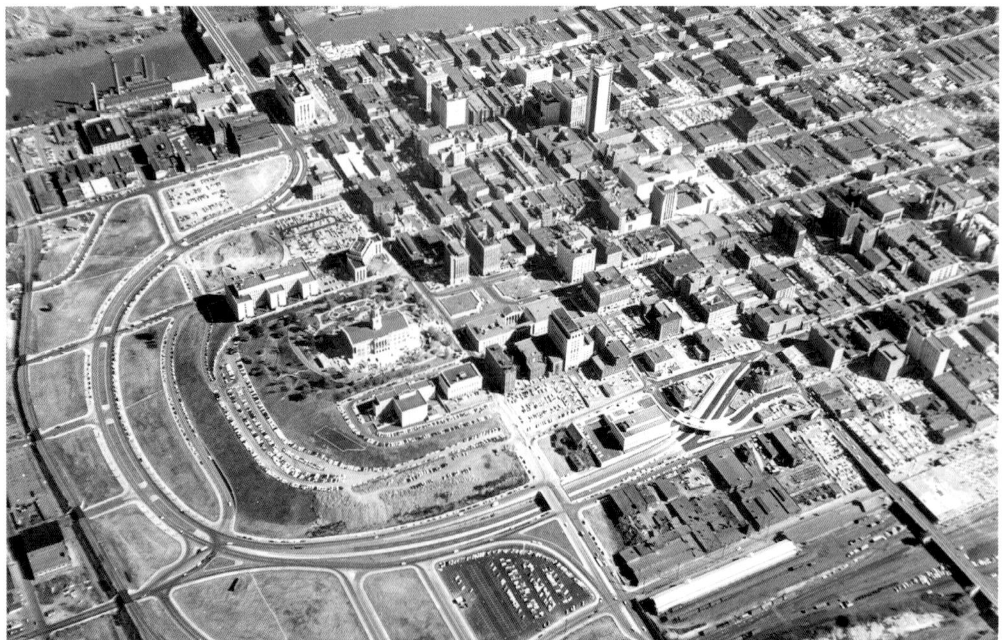

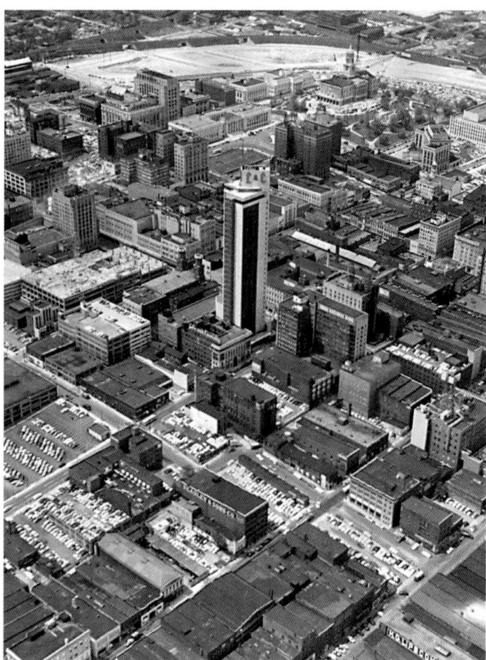

Bottom left: The Capitol Hill Redevelopment Project of the 1950s replaced a shabby African American residential neighborhood and its six historic African American churches with parking for state workers and the six lanes of James Robertson Parkway. Leaders of black communities nationwide dubbed such urban renewal projects "Negro removal." *(ca. 1964: Metro Development and Housing Agency)*

Bottom right: The L&C Tower, designed by Edwin Keeble. When built by the Life and Casualty Insurance Company in 1957 it was the tallest skyscraper in the Southeast. Unlike later exercises in architectural modernism downtown, L&C rests urbanely on its corner at Fourth Avenue North and Church Street, its entrance and lobby retaining a comfortable human scale. *(1957: Courtesy of Special Collections, Nashville Public Library)* transportation—first horses and carriages, then streetcars—departed for homes outside the city, away from the stench and fumes. The laboring classes, who by necessity walked to work, found themselves compressed into slums. Real estate speculators converted old housing stock into tenements while waiting for more lucrative commercial development opportunities. When these came, the poor were also expelled outward.

The lack of public parks in the city was first publicly noticed in 1856, according to Leland Johnson in *The Parks of Nashville*.[3] A year before New York's Central Park officially opened, a local newspaper editor advocated for a park system for Nashville. He suggested that officials begin by purchasing 50 acres surrounding the sulfur spring (the site of the bison's salt lick) just north of the Capitol, a swampy area that had so far resisted development. At that time, downtown greenspace was restricted to the lawns around the Customs House and Capitol. (The public square was the paved site of the farmers' market.) But Nashville was then surrounded by open countryside to which citizens could easily ride or walk, and the recommendation was ignored.

In 1901 Nashville's Park Board held its first meeting, but initially had no funds for land acquisition, relying instead on donations. By this time, however, downtown land had become valuable enough to inhibit potential donors. The board focused instead on the gift of land near a stone quarry in North Nashville owned by Samuel Watkins that became Watkins Park, and converting the Tennessee Centennial Exposition grounds west of downtown into Centennial Park.

After World War I, Nashville's economic mainspring became the banking, insurance, and securities businesses centered on Union Street, self-styled as the "Wall Street of the South." Beginning in the 1920s, rural-to-urban migration, caused by depressed farm prices, brought more workers to Nashville, increasing the market for consumer goods. The city's retail district, which had shifted from the public square to the Arcade and Fifth Avenue North in the early 20th century, expanded along Church Street.

The major long-term impact on downtown, however, came with the automobile and its insatiable demand for space. By 1930 there were over 40,000 vehicles registered in Nashville, and the number climbed inexorably. The cars clogged streets, threatened pedestrians, and required parking for storage.

Garages came to the retail district and Broadway, but the number of vehicles quickly outgrew the numbers of spaces. Downtown retailers, fearing the growing number of suburban shops, pressed for suburban-style surface lots. Many "outdated" buildings were demolished for personal car storage, creating gaps in the street walls that eroded pedestrian interest and endangered walkers with curb cuts. The streetcars could not compete with the car for personal transportation, and ridership declined along with the frequency of service.

The late 1940s saw local officials reaching for ways to stem the tide of commercial migration to the suburbs and the decay of downtown building stock. The strategy they selected was to reconstruct the central city, which was now to be primarily a business district, for the automobile. They would pay for the transformation with federal funds authorized for what was called "urban renewal."

Following the urban renewal of Capitol Hill came the Central Loop General Neighborhood Renewal Plan of 1963 for the rest of the area inside the interstate loop west of the Cumberland River. This plan envisioned a city of wide thoroughfares flanked by tall stand-alone towers surrounded by landscaped plazas, a suburban model sharply distinct from the older shared-wall buildings that form a continuous street wall.

While much of the Central Loop plan was

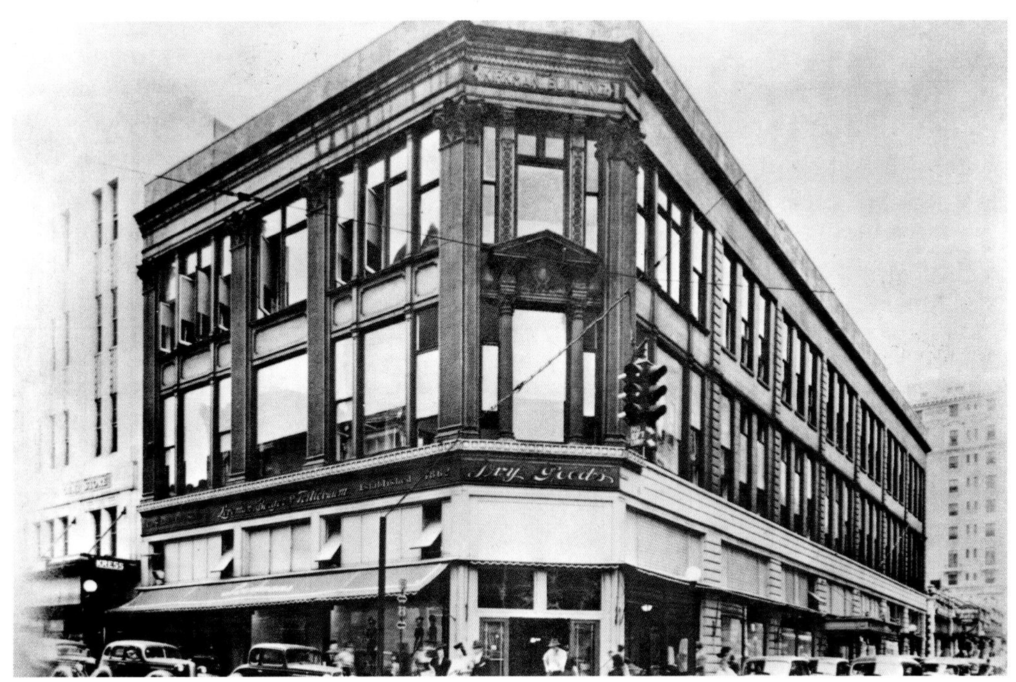

The Kirkman building, constructed at the turn of the 20th century on the corner of Union Street and Fifth Avenue, was home to Loveman's department store, which traced its roots back to 1862. The company constructed a new flagship store in the suburbs in 1951; the downtown building was demolished in 1966.

Tax breaks enticed bankers and insurance moguls to follow government's lead and tear down imposing structures from the early decades of the 20th century to construct large modernist office quarters on Union Street, like the current Tennessee Tower. *(1940s: Courtesy of Special Collections, Nashville Public Library)* fortunately never implemented, the un-urban design philosophy behind it held sway among the city's planners and developers until the 1990s. And the plan's direct impact on downtown between Union and Deaderick Streets, the Metro Courthouse and Eighth Avenue North, was powerful.

The Victorian buildings surrounding the public square were bulldozed for roadways and a tall office tower with the requisite plaza. The square itself, which in 1960 had been the locus of civil rights protests, became a surface parking lot. Deaderick Street was widened to four lanes; its mid-rise buildings and storefronts, many of those near Fourth Avenue North housing black businesses, were replaced by massive stand-alone office buildings on blank podiums; and the Tennessee Performing Arts Center, with its pedestrian-hostile wall on Union Street, was constructed. War Memorial Park became Legislative Plaza, elevated above street grade to accommodate underground parking and state offices.

The arrival of the interstates in the 1960s created a concrete barrier encircling downtown. The

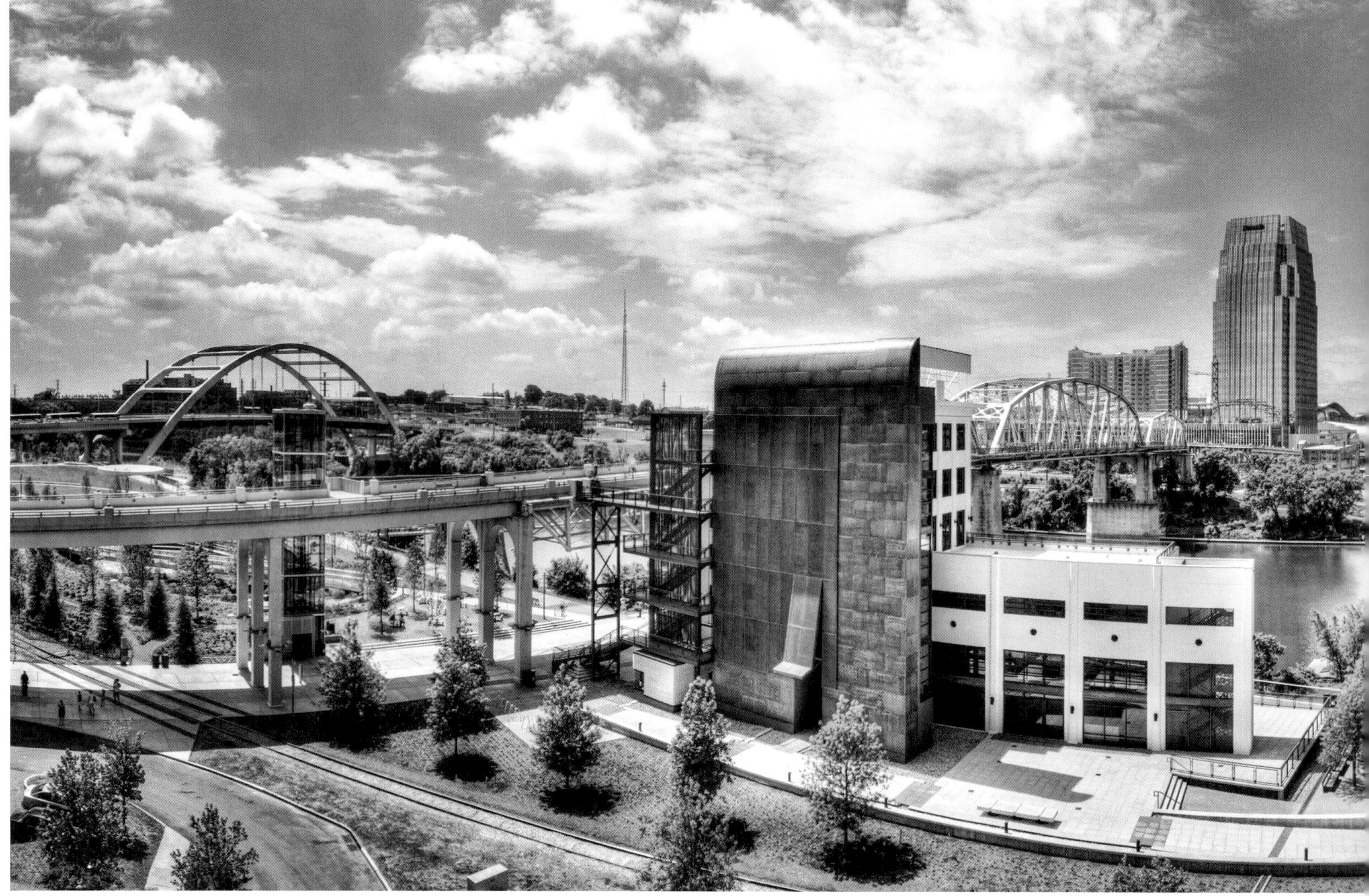

Downtown Nashville, viewed from the East Bank looking across the Cumberland River. The tall buildings south of Broadway indicate the transformation taking place in SoBro. The Nashville Bridge Building, designed by Hastings Architecture, in foreground, received a LEED Platinum rating for its core and shell—the interior was not originally built out. Note how the skyline steps up from the historic warehouses on First and Second Avenues along the waterfront to the skyscrapers beyond. *(2012: Bruce Cain, ElevatedLens.com).*

limited-access highways fractured the network of streets that had connected the core to the first-ring neighborhoods west of the Cumberland and divided the East Bank from East Nashville. Those thoroughfares that fed the interstates became congested corridors hostile to all but vehicular traffic.

The 1974 comprehensive zoning ordinance (COMZO) for what was now Metro Nashville forbade residential construction in the central core. By simplifying the mixture of land uses in downtown to reinforce the core's identity as the central *business* district, Metro's planners and public officials essentially depopulated the central city after working hours.

Given this systematic, government-sponsored assault on the central city's urban character, it is unsurprising that, beginning in the latter years of the 1960s, Nashville's downtown, like many across the United States, went into serious decline. The iconic Grand Ole Opry and businesses like the insurance giant American General, which occupied the skyscraper built with the help of tax breaks that is now the Tennessee Tower, departed for new homes in the suburbs.

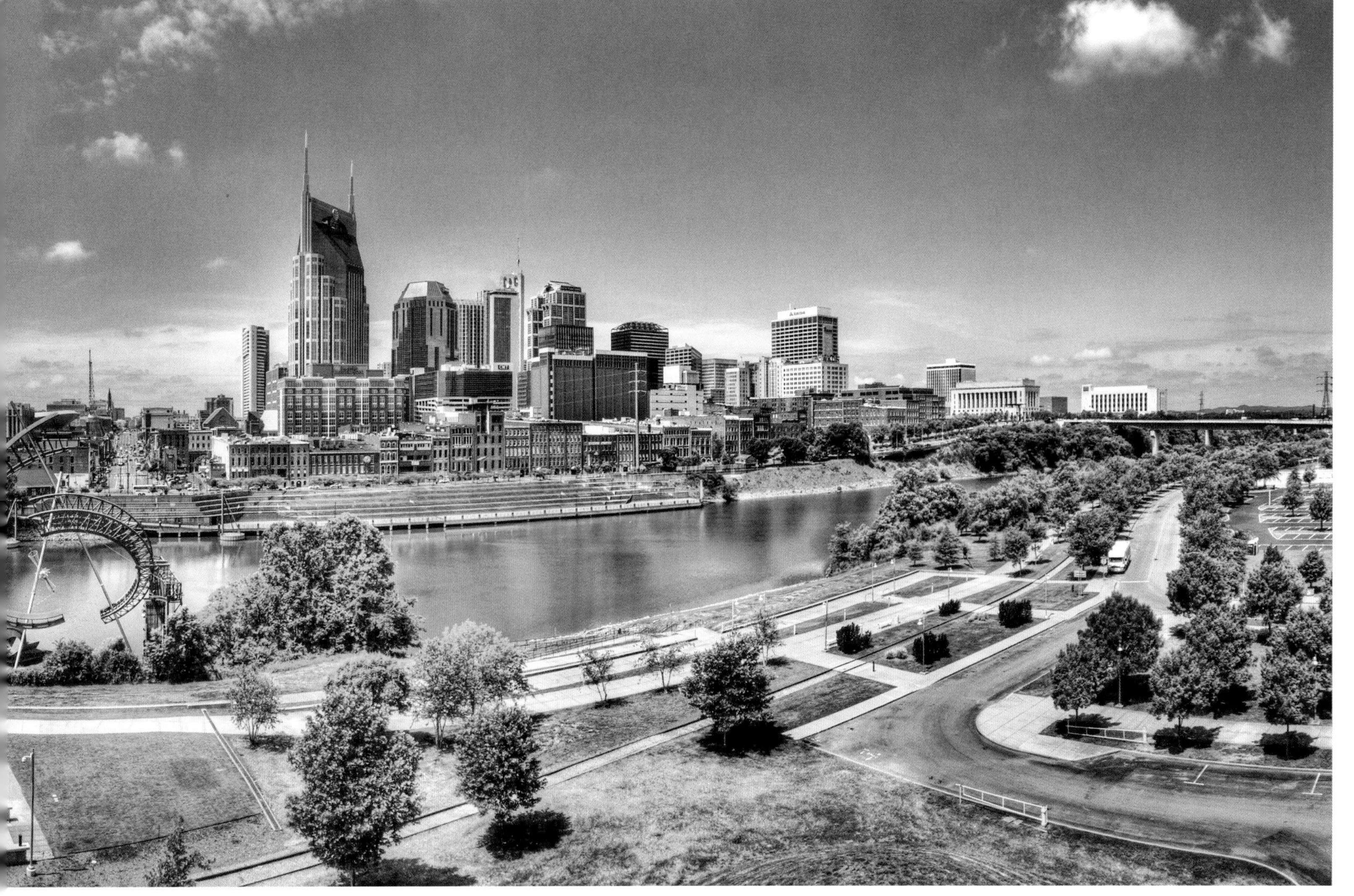

Preservationists had to mount a fierce battle to block the demolition of the Opry's former home, the Ryman Auditorium. The Nashville Convention Center of 1987 was built with its back turned to lower Broadway. Dominated by porno shops and winos, Nashville's "Main Street" had become a source of shame. Church Street, which had been the focus of the movement to desegregate lunch counters, became pockmarked with the surface parking lots that replaced its department stores. An attempt to revive retail on what had been Nashville's historic shopping street, the Church Street Center of 1990, failed within a decade.

The downtown revival began in the early 1990s with the rebirth of Second Avenue, Nashville's original Market Street, as a tourist hot spot. Opryland Inc. brought music back to the Ryman. What is today called Bridgestone Arena was built on a surface parking lot on Broadway, whose honky tonks now attracted natives and tourists alike. In 1994 the central core's zoning was changed to permit residential development. The Cumberland apartments came to Church Street, and the upper floors of old buildings were rehabbed for urban living.

These specific developments reflected changes in the city's planning policies. But among the policy makers were those who still wanted more asphalt for more cars, who failed to grasp the key role played by transportation infrastructure in determining urban form.

In 1995, Metro's planning and public works departments announced plans to demolish the 1909 Shelby Bridge for a new bridge as part of a six-lane corridor south of Broadway linking two interstates. During the long and contentious, but ultimately successful struggle to reform corridor into urban boulevard, downtown south of Broadway became SoBro. The football stadium came to the East Bank. The Shelby Bridge was renovated as a bike and pedestrian connection between the East Bank and downtown.

The early years of the 21st century saw the construction of a new downtown library on the site of the dead mall, Church Street Center. The largely vacant downtown post office became the Frist Center for the Visual Arts. A new Country Music Hall of Fame and the Schermerhorn Symphony Center arrived in SoBro, followed most spectacularly by the Music City Center for conventions.

Less architecturally noteworthy—but equally, if not more, important for the ultimate viability of downtown—has been the growth in residential construction and rehabs. For it is only by returning the central city to a fine-grained mixture of land uses, with enough residents to support the provision of goods and services for daily life, that downtown will become the first among Nashville's neighborhoods.

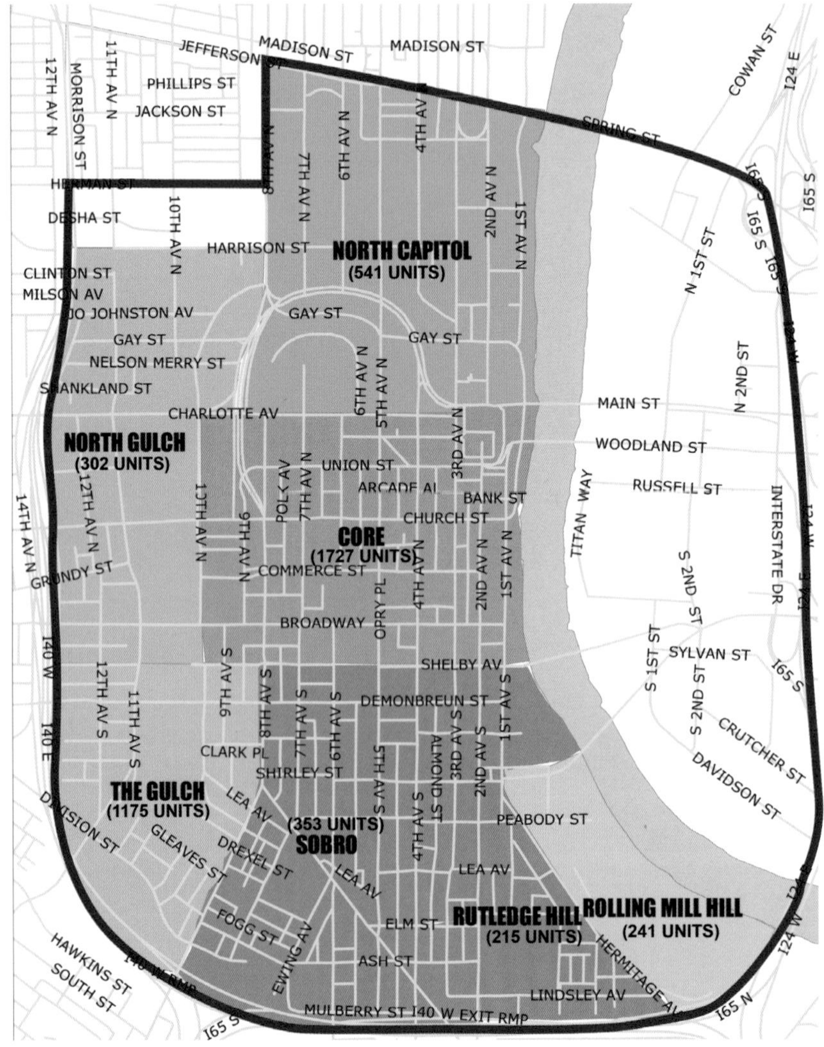

The downtown transect zone's residential population currently dwells in the seven areas within the red outline. These seven districts are delineated by the Nashville Downtown Partnership, which is the source for the number of dwelling units in each. The Partnership also considers Hope Gardens as part of downtown, but this area on the northwest corner of the map lies outside the red line because the neighborhood is defined as part of the urban, rather than downtown, transect zone by Metro's Planning Department.

As if that were not confusing enough, note also that the Partnership's map uses the term "core" for the very center of downtown. Metro's Planning Department defines "core" as interchangeable with "downtown," which is how the term is used throughout this book. *(Map, 2013: Nashville Downtown Partnership)*

DOWNTOWN ZONE BASICS

For planning purposes, the core transect zone exhibits the following characteristics:

- **The most intensely developed of any zone in terms of square footage per acre**
- **A mix of land uses: commercial, office, residential, arts and entertainment venues, local and state government. Individual buildings also often accommodate a mixture of uses, such as residential or office over retail/ restaurant.**
- **Typically high- to mid-rise buildings located within close proximity to one another and often abutting**
- **Mix of modern and historic buildings**
- **The hub of public transportation within the county**
- **A tight network of gridded streets, including sidewalks and crosswalks, to accommodate automobile, pedestrian, and bicycle travel**
- **On-street parking**
- **Formal landscaping, urban street trees, public plazas and small parks, and pedestrian-scaled street lighting**
- **High pedestrian connectivity[4]**

The downtown transect zone covers 1,581 acres[5] housing 7,046 residents in 4,402 dwelling units,[6] a density of 4.45 residents per acre. The approximately 475 acres of the East Bank, which are part of the downtown zone but today contain no residential properties, are included in the average density calculation, diluting the downtown density average by 30 percent.

Even allowing for this dilution, downtown's average residential density is comparable to that in the urban zone, despite the fact that the urban zone features less intense development in square footage per acre than downtown.

Nashville also has a low ratio of downtown residents to overall population. According to a 2012 report commissioned by the Metro Development and Housing Agency, a downtown needs in residence two percent of its metropolitan region's total population to support the goods and services necessary for daily life. As of 2012, however, only 0.4 percent of the population in Nashville's 14-county metropolitan statistical area (MSA) lived downtown.[7] For downtown to reach two percent would require another 18,400 units.[8]

The core's population swells by over 50,000 each day with commuting workers.[9] The public spaces, parks, streets, restaurants, and entertainment venues in the core are not just for downtown's workers and residents, however, but function as resources for residents of the entire region. Downtown is also the hub of Nashville's thriving tourist industry, which in 2013 experienced 12.2 million visitors, with most spending time in the core at some point during their stay.[10]

SHAPING HEALTH IN THE DOWNTOWN TRANSECT ZONE

ANALYSIS AND STRATEGIES

Downtown Nashville has received over $2.1 billion in public and private investment since 2008, a considerable amount given the Great Recession.[11] Several important resources, however, are still missing that are found in the downtown sections of many of Nashville's peer cities, as well as in the urban and suburban transect zones of Nashville itself. Elementary and middle schools, a full-service grocery store, a variety of retail options, and affordable housing units, as well as units that accommodate families, are notably absent in the core. The presence of these amenities would enable downtown residents to walk or bicycle to daily needs and services.

> "The downtown has to be the place where every citizen's heart can sing!"
>
> Joseph P. Riley Jr., Mayor of Charleston, South Carolina, 1975 to 2015

Examples in other cities of amenities that Nashville's downtown lacks *(clockwise from top left)*:

The Riviera 8 cineplex in downtown Knoxville, constructed in 2006. *(2013: Gary Gaston, NCDC)*

School with roof garden in urban Atlanta. *(2011: Perkins+Will)*

Seward Mini Park in San Francisco. *(2013)*

Metreon development south of Market Street in San Francisco features a cineplex, a Target, and a grocery. *(2013)*

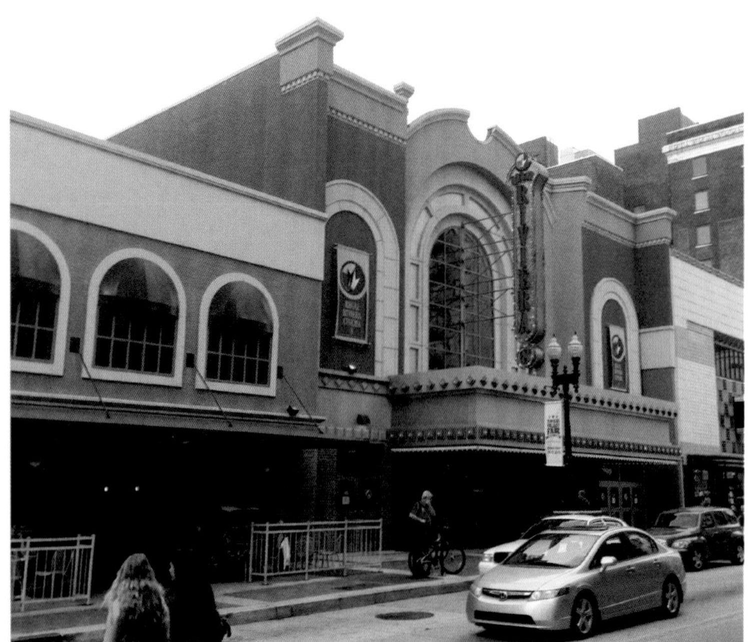

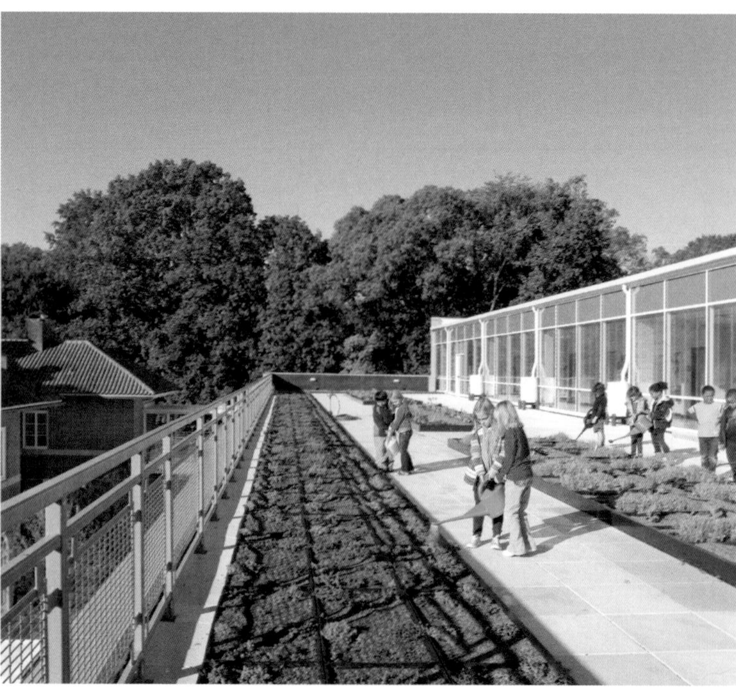

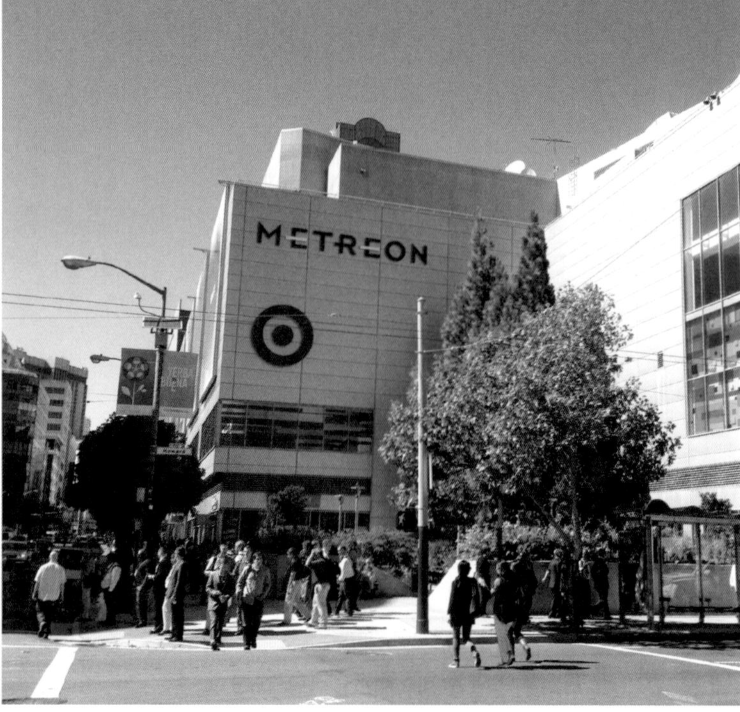

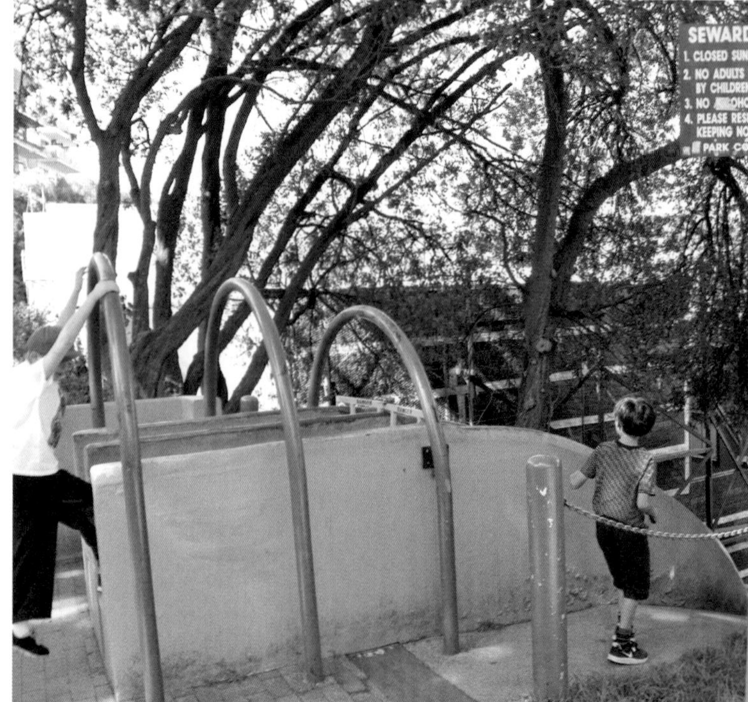

NEIGHBORHOOD DESIGN AND DEVELOPMENT

✓ Health-Promoting

Intense planning and redevelopment in recent years have contributed to the growth of multiple land uses in downtown, expanding from the business-centered philosophy of the urban renewal period. The addition of more social venues—bars, restaurants—and the increase in entertainment and cultural offerings have brought more people to downtown streets, deterring crime and enhancing the pedestrian experience. The development of the core's residential component enables city dwellers to work and play without resorting to cars.

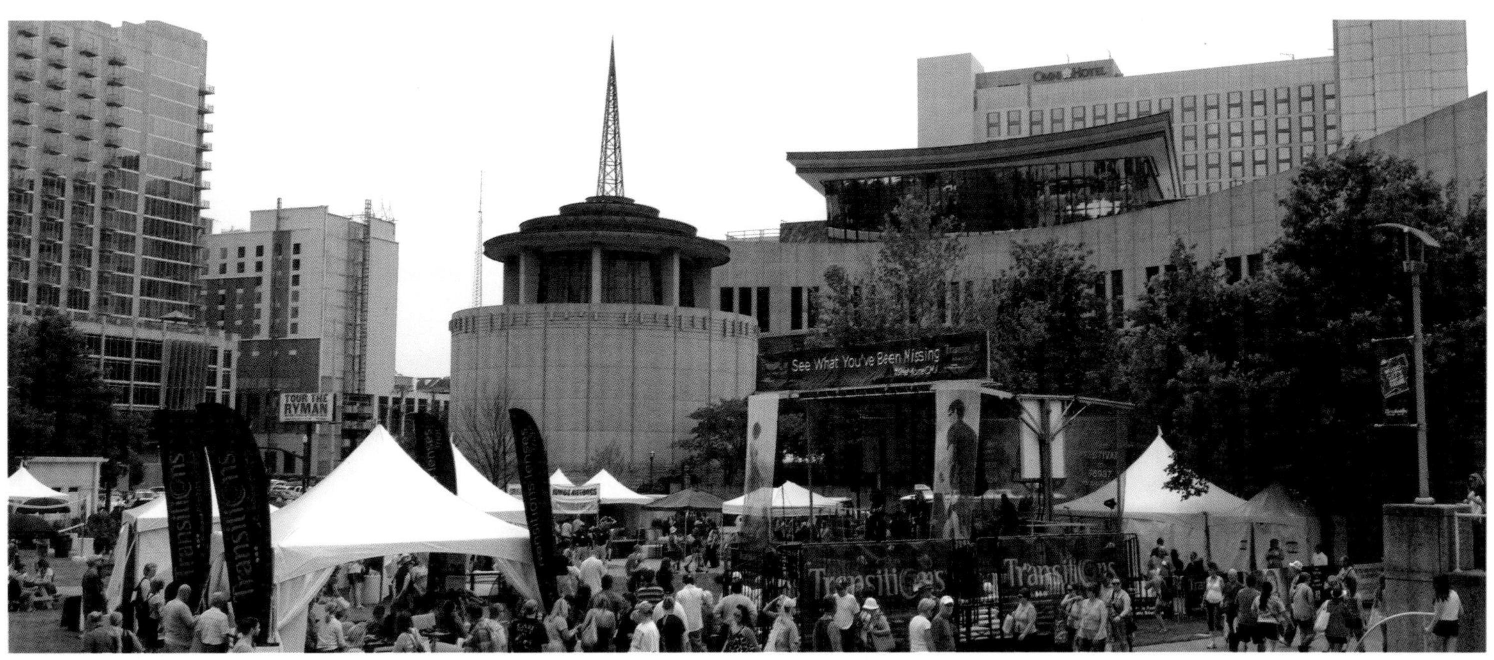

✓ The Country Music Hall of Fame and Museum (background) during the 2013 Country Music Association festival. Relocating the Hall of Fame, designed by Tuck-Hinton Architects, from Music Row to SoBro transformed a drive-to, stand-alone attraction into a walk-to destination integrated with the other amenities of the core. *(2013)*

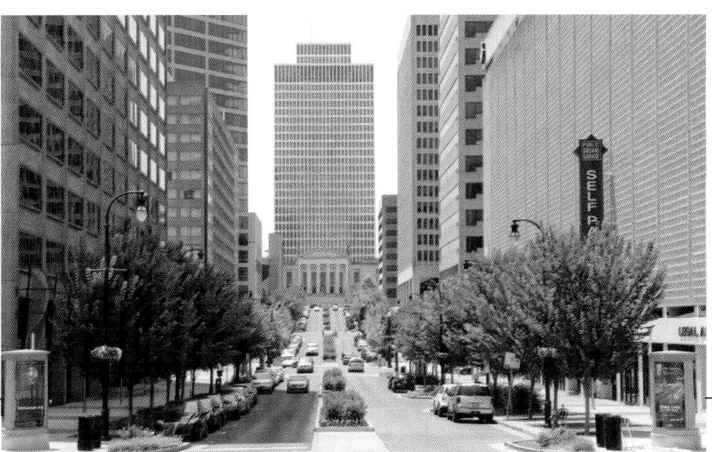

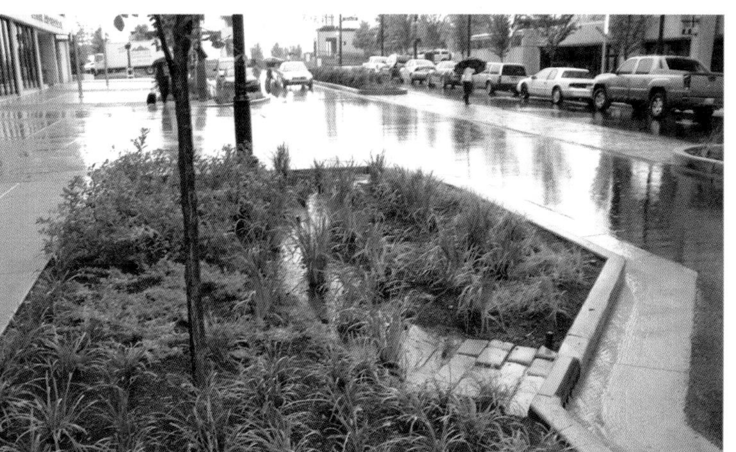

✓ Deaderick Street was the first "green" street in the state.[12] Its design, by Hawkins Partners landscape architects, channels rainwater into bio retention basins that serve as beds for native trees and plants, diverting 1.2 million gallons of water each year from the city's sewer system. *(2012: Gary Layda)*

✗ Health-Defeating

Nashville's core still has many underutilized properties. According to a 2008 study by Metro Planning, 37 percent of downtown property parcels are vacant of buildings; one-story buildings occupy another 25 percent. This leaves only 38 percent of downtown land with buildings of two or more stories.[13] Because the downtown code permits significantly higher densities, there is thus tremendous opportunity for redevelopment. Such redevelopment would build on existing infrastructure and enable the more efficient supply of services, as well as help to achieve the population density necessary for a wider variety of retail.

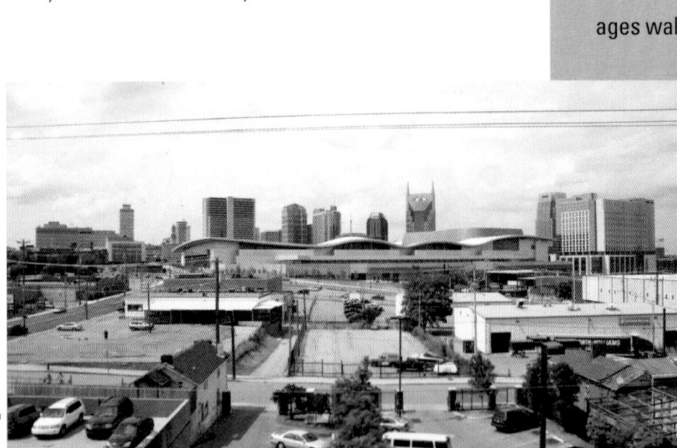

✗ View from SoBro toward Nashville's Central Business District reveals the many surface parking lots and aging one-story buildings still existing within the core. Note also the overhead power lines, which limit the ability to plant street trees and whose poles clutter sidewalks, hindering pedestrians. *(2013)*

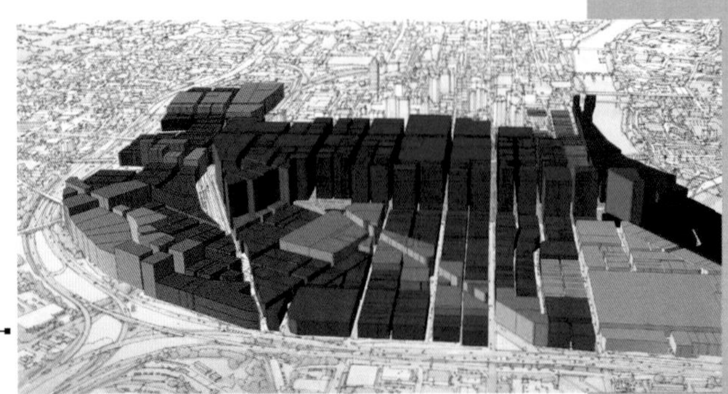

✓ Similar view showing the downtown code's permitted building heights. *(Illustration, 2013: South of Broadway Strategic Master Plan, Urban Design Associates)*

The Downtown Code: A Form-Based Zoning Code

After years of complicated rezonings and variances, Metro Council unanimously approved a customized zoning code for the core of Nashville in 2010. Before the adoption of The Downtown Code (DTC), building heights for much of downtown were capped at five stories; residential uses were prohibited in some locations; and the community had no certainty about the type, form, and character of new buildings. These outdated regulations were holdovers from a time when downtown was relegated to daytime office uses, river- and rail-oriented industrial uses, and adult businesses. The DTC allows greater development rights and a variety of uses appropriate to a city center, while requiring quality urban design.

The DTC creates a built environment that encourages walking as a primary mode of transportation in downtown. Streets are the most plentiful open space in downtown and, as such, the pedestrian experience is prioritized while appropriately accommodating vehicular traffic.

In an urban environment, the street-level design of buildings is of the utmost importance. The activities on the ground floor should enliven the street, making it comfortable, safe, and interesting for pedestrians. DTC standards are based on frontage design—storefront, stoop, porch, industrial, and civic—and address glazing, vehicular access, landscaping, and active uses on the ground level. As residents, workers, or visitors in downtown walk down a wide sidewalk, shaded by street trees, they can window shop, watch passersby, and be enticed to see what is on the next block or around the next corner. Correctly designed, these attributes contribute to safe and interesting streets that result in vibrant neighborhoods and a strong downtown.

In some areas of downtown, open space is appropriately scaled and designed for the envisioned intensity of the neighborhood. Church Street Park, for instance, is a small park, perfect for daily workers to enjoy lunch, or for kids and parents to watch a puppet show. It is also easily accessible to many people who live and work in the nearby buildings. In most areas, however, open space is dramatically lacking. Nearly 2,000 people live in the Gulch, yet there is no public open space for activities or leisure. The DTC identifies quarter-mile radius neighborhoods (about a five-minute walk from edge to center) to show open space deficiencies. To create a desirable, healthy neighborhood, there should be at least a quarter acre of well-designed public open space. The DTC provides standards for the public or private creation of a variety of open spaces: greens, squares, plazas, courts, and pocket parks/playgrounds. The open spaces standards create places for recreation, relaxation, and reflection: much-needed aspects of city life.

By location alone, urban infill creates an environment more conducive to healthy living. By emphasizing mixed-use, walkable neighborhoods within downtown, the DTC ensures that all new development moves toward the goal of a healthy, vibrant, and sustainable downtown.

—JONI PRIEST, Hastings Architecture, former member of the Metro Planning Department

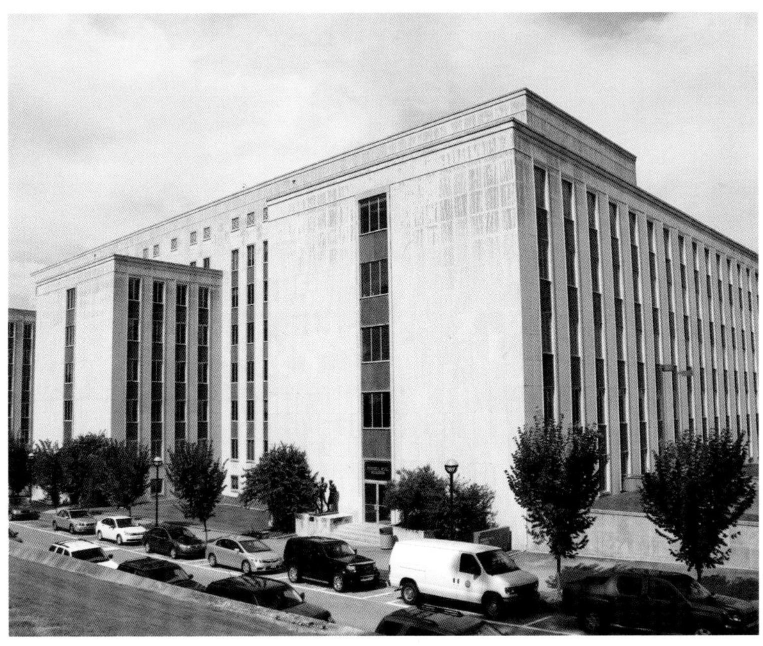

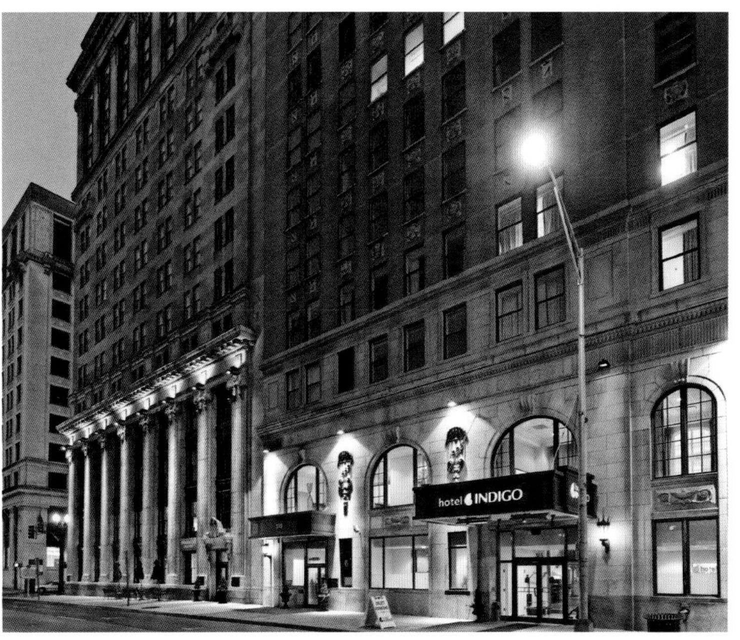

Left: The 1952 Cordell Hull building (shown here) and the former Ben West public library of 1962, both significant mid-century modern structures in downtown, were threatened with demolition in 2013. The buildings were eventually saved after protests by preservationists. That same year the Federal Reserve Bank building (1958) was sold to a private developer for conversion to high-end apartments. *(2013)*

Right: The American Trust (left) and National Trust (right) buildings, both of 1926, are part of Nashville's National Register Financial Historic District and relics of the time when Union Street was called the "Wall Street of the South." In 2010 the structures were renovated into a 97-room boutique hotel. Historic tax credits were a valuable tool for the developer in making the project economically feasible. *(2012: Lineberry Properties)*

STRATEGY: *Make downtown a complete neighborhood.*

STRATEGY: *Promote the renovation and retrofitting of historic structures and the rehab of vacant upper floors in existing structures. A study by the National Trust for Historic Preservation found that reusing rather than demolishing buildings almost always results in lower environmental impacts. In addition, cost savings from reuse are between 4 to 46 percent greater than new construction when comparing buildings of similar energy use.*[14]

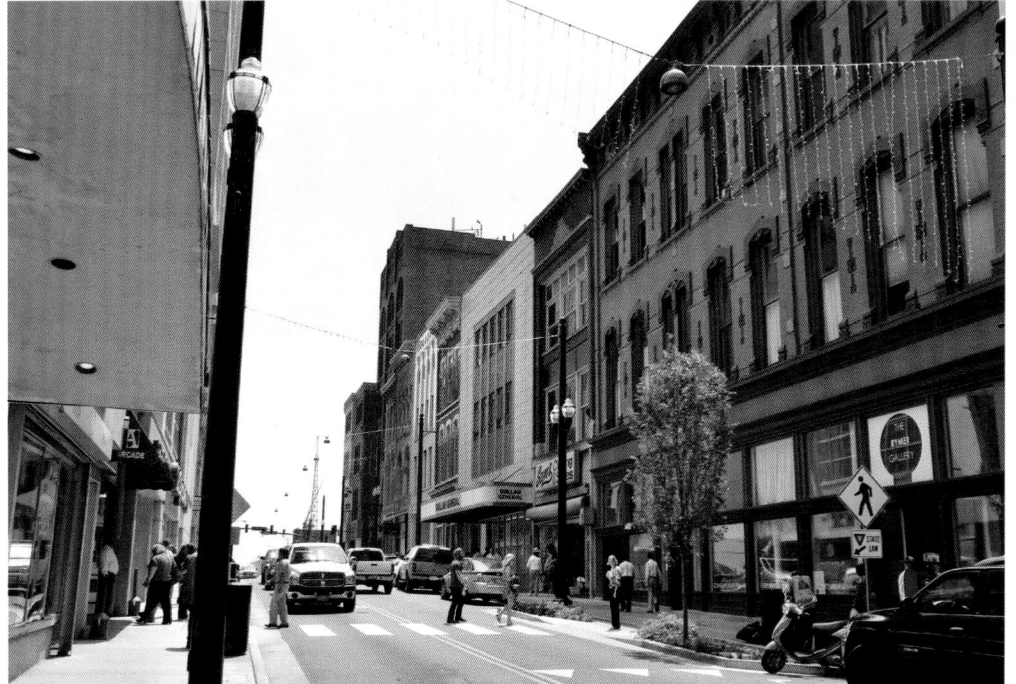

Fifth Avenue North features several buildings whose upper floors have been renovated for residential lofts, but vacant space remains. *(2013)*

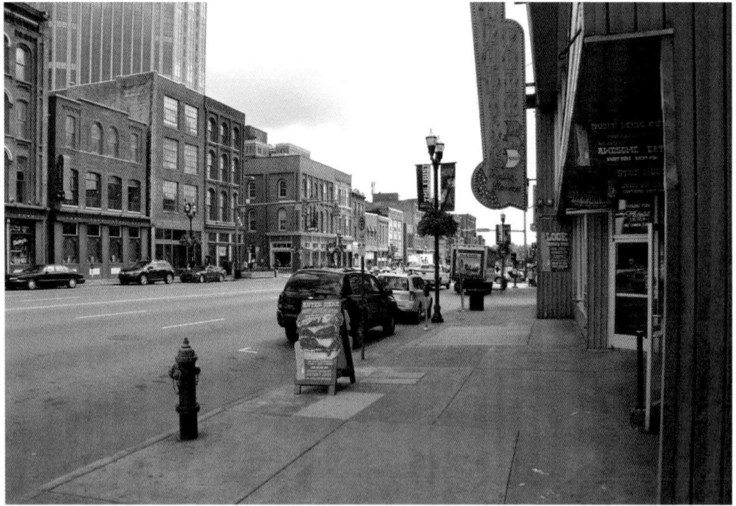

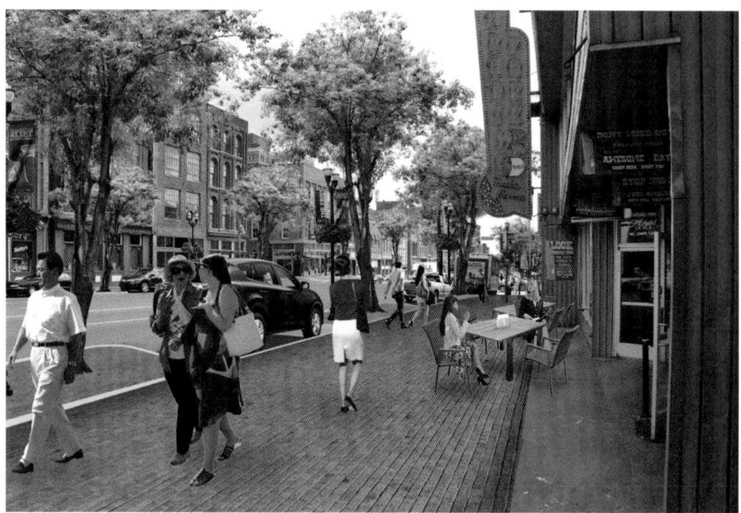

A redesigned Broadway should incorporate wider sidewalks, street trees, and benches. The redesign would create a more pleasant experience for pedestrians, including those walking to the downtown circulator bus, as well as open up space for outdoor cafes. A landscaped median would make the street crossing safer and less difficult. *(Visualizations, 2013: Eric Hoke, NCDC)*

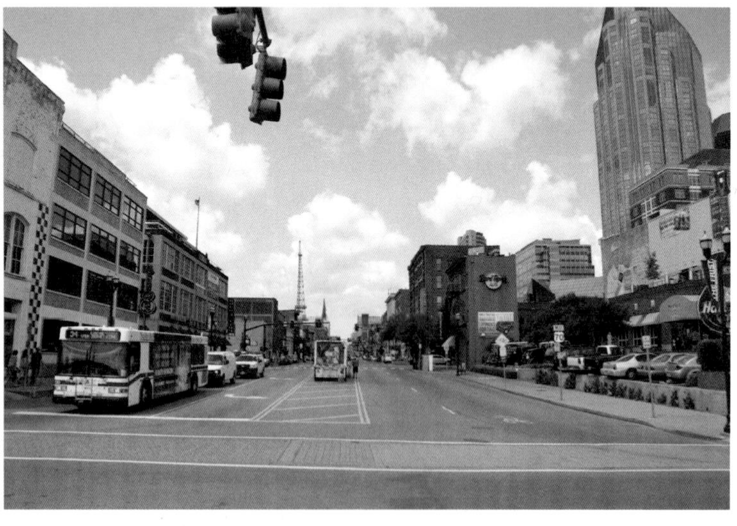

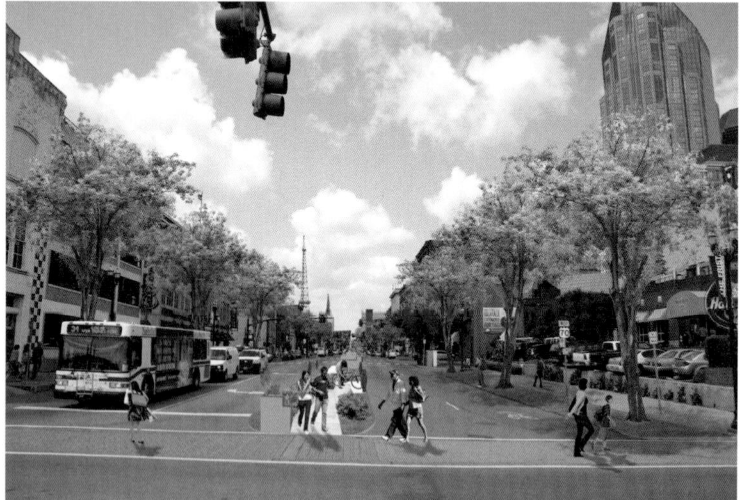

STRATEGY: *Redesign Broadway and Commerce Street as complete streets to balance the demands of cars, pedestrians, and cyclists. Lower Broadway is the busiest street in downtown Nashville for both pedestrian and vehicular traffic. The street's width (more than 100 feet) and six travel lanes, however, make pedestrian crossings challenging. The sidewalks are only eight feet wide.*

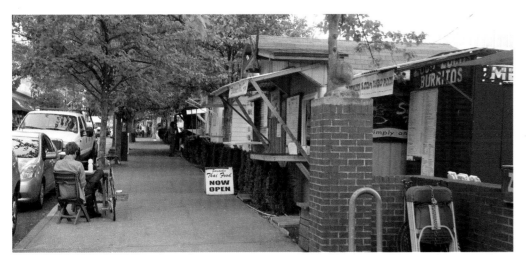

STRATEGY: *Encourage redevelopment of surface parking to create active street uses and increase pedestrian interest and safety. Incentives used in other cities include property tax abatement and tax increment financing (TIF) for redevelopment, as well as increasing property taxes on surface lots to reduce the incentive for demolition of buildings for parking lots. (Currently property owners can decrease the property taxes on underperforming buildings by removing them.)*

Food carts in Portland, Oregon, have become a fixture of downtown, where they line the edges of surface parking lots. Offering an interim use prior to redevelopment, the carts increase pedestrian interest, add variety to food options, and visually shield surface lots. The property owners retain parking revenues while adding the rent from carts, and the city receives the sales tax. *(2010)*

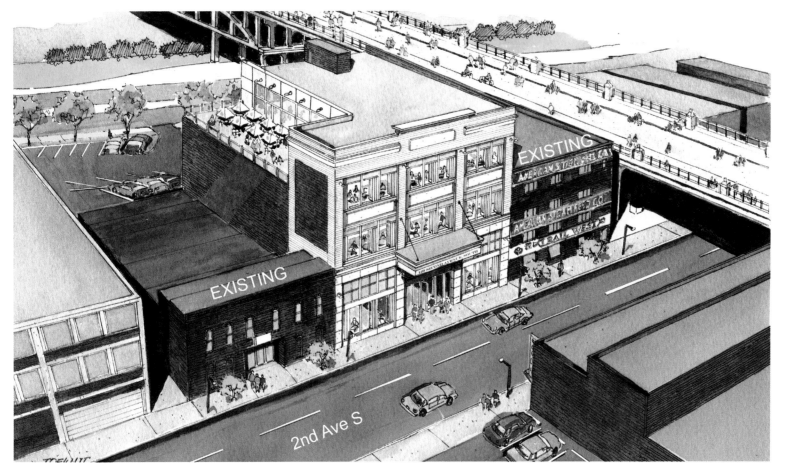

Proposal for a building on an existing 27-space surface parking lot. The new building, which has grown to six stories, will offer active street level uses, restaurant and entertainment venues, a boutique hotel, and a rooftop terrace overlooking the Cumberland River and Shelby Street Pedestrian Bridge. *(Illustration, 2014: Frank May and Mark Robin)*

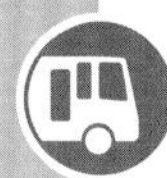

Clockwise from top right:

Passengers from a city bus wait to board the Music City Star commuter rail line at Riverfront Station, located at the foot of Broadway. *(2013)*

The Music City Central bus terminal is the hub of all public transit in the county. More than 20,000 of the system's average of 32,250 daily riders pass through the Center.[15] *(2014)*

Note the green Music City Circuit bus. This free circulator service operates three routes through downtown linking the central city with the Gulch, Nashville Farmers' Market, and the Fulton Metro office campus on Rutledge Hill. The circuit's fleet includes hybrids as well as electric buses; the latter are the result of a $3 million federal grant. *(2015)*

Cyclists are becoming an ever-increasing sight in downtown. *(2013)*

Solar-powered electric car charging facility located on the East Bank. *(2013)*

TRANSPORTATION

Health-Promoting

A wide array of transportation options are available in the core: walking, biking, public transit, taxis, and personal vehicles.

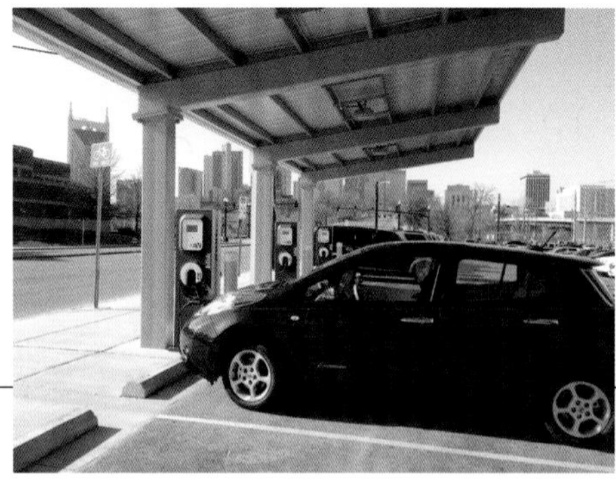

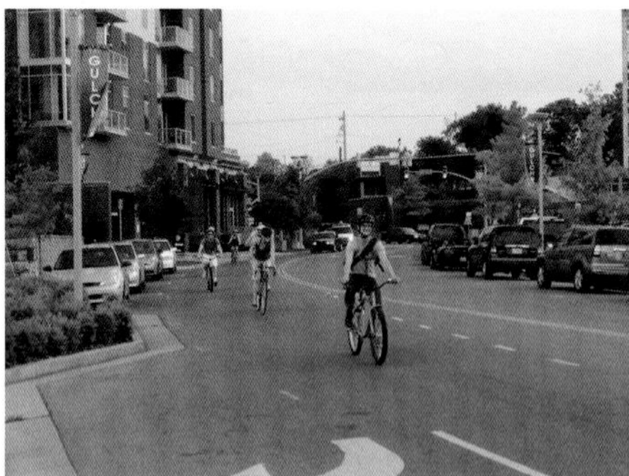

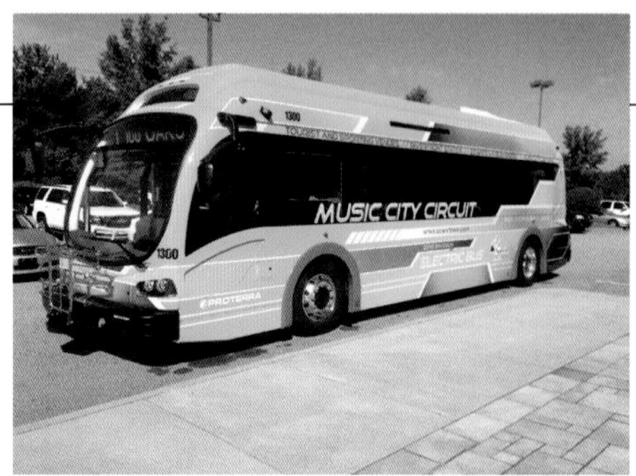

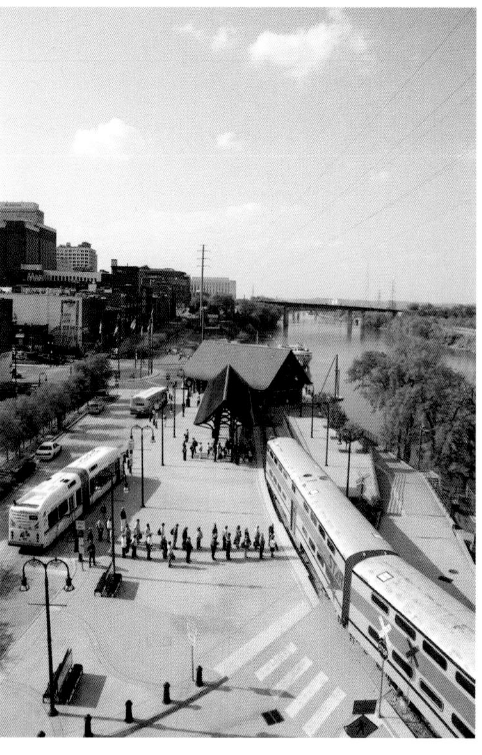

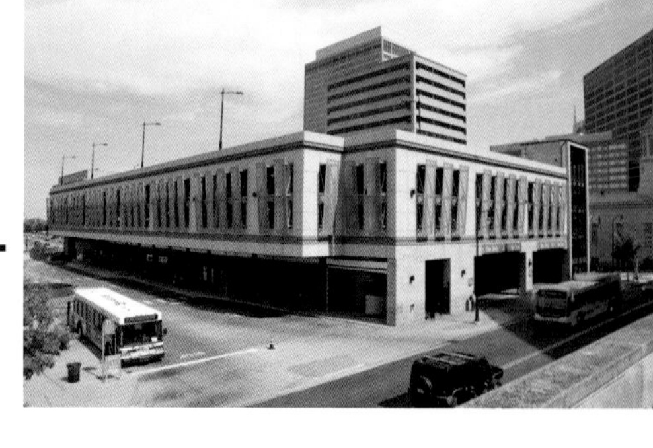

Health-Defeating

While none of the top 20 most congested intersections in Davidson County are in the core transect zone, congestion is nevertheless significant on the streets feeding the interstates during rush hours and throughout downtown on busy event days. Only two percent of Davidson County's citizens use public transportation.[16] Low frequency of buses and limited hours of service for public transit routes limit widespread transit use among the population.

Under the current 2013 plan, the pedestrian/cycling bridge intended to connect the Gulch to SoBro lacks a bicycle ramp, requiring cyclists to dismount and roll their bikes up to the bridge deck using a bicycle groove; those in wheelchairs must use the elevator. This is due to the steepness of the approach and the inability of bridge planners to obtain easements from private property owners.

STRATEGY: *Promote transit ridership through greater frequency of buses and longer hours of service. This strategy will require more funding for Nashville MTA.*

STRATEGY: *Implement a network of protected bike lanes throughout downtown that offer safer alternatives to the current lanes shared by bikes and cars. The network should include clearly defined north/south, east/west routes.*

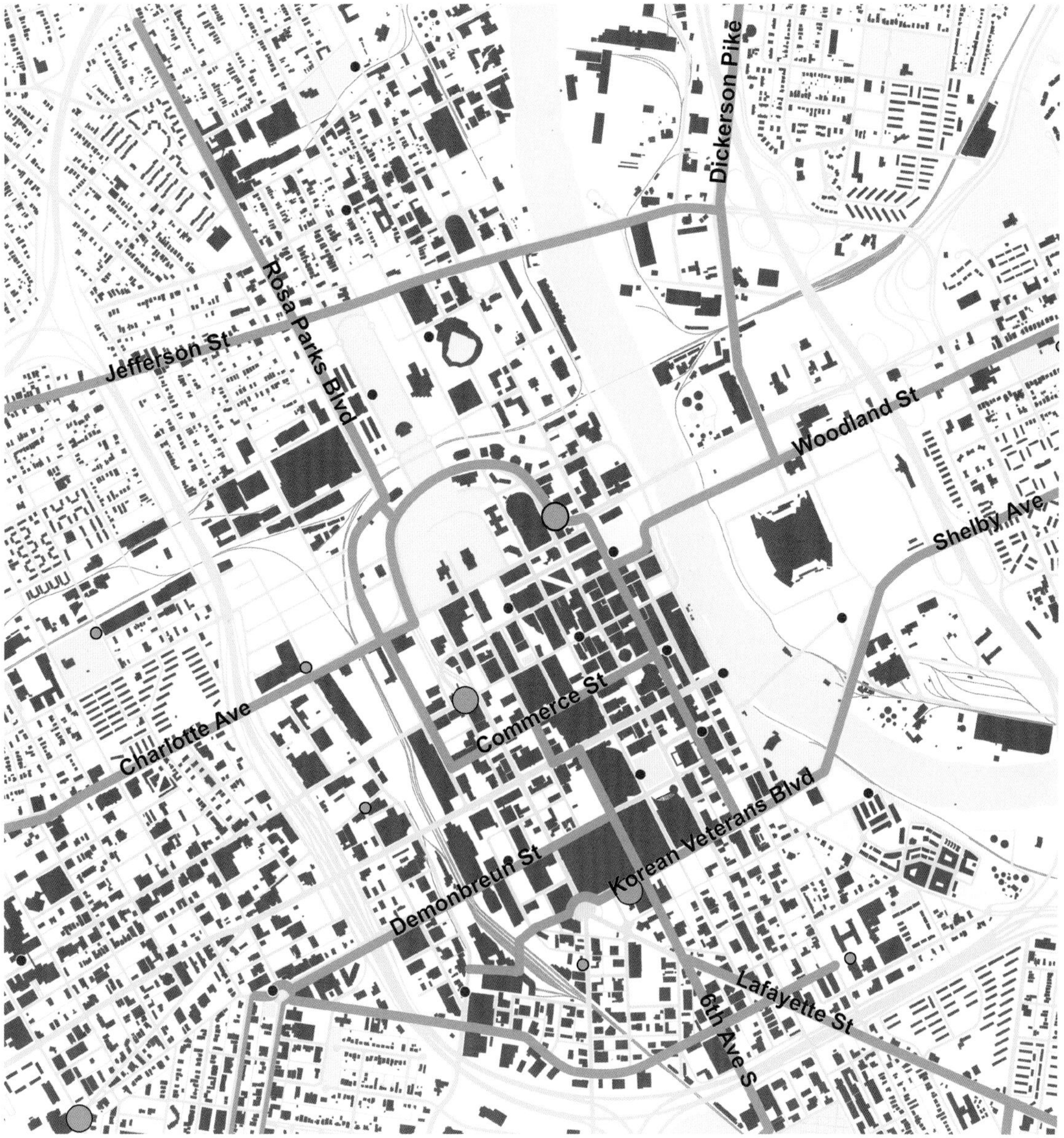

Map of potential protected bike lane network for downtown and beyond the interstate loop. Note that the main east/west route through the central city is on Commerce Street. Downtown currently has some dedicated bike lanes, but none protected by bollards or buffers.

The large blue dots indicate possible locations for bike stations, with showers, changing rooms, and bike storage; small red dots indicate existing B-cycle kiosks, and small blue dots, proposed kiosks. *(Diagram over map, 2014: Ron Yearwood, NCDC)*

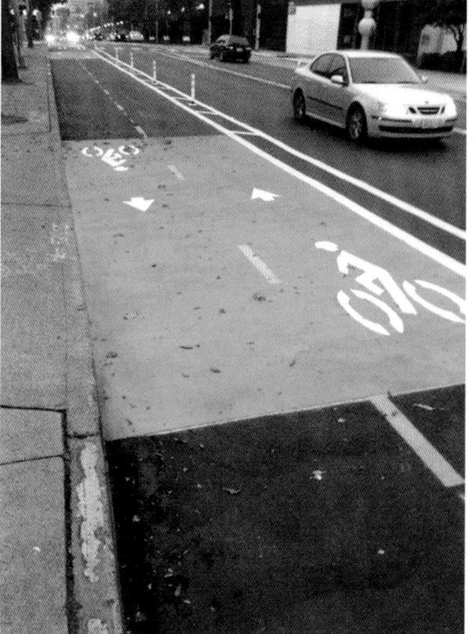

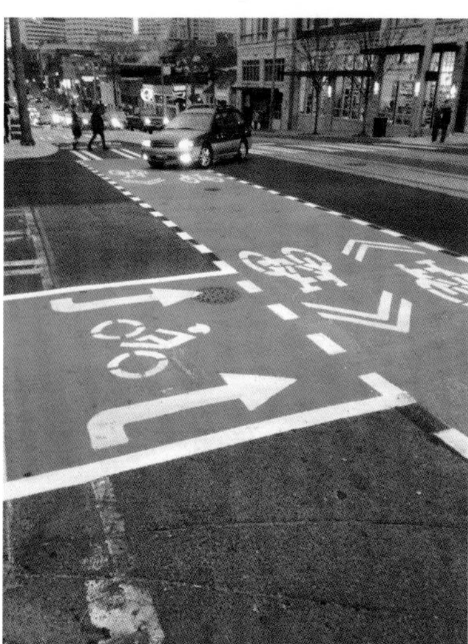

Examples of protected bike lane and crosswalk infrastructure in Seattle, Washington. *(2013: Gary Gaston, NCDC)*

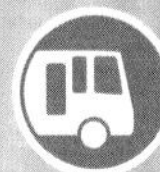

Getting Around Downtown

Over the past 15 years, Nashville's government officials and development community have given considerable focus to strengthening and reenergizing the city's urban core. Through this focus, downtown Nashville has emerged as a popular location to live, work, and play.

The Middle Tennessee region is expected to add more than one million residents over the next two decades. To address the future transportation demands resulting from this expected growth, Metro Nashville recently initiated the "Multimodal Mobility Study." This study will identify a comprehensive and sustainable approach for providing access to, and movement around, Nashville for workers, visitors, and residents.

These newcomers will require access to and from downtown, which will be the study's focus. The goal is to present comprehensive strategies for achieving an optimum balance of transit service, land-use mixture, bicycling, walking, and automobile circulation and parking.

Today, the private automobile reigns as the dominant transportation mode for travel into and out of the core. Recent surveys by the Nashville Downtown Partnership show that 81 percent of downtown commuters drive alone to work, while 8 percent carpool or vanpool. Only seven percent of downtown workers take public transit, one of the lowest ridership levels among the most populous 50 US cities. As Nashville has grown, so has traffic congestion, which has nearly doubled over the past three decades, in large part due to the prevalence of automobile use. Recent traffic counts show that about 140,000 vehicles enter downtown Nashville on a typical weekday. Comparing these volumes to the capacities of the routes into and out of downtown indicates that the core's streets are reaching their practical capacity for accommodating more cars.

To ensure access for the future and accommodate significant downtown growth, Nashville needs to shift from its reliance on the single-occupancy vehicle to a much more robust and comprehensive multimodal transportation system. Public transit is a key component in a multimodal system. In terms of transit service, however, Nashville is behind other peer cities. But recent efforts to improve local bus service and provide more express routes between downtown and the suburbs, as well as the addition of free downtown circulator routes and the emphasis on Bus Rapid Transit (BRT) have Nashville heading in the right direction. Because of its potential to move high numbers of passengers quickly and efficiently, expansion of Nashville's nascent BRT system by implementing dedicated-lane BRT appears to be an especially promising option.

The need for a more walkable downtown is also vital, especially in developing areas such as SoBro, the Gulch, North Gulch, and Germantown where sidewalk infrastructure is not as complete as in the Central Business District (CBD). Just as critical, barriers such as the I-40/I-65/I-24 inner loop need special attention so that safe and convenient connections can be established between the CBD and those neighborhoods that are outside the inner loop but within walking and bicycling distance. Examples of such connections could include repurposing or narrowing travel lanes to provide bike lanes and/or wider sidewalks on existing bridges as well as adding pedestrian-only bridges, such as that proposed for the Woodland Street Bridge in the 2012 Riverfront Master Plan.

Enhancing bicycle access to and around downtown will increase travel options for commuters as well as for downtown residents, employees, and visitors. Currently the bicycle mode share for commuters to downtown Nashville is minimal, approximately one percent. Other US cities such as Minneapolis and Portland have bicycle mode splits ranging from four percent to over six percent, while in European cities like Amsterdam, bike travel exceeds 25 percent.

It is certainly feasible for Nashville to achieve a much higher bicycle ridership. Cities around the world with high bike usage typically have easy connections with transit so that the bike-to-transit-to-bike trip chain works seamlessly. Nashville's buses already have bike racks and the planned BRT systems will also accommodate bikes. Nashville's new bikeshare program allows people to bicycle for short trips within the downtown area and also enhances the trip chain concept. What Nashville needs to focus on is additional bicycling infrastructure, such as dedicated bike lanes protected by curbs or bollards and bicycle-specific traffic signals, so that cycling can truly become a safe, convenient, and efficient travel mode for travel to and around downtown.

Finally, a comprehensive evaluation of innovative parking strategies will be important for downtown Nashville's future. Although additional parking downtown is likely, reducing future demand for parking spaces will be necessary for the downtown area to continue to grow effectively. Options include shared parking, variable pricing by time of day to encourage turnover of on-street spaces, optimal utilization of off-street spaces, and web-based applications that identify open spaces with rates and allow parkers to pay by cellphone. These and other "smart parking" strategies should be utilized to achieve a more effective parking system downtown.

—BOB MURPHY, president, RPM Transportation Consultants and principal-in-charge for the Metro Multimodal Mobility Study

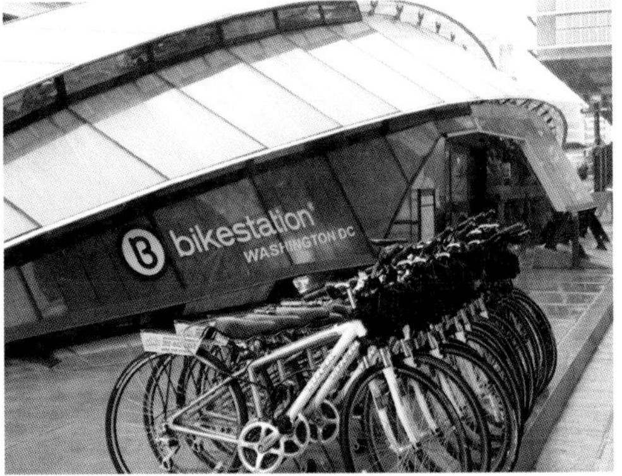

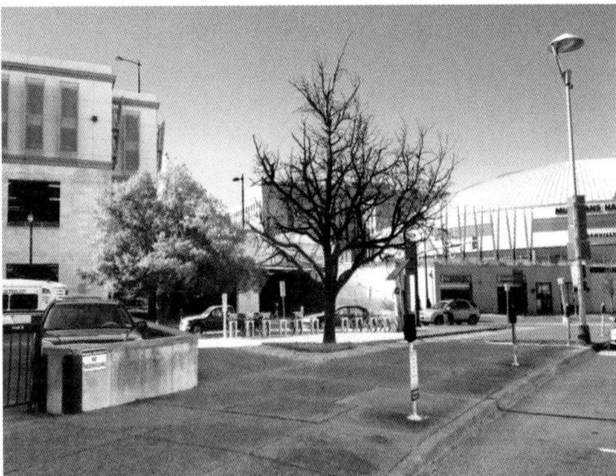

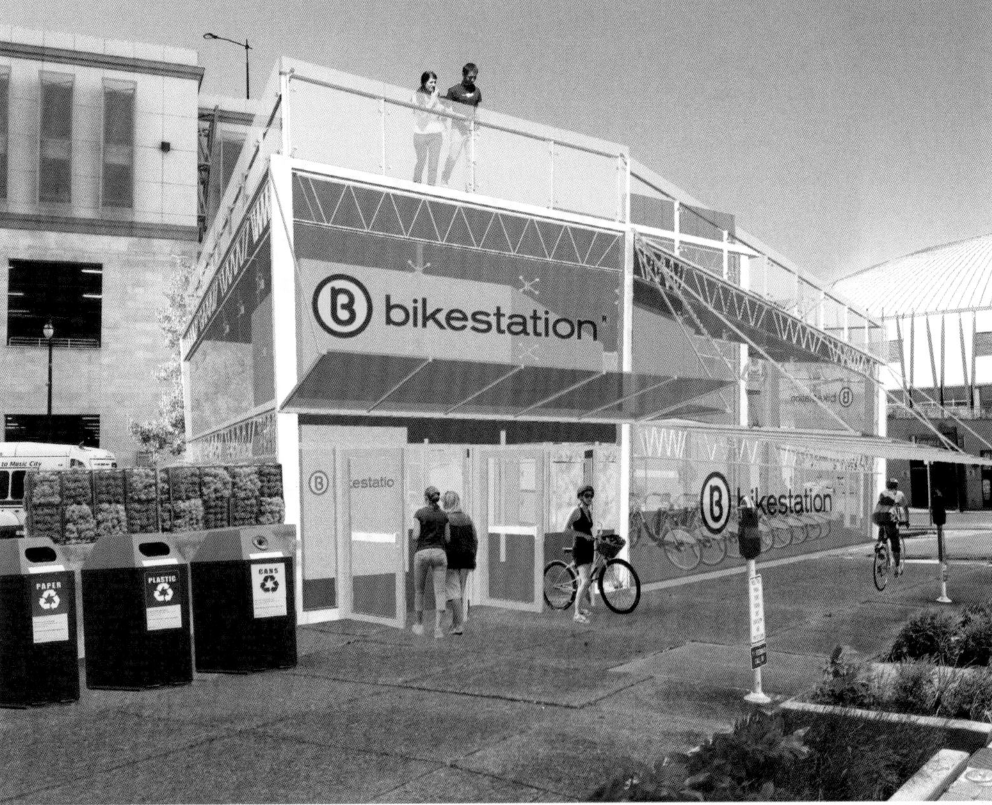

STRATEGY: *Develop a bike center near the Music City Central bus terminal. The center should provide cyclists with secure storage and accommodate commuters with lockers and showers.*

STRATEGY: *Connect the isolated segments of downtown's greenways, particularly the section in the Gulch, to the larger greenway system and attractions such as the Farmers' Market and the Music City Center.*

Bike Sharing

Metro launched B-cycle in December 2012 as a fee-based bike share program with 195 touring bikes. The shiny red bicycles have adjustable seats and are equipped with front and rear lights, a bell, and a shopping basket. The vehicles are available at 31 automated kiosks within a three-mile radius of the core, with 14 kiosks in downtown proper.

The idea behind the program is to make it easy for people to take quick trips without the hassles of parking. A downtown worker, for example, can bike to the YMCA or the library, or to lunch at Five Points, Germantown, or the Farmers' Market

A variety of memberships are available for purchase from one day to annual. Each trip is free for members as long as the bike is returned to any station within an hour; for checkouts beyond an hour, your credit card is charged in half-hour increments of $1.50 each. Annual members can log into B-cycle's web site to see estimates of the number of calories they burned and the amount of carbon emissions they avoided by not taking the trip by car. In its first year of operation, over 23,000 memberships were purchased, accounting for more than 47,000 rides. "It has exceeded our expectations by far," says Keith Rawls, general manager of the Nashville Downtown Partnership that operates B-cycle.

Biking is clean, green transportation that is also good exercise. More than $20 million has been invested in Nashville on bike lanes, bikeways, and greenways during the past six years. These efforts earned Nashville a bronze designation from the League of American Bicyclists for Bicycle Friendly Cities in October 2012.

—AMY ESKIND, NCDC

Left: The Bikestation in Washington, DC, located adjacent to the multimodal transit hub of Union Station, houses over 100 bicycles and is staffed 66 hours per week. Secure bike parking is available to members 24/7. The facility provides a private changing room, day-use lockers for rent, bike rentals, repairs, and retail sales. *(2010: Brian Phelps and Chris Whitis)*

Right: Potential location for a downtown bike center on an unused triangular lot adjacent to Nashville's central bus hub. *(2014)*

A new bike center should provide lockers and showers so that morning commuters can change before continuing to work. Adjacency to transit would allow riders to rent cycles and then continue to destinations throughout downtown. *(Visualization, 2014: Eric Hoke, NCDC)*

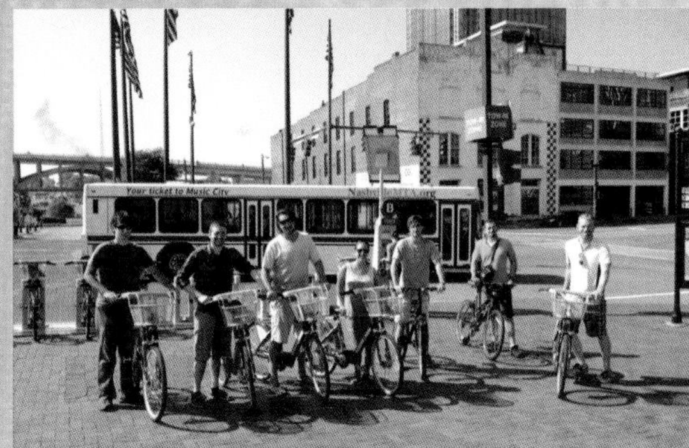

Above: NCDC staff departing from the Broadway B-cycle kiosk on a tour of downtown with summer interns and University of Tennessee College of Architecture and Design students. Additional kiosks should be added to the North Gulch and the area south of the Music City Center as they redevelop. *(2013)*

WALKABILITY & PEDESTRIAN SAFETY

✓ Frequently visited locations in downtown with the 5-minute-walk radius for each.

a. Farmers' Market and Bicentennial Mall
b. Public Square
c. Music City Center
d. The Gulch
e. Metro Government's Fulton campus

(Diagram over map, 2013: Eric Hoke, NCDC)

✓ Health-Promoting

The core is compact and walkable. Pedestrian signage maps were introduced on many downtown corners in 2012 to help visitors navigate to prime destinations.

Efforts are being made to provide better pedestrian access to the Gulch. For example, Gulch Crossing, an office/retail project planned for the former railroad corridor, will have a stairway and elevator connecting the Demonbreun viaduct to 11th Avenue.

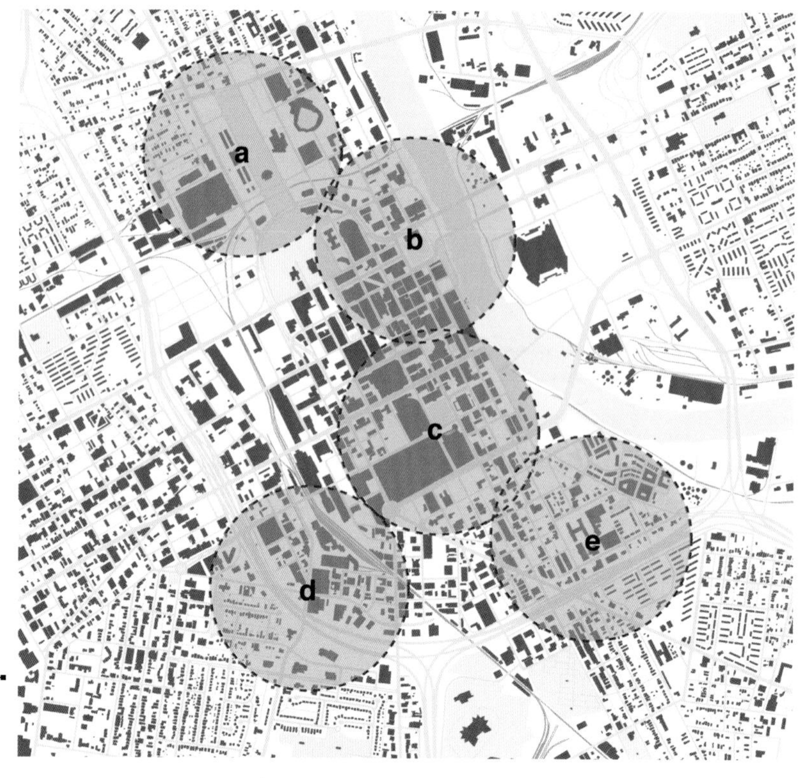

X Sidewalk conditions along Fifth Avenue North in the Sulfur Dell area do little to encourage pedestrian activity. *(2013)*

X In 2013, this intersection of Rosa Parks Boulevard and Church Street was the scene of the death of a 17-year-old junior at nearby Hume-Fogg High School. She was struck by a truck while crossing the street. The police spokesperson said, "Failure to yield to a pedestrian in a crosswalk was a contributing factor to the accident." This intersection is one of the few in the core forbidding right-on-red vehicular turning. *(2013)*

X Health-Defeating

Fragmentary sidewalk networks, high speed limits, and crossing signals geared to moving vehicles—as well as areas with poor street lighting—impede walkability and safety.

Drivers who ignore pedestrian prioity within crosswalks and during right-on-red vehicular turning compromise the safety of walkers at intersections.

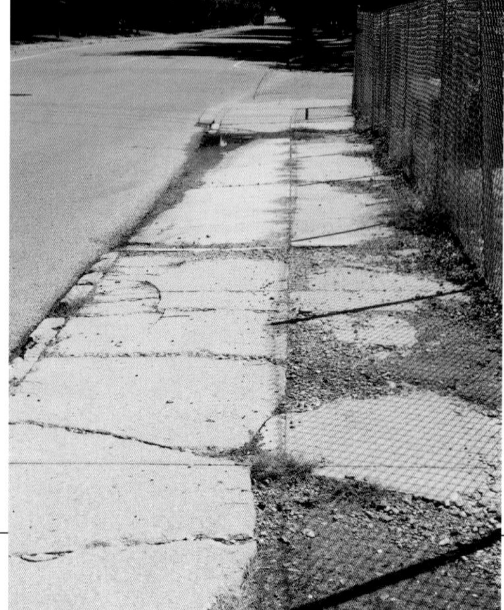

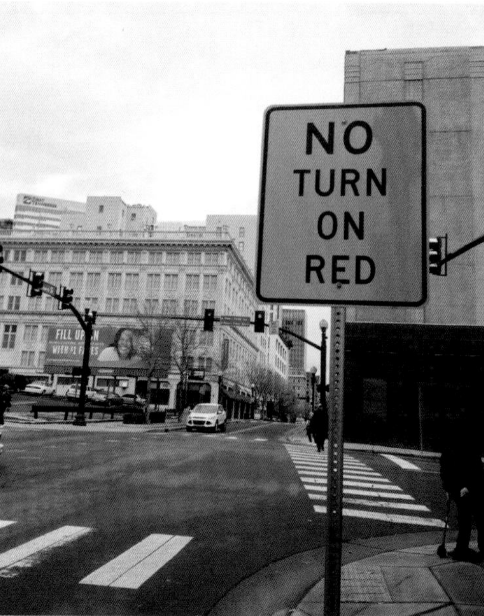

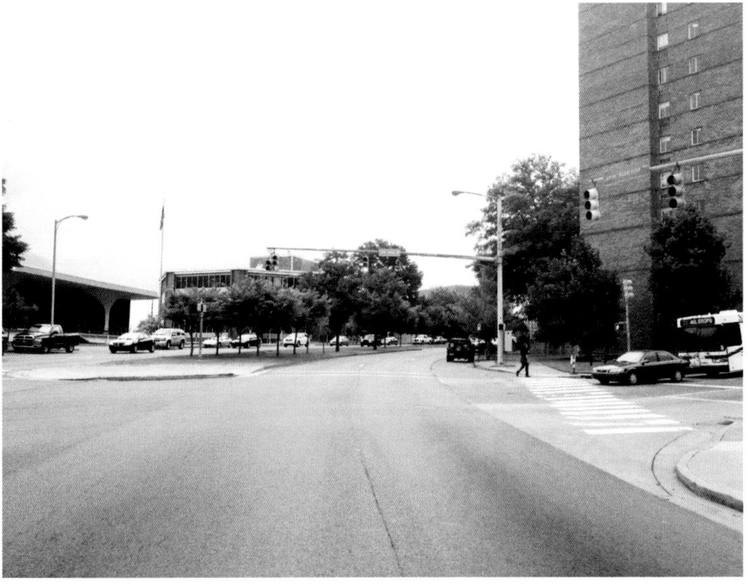

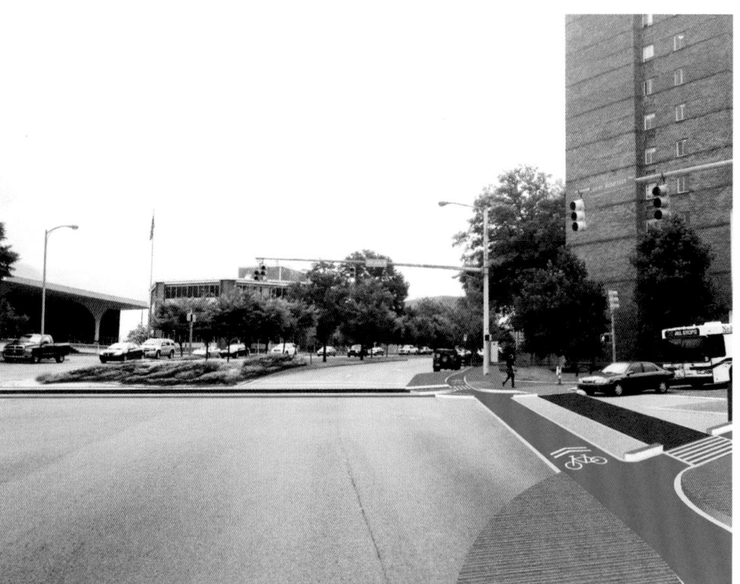

X A pedestrian crossing James Robertson Parkway, where cars are permitted to travel at 40 mph. According to AAA, a pedestrian struck by a vehicle moving at 40 mph has a 79 percent chance of sustaining a severe injury and a 45 percent chance of death. On the other hand, 35 percent of pedestrians struck by a vehicle moving at 25 mph will sustain severe injury and only 12 percent will die.[17] *(2013)*

James Robertson Parkway with protected bike lane and sidewalk curb extensions that work with the existing median to reduce the distance walkers must travel when crossing such a wide street. *(Visualization, 2014: Eric Hoke, NCDC)*

STRATEGY: *Reduce speed limits in downtown to 25 mph and shrink vehicular rights-of-way by installing pedestrian curb extensions and refuge islands/medians.*

STRATEGY: *Give street crossing priority to pedestrians. Time signals for walkers and eliminate right-on-red turns at intersections heavily used by pedestrians. Establish these by pedestrian counts similar to those now used for measuring vehicular traffic.*

STRATEGY: *Develop pedestrian- and bicycle-only events that close certain streets to automobile traffic for special events or during low traffic times, such as Sundays.*

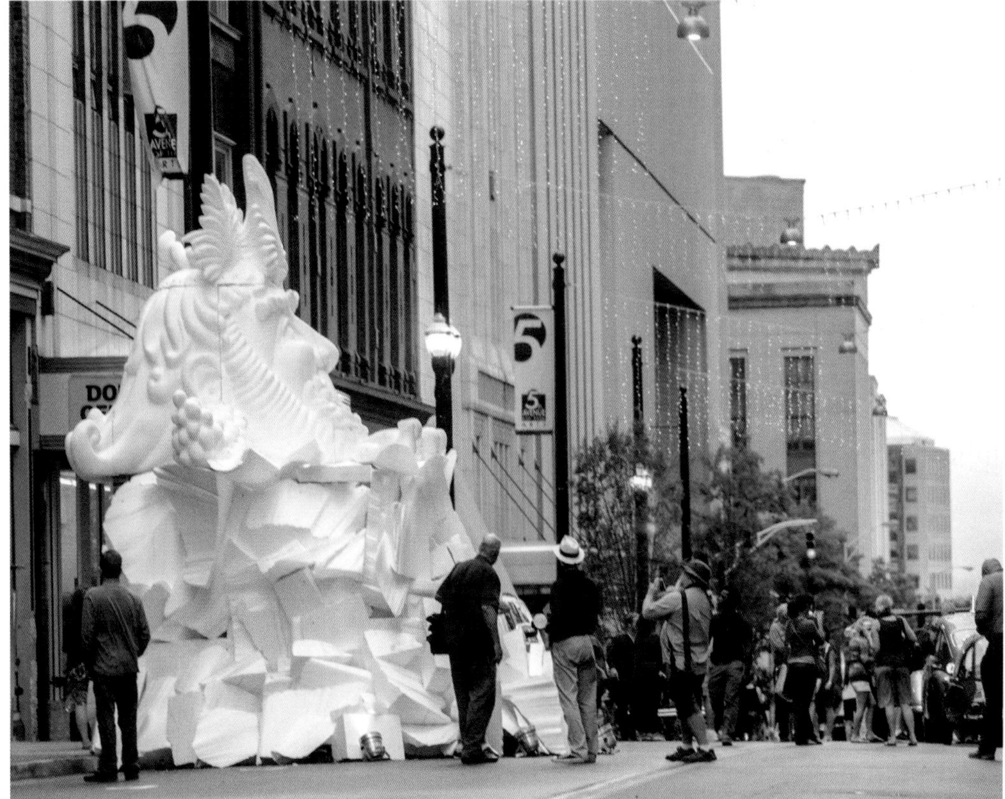

Nashville's "Art Crawl" on the first Saturday of each month draws thousands to downtown galleries. Most of the pedestrian activity happens on Fifth Avenue North, which is closed to cars for the event. *(2013: Metro Nashville)*

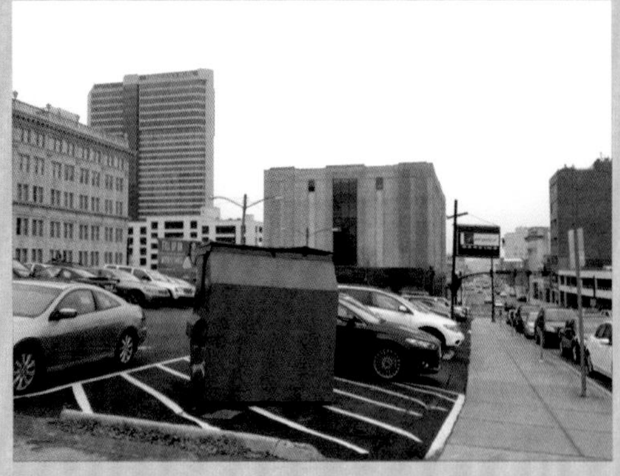

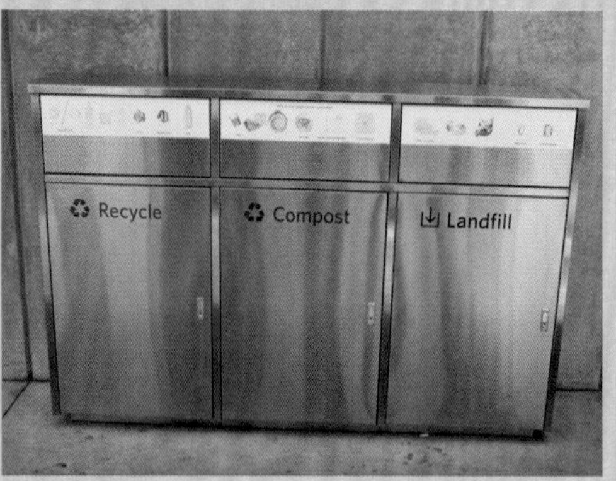

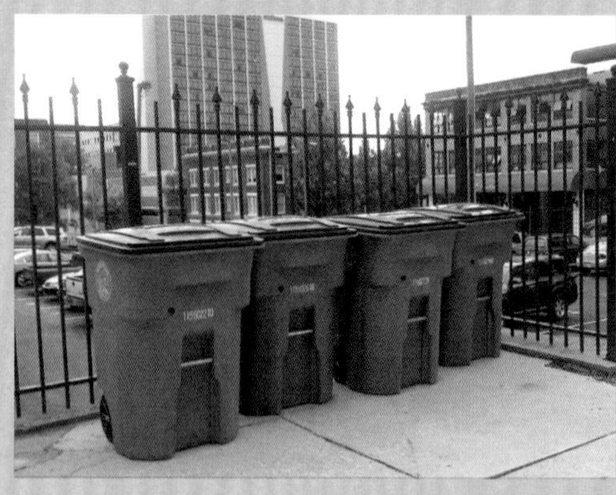

Left: This dumpster for recyclables, decrepit and poorly marked (the signage indicating it takes recyclables faces away from the street), stands near the former Ben West library, a location inconvenient to existing residential properties. It is one of two within the downtown transect zone; the other is on a dead end street near the Bicentennial Mall. *(2014)*

Center: This waste receptacle collective at San Francisco's Academy of Sciences illustrates exactly where trash winds up—buried in the earth—a constant, if subtle, educational tool for the many children that frequent the Academy's exhibits and programs. Nashville's outdoor receptacles should offer the same reminder to our city's natives and tourists. *(2011)*

Right: The city of Knoxville provides these 96-gallon recycling containers in over two dozen locations in its central business district. Each location has between one and six recycling containers for common use, targeted near residential locations. The city also operates an extensive recycling center in a downtown parking lot. *(2011: City of Knoxville)*

Wanted: A Strategic Plan for Downtown Recycling

Downtown Nashville has the densest concentration of people in Davidson County. More people per square foot of building or sidewalk means more garbage produced per square foot. Much of this garbage could be recycled rather than dumped in a landfill. So why is the downtown recycling program so anemic?

Let me explain what I mean by anemic. Downtown residential properties do not qualify for curbside or alley-side recycling pick up. One option is to employ a private hauler, which larger multifamily residential buildings must do for trash as well. Metro requires all commercial trash haulers to also offer recycling pick-up, so those entities willing to pay the extra charge can recycle. The alternative for the individual resident (or small business) is to ferry bagged recyclables to one of the two recycling drop-off dumpsters located in the core or drive to collection centers in the suburbs.

It's understandable that the green recycling carts so visible in urban and suburban neighborhoods on pick-up days would be unwelcome on the highly populated sidewalks of downtown, although the core has an extensive alley network. Less understandable is that downtown businesses small enough to utilize the gray *trash* carts supplied by Public Works—two per business—may place the carts on sidewalks or in alleys as long as they don't obstruct the travel portion of either for free access. Gray carts, good; green carts, bad?

Then there are the pedestrians—workers, tourists, gallery goers, entertainment seekers—strolling the sidewalks who lack sufficient receptacles for their plastic cups and aluminum cans. Currently, only Church Street, Deaderick Street, Korean Veterans Boulevard, and the Arcade entrance on Fifth Avenue North feature recycling alternatives to omnivorous trash receptacles. And so the landfill grows.

When I moved downtown in 2007 to the Quarters on Second Avenue, I didn't flinch at the thought of driving the contents of my personal recycling bin to the Green Hills collection center. After I shed my car, however, things got more complicated. The collective residents of my 30-unit building deemed the cost of private hauling too pricey. Hoarding recyclables until there is sufficient mass to warrant borrowing a car for the drive to the 'burbs is impractical in the typically small units of downtown where space is at a premium and, therefore, expensive.

So I schlepped my recycling, one bag at a time, to the nearest drop-off over a half mile away on my energetic days. When feeling less vigorous, I confess I tossed all in the trash. And so the landfill grows.

In addition, the downtown building in which I've worked for the past four years doesn't offer recycling pick-up, only a dumpster in the basement for trash. Thus whoever among my colleagues draws the short straw takes our latest bag of recyclables home. When it's my turn, "home" is the green cart of my grandmother in Donelson.

Downtown living has come a long way since 2007. It is possible to live downtown—and live well—without a personal vehicle. I can easily get my groceries, a bottle of wine and basic home goods, all within a five-minute walk of my front door. But driving to the 'burbs with recycling in tow defeats the purpose of urban living.

Downtown functions differently from the urban and suburban transect zones. Its very density is an opportunity to capture more recyclables than the average acre outside the core produces. This same density, however, presents logistical challenges to the recyclable collection process.

Metro needs to develop a strategic plan crafted specifically for downtown to take advantage of the recycling potential. Specific strategies needed in the plan:

- Install additional recycling dumpsters in locations more convenient for downtown residents. Sites near large multifamily properties should be prime targets to enable those residents whose buildings do not pay for the collection to recycle. The Gulch and Rolling Mill Hill feature several multifamily complexes and, therefore, offer great recycling potential.
- Offer pedestrians a choice. Phase-in more receptacles for recyclables on downtown sidewalks next to existing trash receptacles. Priority should be given to

those areas where pedestrians are more likely to carry recyclables, such as blocks featuring food, drink, and arts and entertainment venues.

- Create an incentive for business and residential property owners utilizing private haulers to include collection of recyclables. Several cities, including Knoxville, have a rewards program in place called RecycleBank. Points are awarded as you recycle and can be redeemed at grocery stores, restaurants, and other participating businesses.
- Increase funding for expanded recycling in downtown Nashville.

Public Works is to be commended for new general policies that encourage recycling:

- The department no longer issues or replaces more than two trash carts per business or residence. Those that have more than two will be charged a collection and disposal fee for each additional cart.
- As of July 2014, residents and businesses with more than one trash cart must pay a collection and disposal fee. Additional carts and collection for recyclables are available at no cost.
- Public Works now bans yard waste and cardboard from trash carts. Residents with curbside pick-up can place cardboard next to their recycle carts for Metro to collect. Yard waste not composted on site can be picked up during one of Public Works' three annual brush and leaf collection campaigns. As of July 2015, electronics will also be banned from trash containers. Residents should take these items to Metro's household hazardous waste facility.

—RON YEARWOOD, assistant director, NCDC

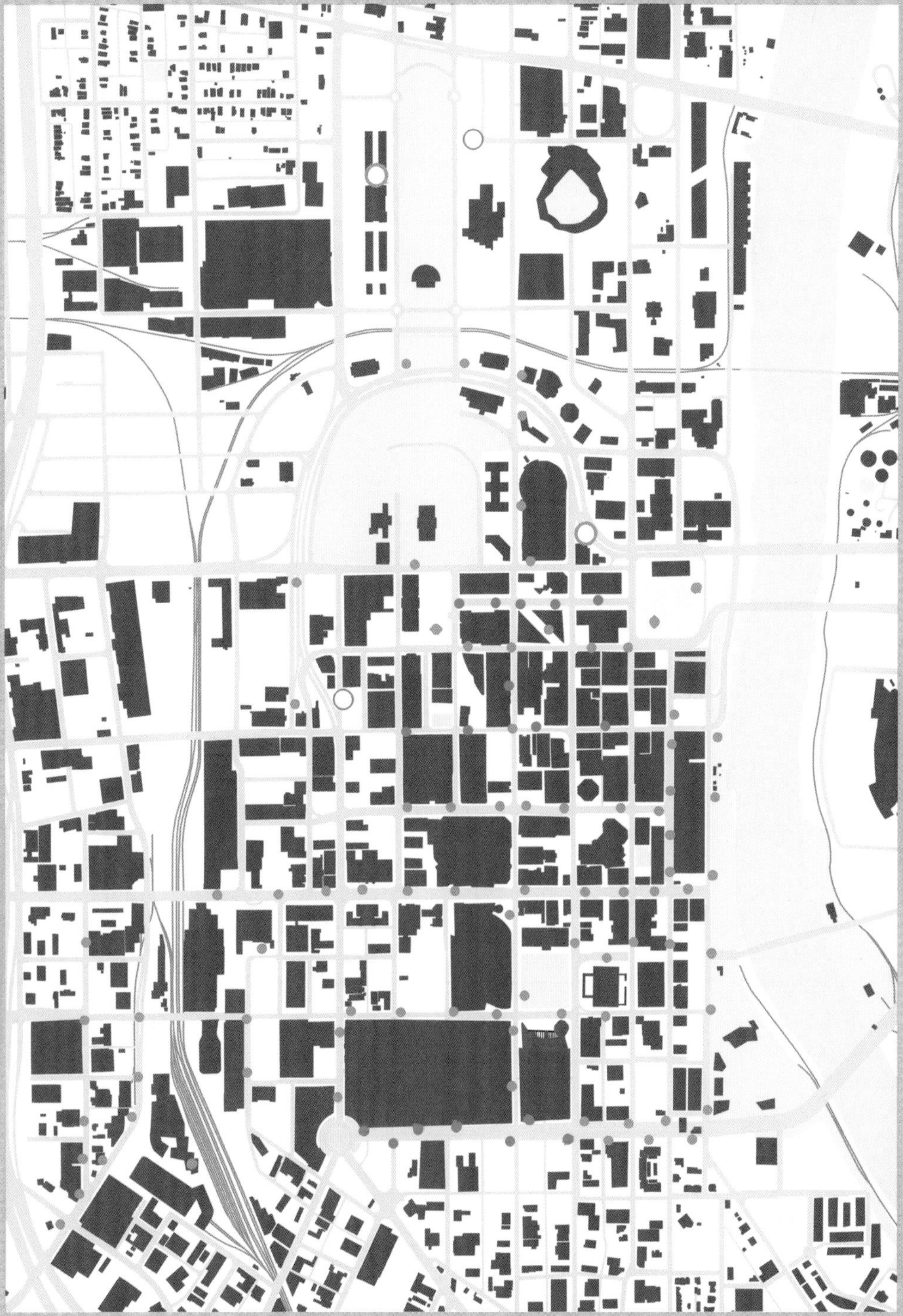

This map of downtown Nashville highlights existing and suggested additional locations for recycling receptacles. Existing bins are shown in green, with recommended additional receptacles in blue. Update: As of December 2015, Metro Public Works replaced 150 trash containers with dual-stream trash and recycling containers along streets with high levels of pedestrian traffic. *(Map, 2014: Ron Yearwood, NCDC)*

FOOD RESOURCES

✓ The Nashville Farmers' Market on Rosa Parks Boulevard is open 362 days per year and features local and regional farmers and numerous restaurants. *(2012: Gary Layda)*

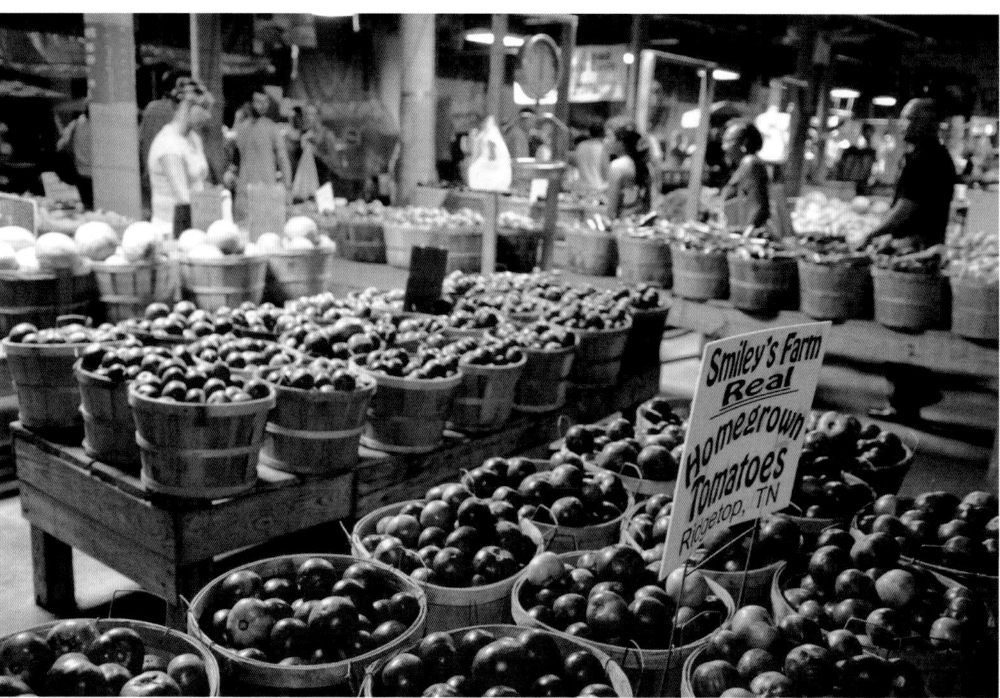

✓ Health-Promoting

The Nashville Farmers' Market just north of the State Capitol, a small grocery on Church Street, and the Turnip Truck Natural Market in the Gulch enable some access to fresh food and healthy take-out items.

X Health-Defeating

The downtown core lacks a full-service grocery store and community gardening options for residents.

STRATEGY: *Secure a medium-sized, full-service downtown grocery store that offers fresh produce—sourced locally whenever possible—with a priority on pricing to meet the affordability needs of all.*

US Census Data indicates that there are an average of 8,800 residents per grocery store nationally, irrespective of store size. The downtown residential population in Nashville is expected to reach that number within five years. When adding the 50,000 workers commuting in and out of downtown each day, the downtown area seems capable of supporting an urban-scaled grocery store—between 10,000 and 25,000 square feet, rather than the 50,000 square feet of suburban stores—especially if located near dense residential development, such as that happening on Rolling Mill Hill and in the North Gulch. (See also "Grocery Rethink" page 159.)

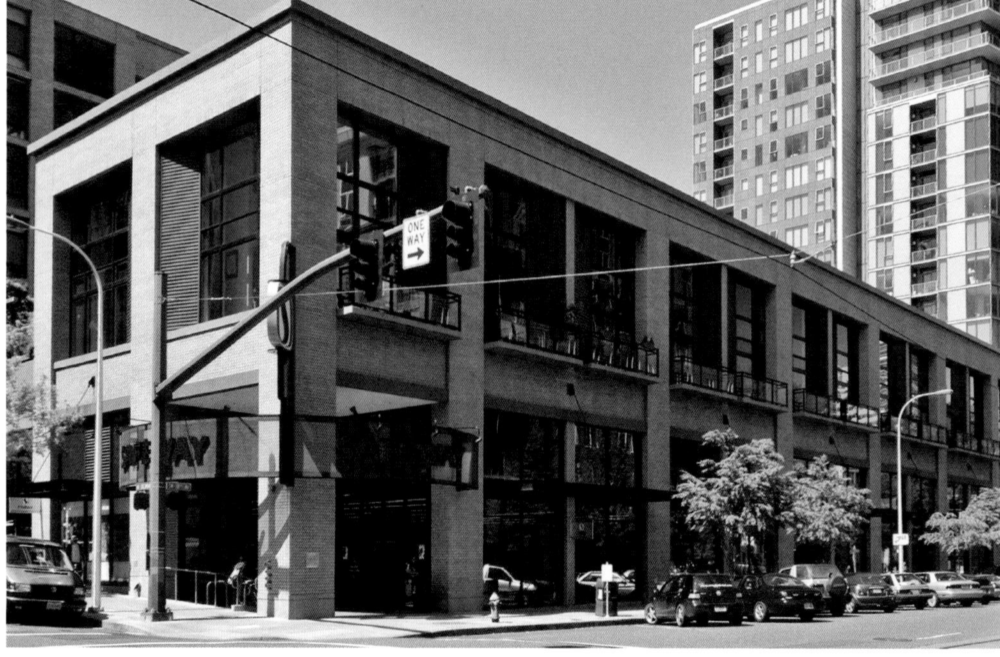

Urban grocery store in the Pearl District of Portland, Oregon, is in a mixed-use building with residential space above. *(2010: Brian Phelps and Chris Whitis)*

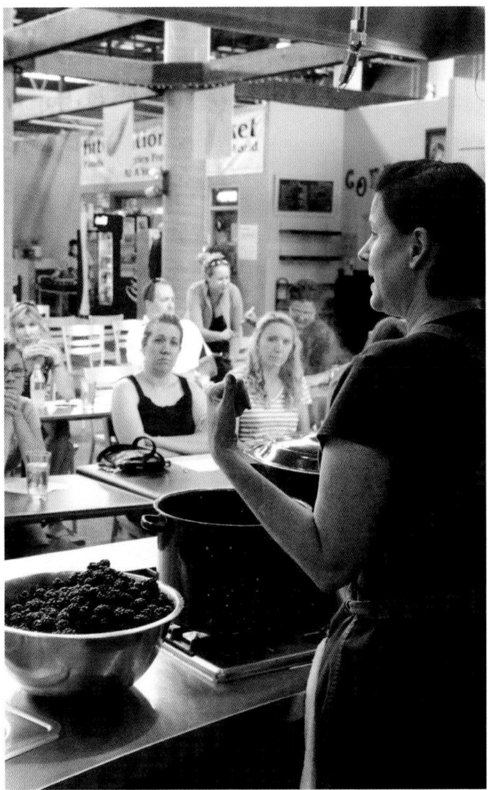

STRATEGY: *Provide more financial and planning support for Nashville's Farmers' Market as the central hub for local food activity. Diversify offerings to include more dairy, meat, fish, and bakery vendors. Consider the market as an amenity for the new baseball stadium and attendant residential/commercial/government office redevelopment nearby to promote market evolution and sustainability.*

STRATEGY: *Create a community garden on city- or state-owned land for downtown residents.*

STRATEGY: *Ensure that healthy food options appear on the menus of food vendors in Metro-owned properties, such as parks, the central bus station, the football stadium, the convention center and the arena.*

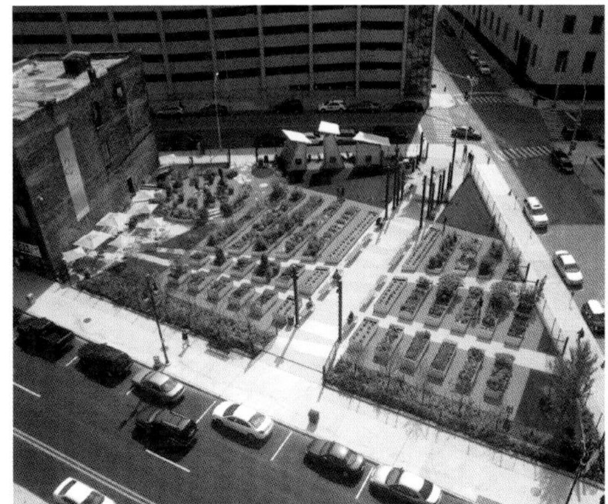

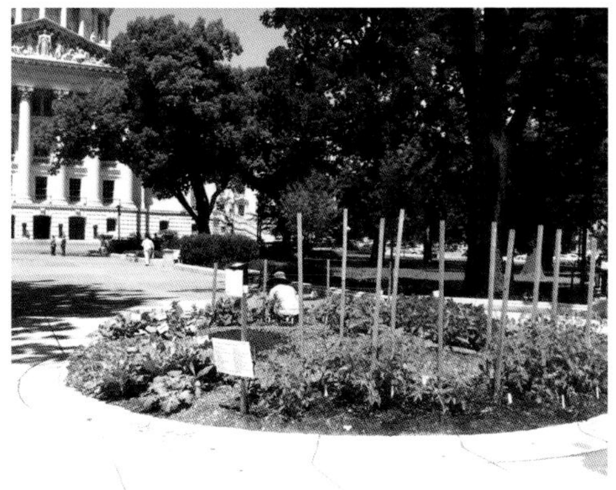

Left: The "Grow Local Kitchen" at the Nashville Farmers' Market serves as a teaching and test kitchen, and as an incubator for local businesses. *(2013: Jolie Yockey)*

Center: Lafayette Gardens (Detroit, Michigan) is operated by a public-private partnership that transformed an underutilized parcel of city-owned land into a productive urban garden in the city center. Detroit has many vacant/abandoned lots in its downtown. Finding a similar space for gardening in Nashville's booming core is more problematic. *(2012: Beth Hagenbuch, Kenneth Weikal Landscape Architecture)*

Right: A small demonstration garden on the grounds of the State Capitol in Madison, Wisconsin. *(2011: Gary Gaston, NCDC)*

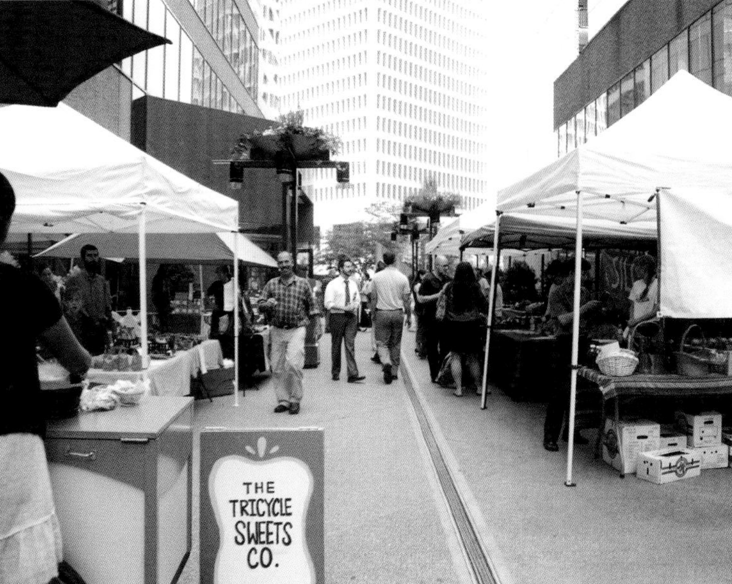

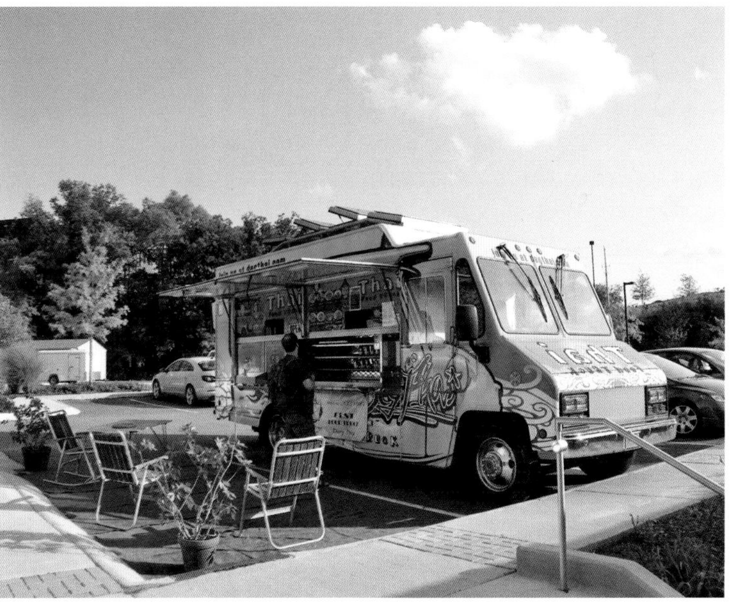

Left: Pop-up markets have spread across the city as ways to bring fresh local food directly into communities. This weekly market occurs during growing season on the plaza of a downtown office tower. *(2012)*

Right: Food trucks, like this one at Rolling Mill Hill, increase dining options in downtown neighborhoods and activate public spaces. In 2012, Nashville passed the Mobile Food Pilot Program to identify eight different locations in downtown for spaces dedicated to food trucks. *(2013)*

HOUSING

The Gulch is a mixed-use neighborhood located in a former railroad corridor that is currently home to 3,000 residents dwelling in various housing types. From left to right: Velocity condos, Pine Street Flats apartments, ICON high-rise condos, and Laurel House Lofts affordable housing. *(2013)*

✓ Health-Promoting

Recent residential development in downtown has drawn an influx of young professionals and "empty nesters." The diverse physical character of different downtown neighborhoods provides opportunities for a variety of residential development types. Nance Place and Ryman Lofts in the Rolling Mill Hill neighborhood are recent examples of affordable rental housing developments.

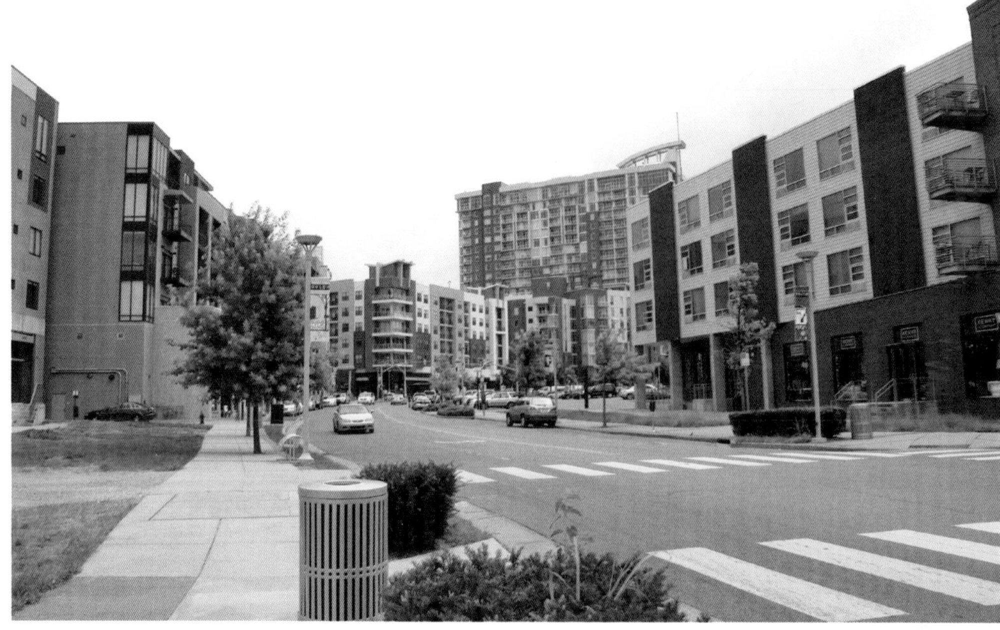

✗ Health-Defeating

Nashville's zoning ordinance did not permit housing in the Commercial Core (CC) district between 1974 and 1994.[18] As a result, Nashville's downtown has significantly fewer dwelling units than our regional peer cities of Memphis, Louisville, and Birmingham.[19] Current residential density is not enough to support significant retail, in particular, a mid-size, full-service grocery and clothing venues. Downtown residents, therefore, must travel outside the core, usually by car, to meet these basic needs.

Two constraints on population diversity are that downtown dwelling units are generally of insufficient size to accommodate families with children and prices that exclude many from the market. Some older structures have environmental hazards related to lead paint and asbestos that require costly renovations for occupation. There is a growing need for a diversity of housing types in downtown, including for-purchase and rental options in all price ranges.

> "Based on anticipated demographic trends, it will be important to build for the needs and desires of baby boomers and generation Y."
>
> Don Klein, retired director of the Greater Nashville Association of Realtors

STRATEGY: *Build more housing in the core to include a wider variety of types and sizes, as well as more affordable units, than currently characterize downtown.*

The Potential of Micro-Unit Housing in Downtown Nashville

For a growing sector of Nashville's population, downtown is a very desirable place to live—if one can afford it. The city core and its surrounding neighborhoods are booming with cultural, arts, and entertainment venues; locally owned restaurants; nightlife; and professional sports. And Nashville's urban neighborhoods each have their own unique character.

Residential density is key to promoting downtown areas as around-the-clock environments, where walking to work and even not owning a car are possible. Young professionals often seek to live in a downtown, but find conventionally sized condominiums or apartments not affordable due to core land costs. Micro-unit housing addresses that equation. Walkable urbanism is an inherently healthy lifestyle choice.

By 2035, the Nashville Metropolitan Statistical Area, now populated by approximately 1.6 million people, is projected to grow by another 1 million. As the large cohort of aging baby boomers retire, and as generation Y enters the workforce, the demographics of the city will shift dramatically. In addition, individuals are marrying later in life than previously and having children later as well. These changes have major implications for housing in Nashville in terms of overall quantity, diversity of type, relative affordability, and proximity to enhanced public transit.

Micro-unit housing (150–400 square feet) is a recent trend that significantly addresses such growth and demographic implications by providing small, adaptable, and affordable units. The small living arrangements of micro-unit housing are enhanced by shared amenities that create a sense of community within the building. If the units are built in convenient proximity to transit and everyday services and activities, micro-unit housing residents can utilize public transportation or walk, rather than relying on the automobile—potentially saving $8,946 a year (on average in 2013 according to AAA) in ownership and operating costs while enhancing their daily physical activity. Micro-units themselves promote low-impact living because of their lean size and density.

Half of American households now have no children in the dwelling, and demographers expect this trend to continue. Because micro-units may not have enough space for a bed, dining table, and sofa, they must be designed to be adaptable during the course of the day, as apartment needs change. Furnishings such as Murphy beds, fold-out sofa beds, tuck-away tables, and compact kitchenettes maximize the use of small dwelling spaces. Clever architecture can make a small space seem more spacious. Maximizing the window wall is very important in extending the space visually. Shared elements—such as fitness centers, roof gardens and terraces, dog grooming facilities, screening rooms, conference rooms, bicycle parking, and bulk storage—all complement the resident's actual unit and encourage a sense of community within the building.

Both the baby boomers and generation Y constitute key potential market sectors for future micro-unit housing in Nashville's downtown. A significant portion of generation Y seems to find suburban environments isolating, car-dependent, and lacking in the entertainment venues and leaner lifestyle that they seek in downtowns. Although micro-housing options exist in such cities as New York, Boston, Denver, Seattle, San Francisco, and Vancouver, as of 2013 no micro-unit apartment buildings existed in downtown Nashville.

In the summer of 2013, the University of Tennessee's Nashville Urban Design Program explored the potential of micro-unit housing as it may emerge in the city. In a design studio based at the Nashville Civic Design Center, ten students focused on five diverse sites throughout the central city. The Nashville Downtown Partnership sponsored the studio and the Greater Nashville Association of Realtors also provided input.

We have built suburban freestanding houses on lots to the point where that demand is met. What is not being met is the market for walkable urbanism in many of our downtowns. It's about providing choices in where and how we might chose to live.

Micro-unit housing could enhance downtown's neighborhoods by being a prime component of walkable, mixed-use development that, in addition to residential, includes retail, offices, entertainment venues, and services. Those desiring downtown living who currently find available options too costly would benefit from micro-units' provision of diverse and relatively affordable housing in desirable infill locations. The concept of micro-units could also benefit the central city by generating urban growth and economic development, increasing density, and enhancing energy on our downtown sidewalks.

As Tamara Dickson, Vice President of Economic Development for the Nashville Downtown Partnership, explains, "With strong demand for various types of downtown housing, affordability is the key to expanding options. Micro-housing offers an appealing alternative to the types of housing currently available downtown."

Micro-unit housing is certainly not for everyone. No one is suggesting such units are an urban silver bullet. Seniors may find the daily conversion of bed to couch cumbersome. It does imply a household with limited accumulated possessions. Micro-units probably provide inadequate space for raising children. A real estate market benefits, however, when it provides choices to meet the needs of various constituencies, including market sectors that may be unrepresented at the moment in downtown. While micro-units may serve a "niche" market, that market promises to be an expanding one. The bottom line is that micro-units, to the extent they encourage another form of walkable urbanism, are intrinsically healthy for adults. Already robustly encouraged in other North American cities, micro-unit housing should be a part of the future development portfolio for downtown Nashville.

—T. K. DAVIS, professor, University of Tennessee College of Architecture and Design

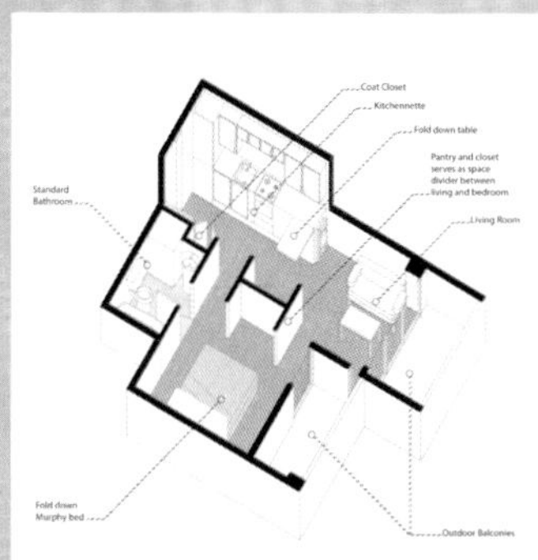

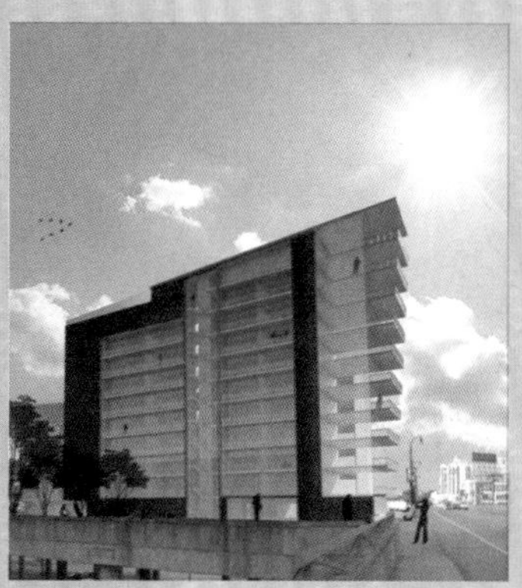

Top: UT students' designs for micro-housing in downtown Nashville include this space-efficient 360-square-foot unit. *(Illustration, 2013: Kaloyan Getev and Sean Miller, University of Tennessee College of Architecture and Design)*

Micro-housing design concept sited on Demonbreun Street adjacent to the CSX Railroad tracks behind Cummins Station. *(Rendering, 2013: Gerry Hogsed and Jamie Schlenker, University of Tennessee College of Architecture and Design)*

PARKS AND OPEN SPACE

✓ Health-Promoting

Public parks are of crucial importance for downtown living because of the dense nature of the built environment in the core. Private open space is largely restricted to balconies and roof terraces. Downtown workers, residents, and visitors are therefore dependent on public open space to experience the outdoors and for civic interaction.

The Bicentennial Mall, a state project that opened in 1996, and the recreation of the Public Square surrounding the Metro Courthouse, dedicated by Mayor Bill Purcell in 2006, are both sizeable open spaces in the downtown zone.

More recent additions include Cumberland Park and a new greenway segment in Rolling Mill Hill.

In 2013, public drinking fountains with water bottle-filling stations and drinking bowls for pets were installed in five downtown locations.

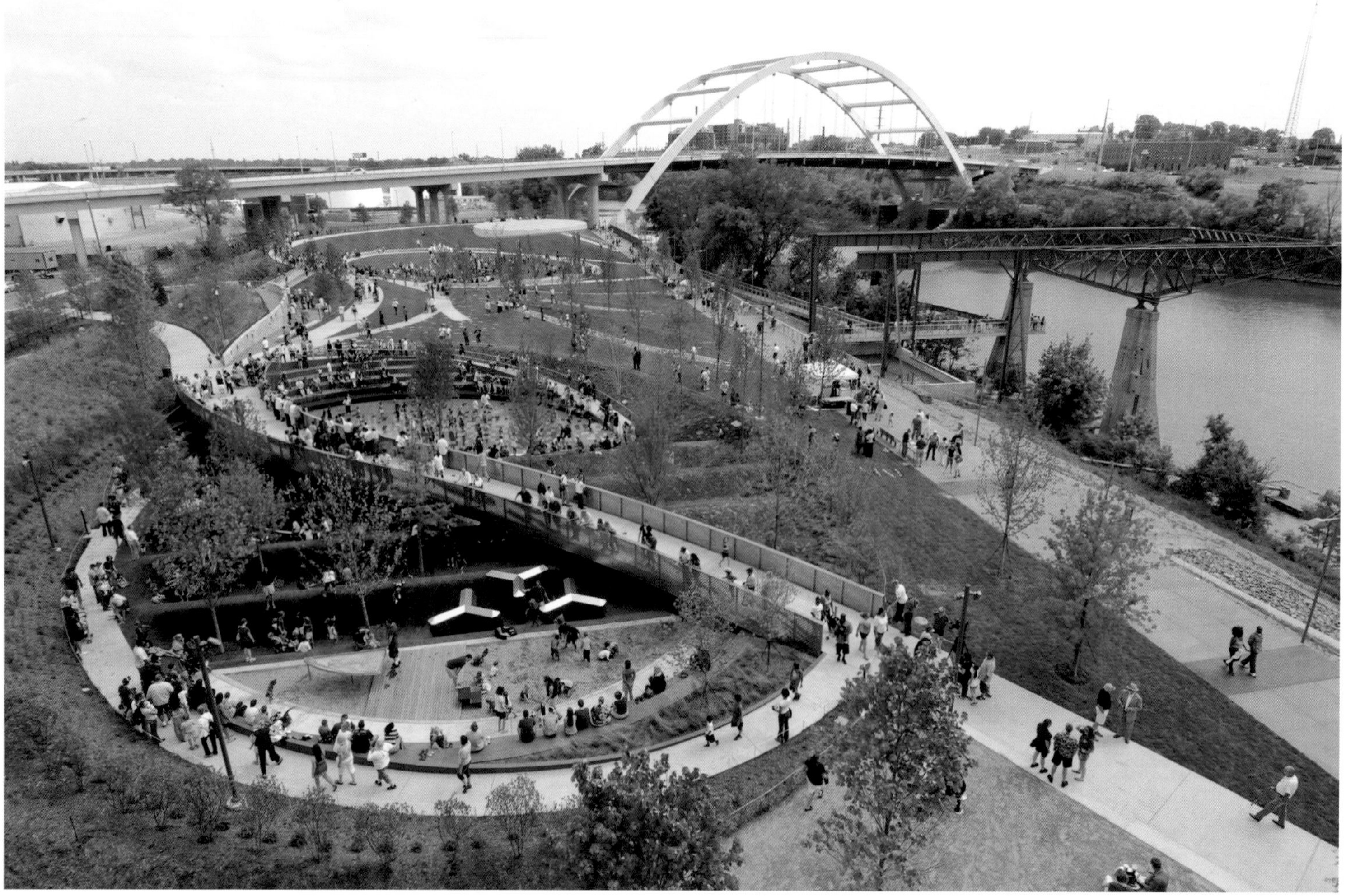

✓ Cumberland Park, opened in 2012, lies on the East Bank of the Cumberland River between the Shelby Bridge for pedestrians and cyclists and the vehicular Korean Veterans Bridge. This interactive play park, once an industrial site that was the scene of barge launchings, has water features, trails, natural play areas, and rock climbing. *(2012: Gary Layda)*

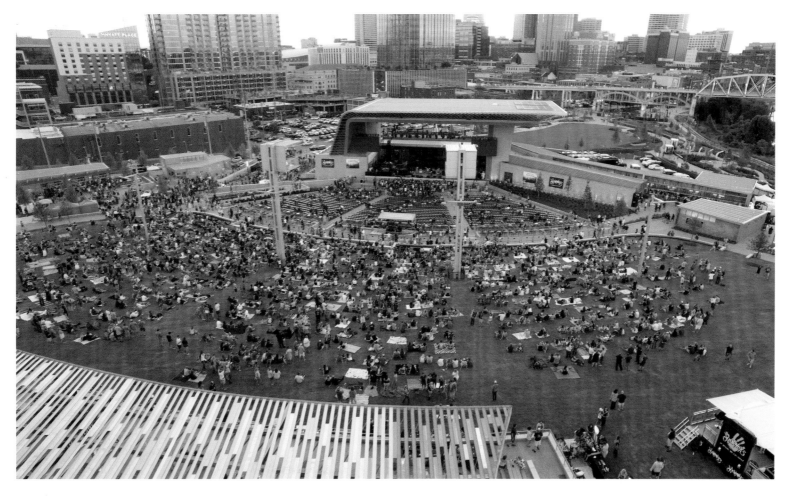

✓ In August of 2015, Mayor Dean opened the West Bank Riverfront Park, which features downtown's first dog park, a one-mile greenway, an arboretum, and the repurposing of the former trash incinerator site for an amphitheater seating up to 6,500 for outdoor performances. The park was designed by Smith Gee Studio and Hawkins Partners landscape architects. *(2015: Aerial Innovations of TN, Inc.)*

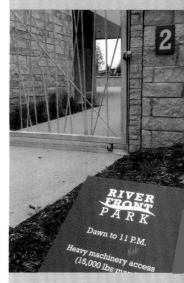

✗ The section of West Riverfront Park housing the amphitheater is often padlocked shut even when no special events are being hosted, limiting usage by pedestrians for daily activity. *(2015)*

✗ Health-Defeating

Existing downtown open spaces lack food/drink venues that would make them more attractive as social space. Some open spaces suffer from poor planning and a lack of programming to activate them. For example, Legislative Plaza, a 1970s urban renewal project to the south of the State Capitol that is mostly hardscape and elevated above street level, really comes alive only for October's Southern Festival of Books. The Walk of Fame Park, even after landscape improvements, still lacks a food/drink venue and public restrooms.

As the residential population grows, more parks will be needed. For example, the Gulch lacks any park space, a significant deficiency given this neighborhood's relative self-containment due to its sunken grade within the context of downtown.

Public restrooms are in short supply in downtown.

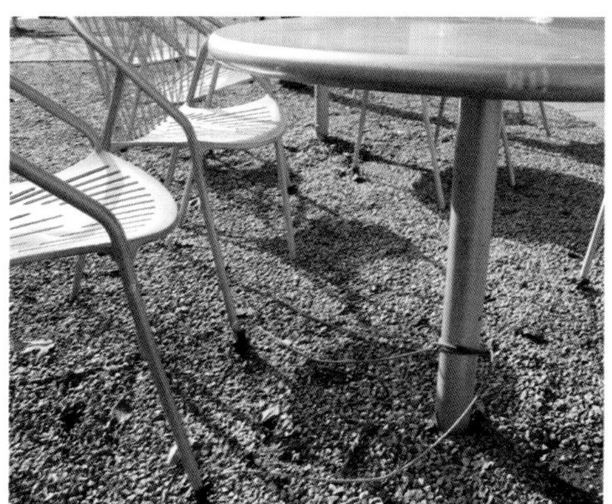

✗ Touted as "moveable" chairs, these examples in the Public Square are chained to tables, reducing their usability and giving users the impression the area may not be secure or safe. *(2013)*

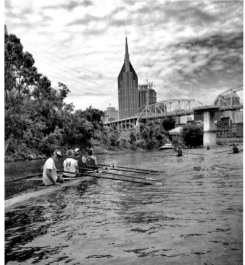

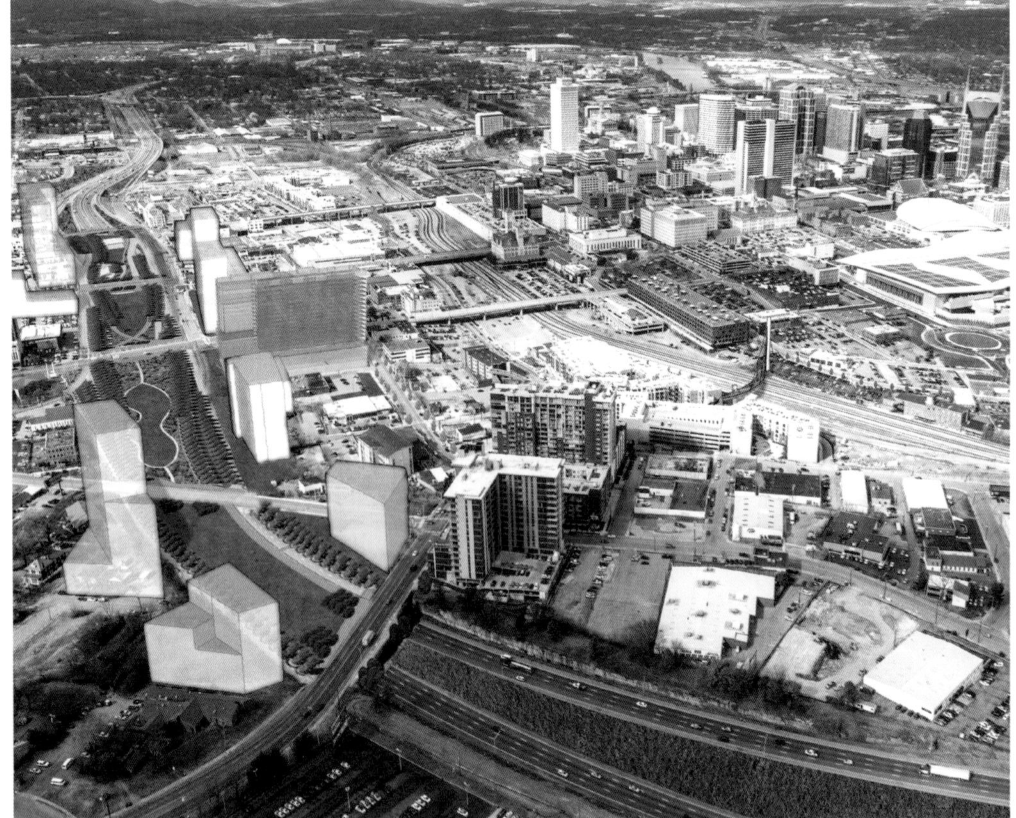

Left: Proposal to "cap" the interstate highway through downtown between the Gulch and Midtown would add park space, as well as create a safer experience for pedestrians and cyclists crossing on and off ramps. *(Design, 2012: Michael Payne, University of Tennessee College of Architecture and Design; Visualization, 2014: Eric Hoke, NCDC)*

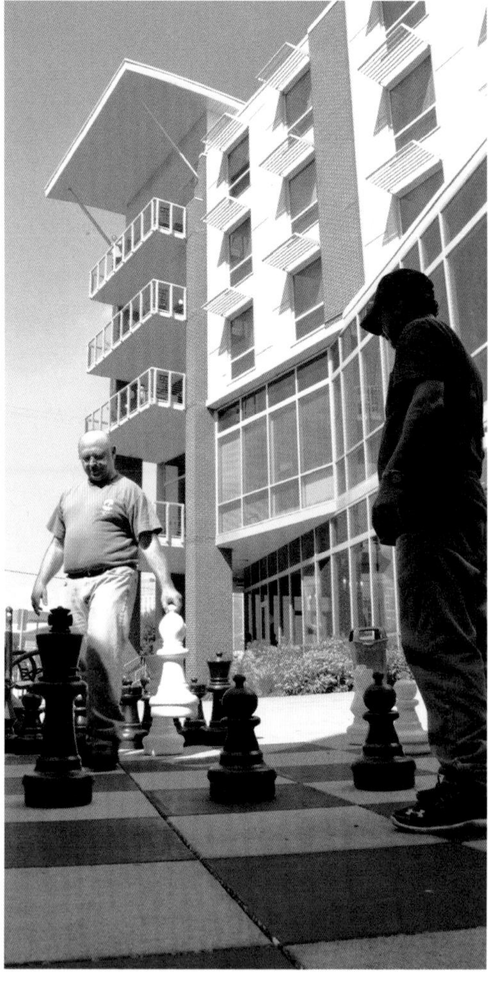

Right: Large-scale outdoor chessboard at the Room in the Inn housing facility provides an active use in a small courtyard space. *(2013: Jeff Moles, Room in the Inn)*

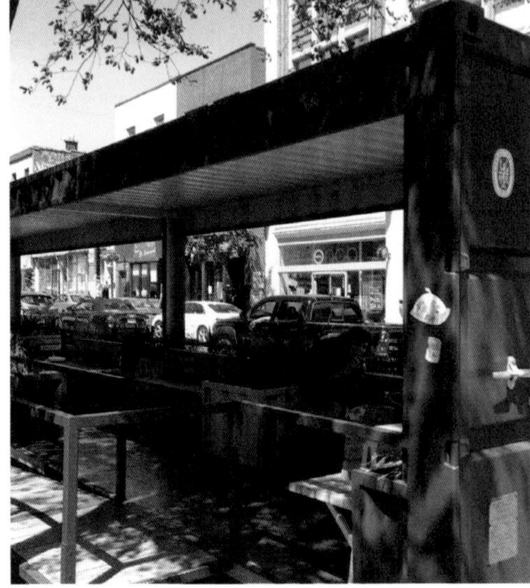

Left: A Montreal "parklet" that utilizes a standard shipping container to provide streetside sheltered seating. *(2013: Miguel Otero)*

Right: Rowers on the Cumberland River passing the John Seigenthaler Pedestrian Bridge. *(2013: Kren Teren)*

STRATEGY: *Create recreational and leisure spaces in the core as active social spaces for all ages.*

STRATEGY: *Exploit the Cumberland River watershed's recreational potential. Construct a city boathouse on the Cumberland River that accommodates nonmotorized boating—rowing, canoeing, kayaking, and stand up paddle boarding—to increase recreational uses of the waterfront.*

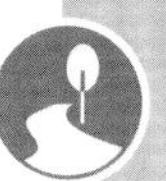

STRATEGY: *Implement a Nashville "blueway": a series of destinations along the Cumberland River from Shelby Park to the Tennessee State University campus that can be reached by a water "path," as well as by greenways on land, offering active transportation in multiple modes.*

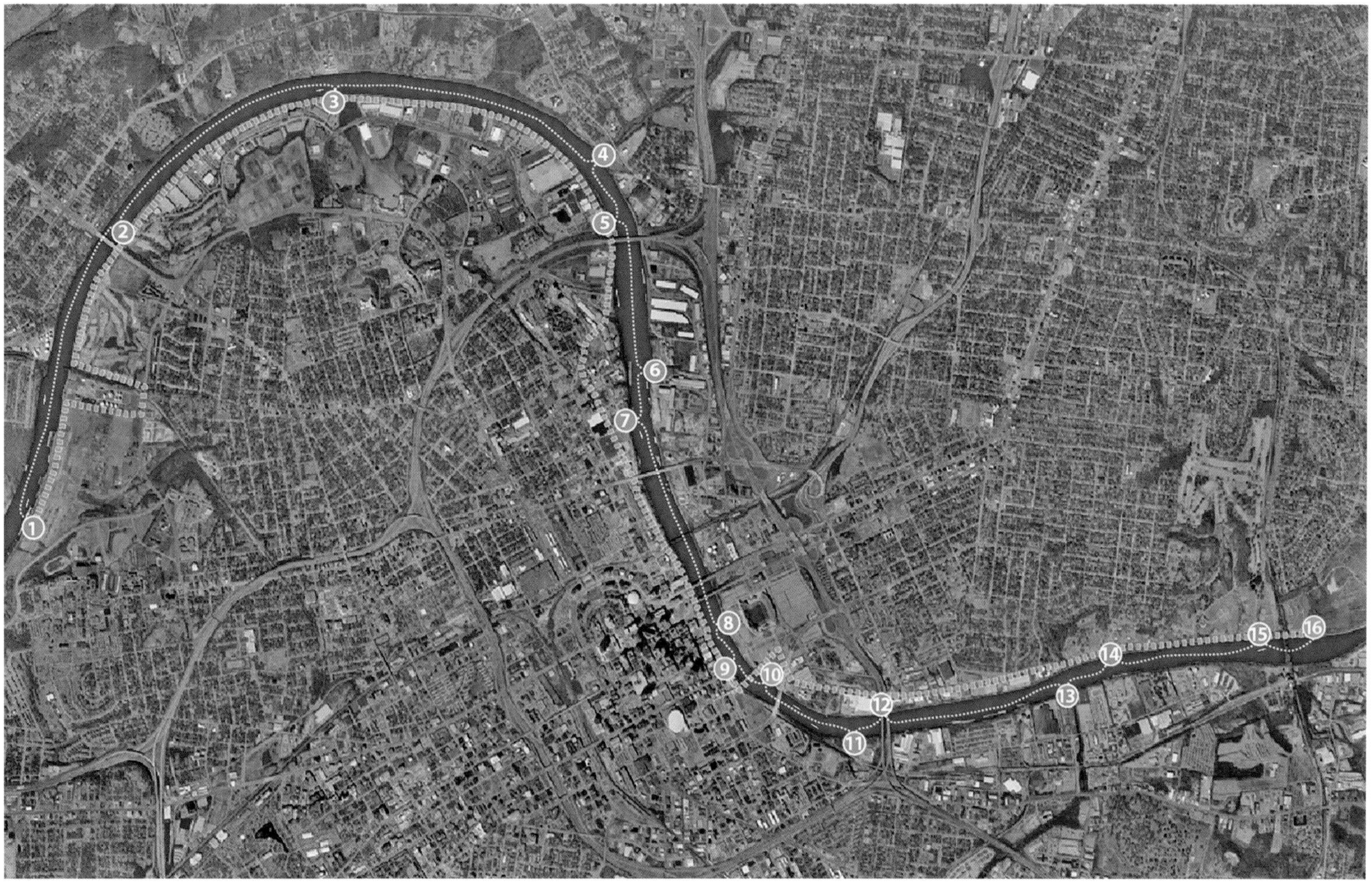

Proposed locations for blueway and greenway access points shown in blue; existing bicycle rental locations are indicated in green. One could rent a canoe at Shelby Bottoms, paddle 9.25 miles to TSU, return the canoe to a rental location, and cycle back along the greenway to Shelby—a physically rigorous round trip of 18.5 miles. *(Diagram over aerial, 2014: Ron Yearwood, NCDC)*

Proposed **canoe and kayak rental locations** in bold.

1. **Tennessee State University**
2. Clarksville Pike Bridge
3. MetroCenter Greenway and Athletic Fields
4. Lock One Park
5. MetroCenter Greenway
6. Cowan Street Boat Launch
7. Neuhoff Complex
8. Titans Stadium
9. Broadway Terminus Cascades Fountain
10. Cumberland Park Dock
11. **Nashville Boathouse**
12. Cayce Landing
13. Brown's Creek Greenway
14. Naval Reserve Dock
15. Shelby Park Boat Launch
16. **Shelby Bottoms Nature Center (currently has bike rentals)**

theBEND
NASHVILLE'S OASIS FOR URBAN RECREATION + HEALTHY LIFESTYLES

Winning entry for Designing Action, the Nashville Civic Design Center's international design competition, depicts a mix of active "alternative sports" uses on the East Bank. Note new pedestrian bridge, multi-use sports fields, skate park, water retention features, and green roofs on mixed-use development. *(Rendering, 2012: Mike Albert and Victor Perez Amado)*

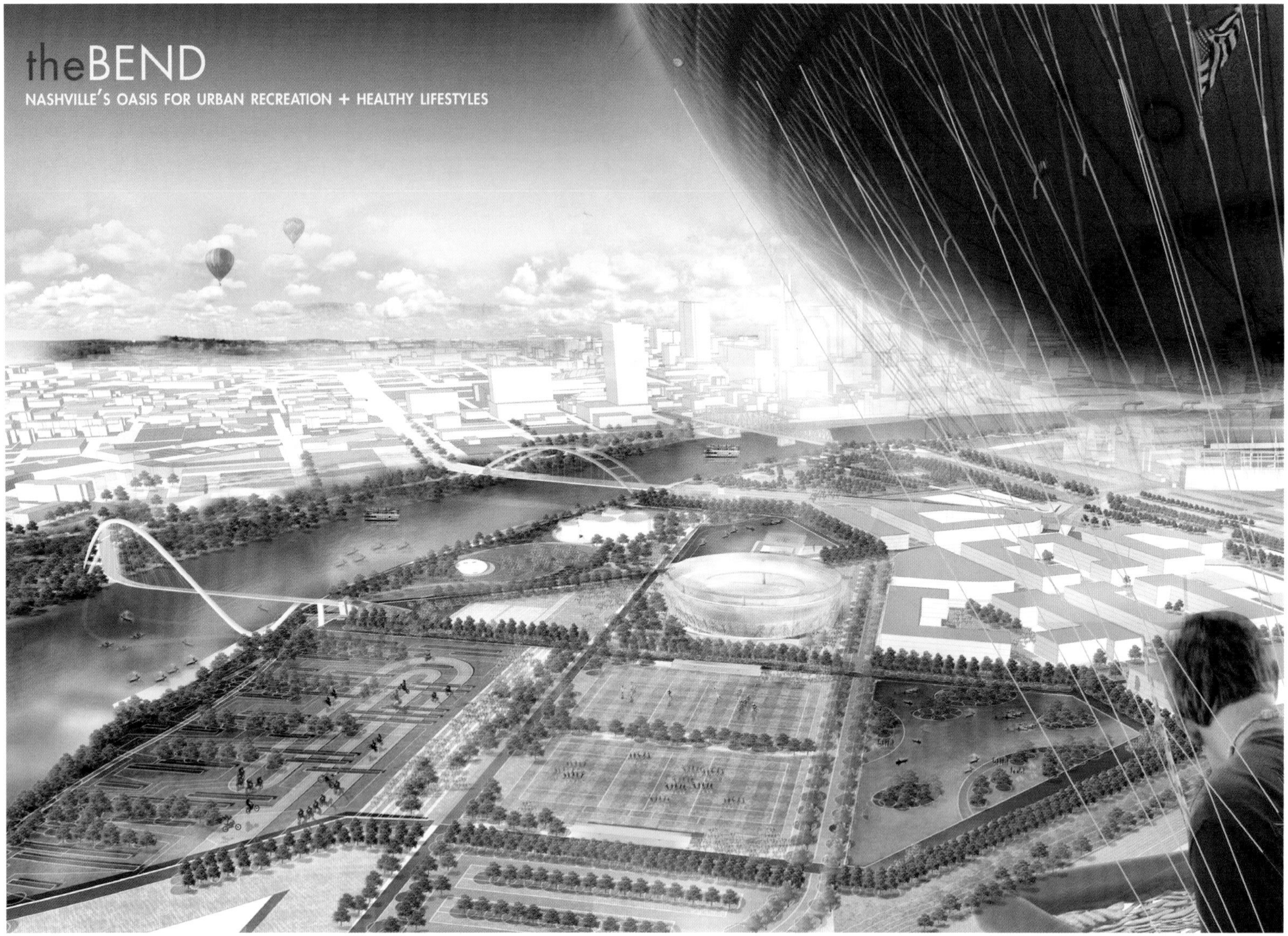

STRATEGY: *Convert the brownfields on the East Bank to more health-appropriate development that engages the riverfront and allows access to the water for open space and recreation.*

STRATEGY: *Provide local food resources and outdoor seating in public spaces. Revenue generated can be used to help maintain the parks.*

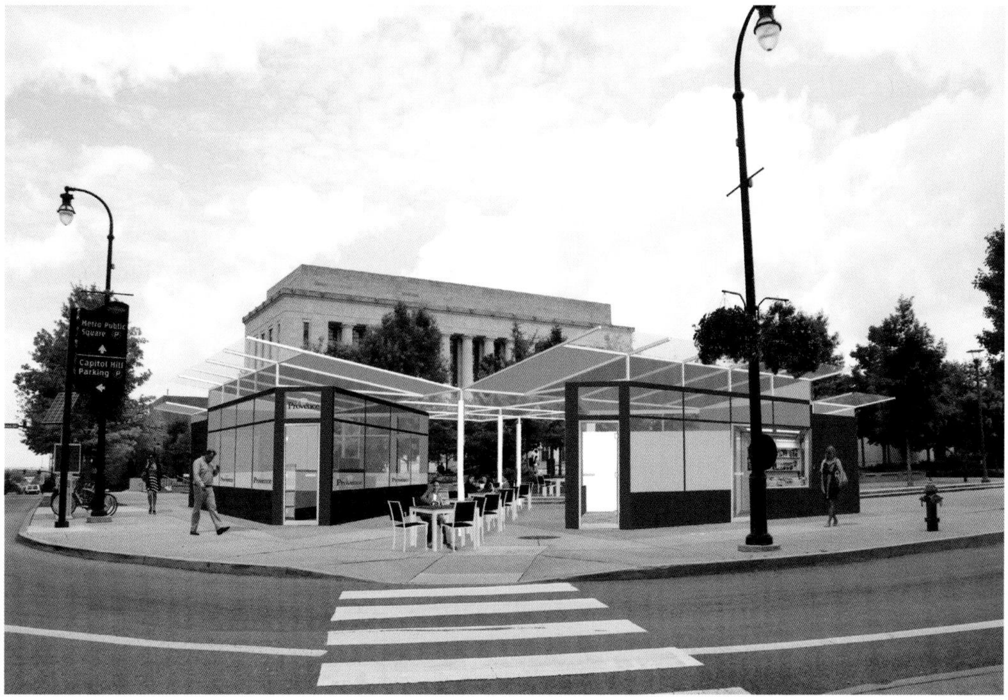

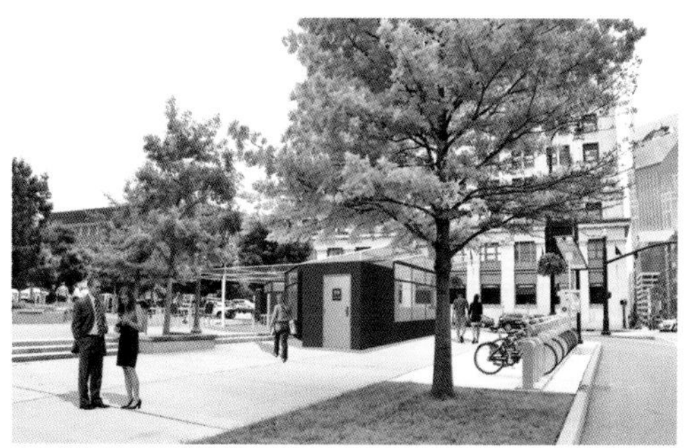

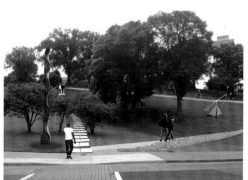

Left and top: The perimeter of the Public Square would support structures because the below-grade parking does not reach to the edge, where there is bedrock underneath. Such structures would help populate this often-inactive civic space by housing a restaurant or café, newsstand, storage area for tables and chairs, and public restrooms. Revenue generated from rents for the café could be devoted to paying for security and upkeep of the Public Square. *(Visualizations, 2013: Eric Hoke, NCDC)*

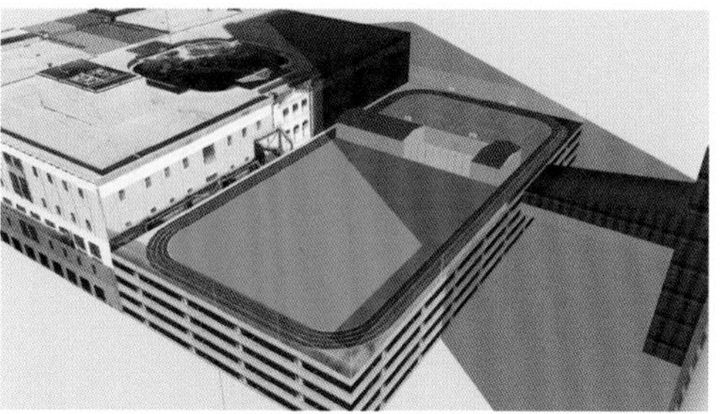

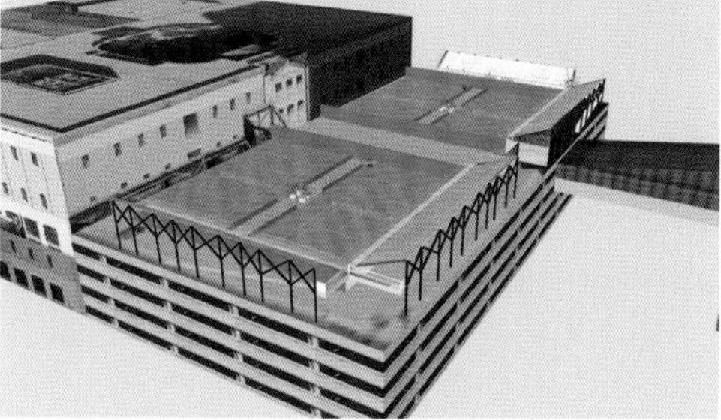

Right: The now-vacant roof of the Main Public Library garage could be enhanced to provide sports fields, tennis courts, or a community garden for the nearby Hume Fogg High School, which currently lacks such amenities. A shared-use agreement could open the facility to the public after school hours and in the summer. *(Visualizations, 2013: Eric Hoke, NCDC)*

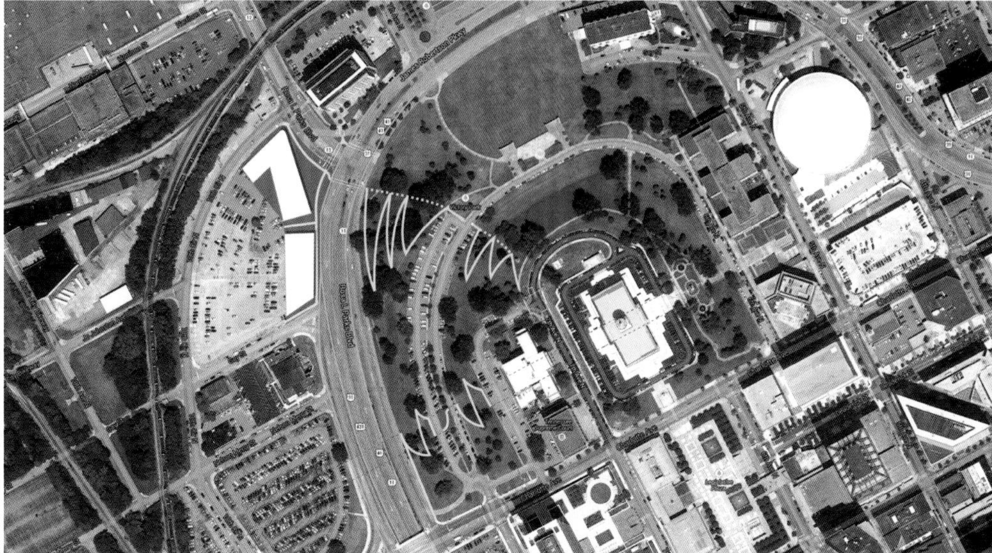

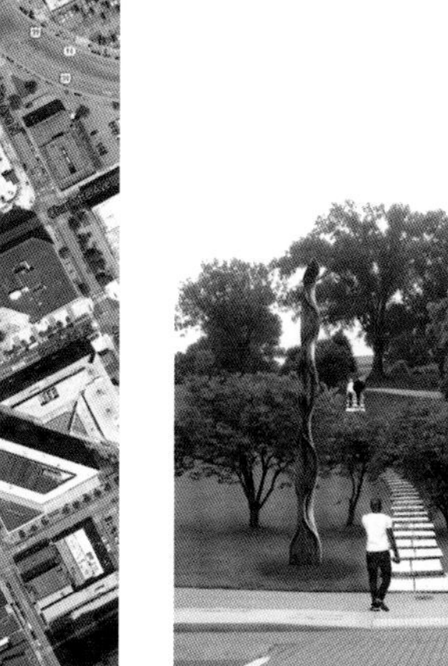

Bottom: Capitol Green Art Trail would provide a pathway for recreation and public art for a currently unused portion of the State Capitol grounds. *(Visualizations, 2013: Eric Hoke, NCDC)*

Battle Academy in Chattanooga.
(2014: Gary Gaston, NCDC)

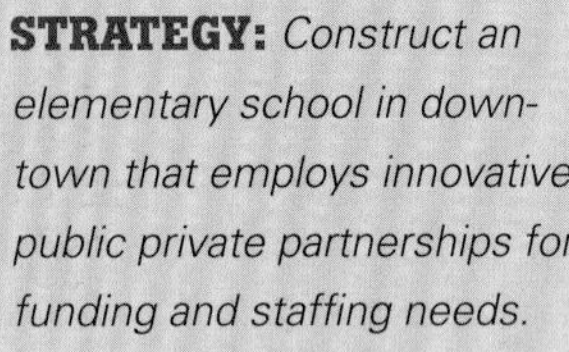

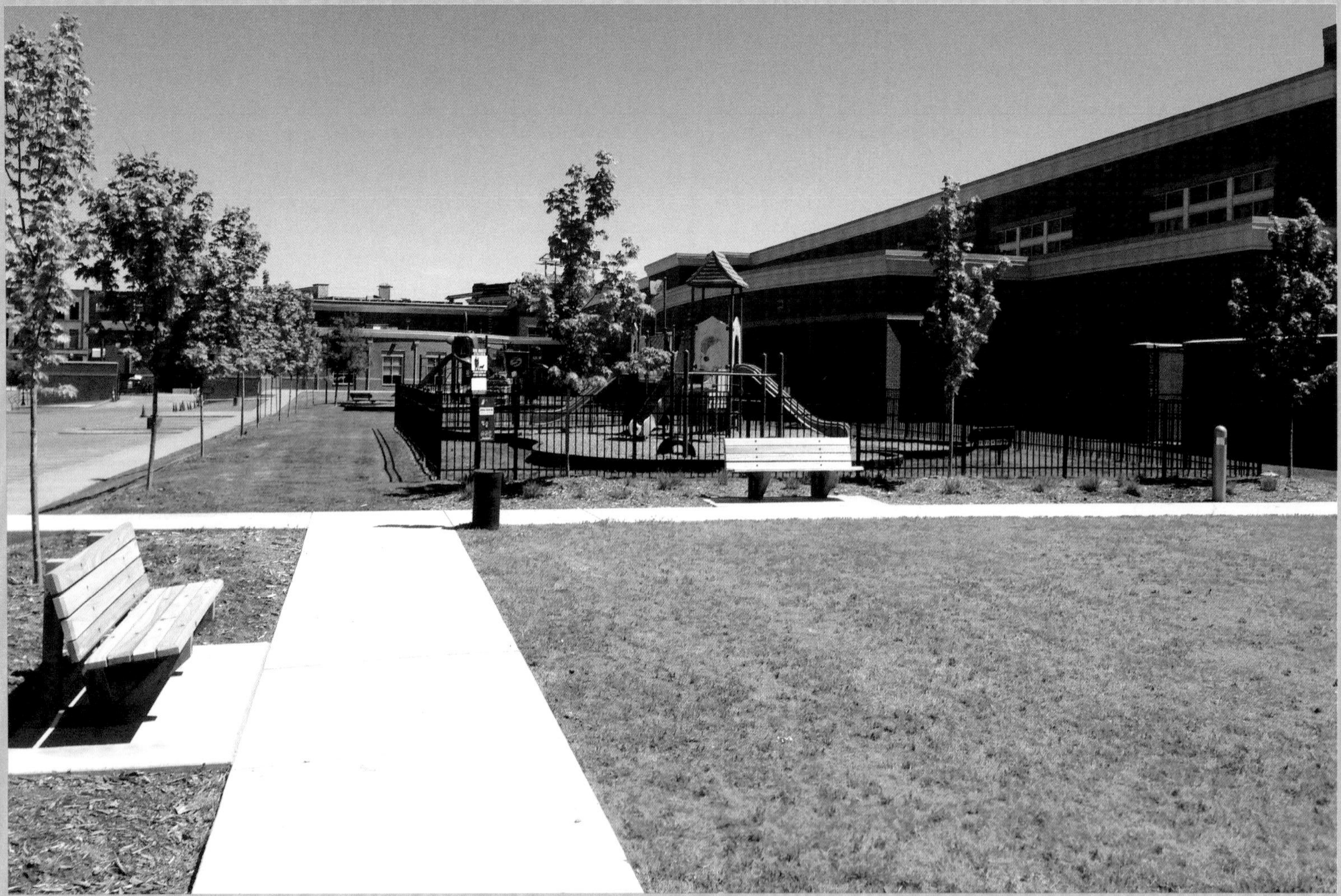

STRATEGY: *Construct an elementary school in downtown that employs innovative public private partnerships for funding and staffing needs.*

Magnetizing Chattanooga

Slump doesn't even begin to describe Chattanooga's situation in the 1970s. Declared the home of the dirtiest air in the nation, the city was suffering from a declining local economy, an empty downtown, and no civic spirit or pride. Two sobering realizations—that you could neglect a city enough to make it unlivable as well as unlovable, and that no one but Chattanoogans could remedy the situation—helped fuel what has become without question one of the most widely recognized urban comeback stories of the last 30 years.

Of course, it didn't hurt that the city had some pretty important assets as well: a stunningly beautiful physical location (when you could see it through the smog), an emerging group of visionary leaders who were willing to take risks, and very generous philanthropic foundations, the Lyndhurst Foundation in particular.

Today, Chattanooga has lots of reasons to boast about redevelopment, such as the Tennessee Aquarium, the historic Walnut Street Pedestrian Bridge, and the 21st Century Waterfront. One story not so well known, even in Chattanooga, exhibits, perhaps more than anything else, the full range of opportunities and challenges ahead for cities and downtowns, while illustrating the importance of Chattanooga's mantra: "Working together works." This is the story of the partnership that built two new magnet public elementary schools downtown years after every other downtown school had closed.

When River City Company, the city's downtown nonprofit development firm, set goals in 2000, one of the major priorities to emerge was to stimulate the market for all types of housing downtown. The hardest nut to crack was housing that would attract families to a place with no schools and housing costs higher than those in suburbia. Children living in or near downtown, many of them in a public housing complex, faced bus rides to other areas for school.

Two important opportunities presented themselves. The countywide school system had funds to build one new elementary school downtown. But it would be full on opening day with children already living in or near downtown, leaving no room for new families. Meanwhile, the University of Tennessee at Chattanooga (UTC) needed to move its on-campus preschool that served faculty, staff, and students to another location, and wanted to improve its teacher education programs with a more active presence in area schools. Where was the win-win for downtown in these scenarios?

Hamilton County Mayor Claude Ramsey called the major players to the courthouse: leaders of UTC, the school system, River City Company, and the Lyndhurst Foundation. The wheeling and dealing began as everyone put their dreams, their needs, and their resources on the table.

Some important principles guided these discussions about downtown schools:

- Downtowns should be for everyone, at every station in life, regardless of income and background.
- Every child has a right to high quality public education, and parents deserve the chance to have their young children nearby while in school.
- A downtown is a classroom—a richer learning environment than can be provided in the suburbs. Museums, celebrations, public buildings, and offices are all places to learn.
- Downtown areas should be complete places where people can work, shop, live, study, play, and engage in civic life.
- Schools are not warehouses for children; they should be attractive community-gathering places that are integrated with the rest of downtown.

Within weeks of the brainstorming, a plan was presented to the River City board, Chattanooga City Council, and Hamilton County Commission, the body that provides funding for the public school system. The idea was to build two new downtown schools instead of one, provide room for new families, site the schools in prominent downtown locations, make them community buildings as well as schools, locate UTC's high quality preschool in both schools, and recruit the best and brightest urban educators to staff them.

The funding mix was crucial. Building schools for students who were not yet living in the area was not typical practice for the school system, so auxiliary funds from outside the system were critical to the plan. The Lyndhurst Foundation stepped up to provide funds for one-half the cost of building the schools, an $8 million commitment from a foundation long involved in both downtown redevelopment and in public school reform. The county provided the cost for the other half.

The city assembled and donated the site for one school; the University of Chattanooga Foundation did the same for the other one. The school system was awarded a multimillion dollar magnet school grant to help pay initial operating costs. Downtown companies and the Tennessee Valley Authority donated funds to equip the libraries, and the Community Foundation helped with playgrounds. UTC funds the annual operating costs of the two on-site preschools, as they also serve as lab schools for their teachers' college.

Both schools opened their doors two years after that first meeting in the courthouse. Ten years later, they are mostly filled with children who live downtown, an indicator that opening the schools attracted more people with children to live downtown, as well as children whose parents work downtown. The two-story, unfenced schools are on tight sites and feature natural day lighting and public art. One has a rooftop teaching garden.

The schools are now in the midst of resurgent communities containing new apartments, townhouses, and single-family homes, in addition to new local businesses. They helped contribute to the fact that Chattanooga's downtown census tracts are growing faster than the county as a whole and becoming more diverse. Best of all, they put children back in the downtown, walking to field trips, walking home or to their parents offices after school, and playing on the playgrounds during the day. These are our next generations of leaders, philanthropists, artists, educators: our young city-builders in training.

— ANN COULTER, A. Coulter Consulting, executive vice president of River City Company from 2000–2005.

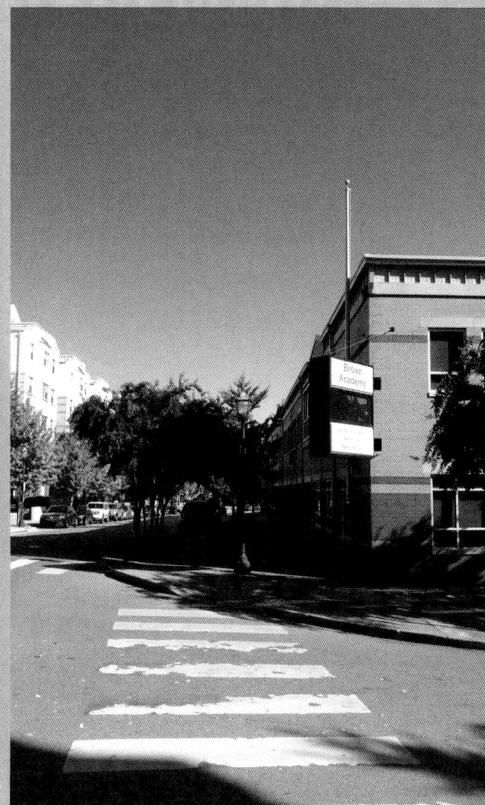

Brown Academy in Chattanooga.
(2015: Ryan Sandwich, Chattanooga Design Studio)

CASE STUDIES

ROLLING MILL HILL AND LAFAYETTE

The SoBro districts of Rolling Mill Hill and Lafayette are located within easy walking distance of one another at the southern edge of downtown, with Korean Veteran's Boulevard as their northern boundary. Yet their infrastructure and development patterns vary significantly. Rolling Mill Hill illustrates how the guiding hand of government, along with significant infrastructure investment, can lead developers in the transformation of a derelict district into a neighborhood-in-the-making. Lafayette-as-neighborhood is still potential waiting to be realized.

Redevelopment planning for Rolling Mill Hill dates to 1996 and has yielded several new and historic rehab housing developments, with more planned for the near future, as well as the conversion of the old trolley barns on the site to commercial space.

The concept of Lafayette neighborhood redevelopment, or even that there could

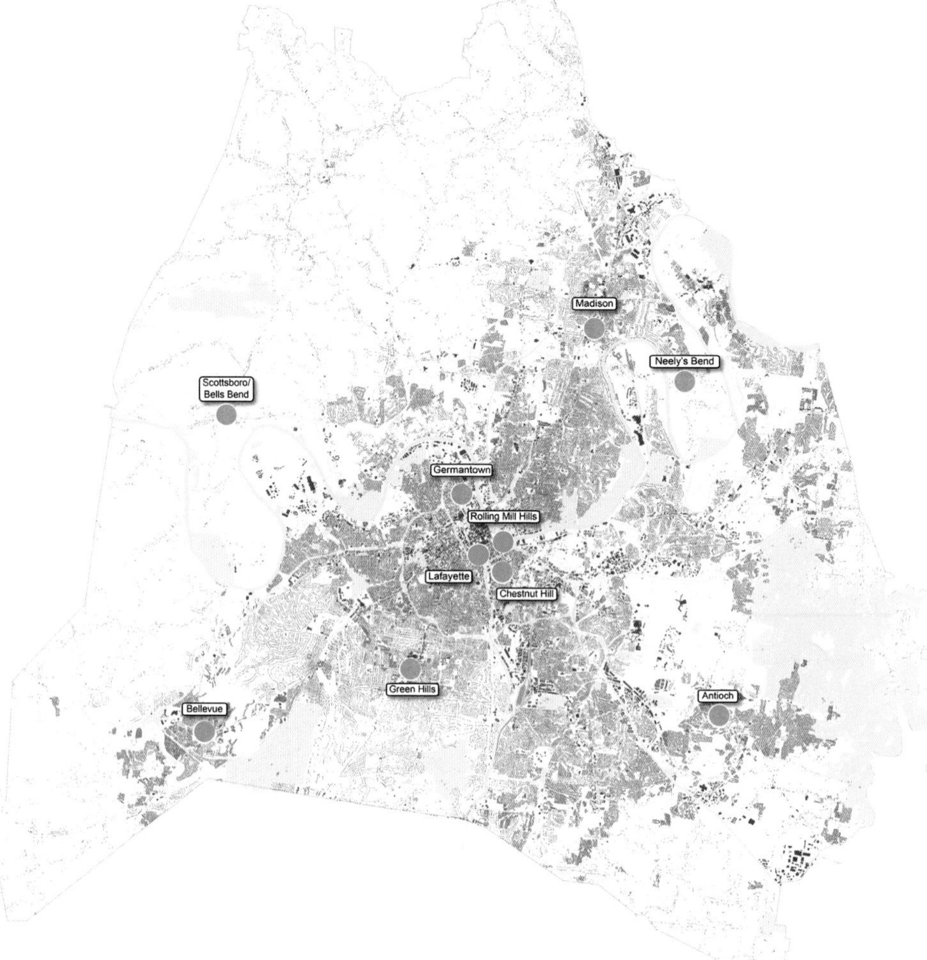

Case study locations.
(Diagram over map, 2012: Eric Hoke, NCDC)

Definition of Family / Non-family

Family = Contains at least two people related by birth, marriage, or adoption. Family households are of two types:

- **Married** = When a married couple is considered the householder
- **Other** = When a single man or woman is considered the householder and lives with other family

Non-family = This may be one person living in a household or multiple people who are not related to each other.

Household Type

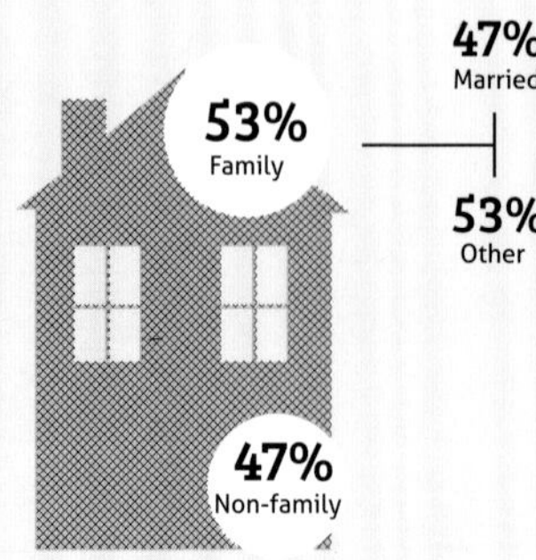

Census Tract 195*

Race

Census Tract 195*

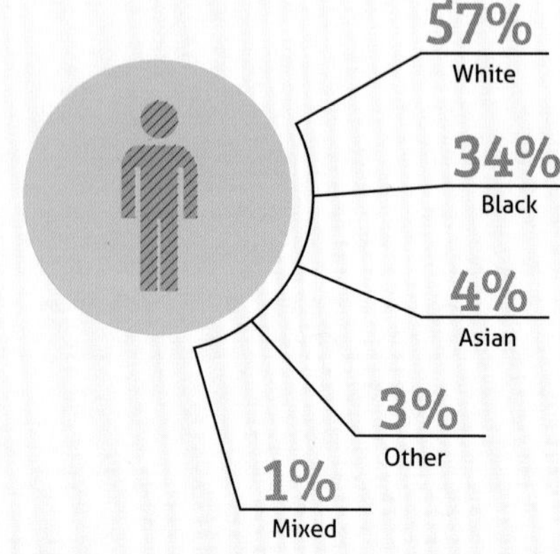

Information graphics, 2013: Ashley Nicole Johnson

be a Lafayette neighborhood, only swam into civic consciousness with the 2006 Nashville Civic Design Center report *Lafayette Neighborhood: Findings and Recommendations.* The *South of Broadway Strategic Master Plan* followed in the wake of the opening of the nearby $623 million Music City Center in the spring of 2013. This mega-space for conventions is expected to spur considerable redevelopment, particularly to the south where Lafayette lies, and the city wanted to plot the nature of the transformation.

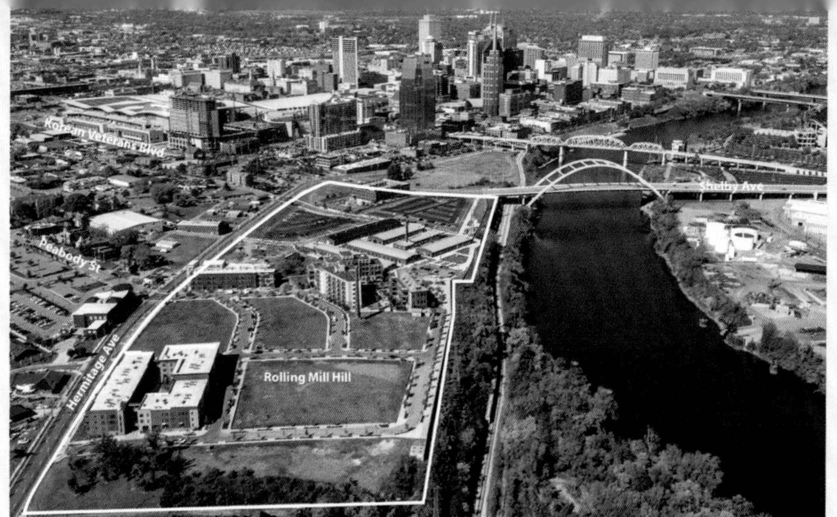

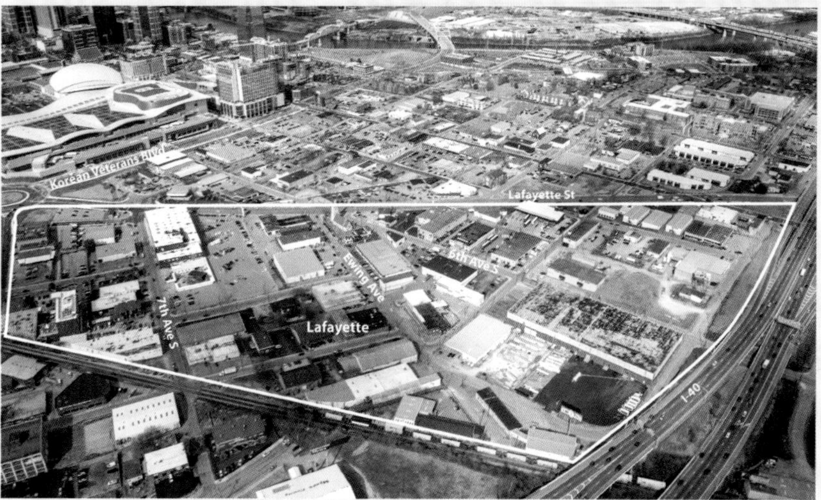

Aerial images of the Rolling Mill Hill and Lafayette neighborhoods (boundaries outlined in white). *(2012: Gary Layda)*

Income

Census Tract 195*

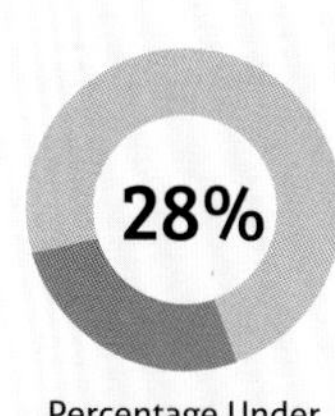

Percentage Under Poverty Level

$42,468
Median Income

Age Demographic

Census Tract 195*

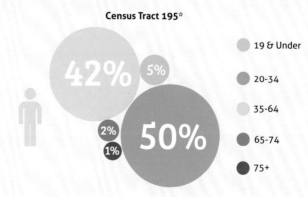

42%
5%
2%
1%
50%

- 19 & Under
- 20-34
- 35-64
- 65-74
- 75+

*Note: Both neighborhoods are located in the same census tract.

Demographic data from the US Census Department's 2010 American Community Survey (5 year estimates). At the time of research for this publication, the 2010 dataset was the most current data available. For the case studies, neighborhood boundaries were identified and data was then collected from the census tracts that best corresponded to those geographic boundaries.

Growing Nashville's Urban Forest

STRATEGY: *Plant trees and maintain existing canopy throughout downtown to offset the urban heat island effect, alleviate stormwater runoff, and create a better pedestrian walking experience.*

"Urban forest" seems a contradiction in terms. We consider urban to be what is characteristic of a city: that habitat constructed to accommodate a dense concentration of the human species.

In a forest, the density is one of trees. In pre-industrial times, tree forests covered almost half of the earth's land area, according to the Earth Policy Institute.[20] Now that figure is roughly 30 percent. Swaths the size of the state of Michigan are lost each year.

Deforestation is a great concern to ecologists and climatologists. "The most dramatic impact is a loss of habitat for millions of species," says *National Geographic*.[21] Deforestation also drives climate change by enhancing extreme temperature swings. Without trees, former forestland can quickly become barren desert. Trees also play a critical role in absorbing the greenhouse gases that fuel global warming.

These issues are remote for the city-dweller vying for a shaded parking space or admiring a tree-lined street during a stroll. Yet the functions trees perform on a global scale are replicated in miniature at the local level.

Physical and social scientists have conducted research on trees and their numerous beneficial effects for society:

- filtering air by absorbing pollutants such as sulfur dioxide, nitrogen oxide, and particulate matter, and oxygen production through photosynthesis
- sequestering carbon as wood biomass, reducing ozone production
- shading homes and buildings from the summer sun and protecting them from winter winds, thus reducing energy consumption and pollutants created from the use of fossil fuels for cooling and heating
- cooling the environment through transpiration, helping reduce the heat island effect
- improving water quality and reducing stormwater runoff[22]

Metro Nashville conducted an inventory of the trees in the public rights-of-way within the downtown "inner loop" of Interstates 24, 40, and 65 that define the city's central core. The report noted the location, size and health of each tree and positioned each on a digitized geographic information system (GIS) map.[23] On nearly 54 linear miles of streets, 2,224 street trees were tallied; in addition, 792 additional spaces were identified where trees could be planted. The tree canopy coverage for this area is only 4.8 percent—the lowest of any area in the county. But it is estimated that downtown could accommodate an additional 16 percent of canopy coverage.[24]

Nashville can do better in regard to its trees, and a plan is currently in place to chart a path for expanding the city's urban forest.

In December 2011, Metro Public Works launched the Metropolitan Landscape Coordination Program. Its purpose is to align the work of different city departments and community stakeholders involved in the management of Nashville's landscapes and green spaces. The program is designed to preserve, develop, expand, and enhance Nashville's natural beauty by supporting ongoing and future projects, ranging from tree plantings to community beautification. The first order of business, the creation of an urban forest management plan, has yet to be completed. The plan will provide a road map to effectively and proactively manage and grow Nashville's tree canopy, and will include multiple stakeholder groups.

Recommendations for Nashville:

- Set a ten-year tree canopy goal and develop a comprehensive implementation plan.
- Identify sources in the government, private, and nonprofit sectors for funding a comprehensive planting and maintenance program.
- Promote the planting and care of trees to homeowners, schools, neighborhoods, and stewardship organizations.
- Create a comprehensive marketing plan that emphasizes the many benefits of trees and explains the care trees need to survive in an urban environment.
- Collaborate with Metro Water Services' Stormwater Division to quantify the value trees provide in lowering the impact of development and work to include trees in ordinances and regulations as a solution to stormwater mitigation and water quality.
- Work with the Metro Health Department to include trees in ordinances and regulations as a solution to air quality problems and to aid in dissipation of smog and mitigation of the heat island effect.
- Review and provide necessary updates at least every five years to the Metro Zoning Code, Chapter 17.24 Landscaping, Buffering and Tree Replacement, and any other section of the Metro Code of Ordinances that relates to trees and landscape.[25]
- Reverse the exclusion of school properties from compliance with Metro Landscape codes; make ROW tree planning near school properties a priority.
- Partner with Nashville Electric Service to limit tree topping and ensure the planting of height-appropriate trees near power lines.

— A. JOYCE KILMER

Special thanks to JENNIFER SMITH, horticulturist, Landscape Coordination Program, Metro Nashville Public Works; and CAROL ASHWORTH, landscape architect, Ashworth Environmental Design

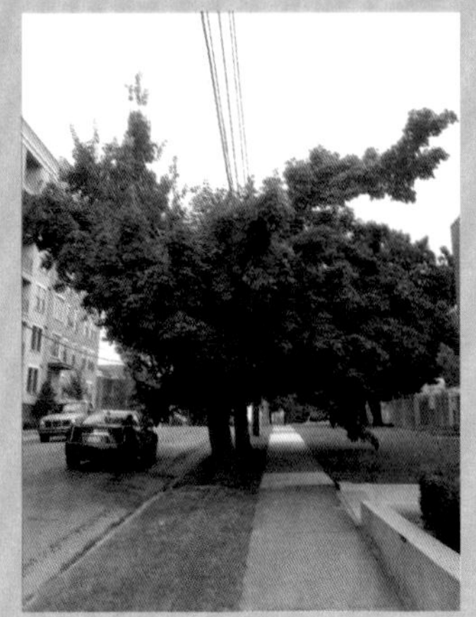

Good and bad examples of urban tree planting. Generous tree planting boxes allow urban trees to grow to maturity. Planting large species under power lines leads to violent pruning, which is detrimental to tree health. *(2013)*

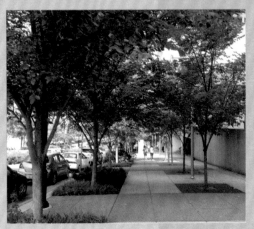

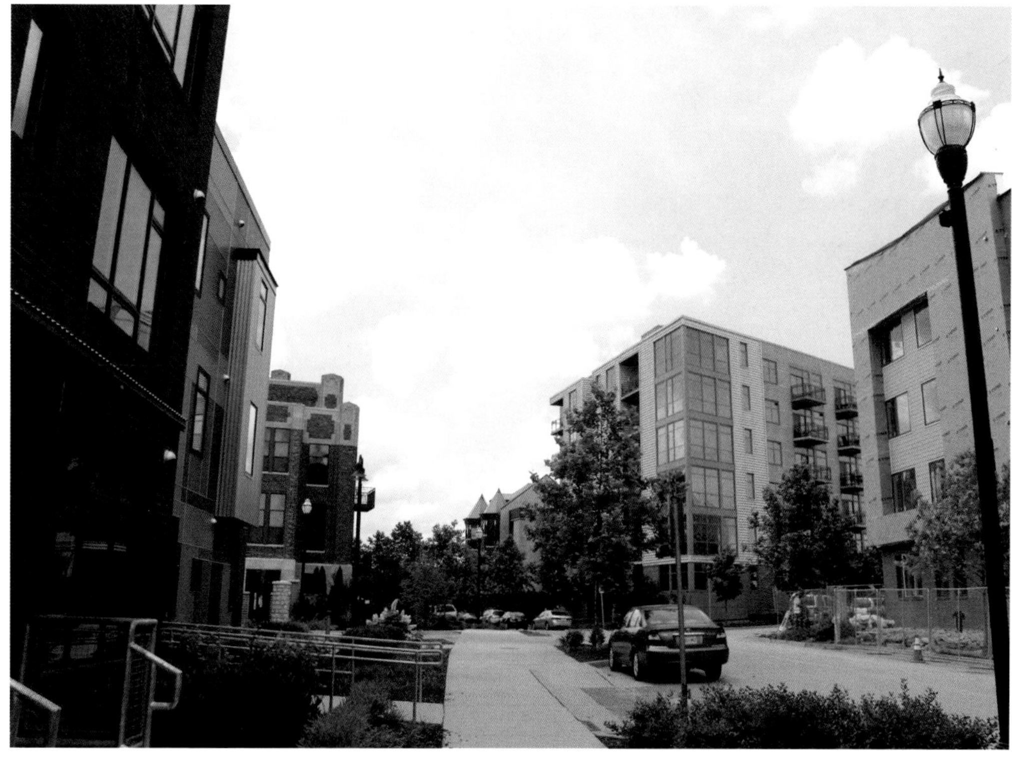

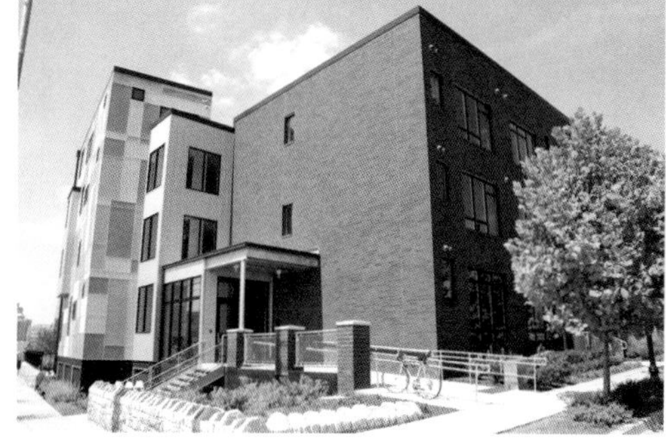

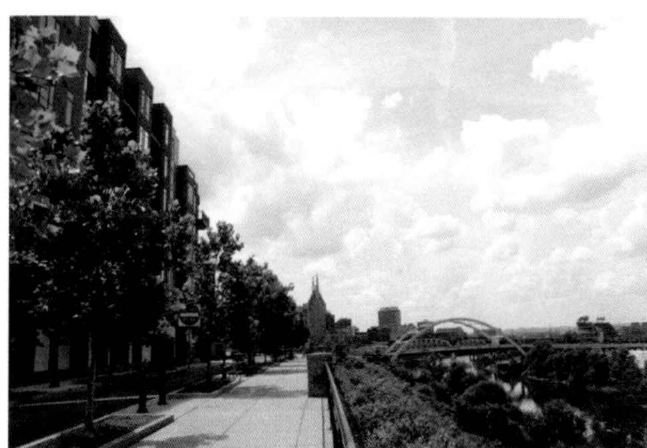

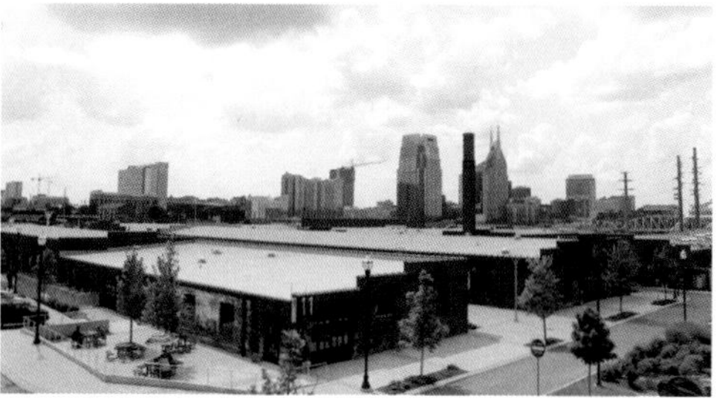

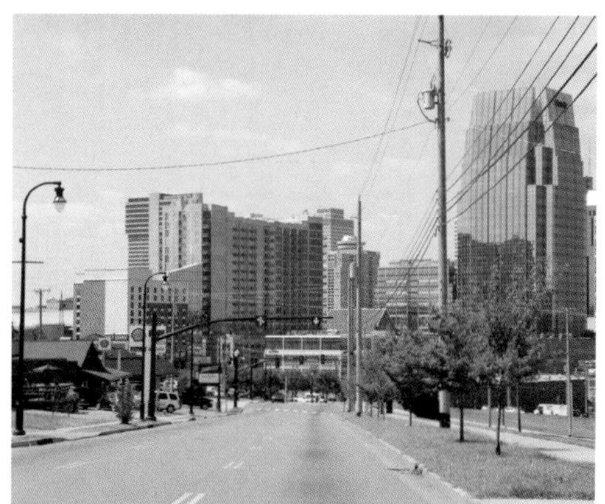

Left: New residential construction, both market rate and affordable, on Rolling Mill Hill; vacant parcels will be developed in future phases. *(2013)*

Right, top to bottom: Ryman Lofts is an affordable housing development for artists located on Rolling Mill Hill. Residents include musicians, painters, and sculptors whose individual annual incomes are less than $28,200. The project was funded by the US Department of Housing and Urban Development's Low Income Tax Credit program for the development of affordable rental housing for low-income households. *(2013)*

A new greenway along the river bluff connects historic Rolling Mill Hill to the heart of downtown. *(2013)*

View from river bluff looking toward downtown. Note the historic trolley barns below, left foreground. *(2013)*

As part of major infrastructure improvements by MDHA, streetscaping along Hermitage Avenue added new sidewalks and street trees in a planting strip. Note the road is designed with three lanes: traffic switches directions in the center lane during morning and evening commute times. *(2013)*

ROLLING MILL HILL

Rolling Mill Hill occupies 35 acres perched on a bluff overlooking the Cumberland River and downtown Nashville. The neighborhood's name derives from the roller mills once located on the hill that turned wheat and corn into flour and meal and led to Nashville's claimed status as "the Minneapolis of the South" at the turn of the last century. The site also housed a stone quarry, the city reservoir, and a water pumping station until the late 1880s, when public water storage moved to Kirkpatrick Hill on Eighth Avenue South. After the departure of milling operations, the hill's tradition of civic use continued with the construction of a campus for General Hospital and brick barns for the city's streetcars, which replaced the city stables. The merger of General Hospital with Meharry Medical College in the 1990s removed medical facility uses from Rolling Mill Hill, which then was used only for storage of the buses that had replaced trolleys.

Planning for the redevelopment of Rolling Mill Hill began in 1996 with a study commissioned by the Nashville Downtown Partnership. In 1998 the Metro Development and Housing Agency (MDHA), the city's overseer for the hill's redevelopment, solicited specific proposals, but market forces halted implementation. Mayor Bill Purcell then determined that the city itself would become the master developer. MDHA commissioned a master plan for the site and invested $25 million in much-needed infrastructure improvements for Rolling Mill Hill and the adjoining Rutledge Hill. The plan included a reworking of Hermitage Avenue to accommodate the area's first stormwater infrastructure, a massive retaining wall, environmental clean up, buried utility lines, and a greenway along the river.

Since then, various private developers have invested over $55 million in the rehab of historic structures and new construction. By the end of 2015, Rolling Mill Hill featured 169 units of affordable housing and 368 apartments at market rate, with an additional 245 units in the design or initial planning stages. The neighborhood units were designed to surround a pocket park, as well as 80,000 square feet of commercial space in the rehabbed trolley barns. MDHA is also exploring the development of additional office and retail space, the latter to perhaps include a grocery. After starting with a dilapidated and neglected site, MDHA is well on its way to building a neighborhood community.[26]

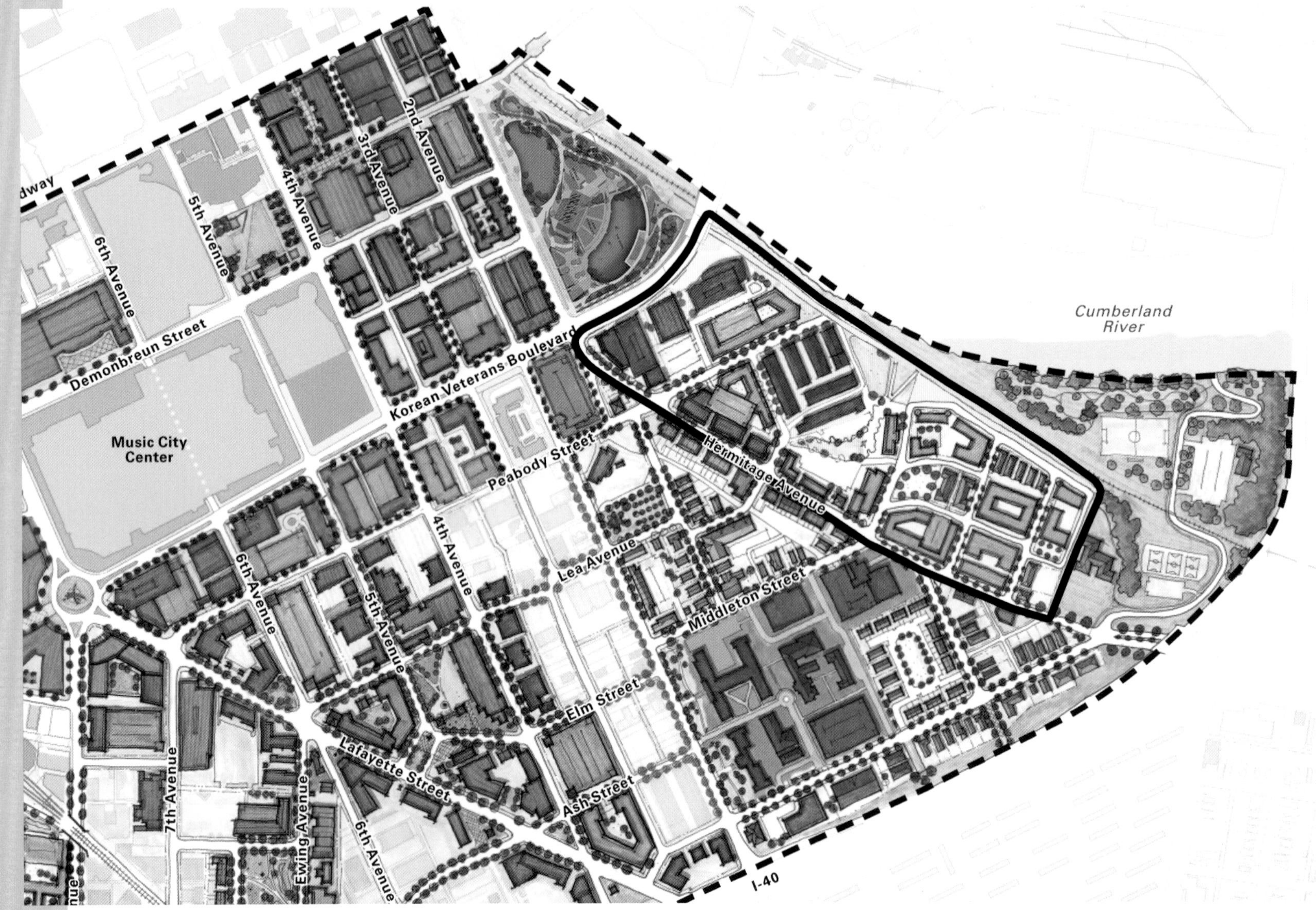

Rolling Mill Hill area indicated within the *South of Broadway Strategic Master Plan.* (Plan, 2013: Urban Design Associates)

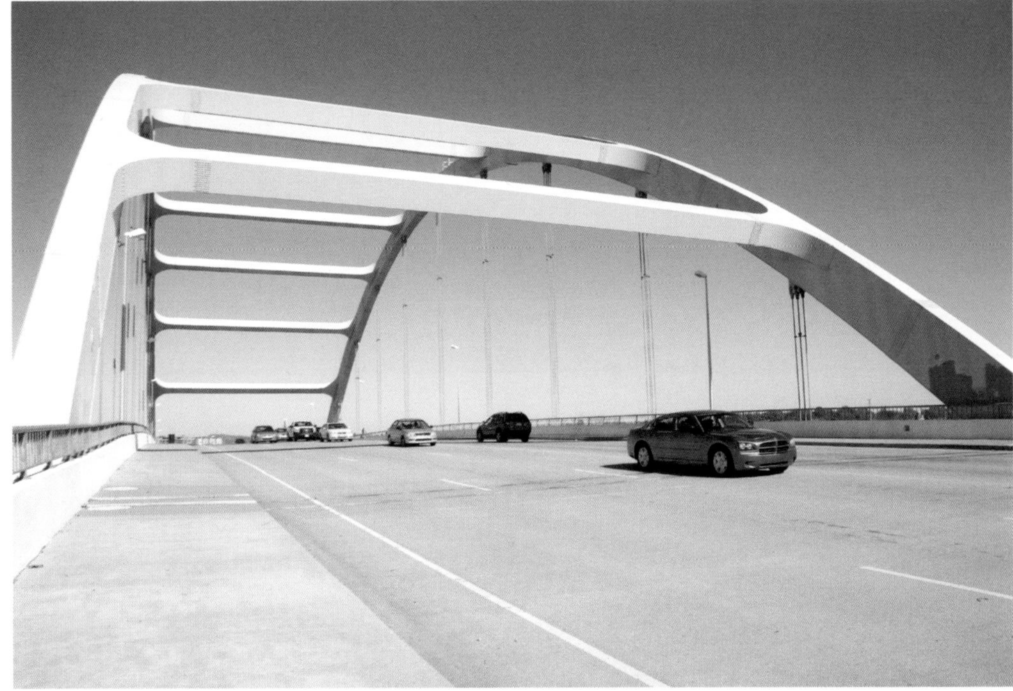

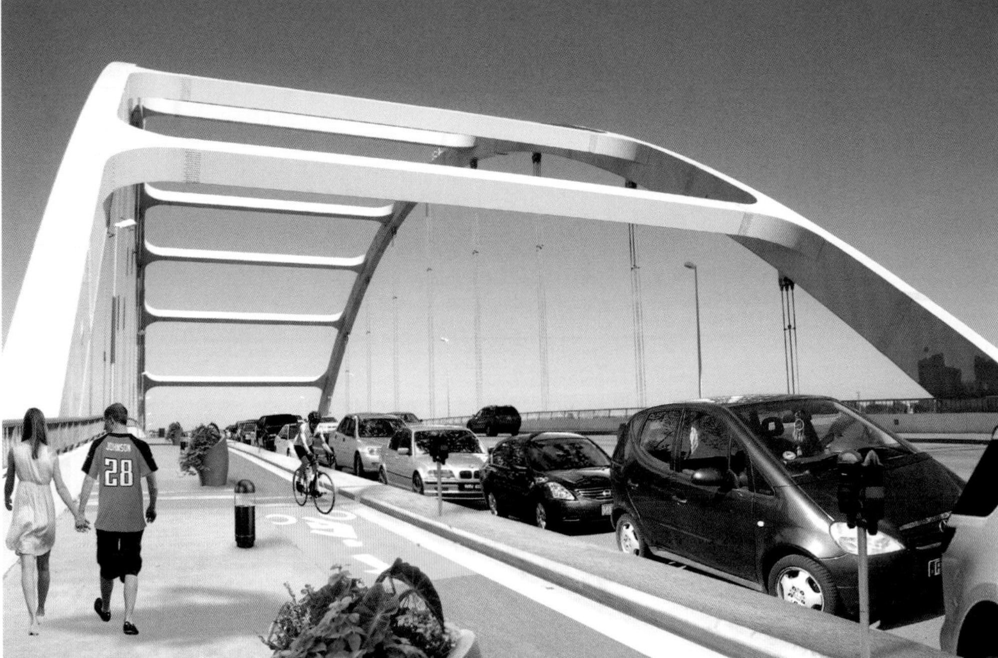

The Golden Gate Bridge in San Francisco is only 90 feet wide, has six 10-foot-wide lanes, a shared bicycle and pedestrian lane, and handles over 100,000 cars daily.[27] Contrast this to the proposed redesign for the Korean Veterans Bridge. *(Drawings, 2013: Eric Hoke, NCDC)*

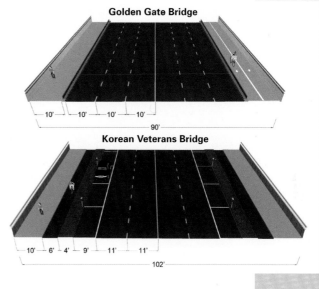

Golden Gate Bridge

10' 10' 10' 10'
90'

Korean Veterans Bridge

10' 6' 4' 9' 11' 11'
102'

STRATEGY: *Implement new streetscaping and traffic calming on the Korean Veterans Bridge. Such improvements to a bridge that has more than enough vehicular capacity could create a direct active-transportation connection between Rolling Mill Hill and the East Bank, with its links to the greenway system.*

Before: The 100-foot-wide Korean Veterans Bridge is currently striped for six 12-foot lanes of traffic that handle approximately 15,000 cars daily.[28] This is much more vehicular capacity than is needed. The posted speed limit is 40 mph, but cars often travel at 50 mph or more due to the interstate-width lane proportions. *(2013)*

After: By performing a "road diet" on the Korean Veterans Bridge that removes one vehicular travel lane in each direction, the right-of-way can accommodate new on-street parking and protected bike lanes. Narrower lanes slow vehicular speeds, which is safer for pedestrians, cyclists, and motorists alike. *(Visualization, 2013: Eric Hoke, NCDC)*

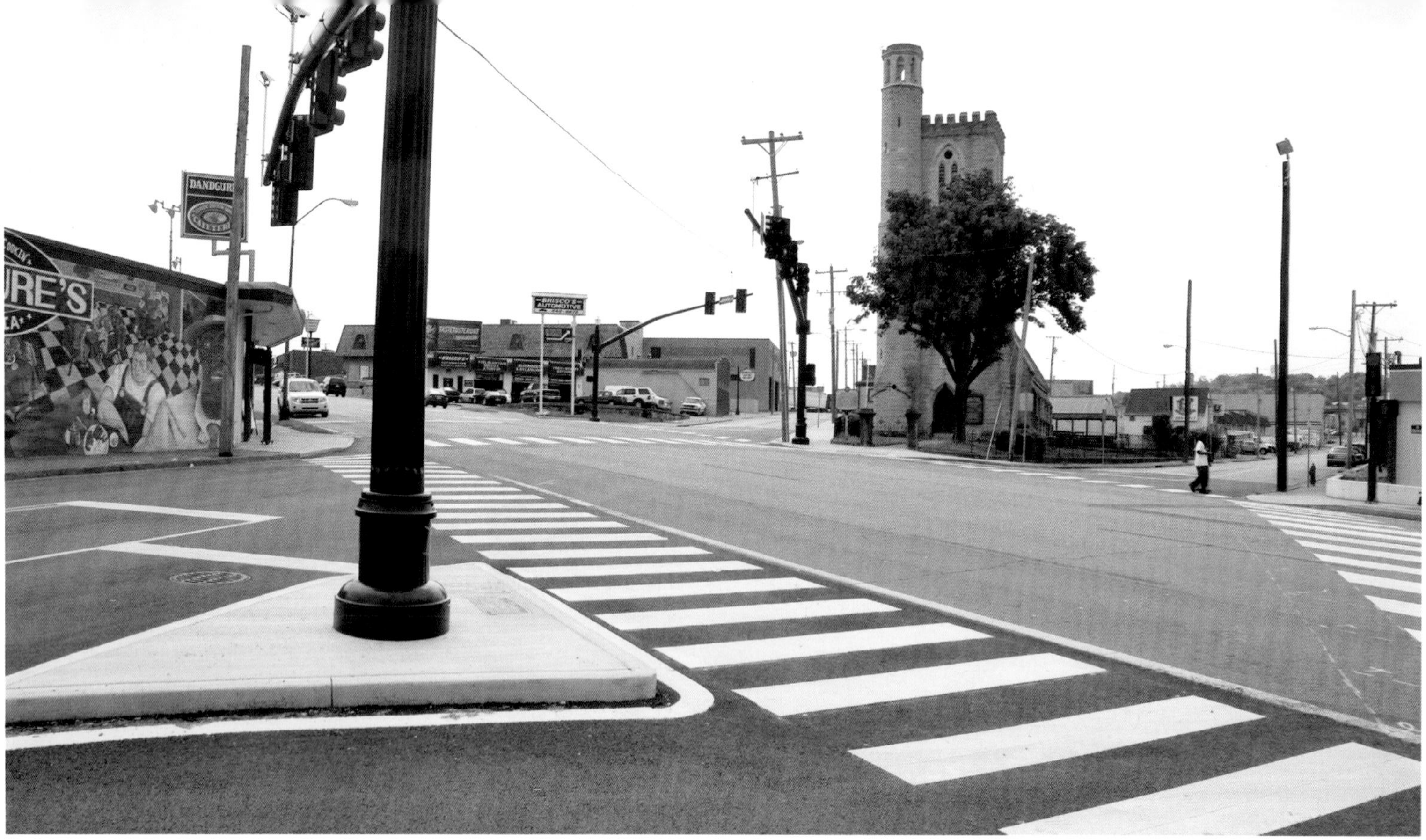

Lafayette Street, the main artery through the neighborhood, as viewed from Sixth Avenue looking south. Note the historic stone Holy Trinity Episcopal Church. *(2013)*

LAFAYETTE

The term "neighborhood" is a bit of a misnomer for the Lafayette area, which, although within walking distance of the bustling entertainment district of Lower Broadway, is characterized by light industrial uses, surface parking lots, significant blight, and lack of residential development.[29]

The primary residents are overnight ones: homeless individuals who take nightly refuge in the Nashville Rescue Mission and Campus for Human Development's emergency shelters. Many of Nashville's primary homeless service providers are clustered in the area. The Room in the Inn opened its $13 million state-of-the-art Campus for Human Development in 2010.[30] The new five-story building features 38 affordable apartments and spaces for classrooms, dining, and support services, and is a model for helping homeless individuals transition into more stable housing.

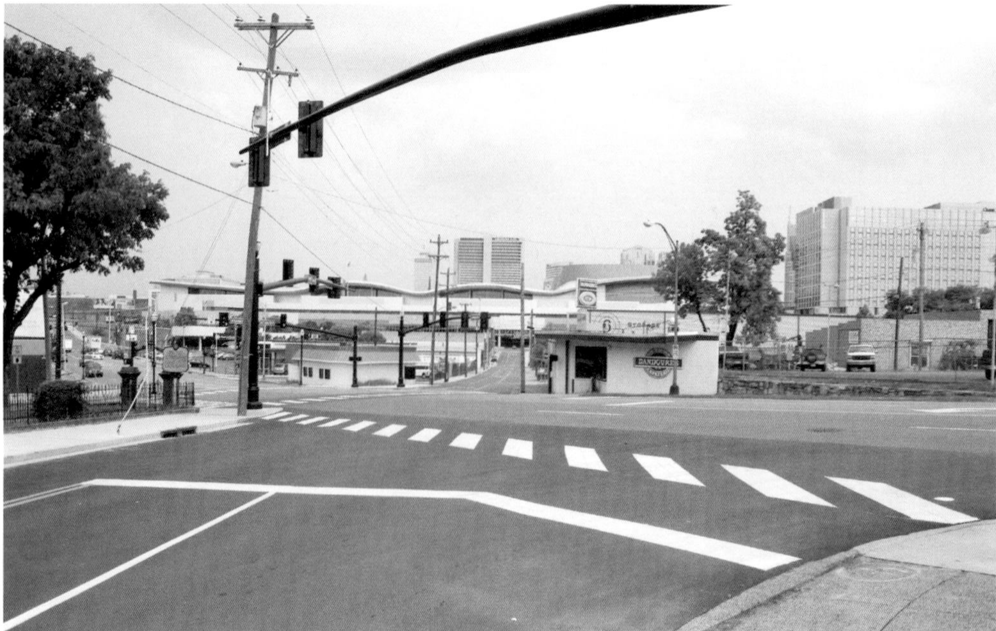

Sixth Avenue crossing Lafayette Street looking north to downtown. *(2013)*

The area's low-density development includes a variety of business types—including artist and photography supply stores, publishing houses, auto repair facilities, and several adult entertainment establishments—with few restaurants and little retail. A new Greyhound bus terminal was built in 2012. The area is home to a several historic churches and Rocketown, a youth-oriented nonprofit that features an indoor skate park and music venue.

A master plan for the entire area south of Broadway to the interstate was completed in January 2013.[31] The plan will guide development and provides strategic initiatives for flood mitigation and sustainability, increased open space and parks, and a better connected street network, all to enhance the private development potential of the area. The plan also encourages improvements to the area's connectivity with the neighboring Gulch, Rolling Mill Hill, and central business districts.

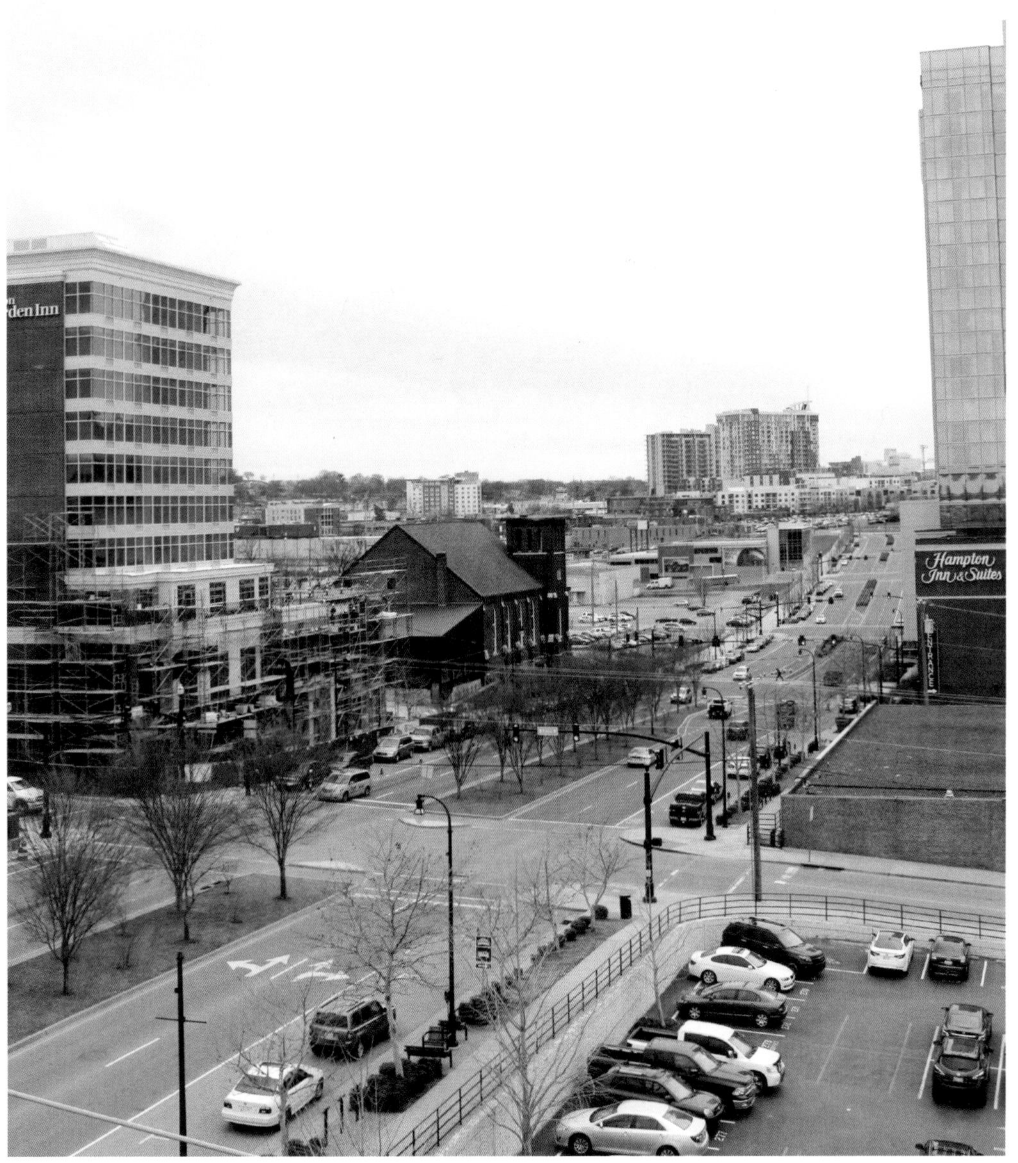

In 1997, *The Plan for SoBro* proposed a roundabout at Eighth Avenue as a way to tame what was then called the Franklin Corridor and turn a high-speed roadway into a boulevard.[32] Fifteen years later the concept was implemented, creating the potential for grand civic space and opportunities for large mixed-use developments at the terminus of what is now Korean Veterans Boulevard (KVB). The boulevard features a broad median strip and street trees. The Music City Center opened in May 2013 on the north side of KVB and has so far spurred significant development, primarily hotels to supply rooms to conventioneers. *(2015)*

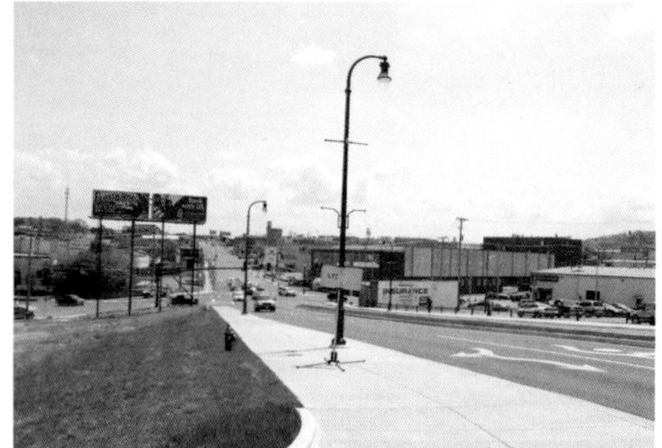

Lafayette Street, view looking southeast from the KVB roundabout. *(2013)*

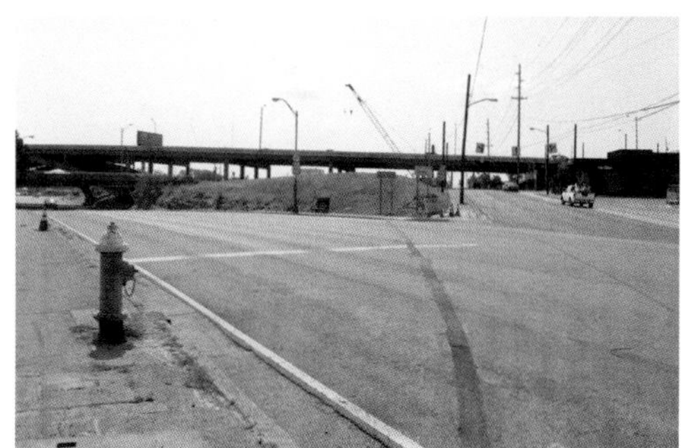

Pedestrian nightmare: intersection of Lafayette Street and Fourth Avenue, looking south. *(2013)*

Map showing the comparable walking distances (approximately 1.2 miles for each) from the Music City Center on Demonbreun Street north to the Bicentennial Mall-Farmers' Market, and south to the Adventure Science Center and Ft. Negley area. Both are easily walkable in terms of distance, but the route to the south is a pedestrian danger zone. *(Diagram over map, 2013: Eric Hoke, NCDC)*

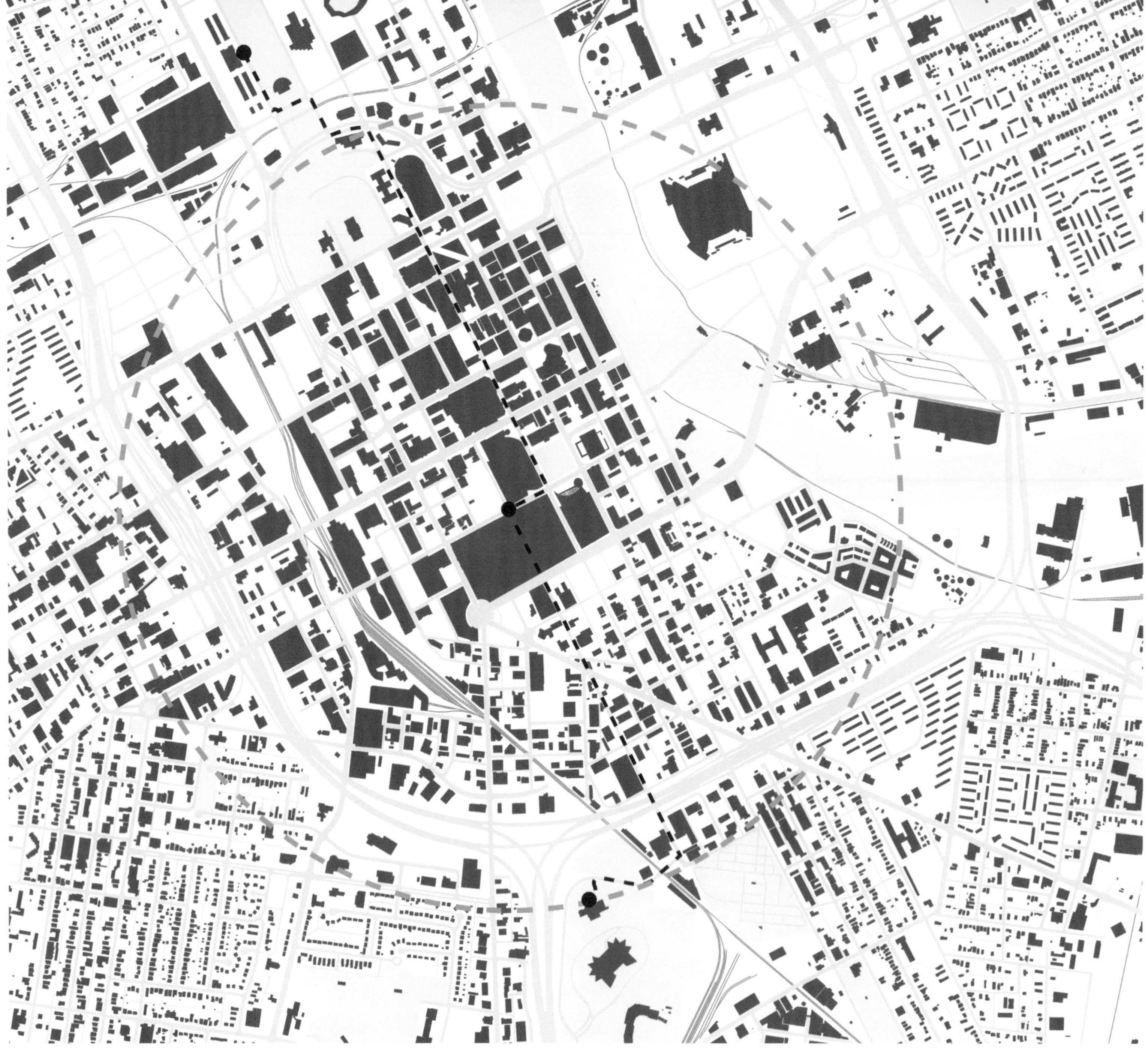

STRATEGY: *Implement new streetscaping along Sixth Avenue South to create a more pedestrian-friendly connection to Nashville's historic City Cemetery and up the hill to the Adventure Science Center and Fort Negley.*

STRATEGY: *Amplify the mixture of land uses in Lafayette. The development of housing in the area would enable it to function as a residential neighborhood; emphasis should be on a diversity of housing types and prices.*

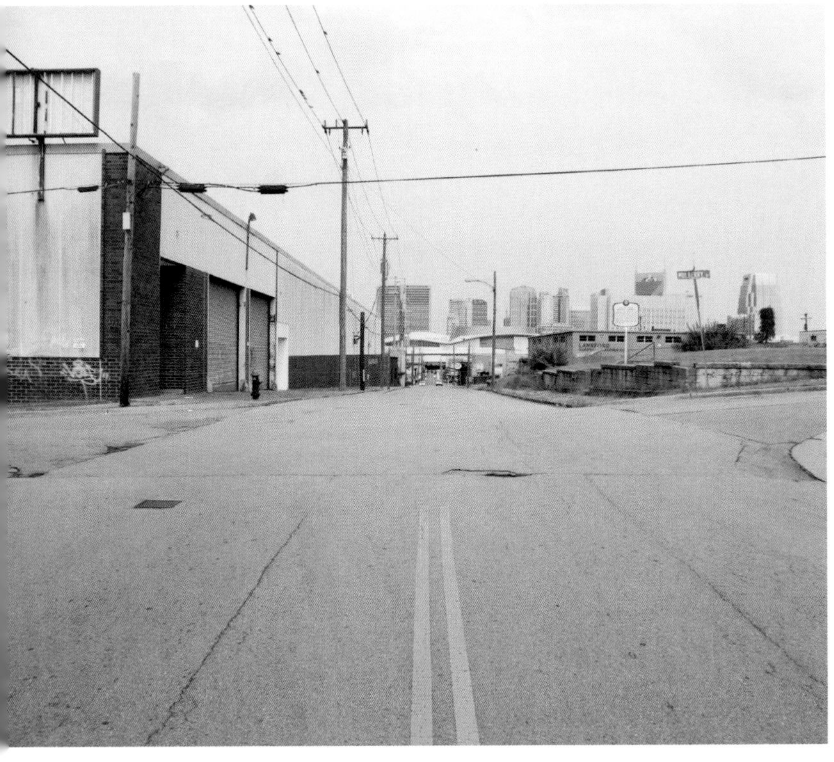

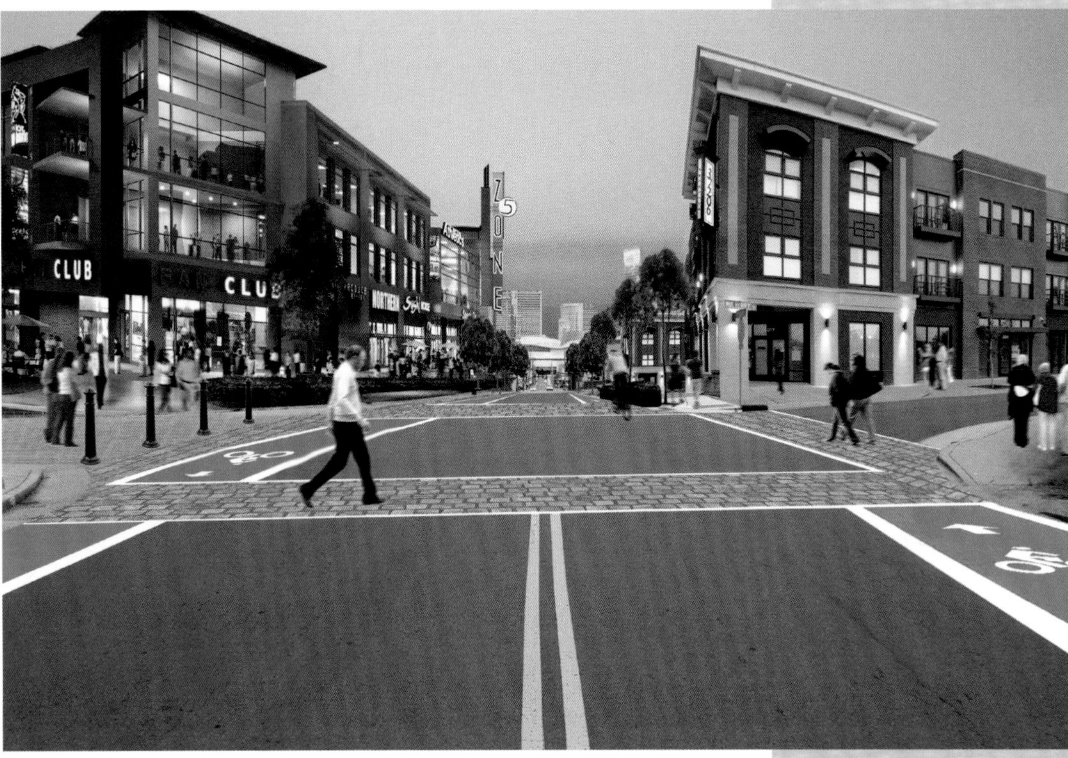

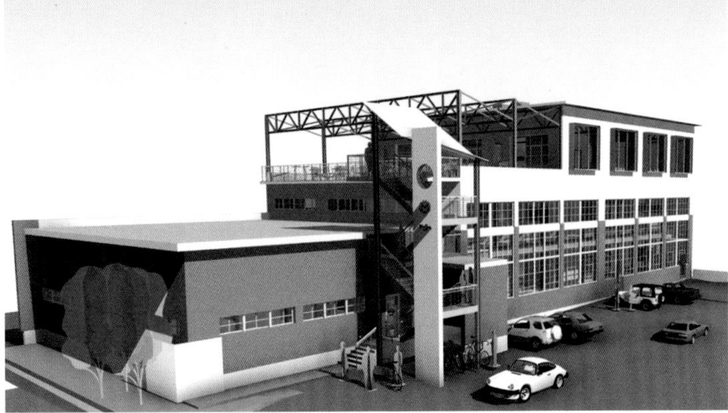

STRATEGY: *Utilize the areas underneath the interstate along the southern edge of the Lafayette neighborhood as public space to mitigate the negative impact on this link to the neighborhoods located to the south.*

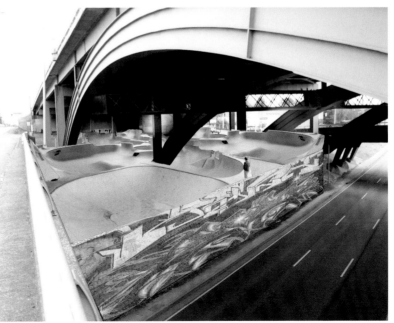

Top left: Existing conditions along Sixth Avenue South; walkers are rare for obvious reasons. *(2013)*

Top right: Pedestrian-friendly streetscaping, bicycle infrastructure, and mid-rise, mixed-use development proposed for Sixth Avenue South. *(Visualization, 2013: Eric Hoke, NCDC)*

Lower left: Plan for the rehab and expansion of a 9400-square-foot former print shop on Ewing Street. Now open, the INK Building houses FloThinkery along with several other creative small businesses, and an event space on the sky deck. *(Rendering, 2014: Manuel Zeitlin Architects)*

Lower right: Concept of turning the currently vacant space under the interstate into a skate park. *(Visualization, 2011: Ron Yearwood, NCDC)*

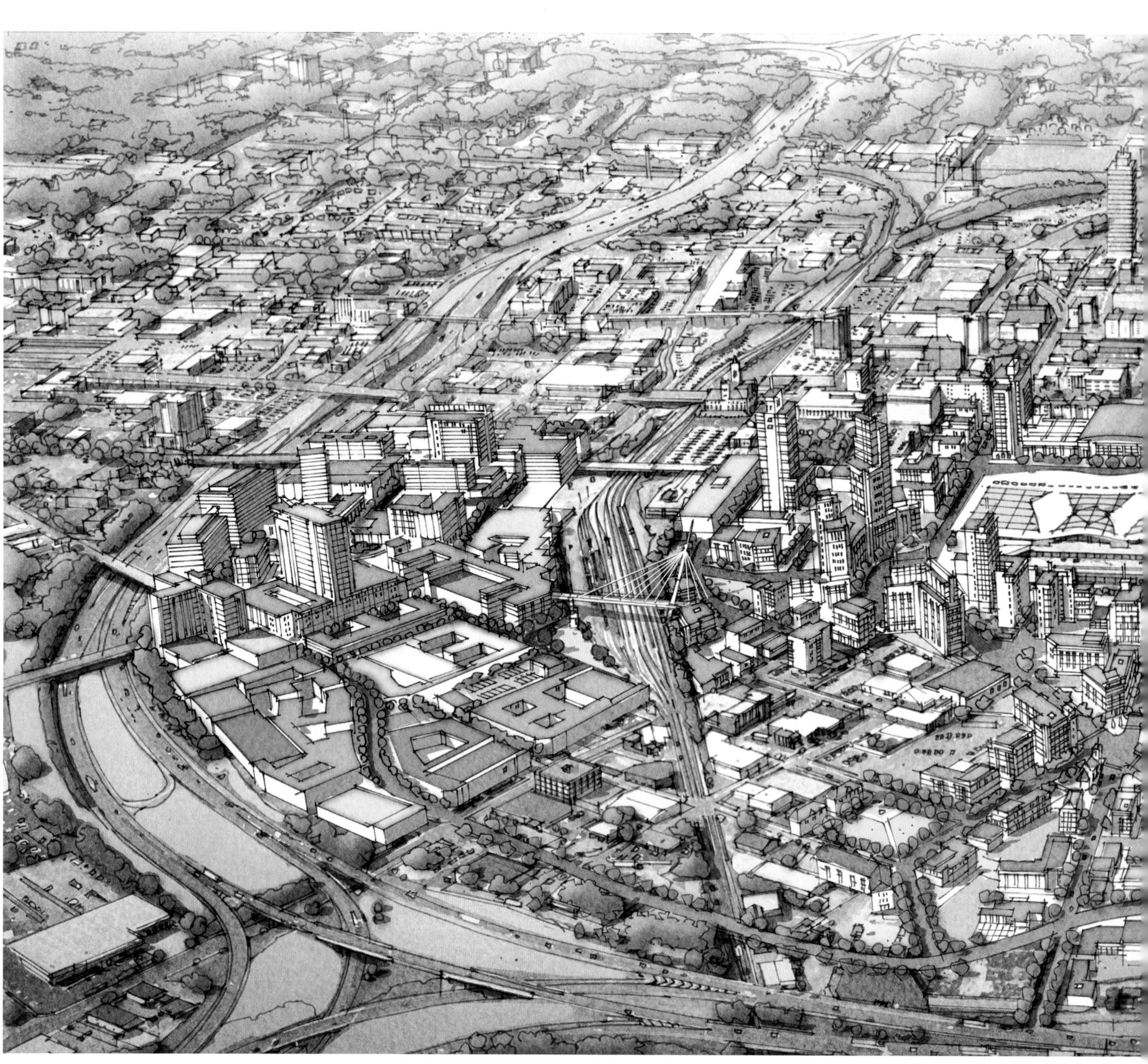

Vision of the area south of Broadway showing a connected street grid, parks, and a multitude of new buildings that create an active, pedestrian-friendly community. *(Rendering, 2013:* South of Broadway Strategic Master Plan, *Urban Design Associates)*

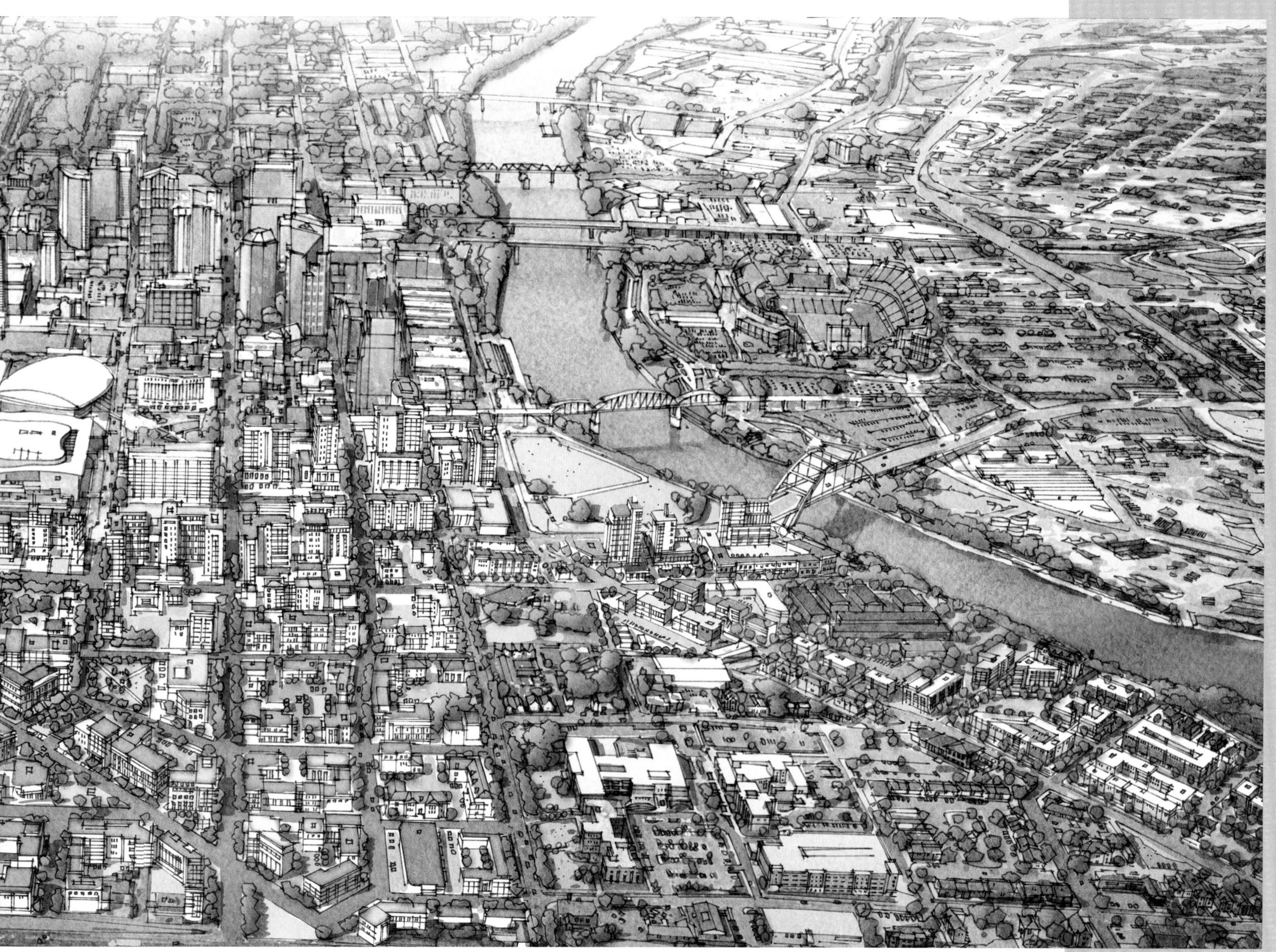

Bottom right; opposite page: Room in the Inn features 38 efficiency apartments and ongoing case management for residents, providing an uninterrupted pathway for homeless individuals transitioning from living on the streets to permanent supportive housing. (2011: Jeff Moles, Room in the Inn; 2010: American Constructors)

Housing the Homeless for Health

"We hold these truths to be self-evident, that all men are created equal, that they are endowed by their Creator with certain unalienable Rights, that among these are Life, Liberty and the pursuit of Happiness." So states our nation's Declaration of Independence, written and published in 1776 and one of the world's most famous assertions of human rights.

Life and liberty, not to mention the pursuit of happiness, are problematic for those who must live outside a regular dwelling. It is difficult to ascertain with precision how many Nashvillians exist in this condition. In an attempt to measure the parameters of this population, Nashville participates in an annual Point In Time (PIT) count. Volunteers canvass the city during a single winter night to record the number of people sleeping outdoors, in campsites, in cars, and in emergency shelters. The count does not measure people who stay in motels or are residing temporarily with family or friends. Each year at least 2,200 people who experience homelessness are counted during one night, providing the city with a snapshot of the overall population.

Experts on homelessness have established a clear link between health outcomes and homelessness. The National Health Care for the Homeless Council (NHCHC), which is headquartered in Nashville, reports that homeless individuals' life expectancy is estimated to be between 42 and 52 years, much lower than the life expectancy of 78 years for the housed population.[33] The mortality rate for people who experience chronic homelessness, according to the US Interagency Council on Homelessness, is four to nine times higher than that of the general population.[34] Chronic homelessness is considered long-term, and is roughly ascribed to individuals who have a disabling condition and have been homeless for one year or longer, or who have experienced four episodes of homelessness within the past three years.[35] Families fall under the chronic category if one family member fits the chronic definition.

Homeless individuals are three to six times more likely to suffer from illness than housed people.[36] In addition, heart disease, cancer, liver disease, skin infections, HIV/AIDS, pneumonia, and tuberculosis are common among people experiencing homelessness.[37] From this census of disease and death we can easily deduce that permanent housing plays a major role in the well-being of people, which is why experts and advocates focusing on solutions to homelessness speak of housing as a major aspect of health care.[38]

Housing assistance is one of the highest needs identified in Davidson County.[39] As rent rates increase and affordable housing units slowly disappear, it is difficult to find housing opportunities for people transitioning out of homelessness. The average rent in Davidson County for a two-bedroom apartment in 2015 was approximately $1,300; for a one-bedroom apartment it was about $1,050, an average increase of 25 percent in two years.[40] If a homeless person receives a rent subsidy under the federal Section 8 Housing Choice Voucher Program, however, he or she must find an apartment for approximately $650, the maximum rental payment allowance set by the local public housing authority.

Communitywide discussions around long-term solutions need to look beyond current services and even beyond linking people who are homeless with existing low-income housing opportunities. We need to determine how we, as a community, preserve and increase our affordable, low-income housing stock. We also need to develop strategies to ensure that people with very low incomes (below 50 percent of the median family income of an area[41]) have a way to maintain their housing. Until Nashville does so, improving health outcomes for this population is not within reach. Cities like Chicago have already started this discussion.[42]

Generally, affordable housing means dwellings on which people spend no more than one-third of their household income on rent. That principle does not work for people who have an extremely low income. For many individuals who have experienced long-term homelessness, their social security and/or disability benefits are their main income. Monthly disability checks average $710 a month.

In Nashville, the Metropolitan Homelessness Commission launched a campaign called *How's Nashville,* which is derived from the *100,000 Homes Campaign,* a national effort to house 100,000 vulnerable and chronically homeless individuals across the country by July 2014. The purpose of the *How's Nashville* campaign is to foster collaboration among stakeholders from the nonprofit, business, faith-based, private, and government sectors. One goal is to improve our local system with regard to the housing placement rate and the retention of housing for individuals and families experiencing homelessness or at risk of homelessness.

Homelessness is a public health issue because it is lethal. Last year, 52 people who died in Nashville while they were homeless were remembered at the annual Homeless Memorial. The local campaign team wants to reduce street deaths in our community by implementing

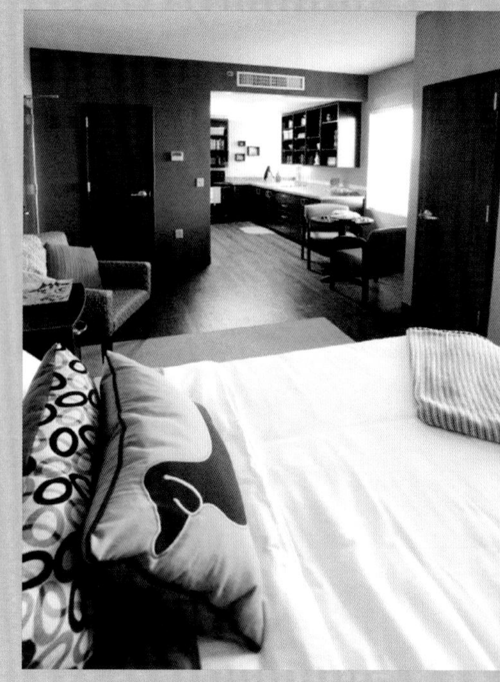

permanent solutions to homelessness. *How's Nashville* partners believe that homelessness can be solved if we, as a community:

- Work together;
- Utilize the resources we already have in a more collaborative and outcome-oriented manner;
- Monitor our progress and become more data-driven;
- Search for more resources using data.

Launched in June of 2013, the *How's Nashville* campaign now has more than 30 partner organizations. Between June and December of that year, our community assisted 356 people who were chronically homeless and/or among the most vulnerable population.

One way we can improve the health and mortality rates for low-income individuals and families is by addressing their housing needs. Nashville has taken the first step by establishing a housing trust fund called the Barnes Fund for Affordable Housing to maintain and expand our affordable housing stock for people with low incomes. It is crucial to expand the resources of this Fund. Another effort underway is the *How's Nashville*'s partners' next goal to implement a coordinated entry system in Nashville, which will create a clearer path from streets to housing. A third objective is to move away from segregated housing developments for low-income residents toward scattered site housing properties. These units will look like regular market rent housing and fit seamlessly into existing neighborhoods.

Now is the time for Nashville's city planners and developers to address how to make our built environment function for all populations, including people with very low incomes. Then we can ensure that all who were created equal have a chance to fully experience their human rights.

—JUDITH TACKETT, communications coordinator, Metropolitan Homelessness Commission

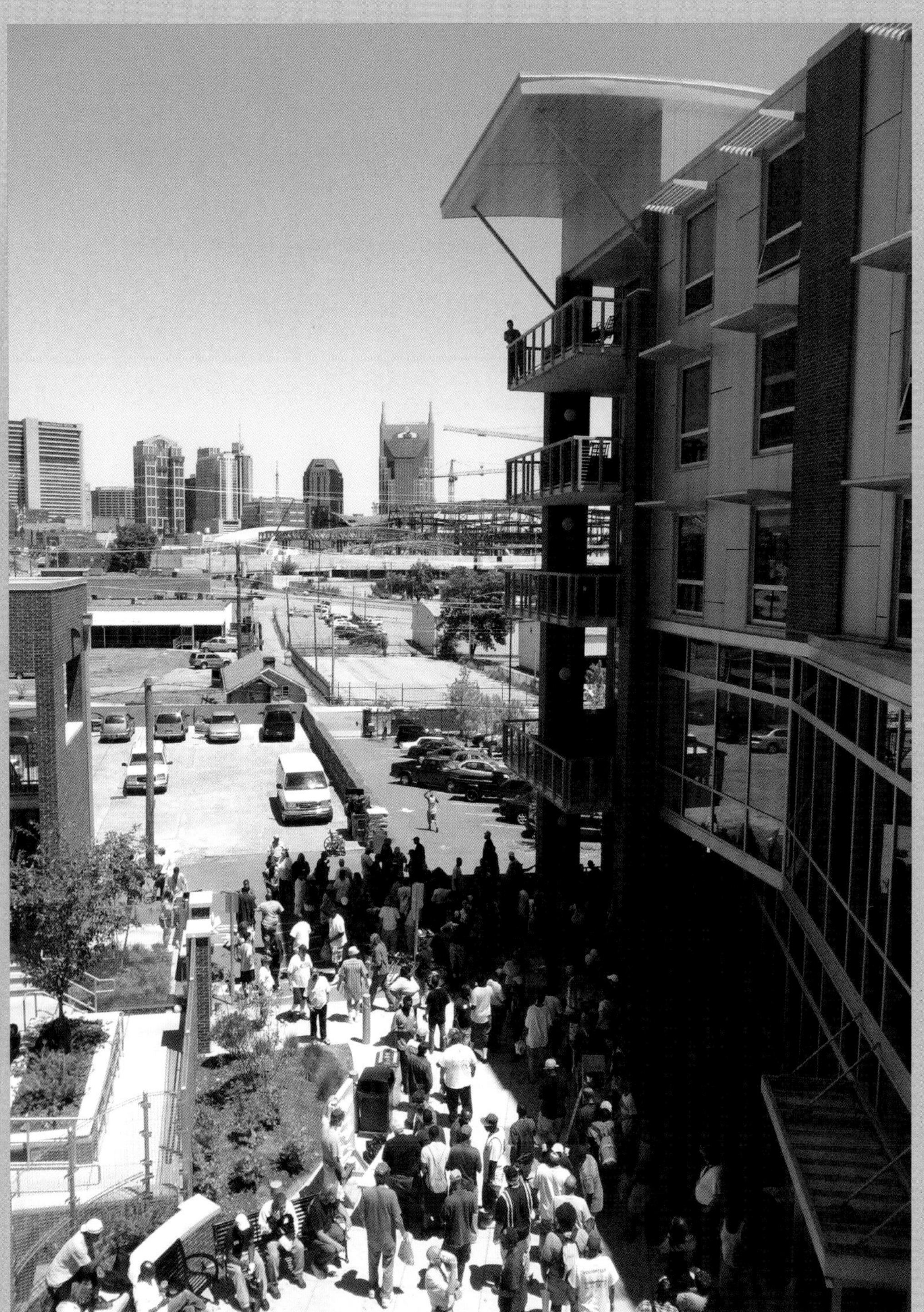

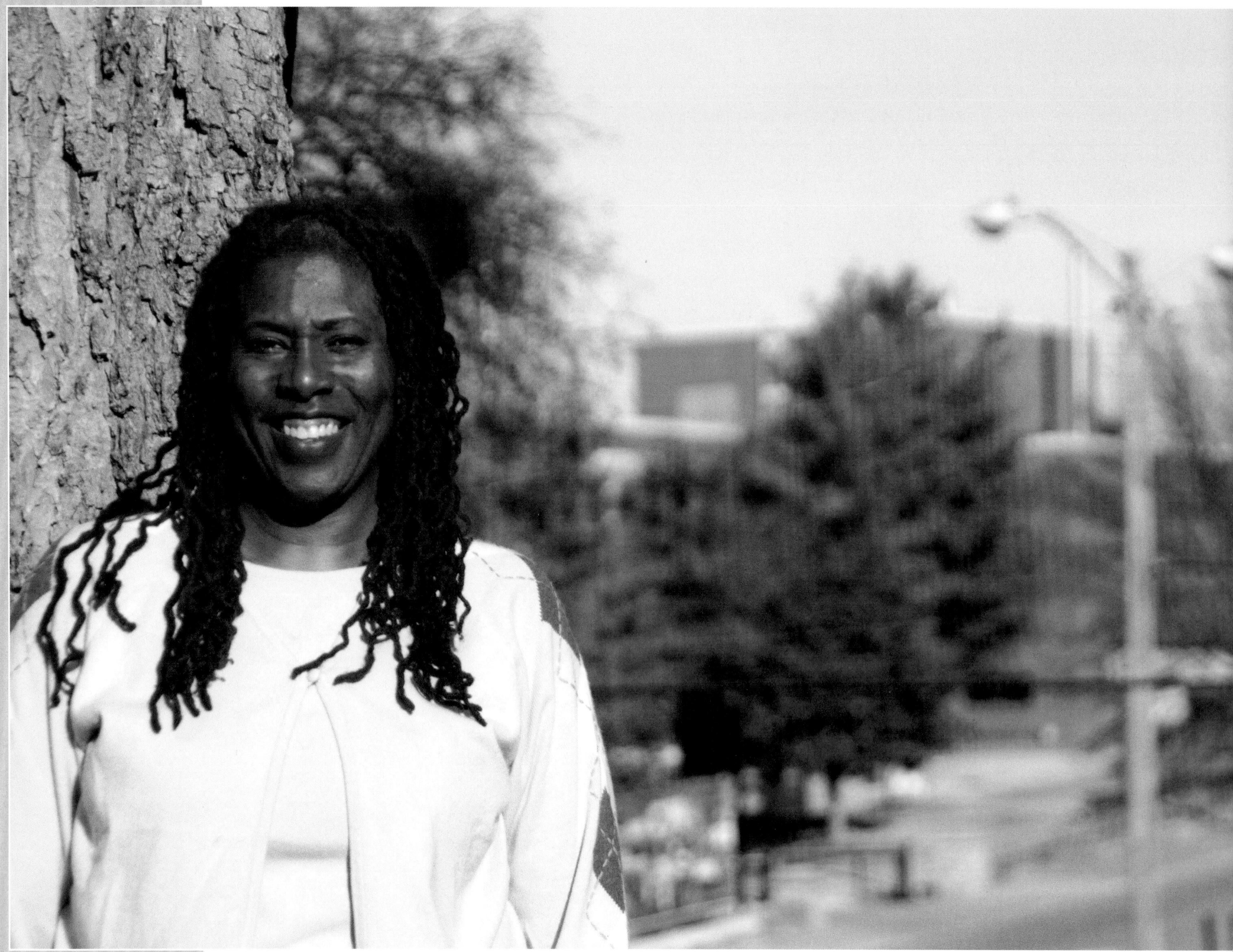

LESLIE SPELLER-HENDERSON

Leslie Speller-Henderson is an assistant professor in the Department of Family and Consumer Sciences of the College of Agriculture, Human, and Natural Sciences at Tennessee State University (TSU). She coordinates the Tennessee State University Nutrition Education Program.

As a wife and the mother of three young adults—two college students and an entrepreneur—Speller-Henderson understands the issues that young people and families face as they navigate through the challenges and rewards of making healthy choices. Her family encourages her work in good nutrition because her children lived all that she teaches and preaches.

Speller-Henderson lived in North Nashville in the Osage–North Fisk neighborhood, about a mile from TSU, for over ten years before moving to West Nashville in 2012. While living in North Nashville, she was able to walk between home and work. "What I liked about my particular neighborhood was it had sidewalks and alleys. I used to walk an hour each morning in North Nashville. People would say, 'I'd join you but you get up too early in the morning.' That's the best time of the day. It's as quiet then as an urban area can be.

"The TSU community garden is in its fourth year. People are growing more tomatoes, peppers, and greens than they could have imagined. There's been a lost generation of gardeners in the African American community.

"Historically, slaves farmed or tended the farms for the master. Then it became sharecropping. Parents told their children, 'Go to college and get an education; never farm again.' Now, we understand that cooking and eating the simple foods that are grown in a garden will get our health back in our hands.

"TSU's main campus is closed to cars. You park on the outside of campus and walk in. The current generation of students has always had cars. They drive from one spot, go to class, get in the car again, and go around campus to the other side. They complain about not enough parking. When I walk on campus students ask me, 'You're going to walk over there?' I say, 'Yeah, it's okay. Wear comfortable shoes!'

"I've seen one or two students at TSU campus biking and skateboarding. It's more a method of getting from Point A to Point B when the car is not working.

"I won't say it's safe biking. You don't see helmets. With hair like mine, which is a lot, it's hard to get a helmet on it. So I don't bike.

"There's also feelings that the community around TSU, Meharry, and Fisk is not safe. Sometimes I think if enough people went outside, say to a park, the people doing things they don't want other people to see would go away.

"What people do with their leisure time is the big question. Are we willing to fit activities into our leisure time? I can't say that we are. There are play areas at the local schools that kids could easily bike or walk to. But I don't see them using the spaces for a pick-up game of football. When you let kids go outside and play it becomes a safe neighborhood once again.

"Tennessee State University has been in the same location since 1921 and used to provide faculty housing in the community surrounding the campus. But then that interstate [I-40] came through and split the neighborhood. The interstate also gave people the ability to move to other parts of town, leaving the older houses vacant. The community has also become run down with Section 8 housing, where tenants do not respect their property or each other, causing a safety issue.

"With suburban sprawl development, there's no requirement to move beyond getting out of our cars in our garages, closing our garage doors, and being at home in our cocoons. TSU has the Ralph Boston Wellness Center; the challenge is getting faculty and staff to use it. If you're going to exercise, you have to plan. And if you're going to eat healthy, you have to plan to cook."

7

Destination Retail District—Includes large retail footprints that are auto-centric in nature, typically surrounded by parking lots.

Employment Center District—Features intense economic activity; can include light industry as well as office uses, along with amenities for workers and often a campus-like setting.

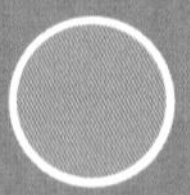

Impact District—Includes hazardous industrial operations, mineral extraction and processing, major transportation terminals, correctional facilities, major utility installations, landfills, large amusement and entertainment complexes, and other large scale land uses that pose some form of safety or security risk.

Industrial District—Includes light to heavy non-hazardous manufacturing, storage, distribution, contractor businesses, and wholesaling.

Major Institutional District—Includes colleges and universities, major health care facilities, and other large-scale community services that pose no safety threats to the adjacent communities.

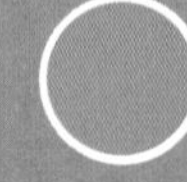

Office Concentration District—Office uses as well as amenities like retail and food for those who work in the area.[1]

THE DISTRICT TRANSECT ZONE

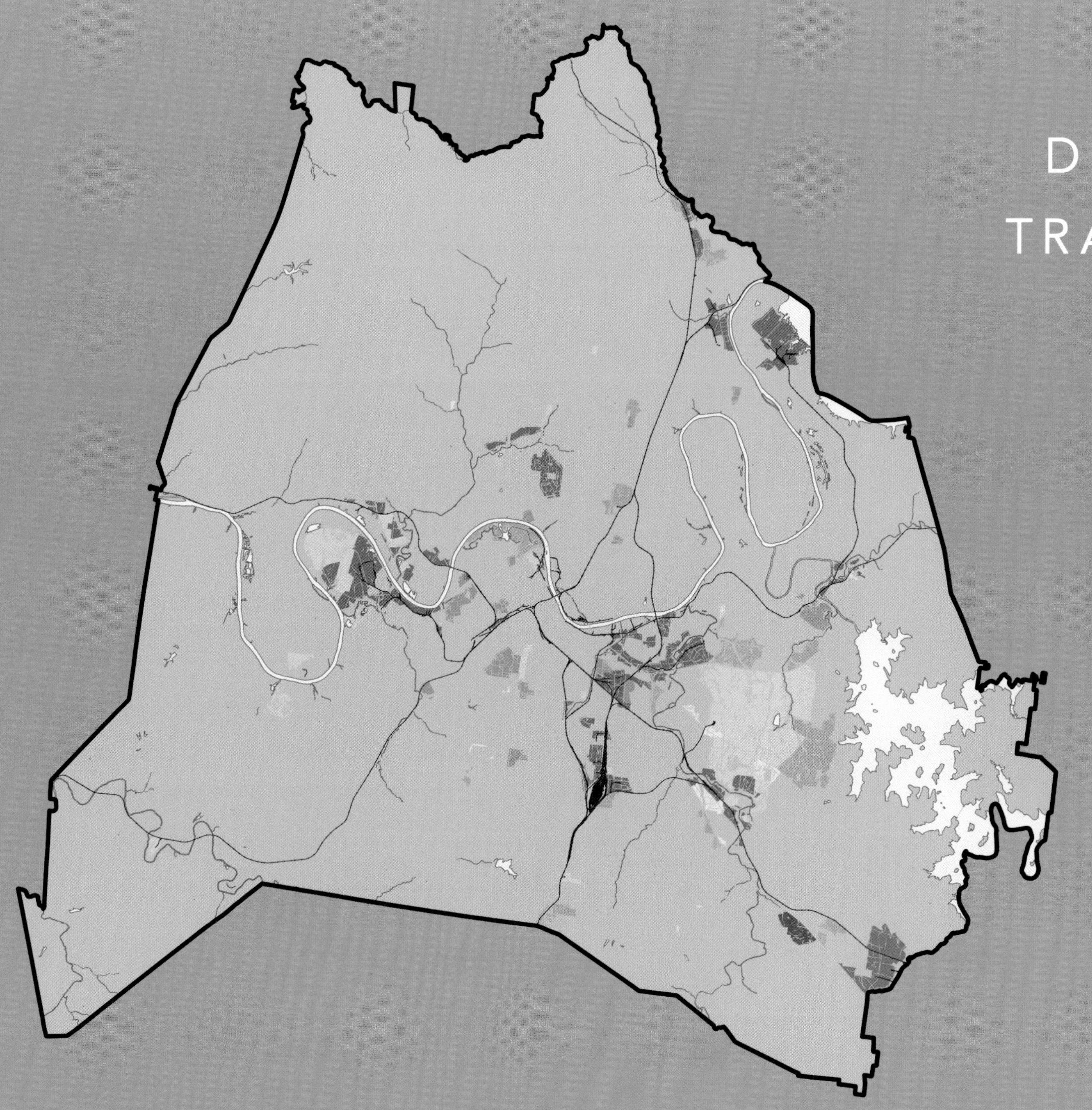

Davidson County with the six district transect subzones highlighted. The district transect zone is comprised of expansive land areas that feature a primary or even single land use. Within Davidson County the district zone occupies almost 30,000 acres—8.8 percent of the county's total land—and houses 6 percent of the total population.[2] Each type of district has its own unique set of characteristics and land usage needs (Map, 2014: Metro Planning Department)

SHAPING HEALTH IN THE DISTRICT TRANSECT ZONE

EMPLOYMENT CENTER AND OFFICE CONCENTRATION DISTRICT

Employment center and office concentration districts feature intense economic activity, can include light industry, and often have a campus-like setting. Both include office use and some amenities for workers, such as retail and food. Residential areas are sometimes located along the periphery but are not fully integrated. Large areas of open space may be provided for employees to use during their free time.

STRATEGY: *Convert office concentration districts to mixed use, live/work communities.*

STRATEGY: *Integrate high-density multifamily housing into employment centers and office concentration districts. Insure that a variety of unit sizes and prices exist to incorporate a range of options. This will provide housing in close proximity to workplaces.*

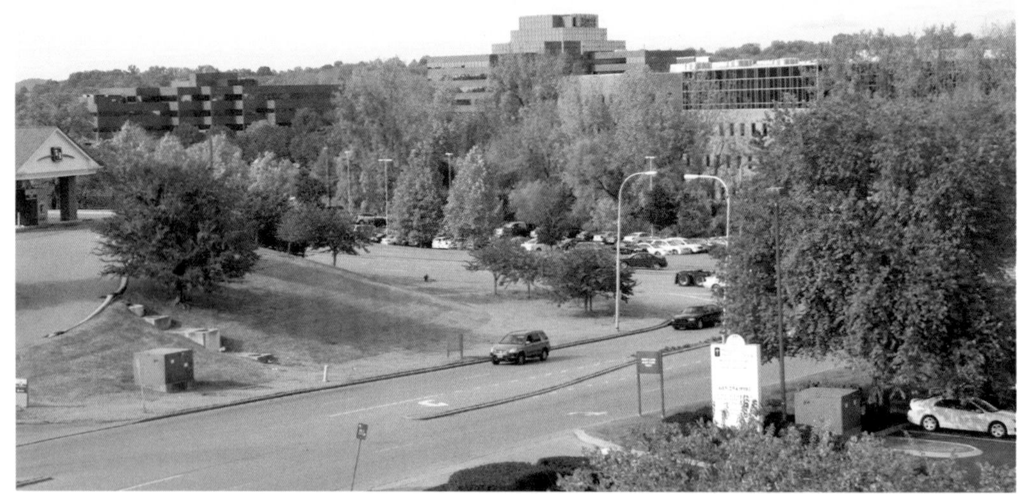

Metro Center, an 800-acre office park north of downtown. It was developed in the 1970s in the Cumberland River floodplain, which is protected by a levee. *(2013)*

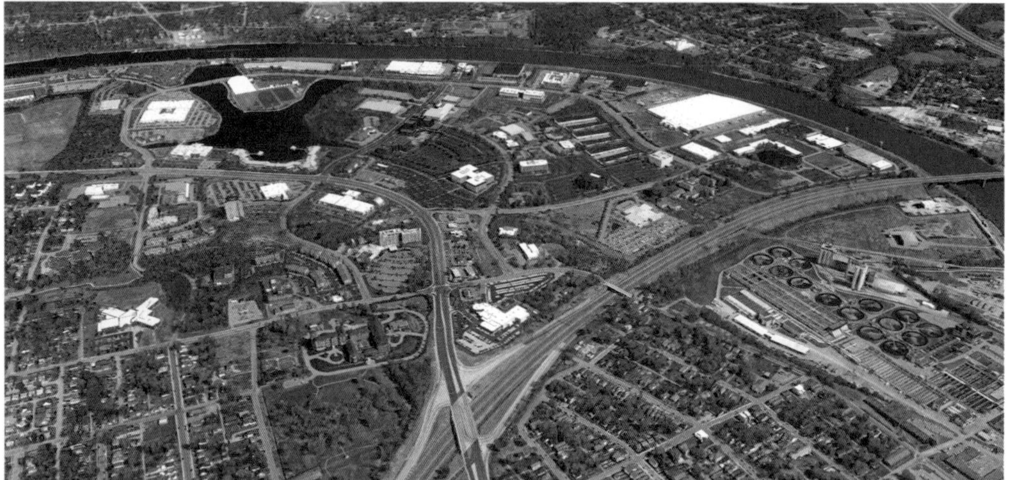

Metro Center: Existing conditions. *(2014: ©Google)*

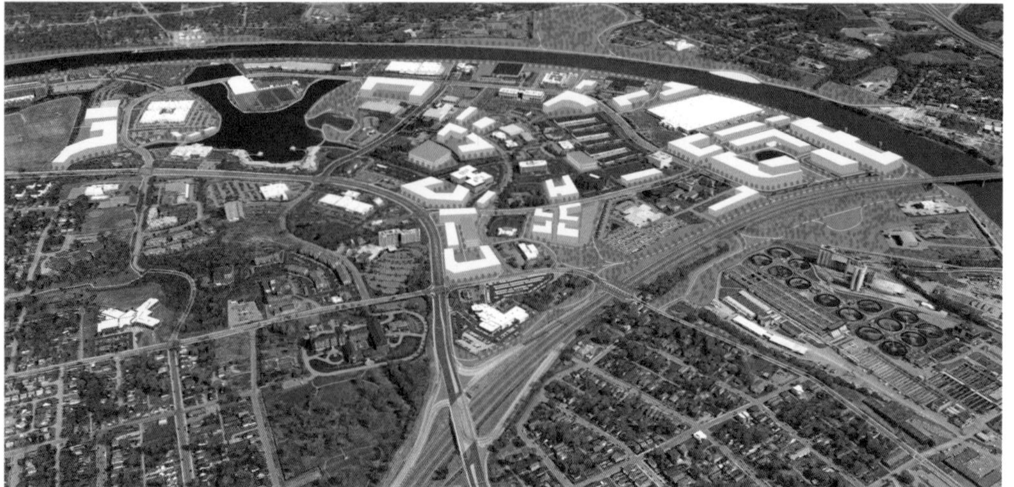

Metro Center with mixed-use infill and significant new residential development on vacant land and parking lots. Note increased open space connectivity via greenways. *(Visualization, 2015: Eric Hoke, NCDC)*

IMPACT DISTRICT

Includes hazardous industrial operations, mineral extraction and processing, major transportation terminals, correctional facilities, major utility installations, landfills, large amusement and entertainment complexes, and other large-scale land uses that pose some form of a safety or security risk.

Buildings are generally low rise—three stories or less—with varying building footprints and occupy isolated sites to minimize negative impacts on nearby development and neighborhoods. Impact districts are located near accommodating infrastructure like railroad corridors and interstates. Industrial and impact districts often require seclusion or sensitive treatment because of their potential for significant negative impact on what surrounds them.

STRATEGY: *Retrofit defunct impact districts as open space and parks. Some areas that were previously used for mining, such as quarries, have been abandoned and could be turned into parks and open space for use by surrounding residents and employees.*

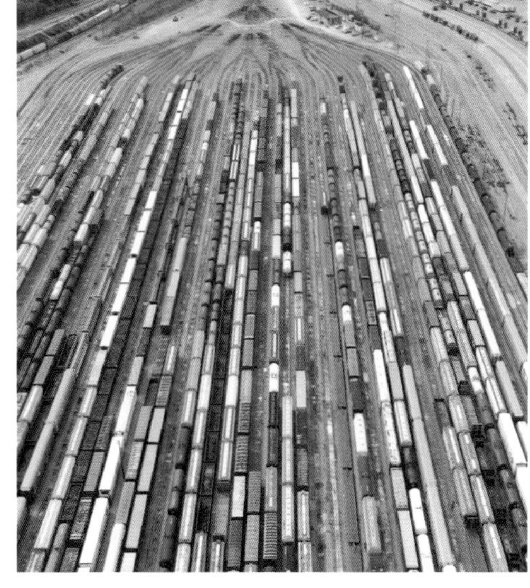

Radnor Rail Yard. *(2008: Gary Layda)*

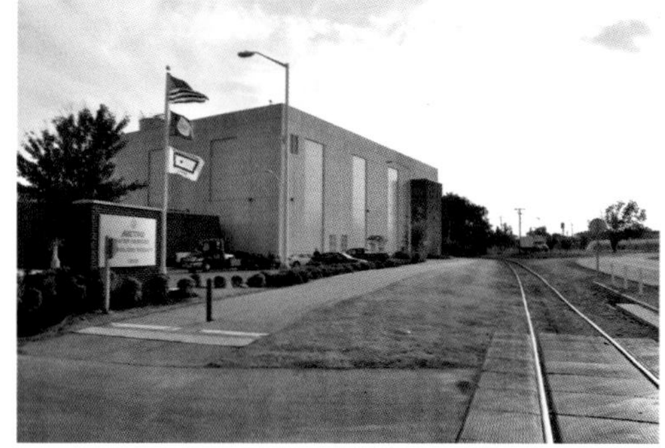

The Metro Water Treatment facility located in an industrial area along the riverfront, adjacent to the Historic Germantown neighborhood. A greenway path parallels its operations. *(2013)*

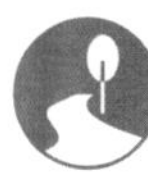

STRATEGY: *Limit the negative effects from impact districts by creating or increasing buffer zones that separate these areas from adjoining land uses.*

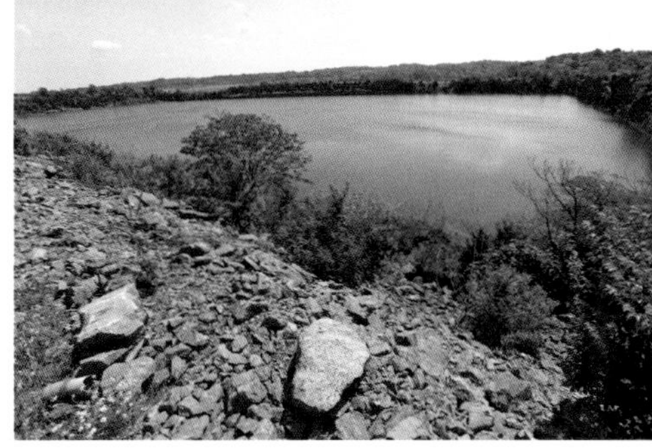

Left: In 2016, the Metropolitan Nashville Airport Authority will complete the largest geothermal lake plate cooling system in North America, located in a former 43-acre rock quarry adjacent to the airport. The system will utilize the cool deep waters of the lake that has formed in the quarry (at 150 feet deep the water is 50 degrees year round) to cool the terminal and provide irrigation to the airport's landscaping. The utility savings for the airport are expected to be $430,000 per year when completed. *(2015: Peyton Hoge Photography)*

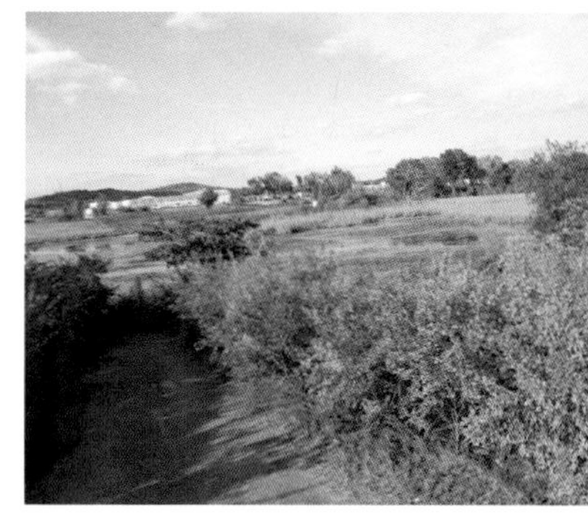

Landscaping and open spaces surrounding the TSU campus, an example of buffer areas for an institutional district or impact district. *(2013)*

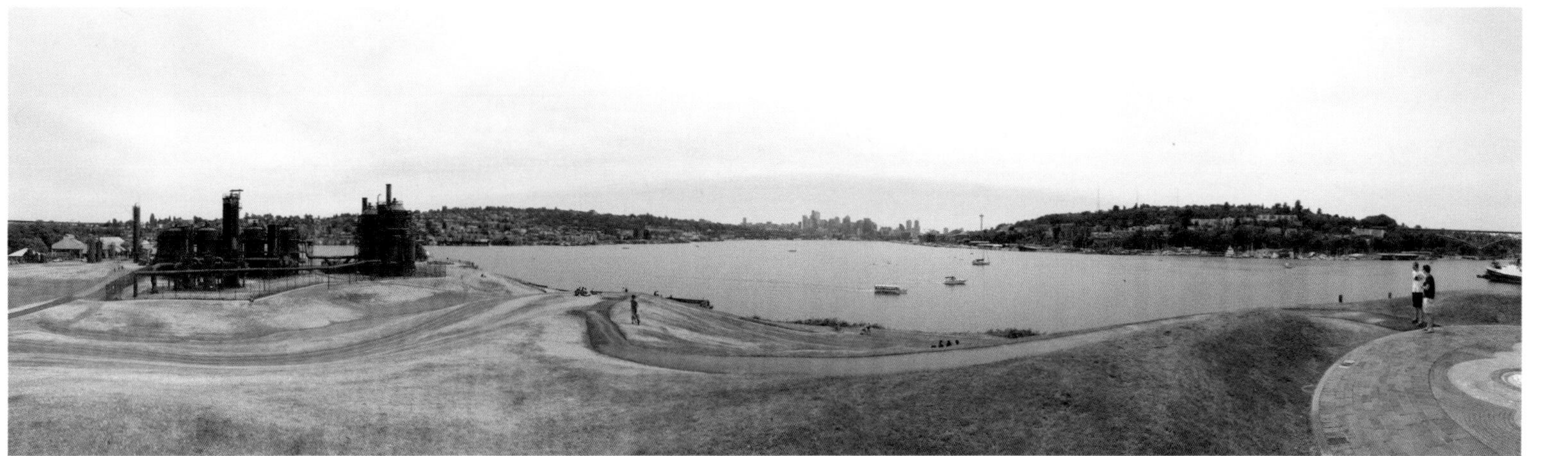

The 20-acre Gas Works Park in Seattle, WA, sits atop the site of an old gas plant. The once heavily polluted site, which was known to ooze tar into the adjacent lake, has achieved safety standards set by the EPA. Note the remnants of the old gas works, which were left as a reminder of the site's history. *(2015)*

INDUSTRIAL DISTRICT

Includes light to heavy nonhazardous manufacturing, storage, distribution, contractor businesses, and wholesaling in generally low-rise buildings. Many industrial areas located across Davidson County are secluded from other land uses. As the county's population grows, however, new residential development may approach existing industry.

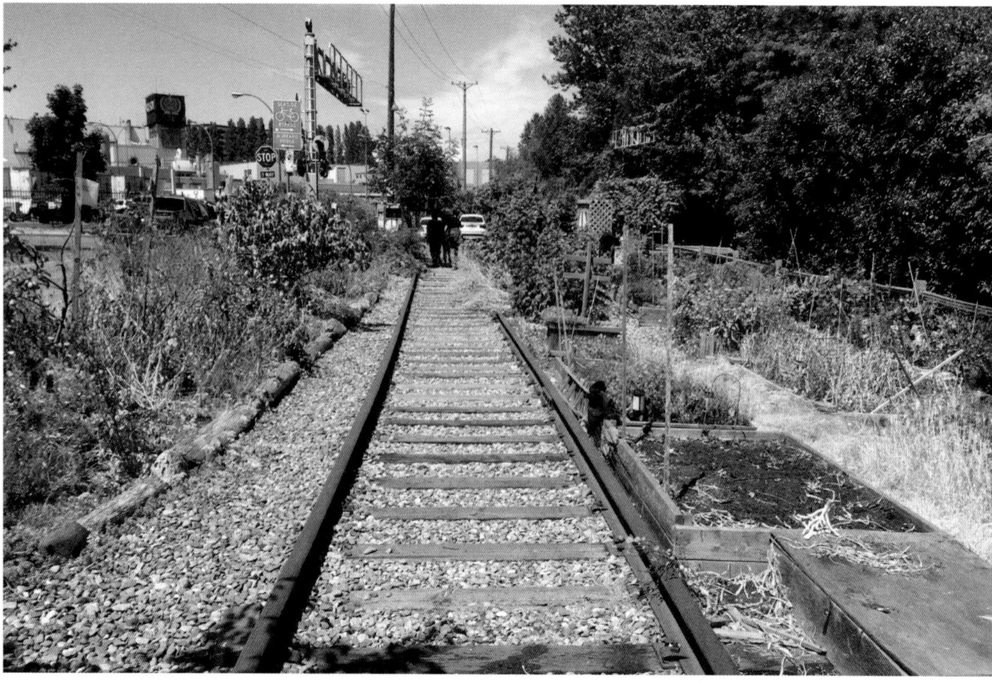

An abandoned rail line in Vancouver, repurposed as a trail with community gardens bordering. *(2015)*

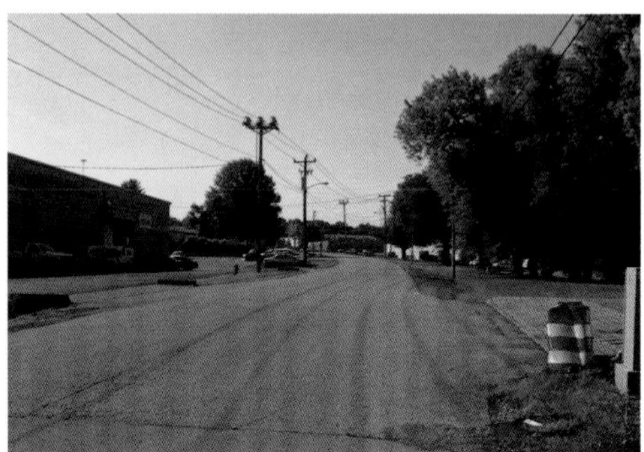

Industrial park located along Elm Hill Pike. *(2014)*

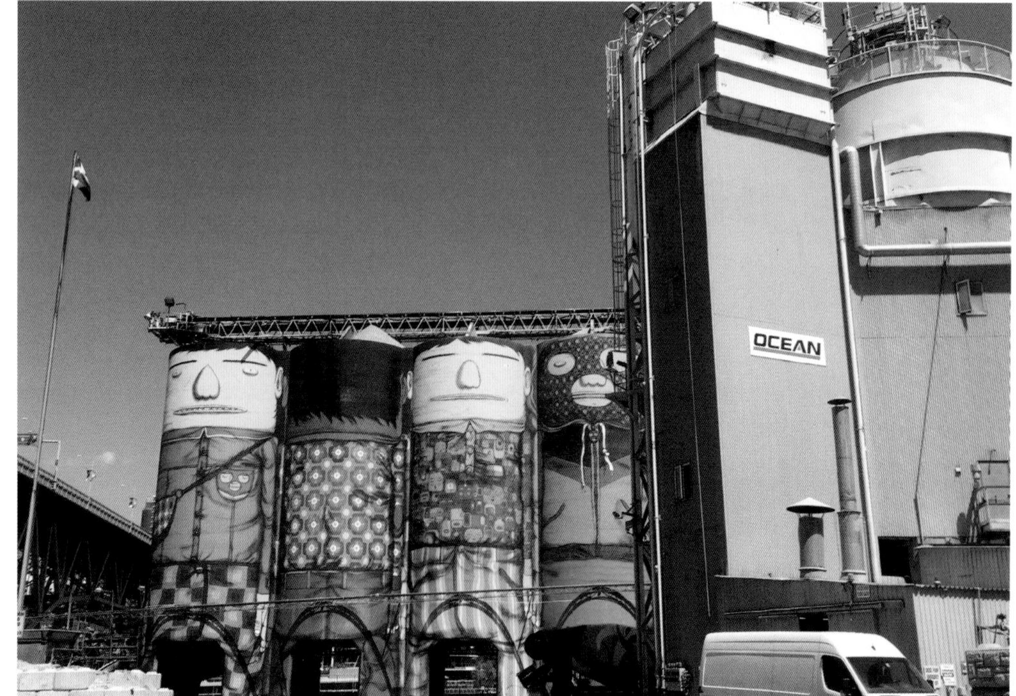

A functioning concrete plant in Vancouver, BC, transformed by public art installations. *(2015)*

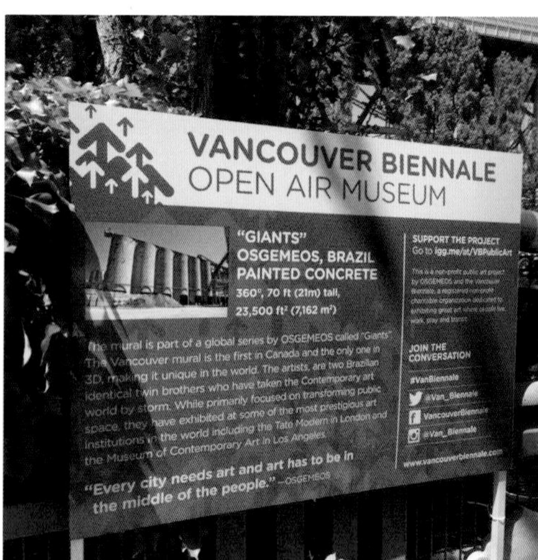

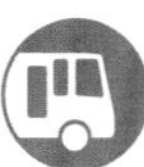

STRATEGY: *Increase connectivity through industrial districts to surrounding communities by means of complete streets, greenways, bike lanes, and multi-use paths.*

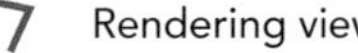

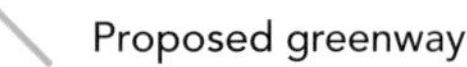

Rendering view

Proposed greenway

Greenways master plan

Existing buildings fronting greenway

Unused space fronting greenway

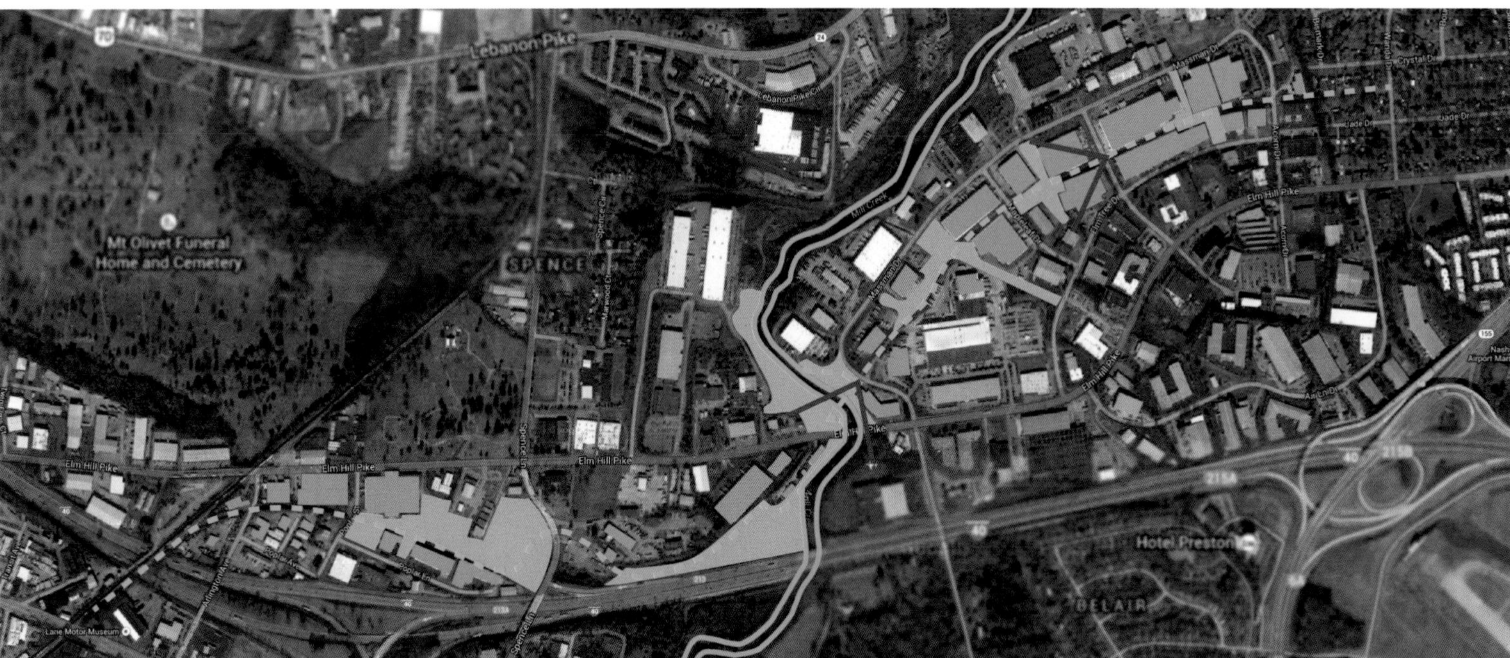

Potential new open space in the Elm Hill Pike area. *(Diagram over aerial, 2015: Eric Hoke, NCDC)*

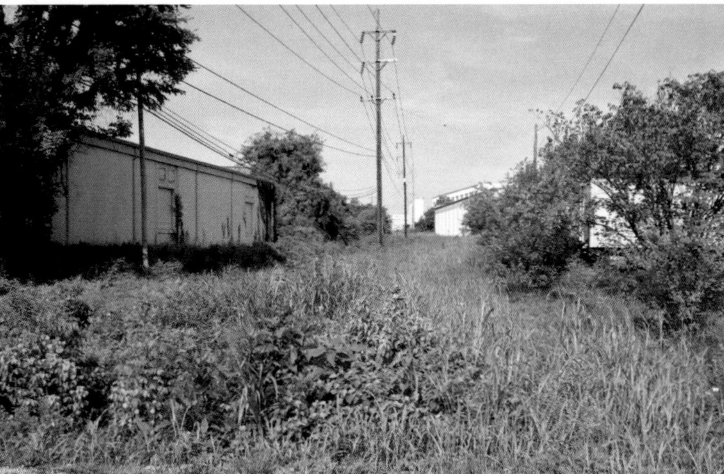

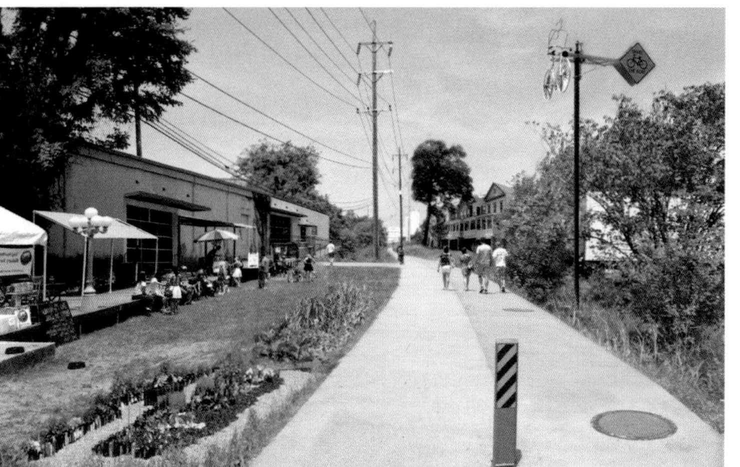

Existing conditions by Elm Hill Pike building. *(2014)*

Activating the same industrial area with a greenway, new retail, housing, community garden, and public art. *(Visualization, 2014: Eric Hoke, NCDC)*

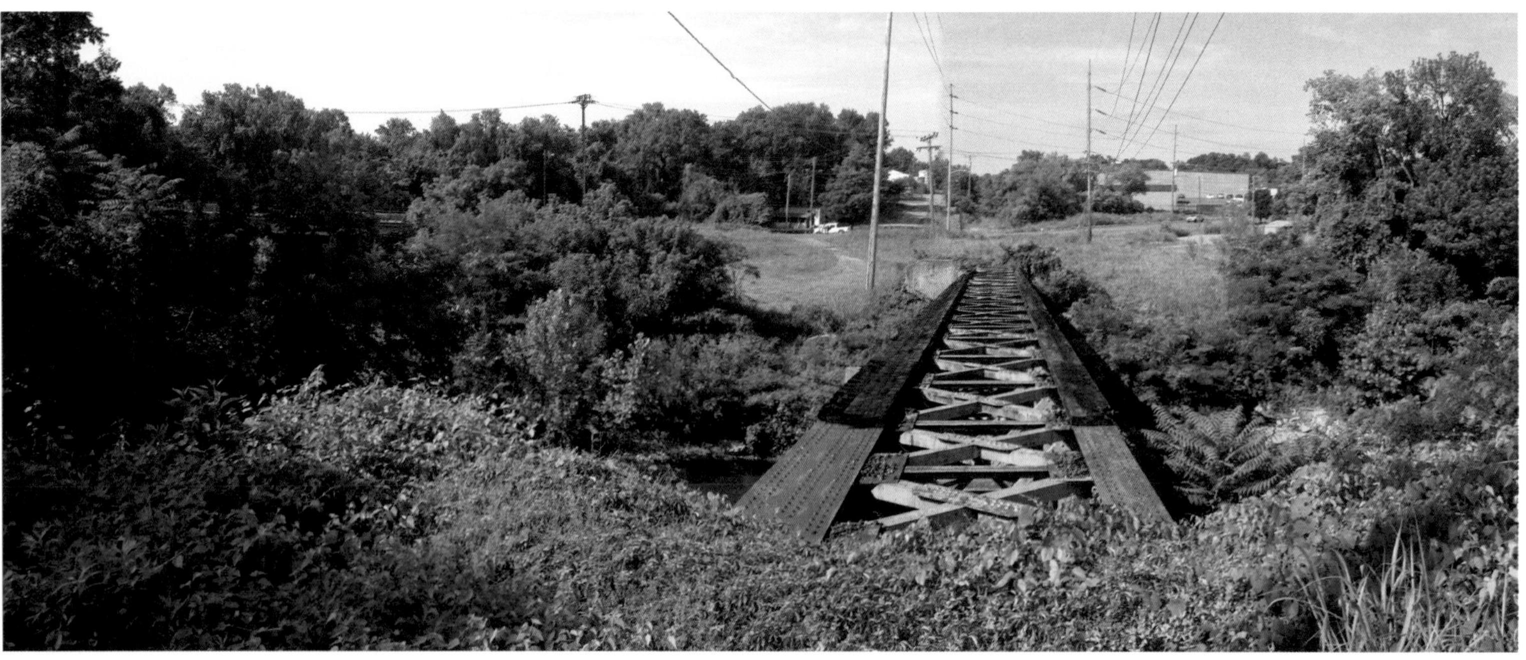

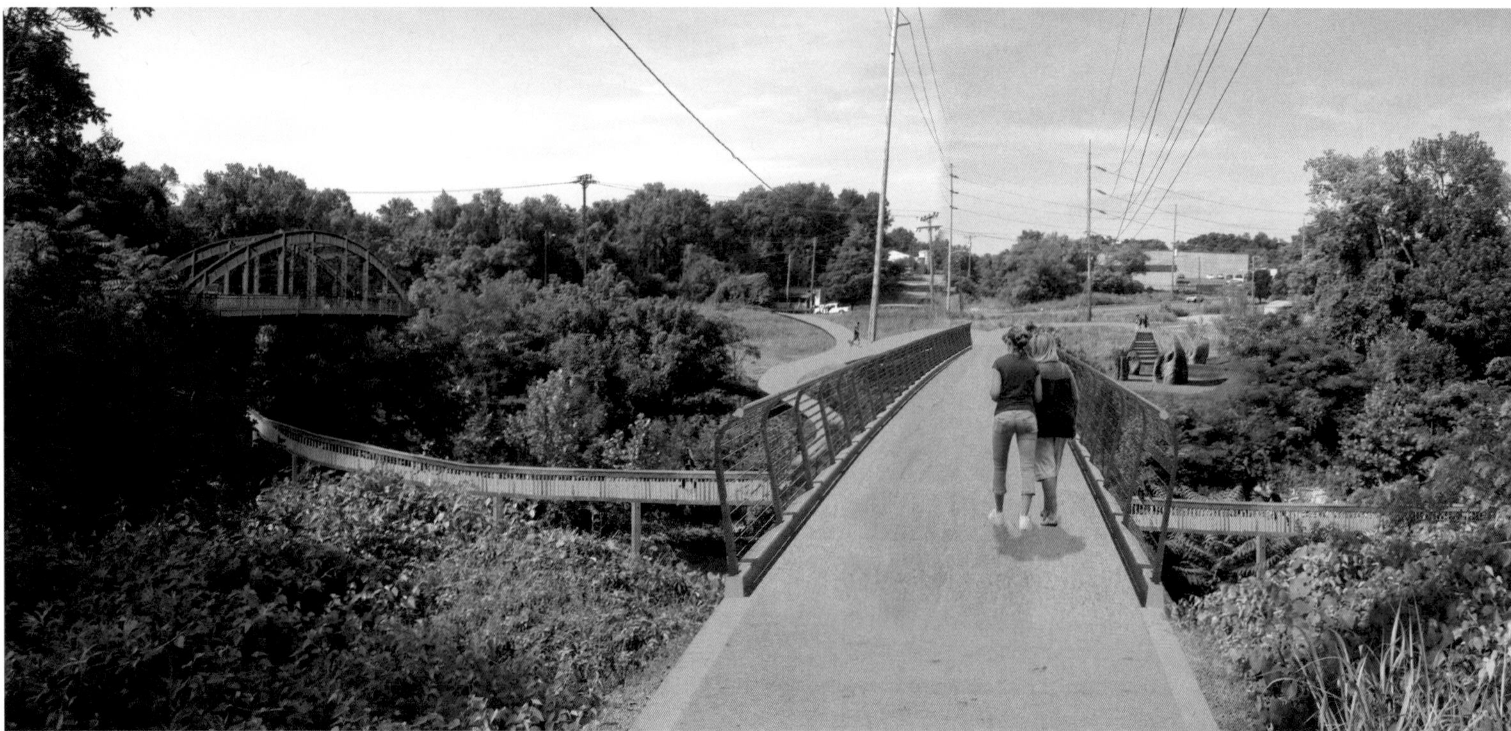

Abandoned rail line in the Elm Hill Pike area. *(2014)*

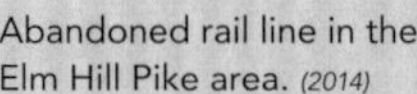

Proposed pedestrian bridge and greenway using previously abandoned space. *(Visualization, 2015: Eric Hoke, NCDC)*

MAJOR INSTITUTIONAL DISTRICT

Includes colleges and universities, major health care facilities, and other large-scale community services that pose no safety threats to the adjacent communities. In contrast with impact and industrial districts, major institutional districts are located in close proximity to residential neighborhoods, centers, and corridors, enabling the surrounding community to share some of the amenities these institutions offer.

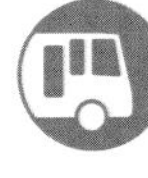

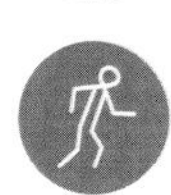

STRATEGY: *Make major institutional areas more permeable to surrounding communities by means of complete streets, sidewalks, greenways, bike lanes, and multi-use paths.*

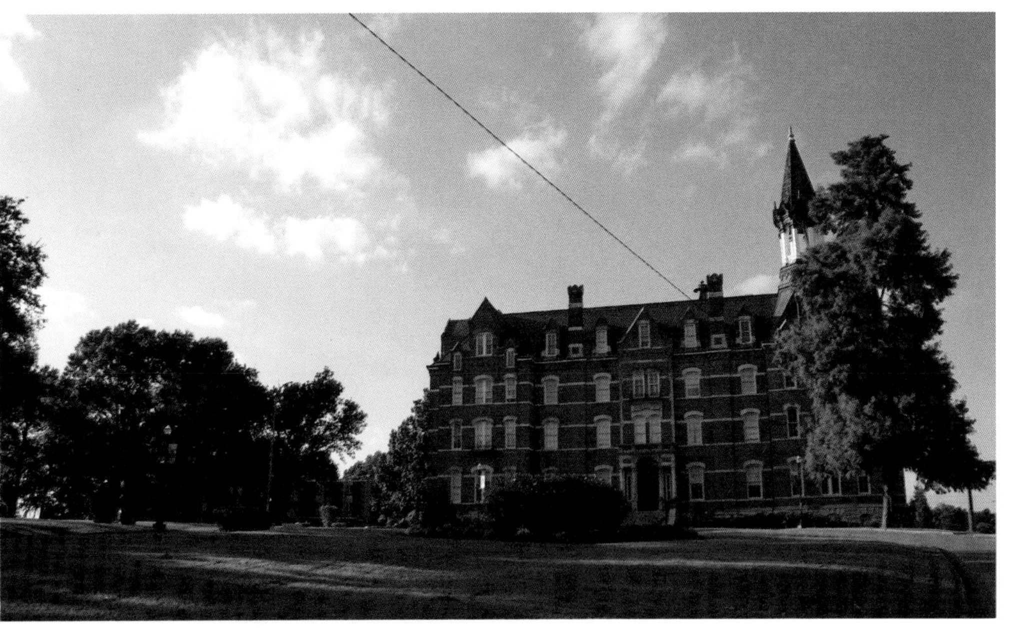

The Fisk University campus, including historic Jubilee Hall, lies along Jefferson Street in North Nashville. *(2013)*

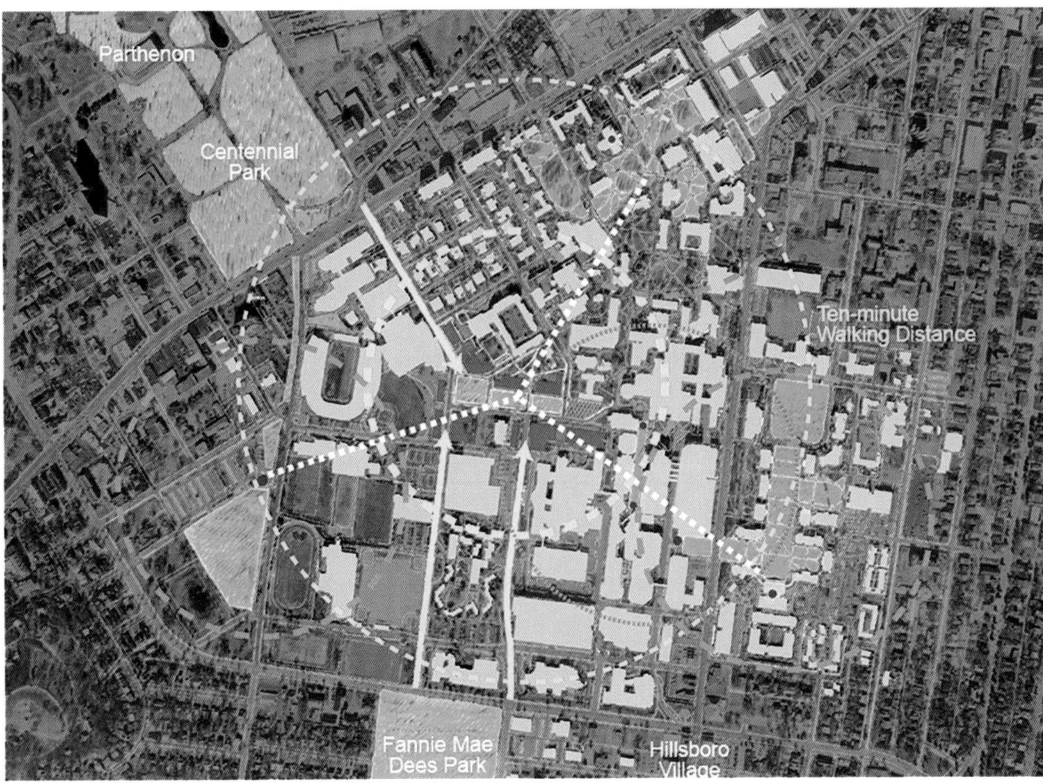

Vanderbilt University's 2001 land-use study projection. The study by Sasaki Associates prioritizes strengthening the relationship between the campus and surrounding urban communities. Strategies include increased walkability to campus-adjacent open spaces. Note that no area on campus is more than a ten-minute walk from the center.[3] *(Diagram over aerial, 2001: Vanderbilt University)*

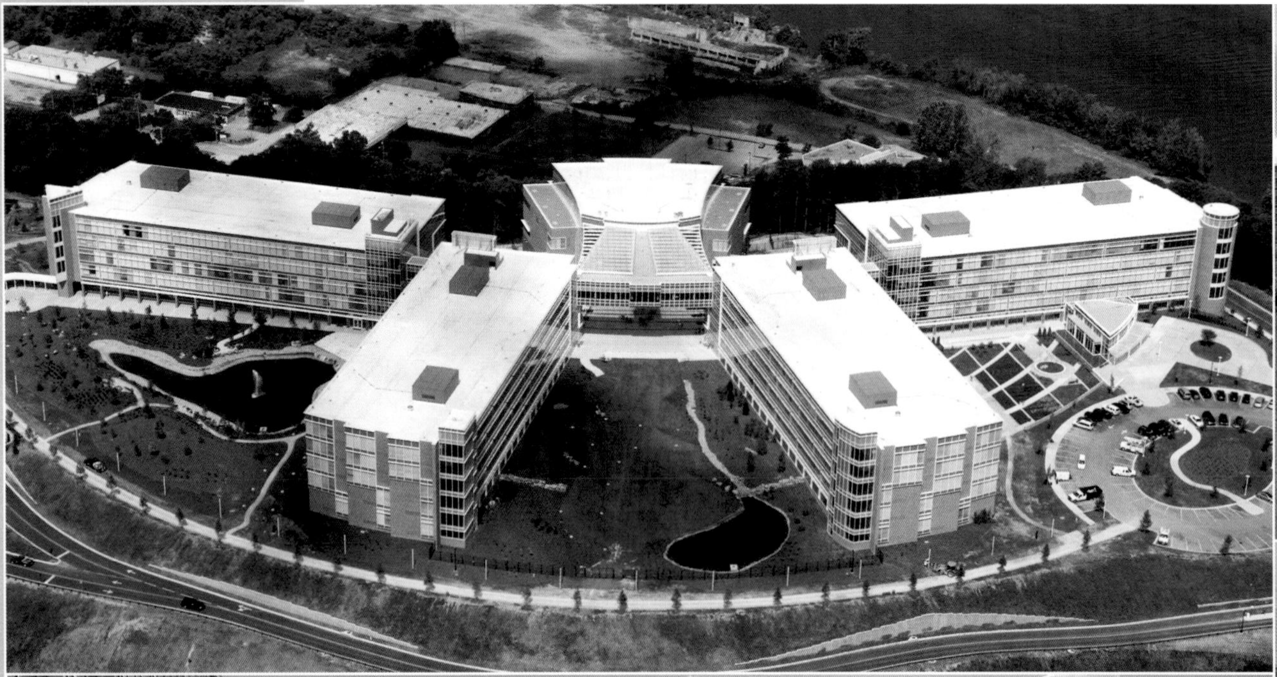

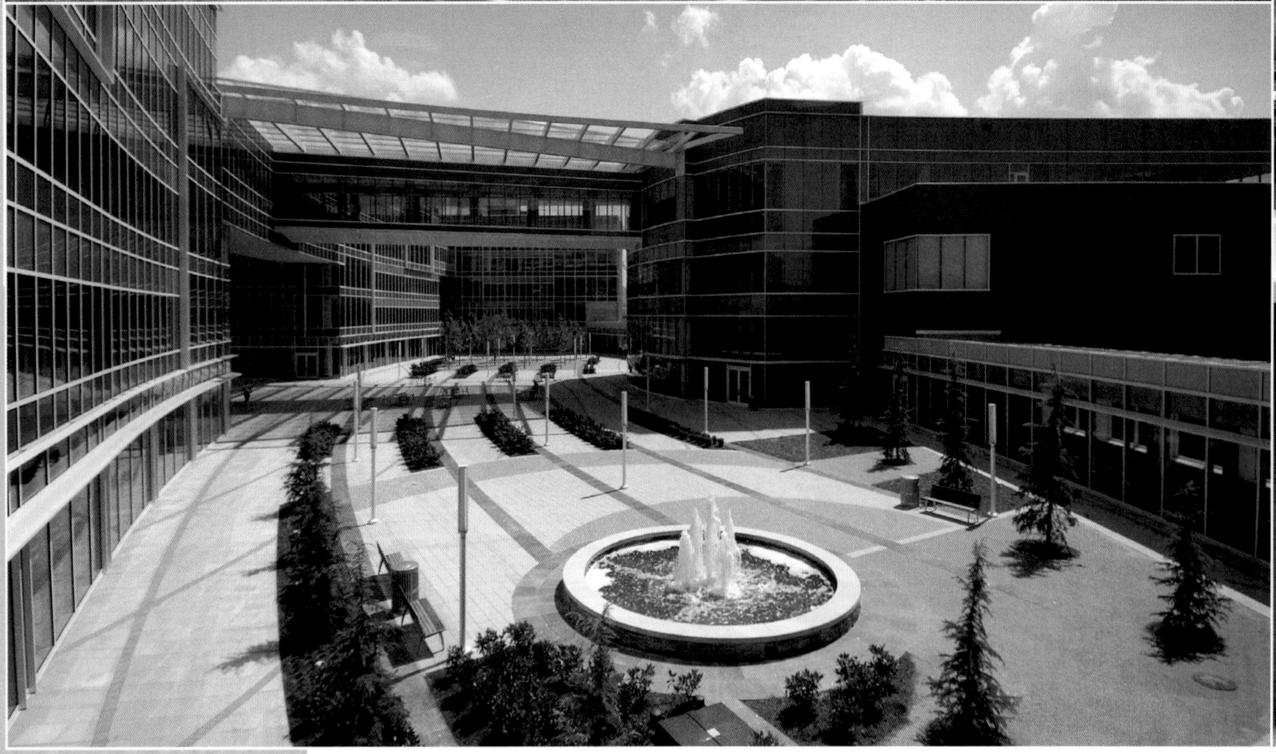

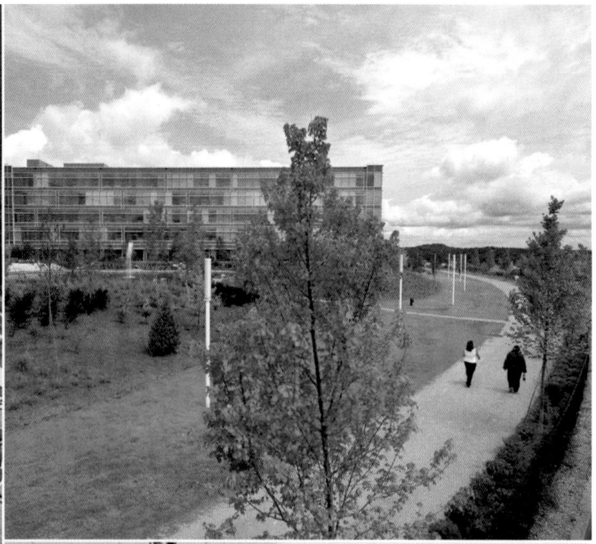

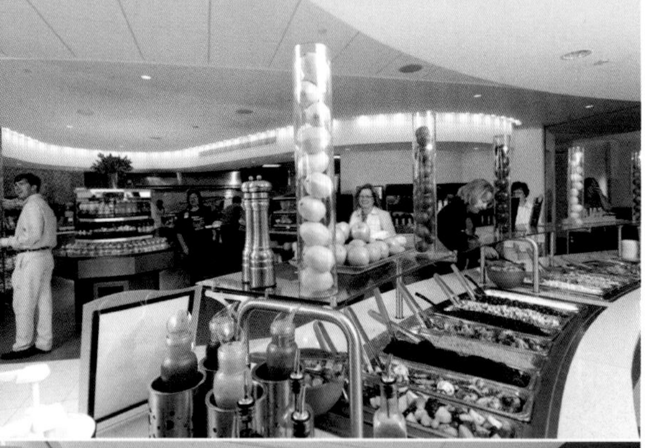

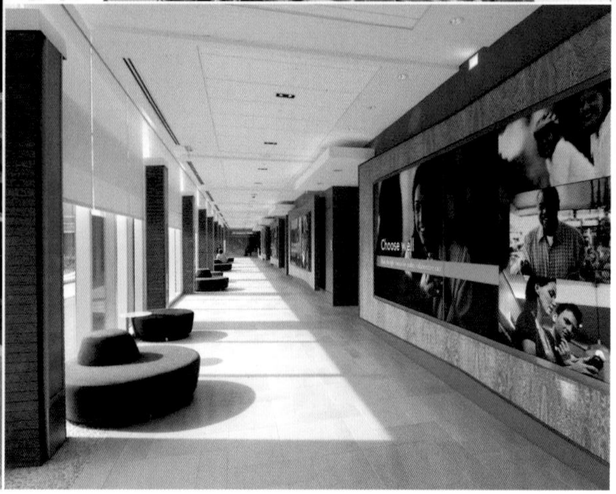

BLUECROSS BLUESHIELD OF TENNESSEE

BlueCross BlueShield of Tennessee (BCBS) formally opened a new facility in 2009 whose design focuses on both the health of the environment and the health of its employees.

The LEED (Leadership in Energy and Environmental Design) Gold-certified headquarters consists of five connected buildings strategically positioned on a hilltop within the 52-acre site. Glass curtain walls offer views of downtown Chattanooga and the Tennessee River. Since moving in, BCBS claims, the company's healthcare costs have risen less than one percent, unlike many companies that average double-digit growth each year.

According to John Hawbaker of BCBS, after relocating to the new headquarters, its 3,700 employees have taken a greater interest in their personal health. Ninety-one percent of full-time staff have participated in the wellness program, 56 percent reported an increase in physical activity level, 47 percent improved their nutrition, 39 percent lost weight—a 12-pounds-per-employee average—and 27 percent quit smoking. The annual savings per employee for medical and pharmacy claims is $1,000.

Improving employee health was one of the main objectives that influenced the planning and design of the facility, as well as staff programs and services. Many features were selected from the LEED list of accreditation criteria to make the building environmentally sustainable as well as promote a healthier lifestyle for the buildings' users. LEED design elements include walkability, an emphasis on natural lighting, use of low-emission paints, environmentally friendly cleaning agents and pest control, fitness and nutrition centers, bike sharing, bike parking, improved air quality with a more efficient under-floor air distribution system, and ventilation rates that are 30 percent higher than required by local building codes.

While most BCBS employees sit at their desks throughout much of the day, the layout of the five different buildings within the headquarters promotes walking, with floor-to-ceiling windows that highlight long hallways and emphasize stairways over elevators. Another strategy used to increase pedestrian activity is the location of the parking lot, which is approximately one-quarter mile from car to desk, for an average walk of a half-mile per day. A 0.6-mile walking trail encircles the headquarters, providing staff with a pleasant ambulatory setting for breaks from their desks and computer screens. When weather does not permit outdoor activities the employees have access to an indoor 0.2-mile circular track in the basement.

BCBS also offers a gym for its employees' use, with professional trainers who lead free classes in yoga, Zumba, boxing, and spinning. Amenities include day-lockers, changing rooms, showers, and towels. Managers are encouraged to schedule flexibly and allocate at least 30 minutes per day for physical activities. In conjunction with the exercise classes, BCBS offers weight support groups and instruction in healthy eating and grocery shopping habits. Employees may also request a treadmill desk in their office for individual use.

"The training is very encouraging," says DeLeslyn Mitchell, 38, who works in the marketing department. "We laugh a lot." With a co-worker Mitchell trained and completed the Iron Man competition in November of 2013, evidence of a major transformation. "I was 243 pounds. I was depressed, suicidal. I was so tired by lunch I would take a nap in my car," she says. "I would get angry when people would ask me to do my job." Mitchell says her new active lifestyle helped her lose 85 pounds and saved her life. "I'm grateful that I get to do my strength training during the day."

To encourage good nutrition, a cafeteria presents healthy, made-from-scratch lunch entrees under 600 calories and displays nutritional information at each serving station. A weekly farmers' market at the headquarters offers fresh produce and grass-fed beef for take-home as well as lunch-and-learn classes to promote healthy eating outside the workplace.

Design features to reduce work-related stress include relaxation areas: ponds, fountains, small parks, vegetable and herb gardens, and outdoor courtyards. Services such as scheduled chair massage by licensed professionals and an on-site clinic and pharmacy provide quick remedies to keep ailing employees productive and healthy.

The proof that employees have responded to BCBS healthy initiatives can be found in the before-and-after photos lining the walls.

BlueCross BlueShield Headquarters, Chattanooga, TN. Duda Paine, design architect; HKS, architect of record; TVS Interiors, HGOR, landscape architect. *(2009: Alex McMahan Photography)*

STRATEGIES

Design ground floors of buildings to be as "extroverted" as possible. Transparent glass at street level, for example, allows pedestrians to see interior activity.

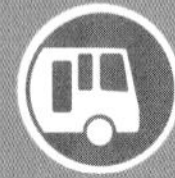

Design buildings to encourage use of active transportation options. Rather than focusing on convenient car parking, prioritize accommodation for transit users and cyclists—including showers and lockers—whenever possible.

Design buildings to enable growing food for both people and wildlife: green walls, rooftops, and gardens.

Design with nature. Orient buildings and sites relative to the sun; respect the body's need for natural light and vegetation. This saves energy while increasing comfort.

Make the staircase an obvious and attractive choice, while backgrounding the elevator.

Build with materials that protect indoor air quality.

Design ample opportunity for children's imaginative, physically active play.

Implement principles of Universal Design to allow anyone and everyone, regardless of age or ability, to use public and private interior environments safely and optimally.

ACTIVE BUILDING AND SITE DESIGN

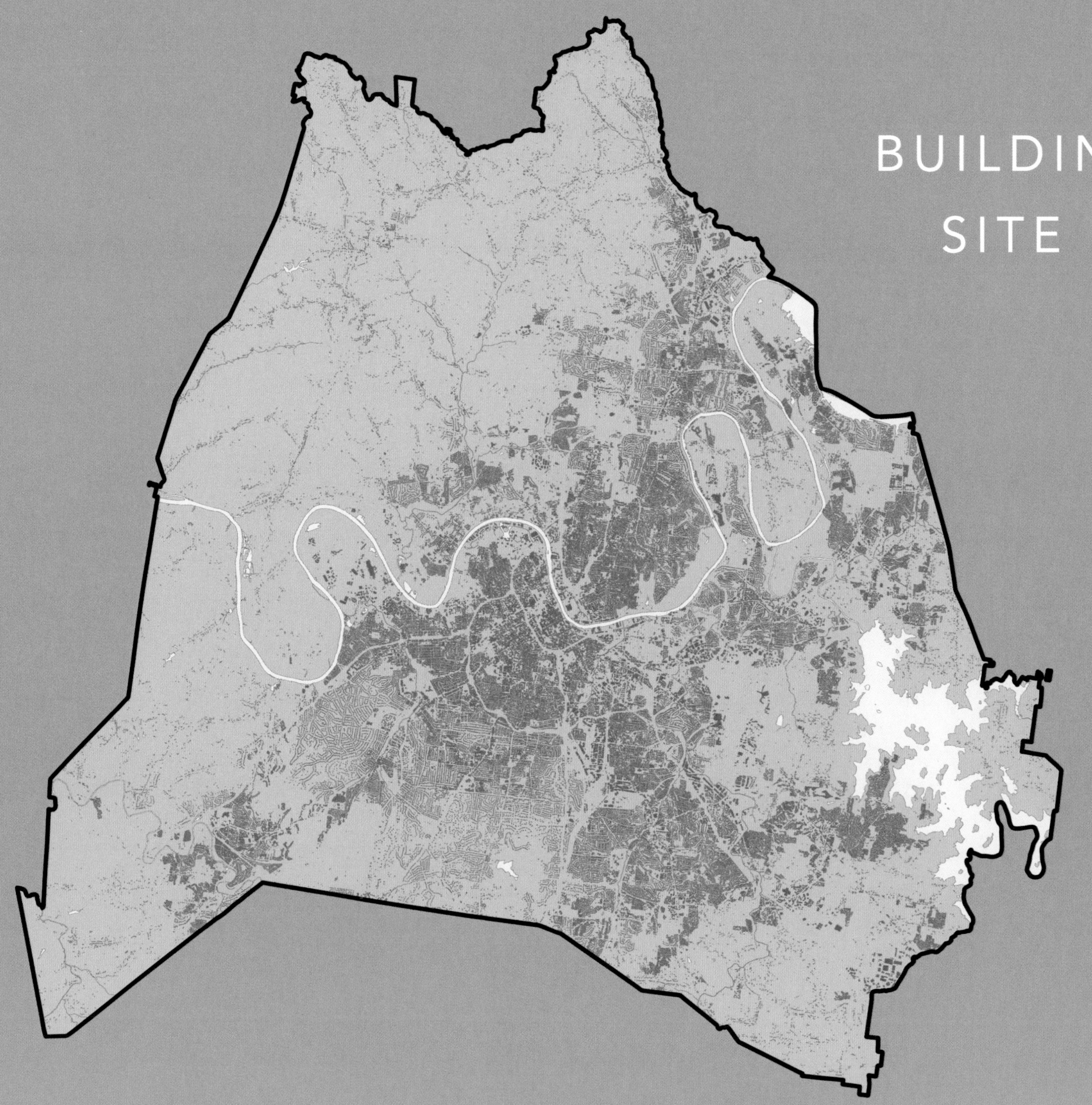

A figure-ground map of Davidson County depicts the footprints of individual structures. Built space is shown in gray, water in blue. The map illustrates how densely built the core transect zone of Nashville is relative to the suburban and rural zones where structures are fewer and farther between. (Map, 2014: Metro Planning Department)

CREATING HEALTHY SITES AND BUILDINGS

by DAVID KOELLEIN, real estate and urban design specialist; NCDC Board of Directors, 2009–2015

ANALYSIS AND STRATEGIES

The definition of any particular transect zone is determined by the configuration, density, and height of structures within the zone.[1] More often than not, these structures are designed and built individually. The opportunity to design, let alone construct, entire blocks of buildings simultaneously and as a group is rare. The aggregate impact of urban design on health is thus highly dependent on the design of discrete sites and the buildings that occupy them. The cooperation of the architect, interior designer, and landscape architect with the health goals of the urban designer and planner becomes paramount in ensuring that sites and buildings are designed in ways that promote walkability, access to open space and nutritious foods, and other health-supportive strategies.

Further, the conscientious designer of the individual structure must assume substantial responsibility for health, recognizing that most people spend as much as 90 percent of their days indoors.[2] Indoor time is largely passed sedentarily, but strategies for individual buildings can effectively get people up off of their perniciously comfortable chairs and sofas and put them in motion.

For instance, research has shown that an increase of two minutes of climbing stairs per day can result in over 1.2 pounds per year of weight loss. This offsets the estimated one-pound of weight gain averaged each year by Americans.[3] Thus, a building with easy to use, highly visible stairs becomes a health benefit to its users. Enclosed fire stairs with harsh lighting and stark material finishes are not the most inspiring physical motivators.

In the past, addressing health through building design had much to do with protecting occupants' lungs by measuring indoor air quality and quarantining smokers, strategies that remain important and are specifically addressed in LEED ratings systems for new construction. Today, though, addressing health issues in buildings is increasingly reactive to skyrocketing obesity, diabetes, and heart disease rates by shifting toward design that invites movement and discourages daytime inactivity, both at home and at work.

ACTIVE MOBILITY: BUILDING DESIGN TO ENCOURAGE WALKING, BIKING, AND TRANSIT USE

Insofar as health improvements are tied to urban design strategies, buildings can play a decisive, if paradoxical, role by encouraging people to get out of the building, preferably on foot, in order to participate in the active life of the city. Walking and biking become more obvious modes of travel when buildings are orientated to the sidewalk rather than to the garage. When a person exits an office or an apartment located in a large structure, the building's front door—or the pathway leading to it—should offer an immediate and visible connection to the sidewalk, while connections to the garage should be de-emphasized.

STRATEGY: *Design ground floors of buildings to be as "extroverted" as possible, offering active peripheries that engage sidewalk users.*

The attractiveness of using a city's sidewalks is related to the ways in which individual building design provides visual interest to the pedestrian. The design of a building's first floor, then, deserves particular attention. The interior program of space should make maximum use of storefront windows, offering glimpses into the life of a structure and packing the pedestrian experience with action. Busy lobbies, restaurants full of diners, and engaging displays of merchandise should be located as close to the storefronts as possible. By the same token, plans should position such spaces as storage rooms, empty corridors, bathrooms, and other back-of-house functions deep within the floor plate.

On the exterior, the rhythm of storefronts, especially an emphasis on vertical lines—pilasters, columns, and other details that define increments

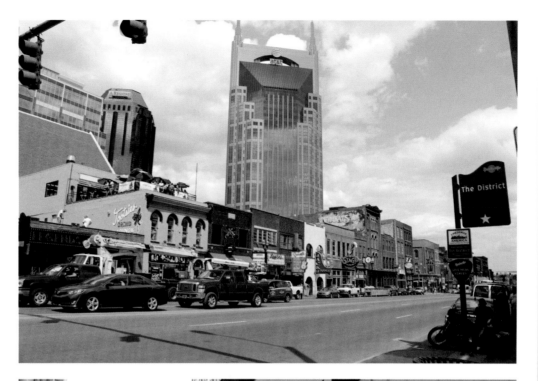

Broadway in downtown Nashville exhibits storefronts with interior activity visible from the street. *(2015)*

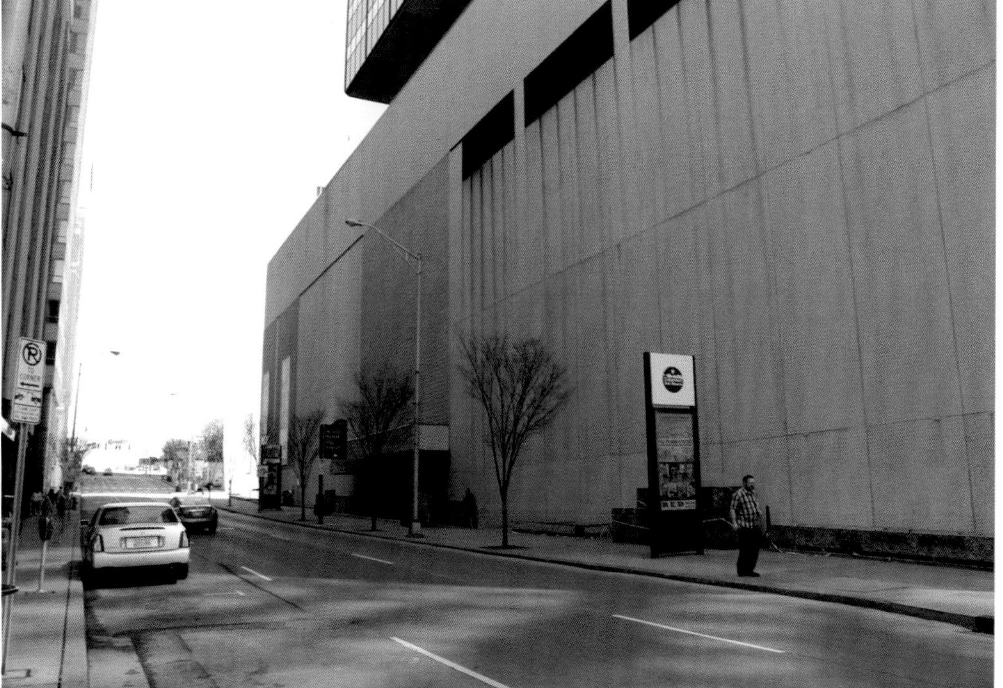

The blank wall of the Tennessee Performing Arts Center on Union Street is a hostile gesture to pedestrians. Features that could help improve this condition include public art installations, murals, and vegetation. *(2015)*

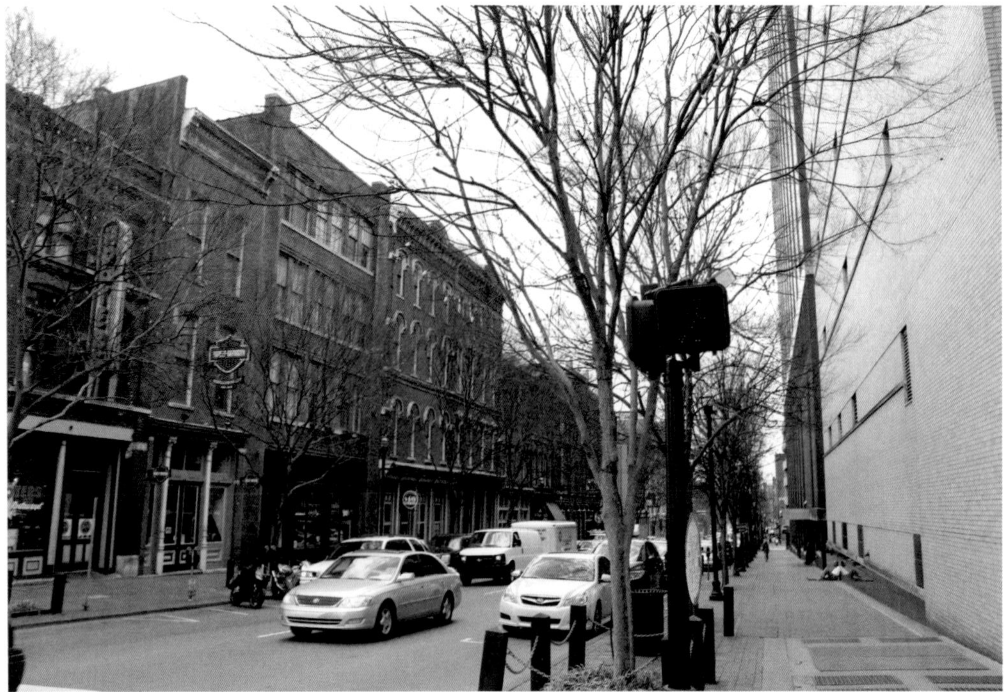

Which side of the street would you choose to walk on? A transparent street façade versus a largely masonry façade with recessed entrance stand opposite one another on Second Avenue North in downtown Nashville. *(2015)*

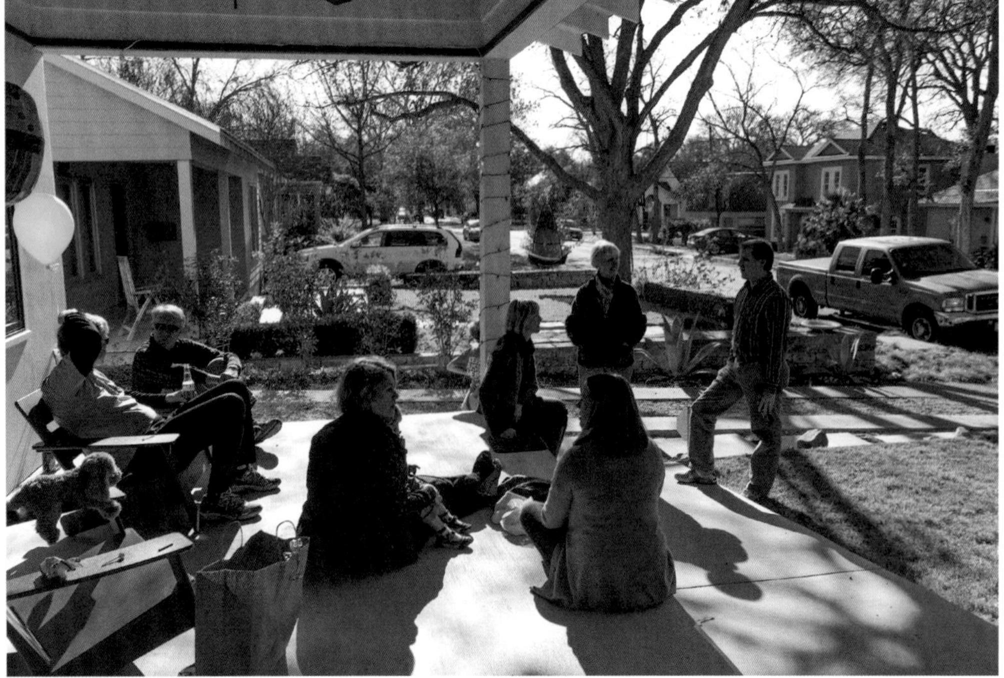

Front porches with a depth of six to eight feet have enough space to adequately accommodate users and porch furniture—and encourage social interaction with neighbors. *(2013: Lars Plougmann, Wikimedia Commons)*

of distance—can motivate a pedestrian to continue taking the next step. By contrast, blank, nontransparent exterior walls (e.g., the Tennessee Performing Arts Center) and deep building setbacks ignore pedestrians, leaving them disengaged. Studies have shown that pedestrians are willing to walk farther distances if the route is visually engaging and feels safe; distances of over a half-mile or more are not unusual.[4]

Overhead canopies, awnings, and other projections reaching from a building over the sidewalk, particularly above entryways, make walking a more comfortable, sheltered experience. In residential zones, porches and stoops bridge the distance between the front door and sidewalk, encouraging arrival and departure on foot. Stoops raised six to eight inches from grade are required in many municipalities to help separate the "public" sidewalk area from the "private" residential zone to protect residents' privacy and allow windows on the front to be less covered and so admit more natural light.

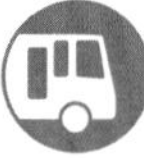

STRATEGY: *Design buildings to encourage active transportation options. Rather than focusing on convenient car parking, prioritize the less expensive accommodations for transit users and cyclists—including showers and lockers—whenever possible.*

For the last seven decades, building and site design have assumed that a building's occupants are car drivers, not cyclists or pedestrians.

For commercial structures, the typical priority of allocating 350 square feet to store each vehicle of practically every one of a building's users challenges both development budgets and the efficient use of space. Enormous amounts of precious real estate would be recovered if this were not so.

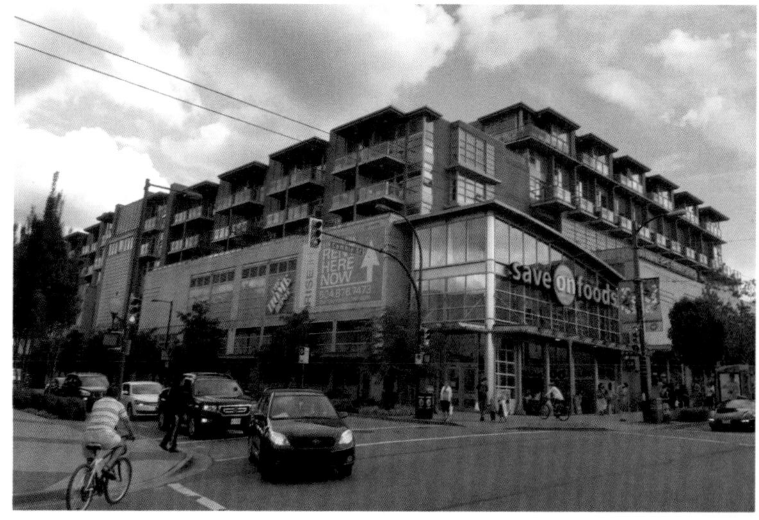

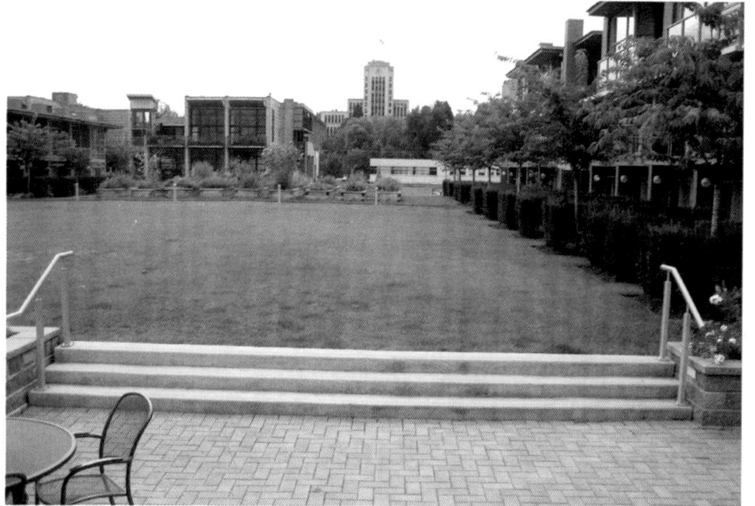

This mixed-use project in Vancouver features a Home Depot, a grocery store, over 90 condos, townhomes, and underground parking within the same structure on a 2.3 acre site, enabling people to walk between destinations rather than the typical suburban shopping pattern of drive-park. Residents also enjoy a 20,000 square foot green roof that serves as a park and community garden. *(2015; 2015: Grosvenor, Ltd.)*

The median construction cost per parking space in a car garage is approximately $15,783 in Nashville.[5] This price tag is astronomical relative to bicycle racks, one of which provides storage for several bikes and can be installed for no more than a few hundred dollars. Yet office designers and developers prioritize car parking due to what they perceive as tenant demand.

Significant incentives are lacking to do otherwise. Metro Nashville does not currently offer any density bonuses for providing bicycle infrastructure. The LEED rating system offers merely one point for providing bicycle facilities in a building: LEED Neighborhood Design (ND) provides up to two points.

The preeminence of the car is often supported by municipally mandated minimum parking ratios. A retail location in the suburbs, for example, may be required to provide ten parking spaces for every 1,000 square feet of floor space; that is, a typical 40,000-square-foot big box store would have to provide 400 parking spaces. That this number is excessive is illustrated by the fact that more than 50 percent of such parking spaces are often unused, except during the Christmas shopping season.[6]

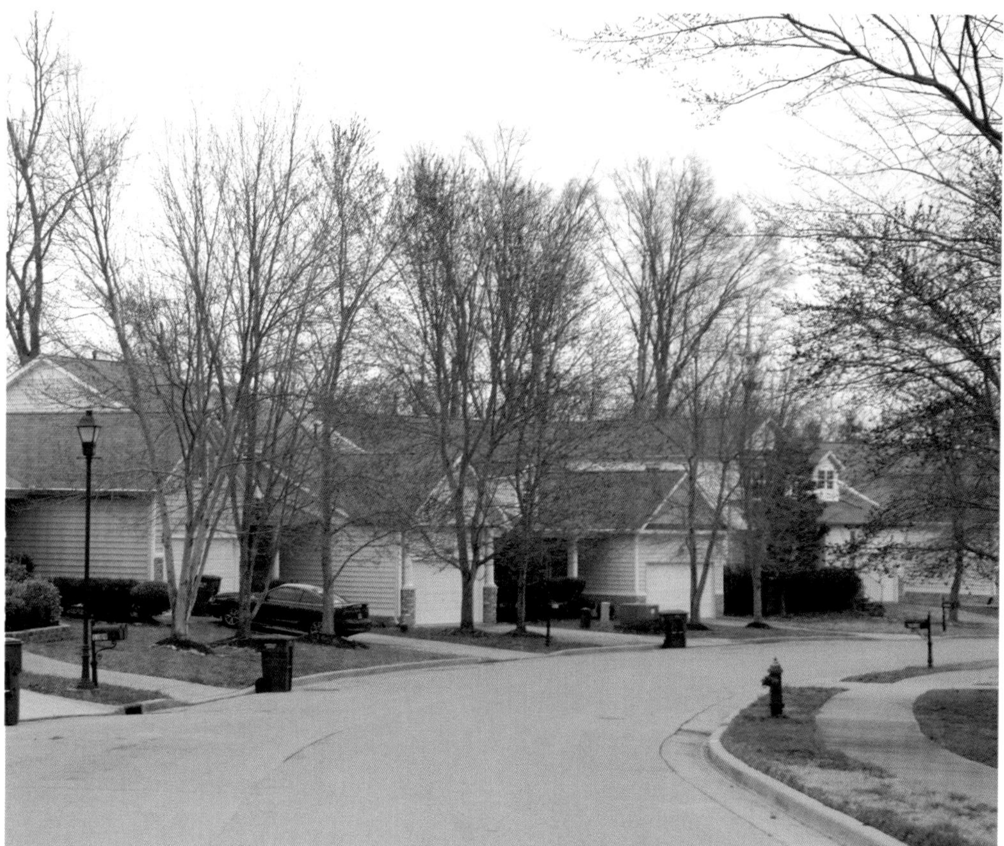

Single-family homes are also often designed to privilege travel by automobile. The common "snout house" projects the garage toward the street, giving the door for cars primacy of place. In this layout, the traditional front door is recessed into visual insignificance and rarely used. *(2013)*

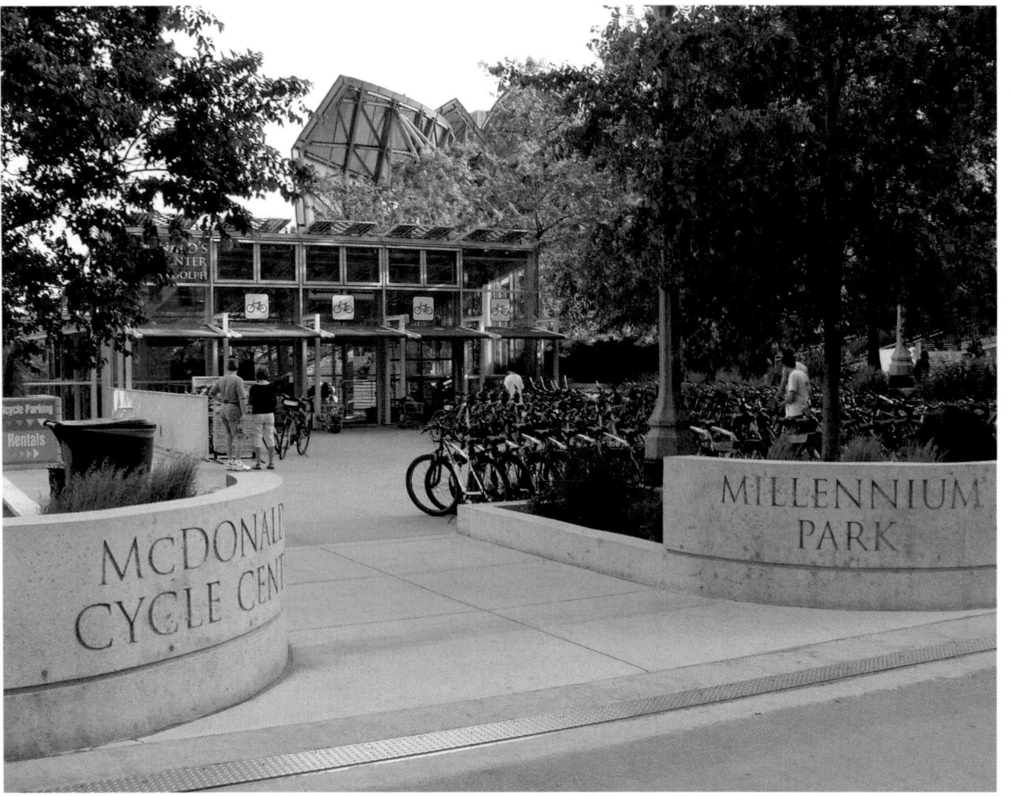

McDonald's Cycle Center in Chicago's Millennium Park offers cyclists a safe, indoor place to store their bicycles during the day. The center also provides lockers, showers, a snack bar, bike repair, and bike rentals for commuters. *(2008: Torsodog, Wikimedia Commons)*

To support biking as a mode of transit, buildings must provide convenient bicycle parking. For employees in office buildings or residents in multifamily buildings, bike racks should be located in secure, preferably covered, facilities. For visitors to buildings, dedicated bike parking out front is optimal.

Racks are more easily anchored in concrete pads than in pavers or asphalt. Stairs cyclists must navigate with their bikes to store their machines are a major deterrent. Washrooms and lockers adjacent to bike parking support end-of-trip needs, and power supplies serve electric bike options.[7]

In multifamily housing, using a bike often requires lugging it on elevators or up flights of stairs, finding a place to store it in one's typically small apartment, or leaving it vulnerable to theft and corrosive weather outdoors. All of these conditions are major handicaps for cyclists.

Efficient and comfortable transit options are critical to entice people to forsake their personal vehicles. Thus the design of transit facilities is important to health. Bus stops must be designed

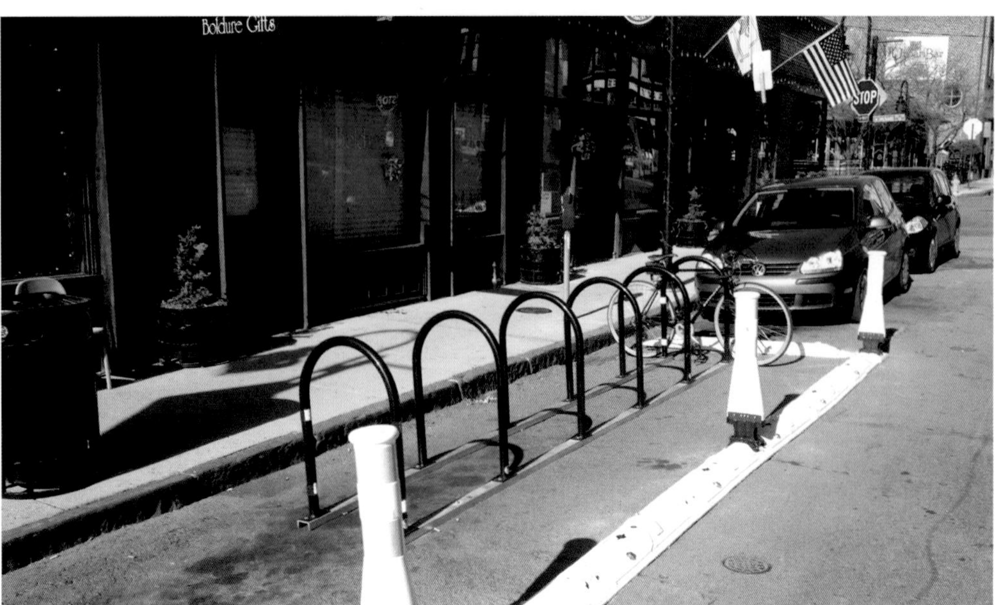

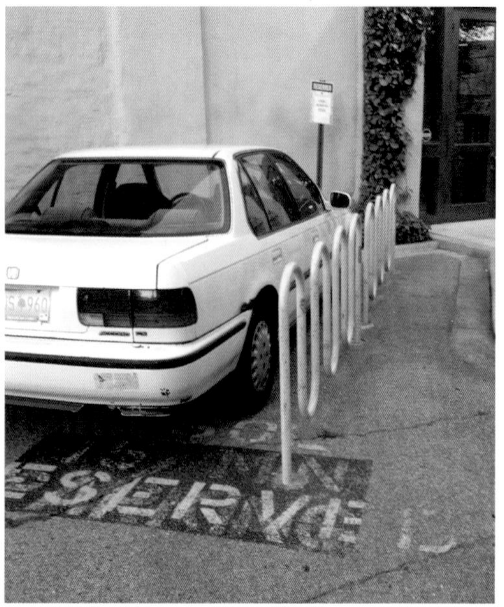

Bottom left: This "corral" for bicycles in Knoxville's Old City replaces a space for car storage and provides racks protected from cars in a location convenient for visitors to nearby stores and offices. *(2012)*

Bottom right: Bike parking outside a Charleston, SC, development is rendered unusable by a careless driver. *(2014)*

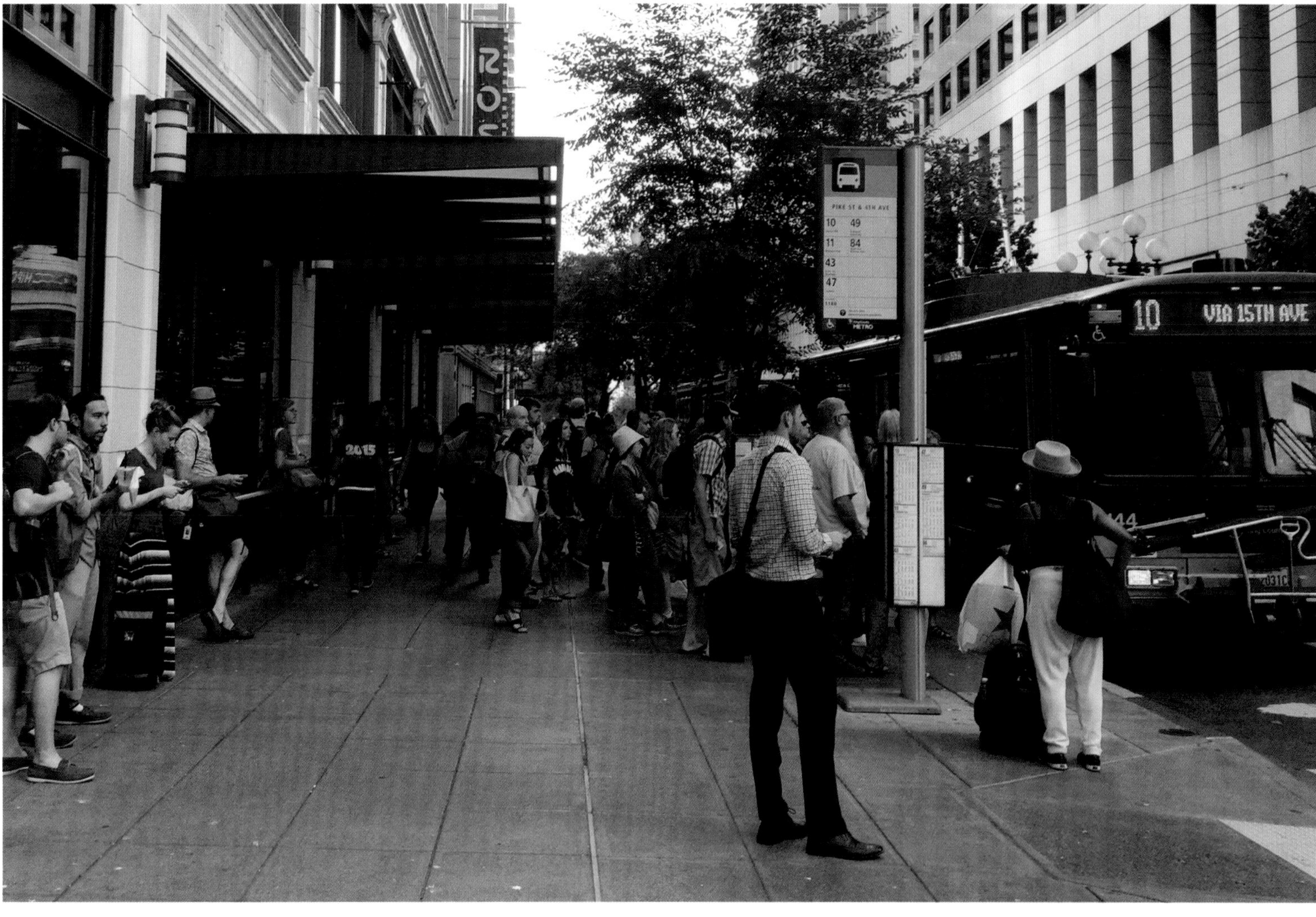

Designing bus stops with the comfort of commuters in mind has become increasingly important in attracting riders. This version in Seattle features a canopy for protection in inclement weather and leaning bars along the building facade. *(2015)*

to give users a pleasant experience while waiting. Transit maps and schedules should be posted, and the arrival time of the next bus or train should be made clear using passenger information systems. Stops should have roofs to protect riders from the elements. Shade trees reduce summertime heat. Too frequently, bus stops are mere benches whose designs are better suited to advertisers than transit users. Restrooms, food and beverages, retail outlets, and artwork can make a larger transit station attractive to riders.

While it is nearly always assumed that bus stops—whether defined by signage, benches, and/or small shelters—are street furnishings, just like street lamps and trashcans within the sidewalk space, there is precedent for the placement of transit shelters in the interior of buildings on the ground level. In this configuration, the transit stop is much like a small lobby built into an office or residential building, offering a handy transportation amenity to the building's users as well as the public. Riders enjoy conditioned, comfortable space while they wait and are alerted when their bus, trolley, or train arrives.

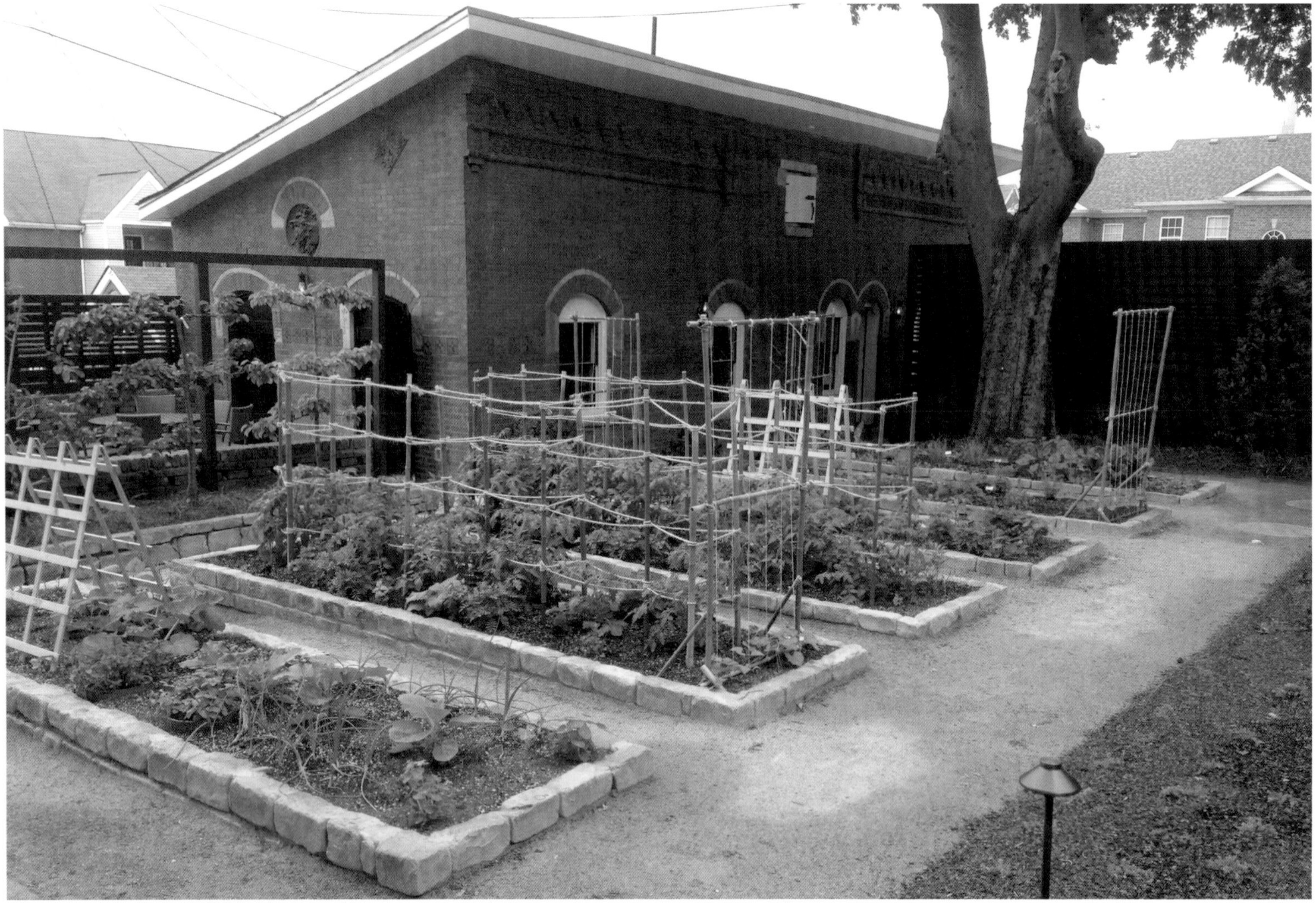

Husk Restaurant in Nashville's Rutledge Hill neighborhood features a small herb and vegetable garden. *(2013: Gary Gaston, NCDC)*

BUILDING DESIGN FOR GOOD NUTRITION

STRATEGY: *Design buildings that allow for growing food for both people and wildlife: green walls, rooftops, and gardens.*

Along with corner grocery stores, the farm-to-table restaurant or other slow (as opposed to fast) food experiences should be important aspects of walkable neighborhood composition. In 2009 the Metro Council passed an ordinance legalizing community gardening in Nashville, eliminating a major roadblock to growing food in the city.[8]

The next step is to make sites and buildings themselves into food production facilities. The site design of many restaurants can incorporate vegetable gardens, eliminating the distance between the harvest of fresh food and the plate on which it is served. In urban settings, small side or back yards or rooftops can serve this purpose. Vertical hydroponic and aquaponic systems may be particularly appropriate ways to grow food in the city, as they occupy very little space.

Aquaponics: The Future of Farming

The more we became aware of the way food is grown and processed in America, the more we sought a different path. The liberal use of toxic herbicides, pesticides, and fertilizers; the widespread cultivation of genetically modified crops; and the cocktail of hormones and antibiotics being pumped into conventional American meats were more than we could stomach. We became highly motivated to grow affordable, clean, nutrient-dense food like our grandparents used to know and enjoy. We're not alone in this food renaissance. Middle Tennesseans have embraced local, sustainably grown food, and we have high hopes to see urban agricultural play a large role in shaping our community's future.

Aquaponics is an exciting technology that has the potential to revolutionize the way we grow food. It is the marriage of aquaculture (fish farming) and hydroponics (growing plants using water and nutrient solutions, but no soil). Put simply, aquaponics is a closed-loop system containing both fish and plants. Fish are raised in a large tank adjacent to a hydroponic system designed to grow large amounts of food in a small area. The wastewater from the fish tank is pumped through the hydroponic system, providing readily available nutrients to the plants. As the plants take up those nutrients, their roots clean the water. That clean water returns to the fish tank and the closed-loop cycle starts again. As a result of this process, premium organic food is grown in only 40–60 percent of the time, using just 3–5 percent of the amount of water it would take to grow the same amount of food in soil.

Lettuce, kale, basil, and other leafy greens and herbs grow like wildfire in these systems. They are far from the only plants that do well in aquaponics, however. Fruiting plants like tomatoes, peppers, and cucumbers—just to name a few—also thrive. There are even aquaponics farmers experimenting with corn and grains. Not only are there abundant harvests of vegetables, but there are also occasional fish harvests. Tilapia, yellow perch, and Chinese catfish (even trout in some cases) are all commonly used as the nutrient source in aquaponics.

We ultimately decided to pursue a personal aquaponics greenhouse because of the health, financial, and environmental benefits. Our 90 square foot starter greenhouse cost $4,000 in materials and $3,000 in labor (plus a LOT of research time). Accessory structures less than 100 square feet do not require a building permit, but you will need a level site and access to electricity and water. Now that we've invested our money, time, and energy, we're set up to reap the benefits for years to come.

The greenhouse was designed with passive building design in mind, greatly reducing our need for fossil fuels for heating and cooling. While our greenhouse is designed to produce food year round, a less expensive option is an outdoor aquaponics system, operating only in the summer months. Our steady stream of organic produce—for smoothies, salads and flavors galore—will save us anywhere from $50 to $100 per week on premium nutrition and provide us with the occasional fish fry.

While this technology has roots tracing back to the Aztecs, the potential for modern-day applications is extremely exciting. The United Nations predicts that by 2050 nearly 70 percent of the world's population will be living in urban centers. Because of this, effective urban agriculture will become more and more important. The possibilities for aquaponics in urban infill abound. Aquaponic farms present a solution to what many view as problems. They are the perfect tenants for unoccupied rooftops and abandoned or vacant lots and warehouses. Acquaponics is an opportunity to provide Nashvillians with hyper-local, quality food, while enabling our region's nonrural residents to reconnect with the sources from which their food comes.

— BETSY MASON AND AUSTIN LITTRELL,
founders, Green Leaf Aquaponics

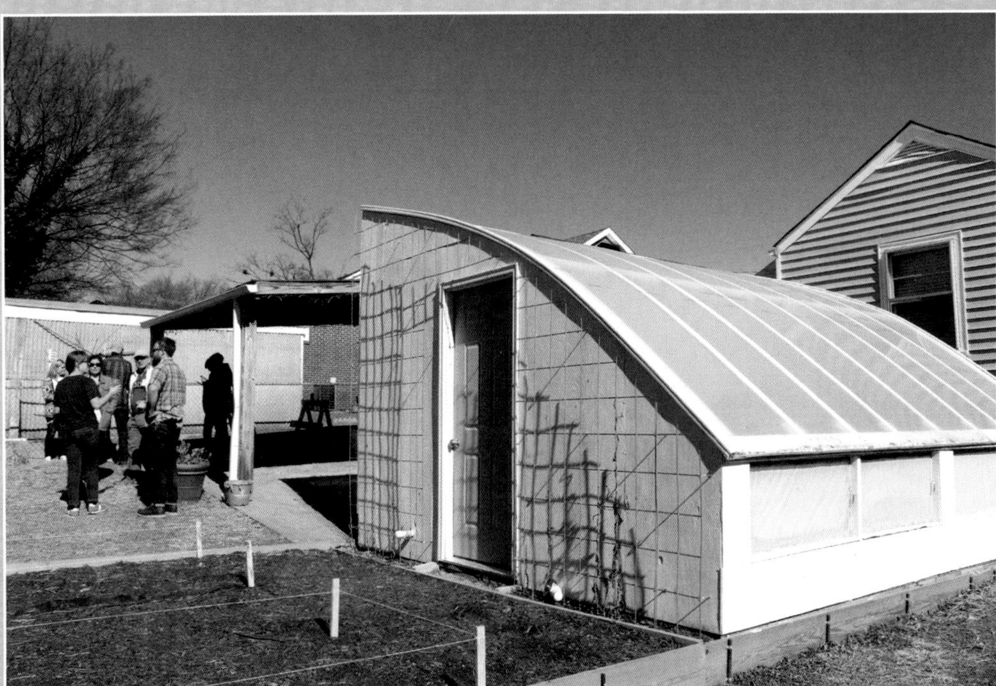

Green Leaf Aquaponics greenhouse in Nashville's Wedgewood-Houston neighborhood. *(2015)*

DESIGN WITH NATURE

STRATEGY: *Orient buildings and sites relative to the proper sun angles; respect the body's need for natural light and vegetation. This saves energy while increasing comfort.*

Building orientation is a critical factor in passive solar cooling and heating. Buildings should have their longest facades oriented within 30 degrees of true north-south, allowing the south façade to be exposed to direct sunlight between 9:00 a.m. and 3:00 p.m. Rooms that require the most heat and light, such as living and work areas, should also be located on the south face of the structure, while less used spaces should be located to the north. Vents that open at night, allowing hot air to

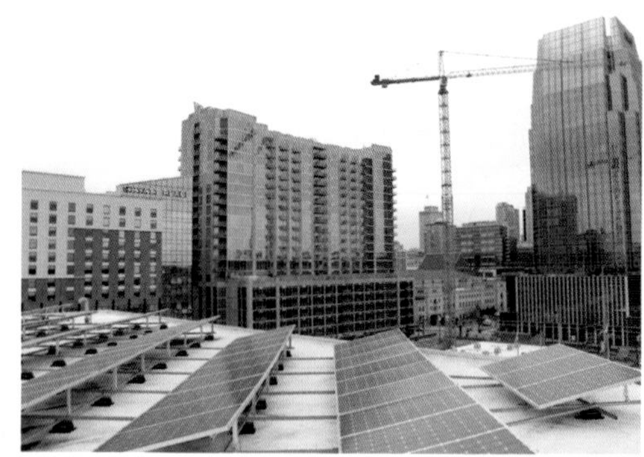

Top right: The Ragland Building in downtown Nashville has a white roof and solar panels. *(2015)*

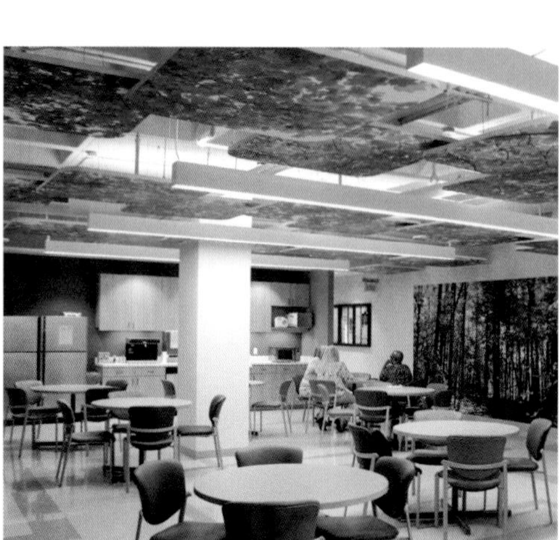

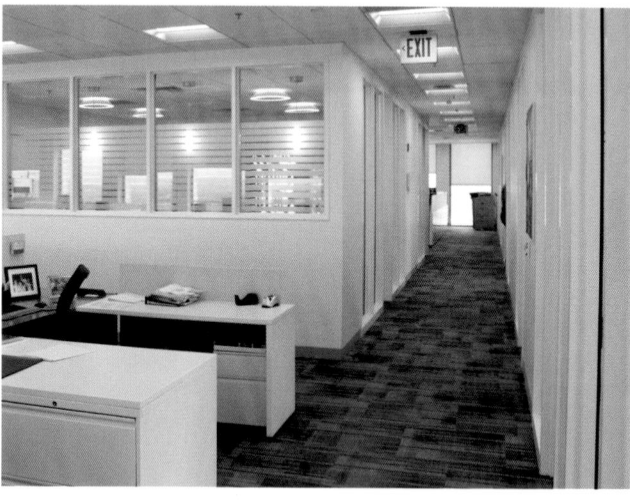

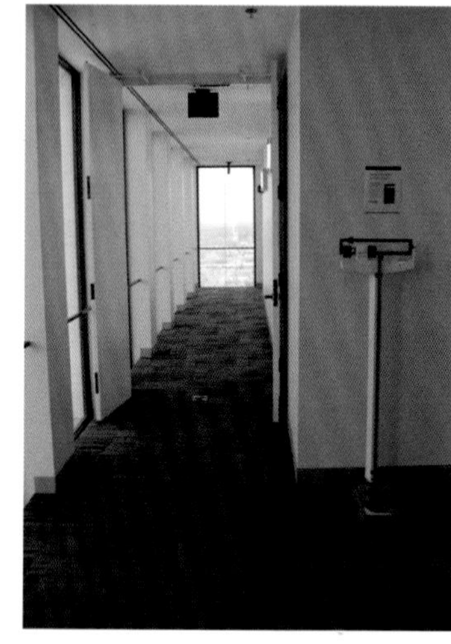

Center: A recent renovation features an open and airy design for the Tennessee Department of Environment and Conservation (TDEC), located in the Tennessee Tower office building's basement level. Modifications include uplighting, large photographic mural panels and a variety of meeting spaces. The State architect's office features a more open layout with flexible workspace and shared, private meeting rooms. The top mechanical floor now features a walking track around the perimeter with information promoting healthier activities and a scale to track progress. *(2015: Courtesy of TDEC)*

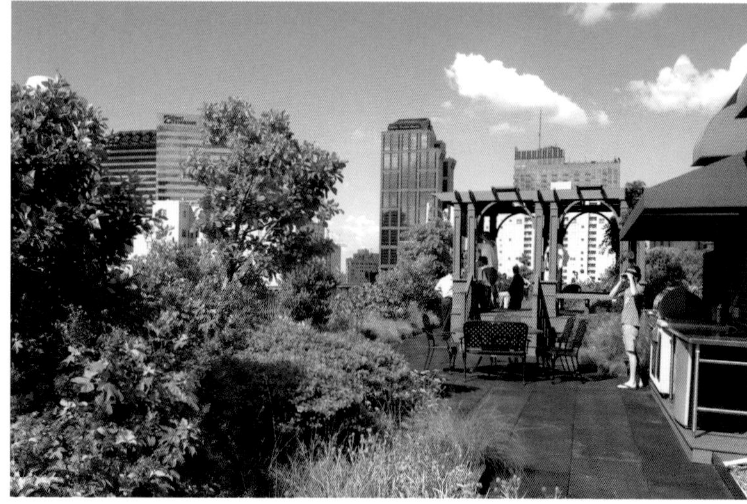

Bottom left: Westview residential complex, in downtown Nashville on Rosa Parks Boulevard near Church Street, offers residents a large green roof for relaxing and gardening. Especially in highly urban environments, the roofs of buildings, often ignored by designers, can be planted with grasses and small shrubs or even, if structurally accommodated, with trees. Small green roofs can provide moments for socialization and relief from the "concrete jungle." They also capture pollution and can improve air and water quality. *(2013)*

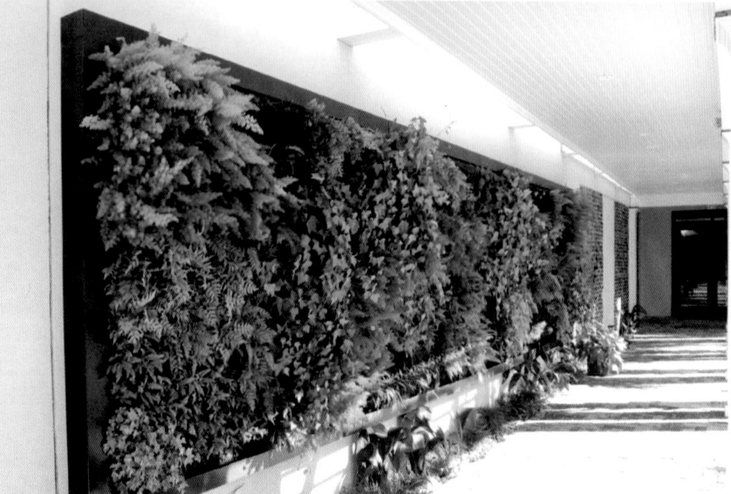

Bottom right: Vertical garden incorporated into an event space located in Charleston, South Carolina. *(2014: Living Roofs, Inc.)*

escape and cool air to enter, should be installed to aid in passive cooling during warmer months.[9]

The value of open space to individual health is in its sunlight, fresh air, and connections with nature. Yet building interiors too often offer the opposite, biophobic sort of environment.

The office cubicle "farm" is an example in biophobic design. Such cubicles—often buried deep in a building's floor plate, with their reliance on fluorescent lighting, conditioned and stagnant air segregated from enlivening outdoor breezes, and the total absence of indoor vegetation—insist on the interiority of interiors.

Biophilia, by contrast, is the notion that an innate human affinity for nature is manifest in health benefits—especially mental health benefits—accrued through contact with natural elements.[10] Biophilic design introduces the characteristics of parks and open space to the indoors. Gardens—including grasses, flowers, and trees—in planting beds, in pots, or even climbing on walls offer the visual and aromatic presence of nature and have been shown to reduce stress and speed healing processes. Strategically placed windows can offer views of trees or meadows, and the visible use of natural building materials such as wood and stone in interior space can have similar effects.[11]

Of the approximately 291,000 buildings in Davidson County, fewer than 35 have green roofs. Building roofs are largely wasted space, typically black in color, absorbing heat that contributes to stifling summer conditions. Short of converting roofs to gardens, painting them white reflects sunlight and avoids heat capture, with benefits realized in reduced air conditioning bills—up to 40 percent at peak demand periods. HVAC units are far more efficient when mounted on white roofs, where the air intake on hot days can be as much as 70°F cooler than on dark surfaces.[12]

DESIGNING THE HEALTHIER OFFICE

STRATEGY: *Make the staircase an obvious and attractive choice while backgrounding the elevator.*

The way in which the 40-plus hours per week are spent at work has much to do with overall health patterns, starting with how a worker navigates through the office upon opening the front door. The elevator is too often the assumed form of inter-floor transportation in taller structures. Finding the staircase, by contrast, requires a deliberate hunt.

Within a multistory building, the staircase should be a prominent and attractive feature. In many buildings, the only alternatives to the elevator are the enclosed and stark stairwells that serve as fire escapes and are invariably located on the perimeters of floor plates. Open, generous, and attractively designed stairs should greet employees and visitors in any lobby, relegating the elevator to the fallback choice.

Even in multistory tenant spaces, getting from one co-worker's office to another frequently necessitates a visit to the elevator when someone could so much more logically, easily, and healthily take the stairs. An average person who weighs 160 pounds burns about 4.5 calories per flight of stairs, while he burns less than one calorie waiting for an elevator. Climbing stairs promotes cardiovascular health, builds muscles, strengthens bones, and increases the rate at which the body burns calories.[13]

In office buildings, spaces should be designed to allow employees to move about without compromising productivity. Desk heights almost always assume a seated posture for working, though simply standing while at work has been shown to improve metabolism and circulation, support good posture, burn calories, and increase

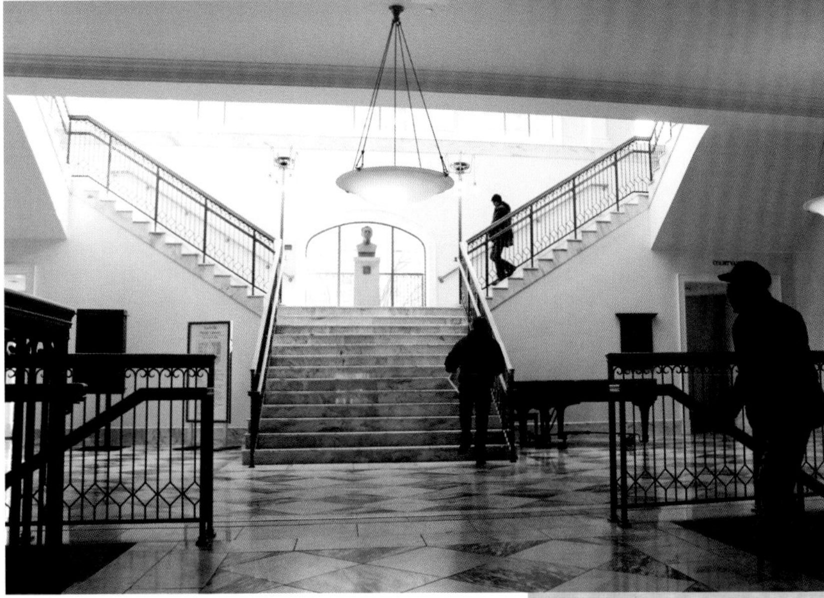

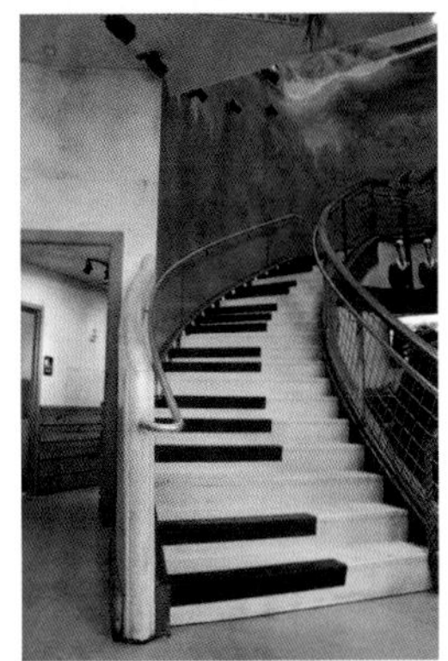

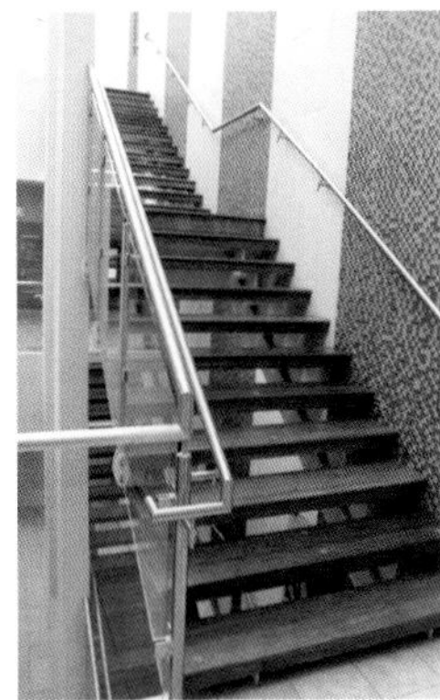

Examples of "good stairs" in Nashville: Downtown Public Library, Margaritaville Café where the stairs play piano notes, and Metro's Howard Office Building. (2015)

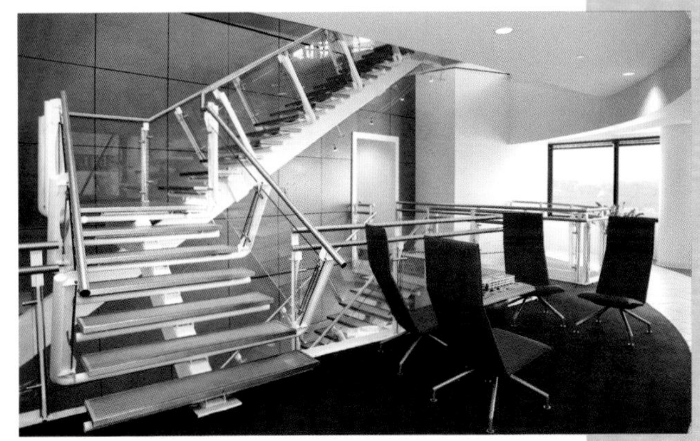

Nashville headquarters of Gresham Smith and Partners architecture firm. (2014, GS&P)

Walking the Walk: The Lentz Public Health Center

The Metro Public Health Department's mission is "to protect and improve the health and well-being of all people in Metropolitan Nashville." It is thus appropriate that the department designed its new headquarters to promote physical activity in the workplace, engage the customers of the department, and connect to the surrounding neighborhood.

The Lentz Public Health Center, named after Dr. John J. Lentz, who became the city's first public health officer in 1920, was planned to reflect six guiding principles established collectively by designers from Gresham Smith and Partners and a leadership committee from Public Health. One principle specifically targeted a proactive approach to health: "Set an example for healthy living to support and promote the health and well-being of people and employees."

Taking advantage of the large site, a quarter-mile walking track is incorporated into the perimeter of the parking lot. The building's north façade opens to views of this track, which is well lit and monitored by the building's surveillance system. Emergency phones are available along the track, creating a safe place for neighbors from the surrounding community to walk and improve health. The site also features road frontage with a bike lane and bike racks to encourage the use of active transportation. The Metro Arts Commission recently completed a competition for artistic bike racks whose theme was "healthy, active, and green." The Lentz site incorporates racks with a form that suggests movement—abstracted walking legs—at its street-facing entry plaza.

Inside the new facility is a fitness and showering facility for staff with some of the best views of downtown Nashville available in the building. The third floor includes a perimeter walking loop that enables staff to stage walking breaks and walking meetings.

Some design elements promote physical activity less obviously. As part of the healthy workplace strategy, copiers and break rooms are centrally located, and there are opportunities for stand-up meetings and flexible collaborative work areas. These features encourage employees to get out of their cubicles and onto the floor rather than spend long hours at their desks.

The design also features a monumental stair, connecting all three of the building's floors, as a central focus of the atrium lobby. This placement encourages its use as the primary way to circulate from floor to floor. Elevators (the slowest on the market!) are tucked around the corner in a less conspicuous location. Adding to the stair's dynamic, the Metro Nashville Arts Commission selected the monumental stair for an interactive artwork that responds to motion on the steps.

The design of the built environment can make healthy choices easier and more obvious for regular instances of physical activity. The Lentz Public Health Center embodies the Public Health Department's desire to advance strategies for wellness, rather than treat diseases that stem from unhealthy lifestyles.

— ANN S. TRENT, AIA, LEED AP, and LAUREN COMET, Gresham Smith and Partners

The new Lentz Public Health Center, located on Charlotte Avenue in Nashville, has a highly visible street presence with accommodations for public transit, a bicycle station, and outdoor seating. The interior features a centralized staircase that functions as an interactive public art component that lights up when people utilize the stairs. Note the upper floor circulation also doubles as a walking track. *(2014: © Chad Mellon)*

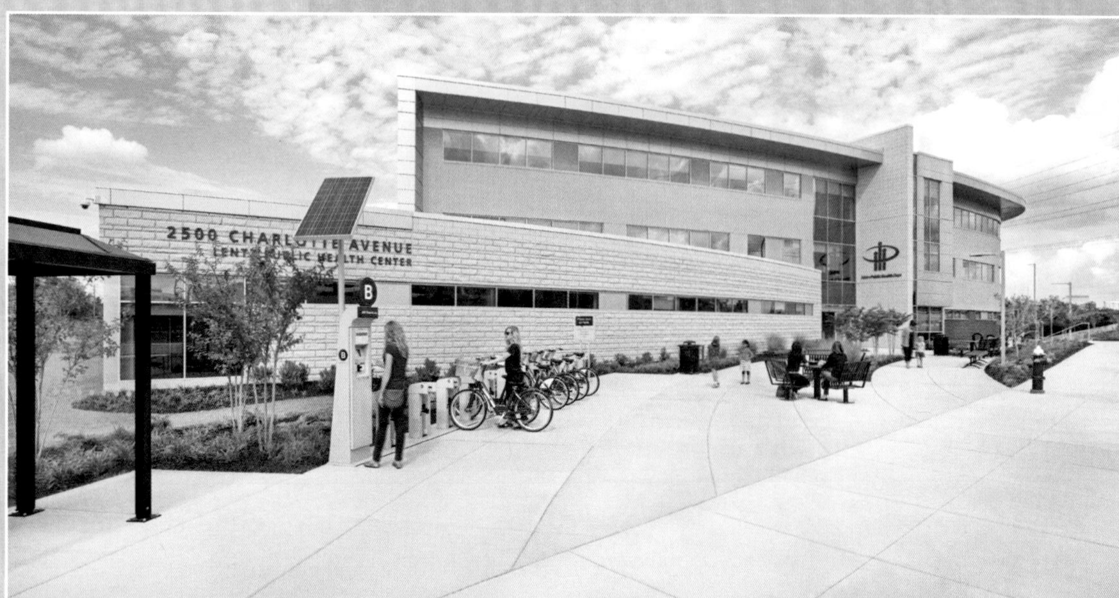

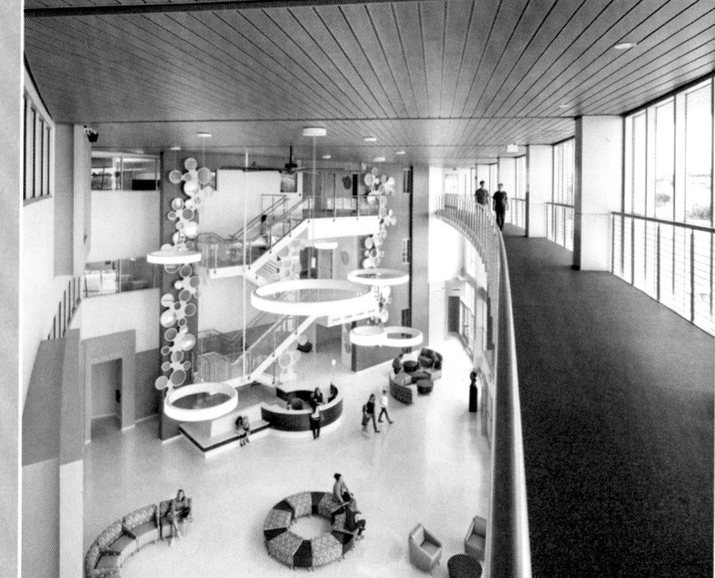

energy.[14] Office furnishings can be chosen to take this into account by allowing employees to use standing desks, treadmill desks, and balancing ball chairs, which have been shown to boost productivity, focus, and energy levels, in place of standard office chairs.[15]

The body harmonizes with the spectrum of sunlight, according to research by environmental psychologist Sally Augustin.[16] Any environment that exposes workers to natural light is much preferred to ones that rely heavily on artificial illumination. Offices flooded with sunlight have been shown to reduce absenteeism, increase productivity and mental performance, raise morale, and reduce headaches. Particular improvement occurs during the post-lunch, afternoon energy "dip."[17]

STRATEGY: *Build with materials that protect indoor air quality.*

Volatile organic compounds (VOCs) are increasingly regulated due to their health effects but are commonly found in synthetic building products, adhesives, paints, and upholstery. VOCs are emitted as gases at room temperature and, in spaces that are poorly ventilated, can cause headaches, allergic reactions, dizziness, and nausea. Some VOCs are linked to lung and eye irritation, and in the long term may harm the liver and nervous systems and cause cancer. Designers and contractors should use paint, fabric, and natural building materials that are certified as low emitters of VOCs.

The GREENGUARD Environmental Institute evaluates the chemical and biological effects of building products to help ensure a healthy interior environment. GREENGUARD Certification helps manufacturers create and buyers identify interior products and materials that have low chemical emissions, thus improving the quality of the air in which the products are used.[18]

While the tendency in office environments is

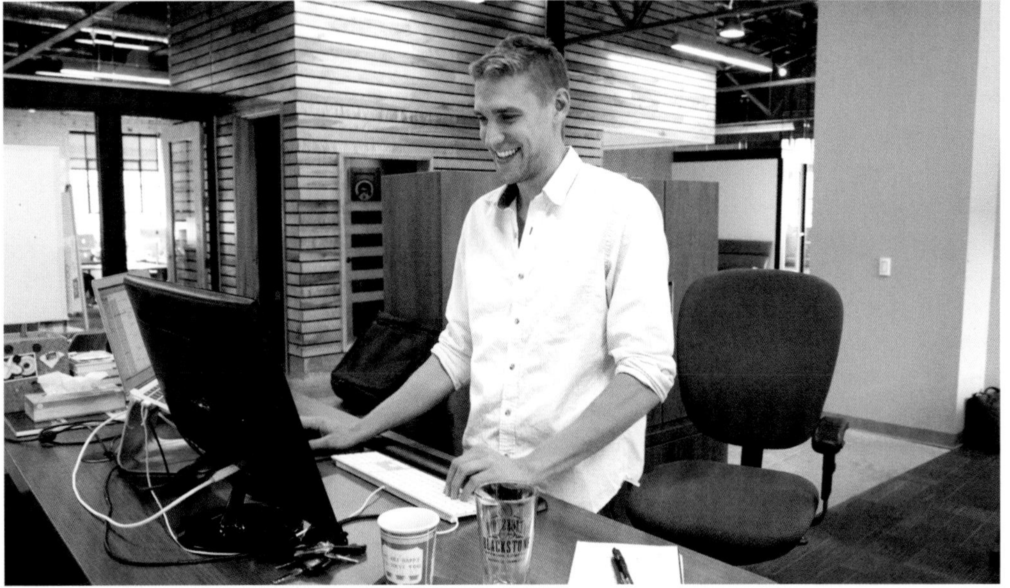

The stand-up desk offers an alternative to the sedentary work-style. Famous users include Leonardo Da Vinci, Benjamin Franklin, Thomas Jefferson, Ernest Hemingway, Winston Churchill, and Frank Lloyd Wright. *(2014: Emma)*

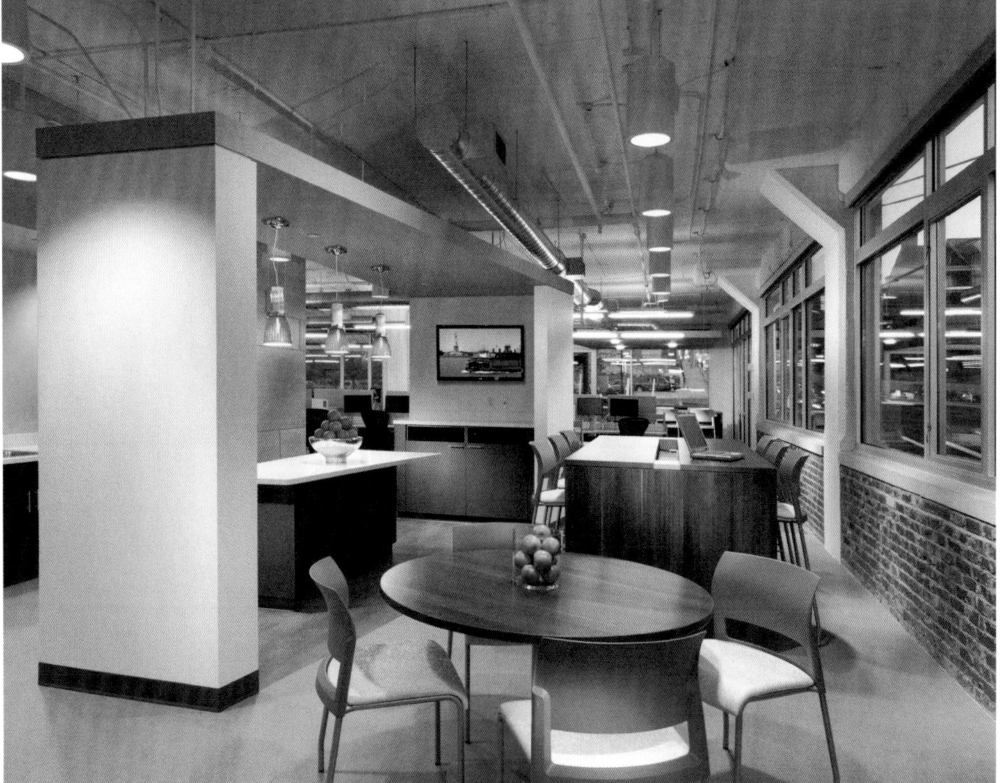

The headquarters of Asurion on Second Avenue South in downtown Nashville was specifically designed to maximize daylight. The interior layout allows employees to step away from desks and work at a variety of different types of spaces. *(2014: Hastings Architecture Associates, LLC)*

Top right, clockwise: Off-gassing of dangerous VOCs occur in many common house-hold items, including paint, new furniture, cleaners, ink-jet printers, and new carpeting. *(2007: Imagery provided by Tom Murphy VII from Wikimedia Commons, 2008: Ashe, Flickr, 2008: Binghamton University, Flickr, 2010: Keith Williamson, Flickr, 2005: Joseph Barillari, Wikimedia Commons)*

to plan for greater efficiency in the use of space, as characterized by densely populated partition mazes, *The Handbook of Work Stress* presents evidence that the "open office" concept may have significant downsides for health.[19] While ostensibly more productive due to the increased capacity for collaboration, open offices can contribute to significant stress as the workplace becomes crowded and louder and makes focus on tasks more difficult to sustain. Returning to vogue are the historic assumptions that work is more effectively completed behind closed doors and without distractions. Even in open office spaces, sound deadening textures and devices can create a more relaxed atmosphere, and intimate furniture arrangements can offer opportunities for individual workers to find a calming sense of personal control and privacy.

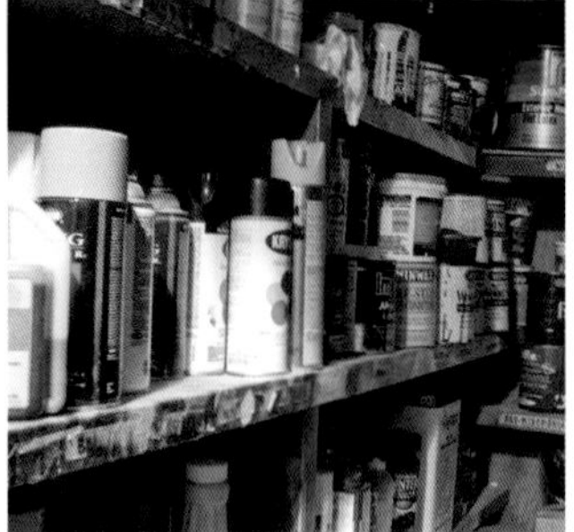

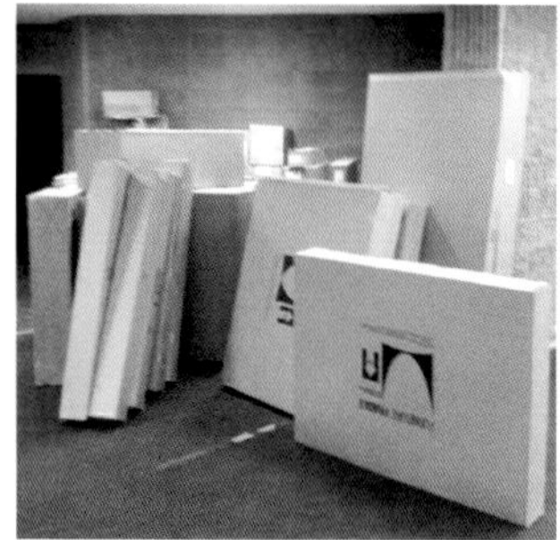

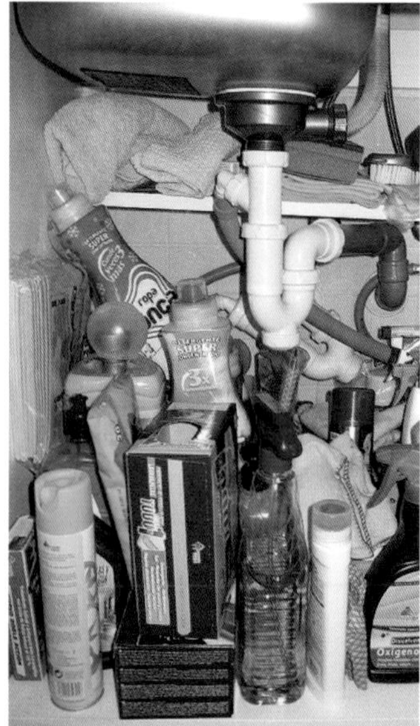

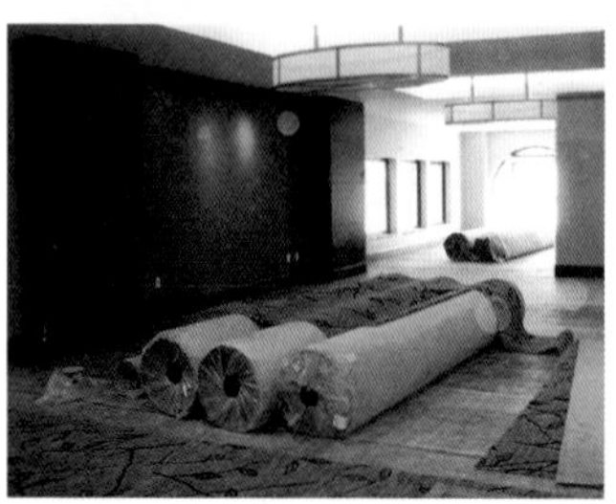

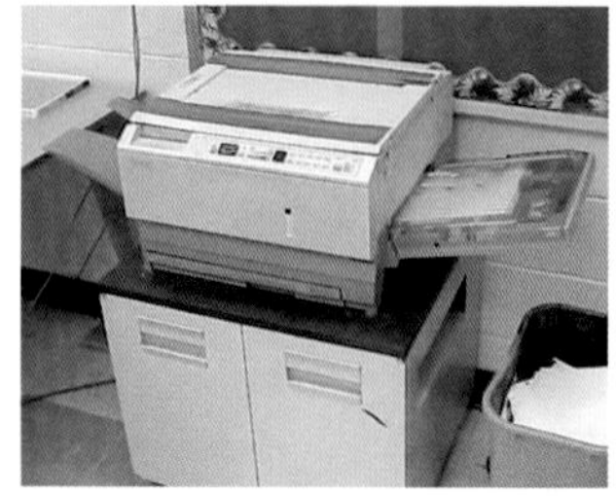

Email marketing company Emma in Nashville has an open plan design, but with a variety of work spaces. Creative breakout areas are for worker comfort and increased collaboration. *(2014: Emma)*

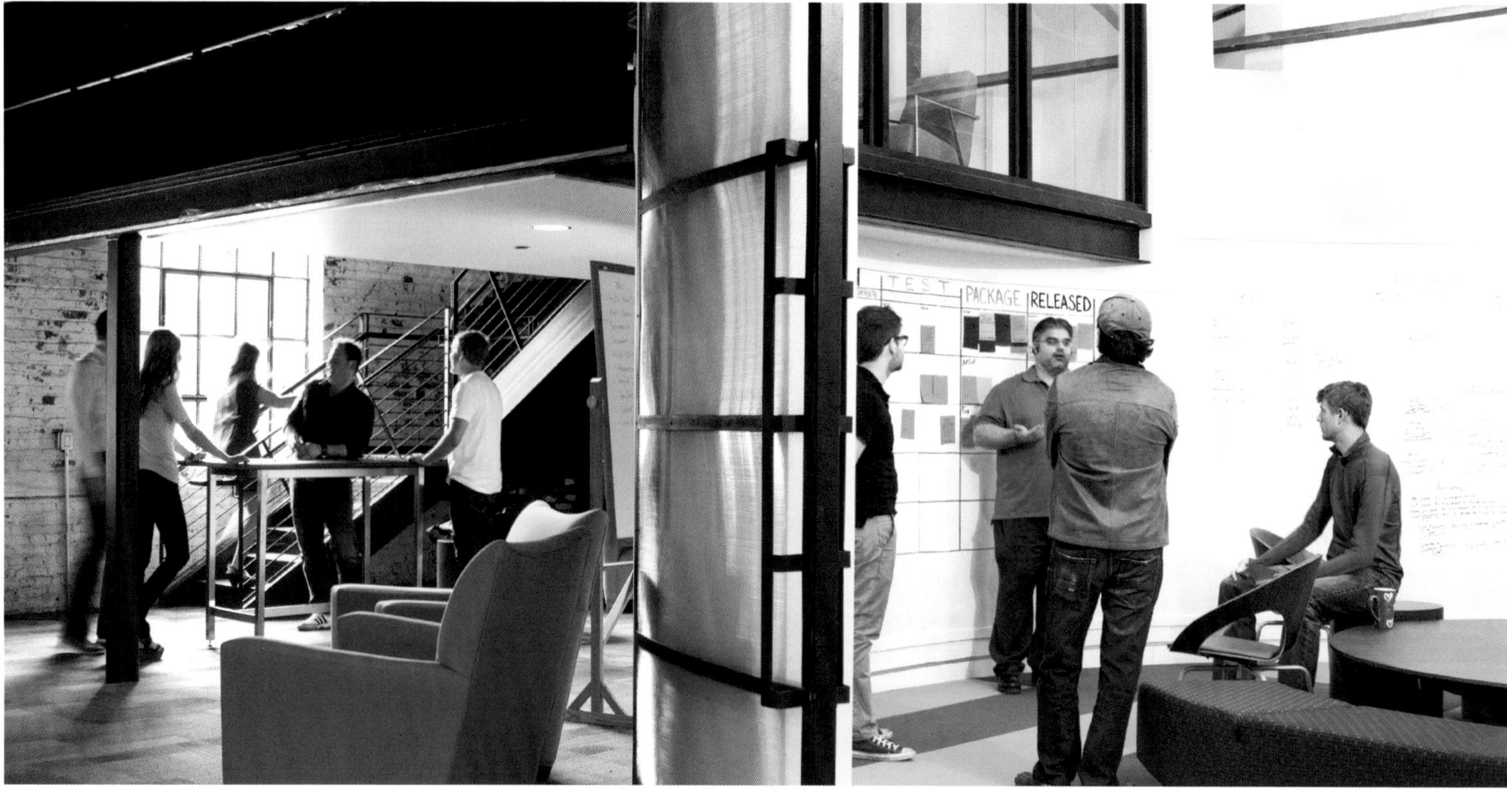

Case Study: Metro's Fulton Campus

When it comes to the design approach for retrofitting buildings, a lot can change in just a few short years. Take Metro's Howard Office Building and the Metro Office Building, for example. Both historic structures are located within Metro Nashville's Fulton Campus on Second Avenue South. Renovations of both were led by the Metro General Services Department and took place a mere five years apart. Both represent the recycling of older structures, a practice more environmentally sustainable than demolition and new construction. But the buildings stand in stark contrast in their respective design philosophies and illustrate how far designers and building managers have evolved in creating buildings that induce physical activity and interaction.

The Metro Office Building, a former hospital turned juvenile detention center, had been shuttered since 1995[20] prior to its renovation and the addition of a new wing, which opened in 2006. Its interior plan and design is that of a bygone era: a lobby with no visible stairs and one lonely elevator that often leaves occupants waiting for up to five minutes. Contrast that with the LEED Silver-certified Howard Office Building, which opened in 2010. Here General Services implemented multiple strategies to reduce energy costs as well provide a healthier interior environment for employees and encourage activity among staff and visitors.

—WHITNEY YOUNGBLOOD, NCDC

METRO OFFICE BUILDING

- No visible staircase upon entering building (rather, staircases located at either end of building with no directional signage and accessed through a welter of cubicles)
- Central elevator visible upon entering the building
- No workout facility
- Confusing indoor layout undermines a pleasant walking experience

HOWARD OFFICE BUILDING

- Prominent central staircase visible from main entrance that appeals to the senses
- Elevator hidden from direct sightlines at the main entrance
- Workout facility with lockers and showers inside building
- Open indoor layout easy to understand and thus conducive to walking
- Transoms bring natural light to interior spaces

DESIGN FOR DOWN TIME

All open spaces are not created equal. Many are not intended to be recreational but social in nature. Poorly designed, such civic space can simply waste real estate. Large, empty, windswept plazas, the result of misguided efforts by planners to create more downtown open space by awarding density bonuses to developers in return for public plazas, are among the worst offenders. Their designs exhibit no grasp of how people interact in public places and frequently inhibit activity and social interaction: nothing to play on or with, no shade, no visual interest or sense of spontaneity.

Where playgrounds are available, especially in parks, schools, hospitals, and daycare facilities, they often prescribe children's use of the equipment—slide here, swing on these, use this for

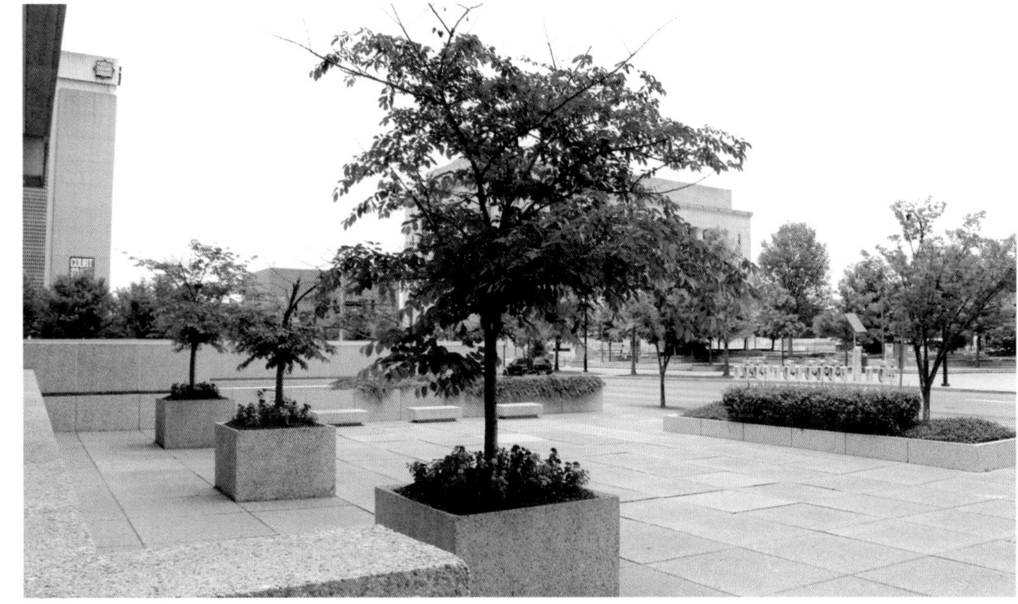

Barren and unused plaza at the UBS Building in downtown Nashville misses an opportunity to activate prime public space located opposite the city's courthouse and public square. *(2015)*

STRATEGY: *Design ample opportunity for children's imaginative, physically active play.*

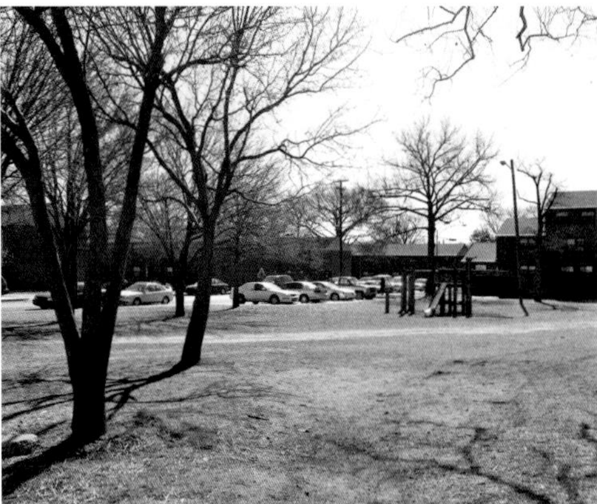

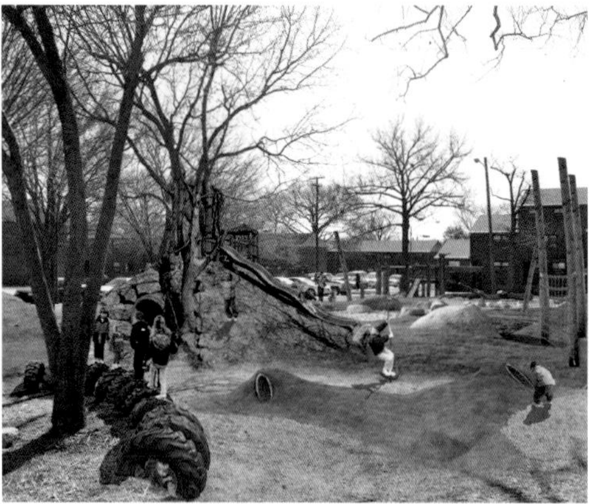

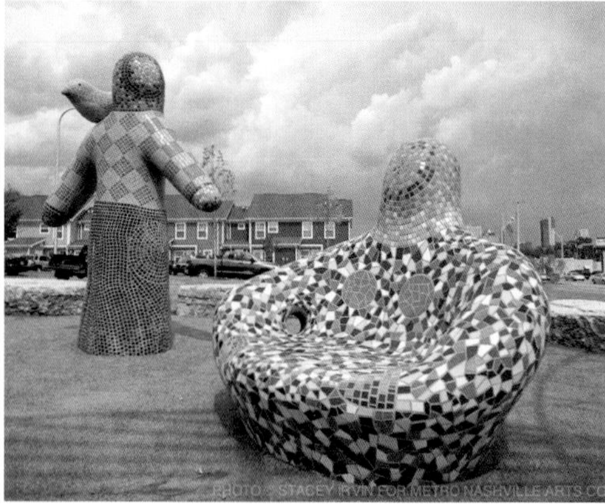

Left, center: An existing playground at the Tony Sudekum Apartments, redesigned as a natural playground that incorporates creative play features. *(Visualization, 2010: Ron Yearwood, NCDC)*

Right: Edmondson Park on Charlotte Avenue is Nashville's first art park. It is named after Nashville's William Edmondson, a self-taught sculptor who in 1937 became the first African American to have an exhibition at the Museum of Modern Art in New York. The original park was not much more than open lawn with a marker about Edmondson. The redesign, which incorporates significant community input, was done by landscape architecture firm Hawkins Partners. It features artworks by internationally recognized Thornton Dial and Lonnie Holley, which were installed by the Metro Arts Commission in 2014. In addition, *The Gathering*, a mosaic sculpture by Bell Buckle, Tennessee, artist Sherri Warner Hunter was relocated to the park. *(2014: Stacy Irvin, Metro Arts Commission)*

teeter tottering—failing to cultivate imagination and serving only the shortest of attention spans.[21] Some also promote competitive rather than cooperative behavior.[22]

It takes very little to induce imaginative children to be active. On-site playgrounds or even interior lobbies or waiting rooms in individual buildings can offer the space for the exploration of objects or equipment to use. Climbing—on, around, into, beneath, over, through—can be encouraged by creatively situating objects in relationship to each other and to surrounding activities.

Strategy: Universal Design

Universal Design supports usable spaces for those of all ages and abilities. The intent of Universal Design is to allow anyone and everyone, regardless of age or ability, to use public and private interior environments safely and optimally, without the need for adaptation or specialty design. Public spaces that use tactile paving, for example, can be more easily navigated by the visually impaired.

Aging-in-place design features also fall into this category: no-step entries, one-story living, wide doorways and hallways (minimum of 36"), nonslip surfaces on floors and in bathtubs, grab bars and handrails, wall-mounted sinks, thresholds that are flush with flooring, good lighting levels, and lever door handles and rocker light switches instead of knobs and standard switches.[23]

—WHITNEY YOUNGBLOOD, NCDC

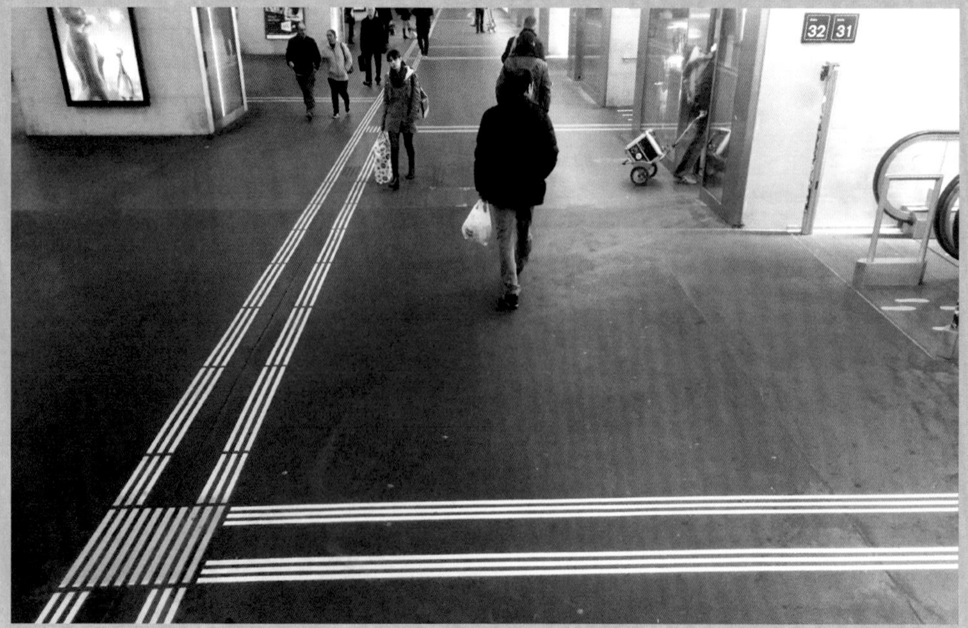

These raised lines and squares in the train station in Zurich assist pedestrians who are blind or visually impaired in moving between trains and to other public facilities. Tactile paving is found in many public buildings and on sidewalks in Switzerland. *(2014)*

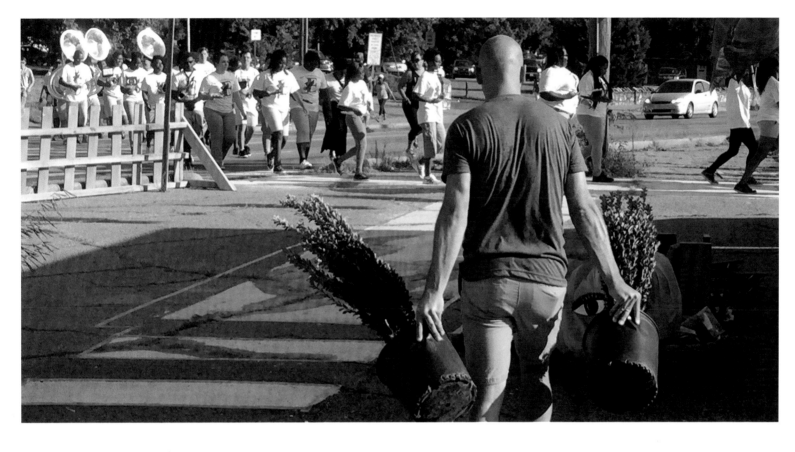

Public space installation by Tactical Urban Organizers during the East Nashville Tomato Art Festival. The group stages temporary enhancements of public spaces to call attention to the need for permanent improvements. Here a high school band uses a crosswalk installed near Five Points to make the area more pedestrian friendly. *(2015: Michael Kenner)*

STRATEGIES INTO REALITY

For *Shaping the Healthy Community: The Nashville Plan (SHCN)* to be more than just another book on a shelf, it must be implemented by means of a systematic approach to the recommendations and design strategies within it. This will require leadership from the Nashville Civic Design Center as well as our partners in the design and development communities, city and state government departments, nonprofits, neighborhood and community groups, and concerned citizens.

PARTNERSHIPS

Much is already being done to lay the groundwork for implementation. The Metro Nashville Planning Commission's adoption of *NashvilleNext* in June 2015 provides a citywide platform for many of the concepts in *SHCN*. This general plan will serve as the blueprint for Nashville's development over the next 20 years; it contains an action plan that includes near-, mid-, and long-term recommendations for implementation. Health is an explicit focus of the plan, with an entire chapter dedicated to "Health, Livability & the Built Environment."[1]

In addition to *NashvilleNext*, several other major planning processes are underway that can incorporate *SHCN* strategies to enable healthier communities. These include the Nashville Area

> Good ideas are common—what's uncommon are people who'll work hard enough to bring them about.
>
> Ashleigh Brilliant, *All I Want Is a Warm Bed and a Kind Word and Unlimited Power: Even More Brilliant Thoughts* (1985)

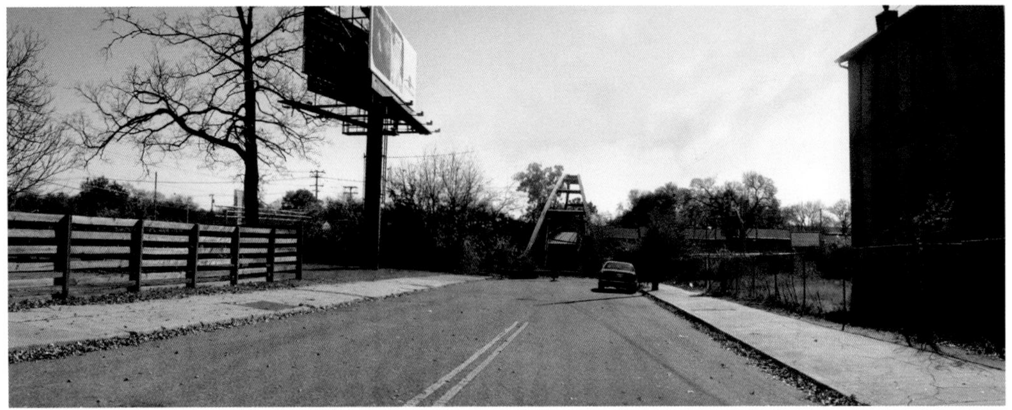

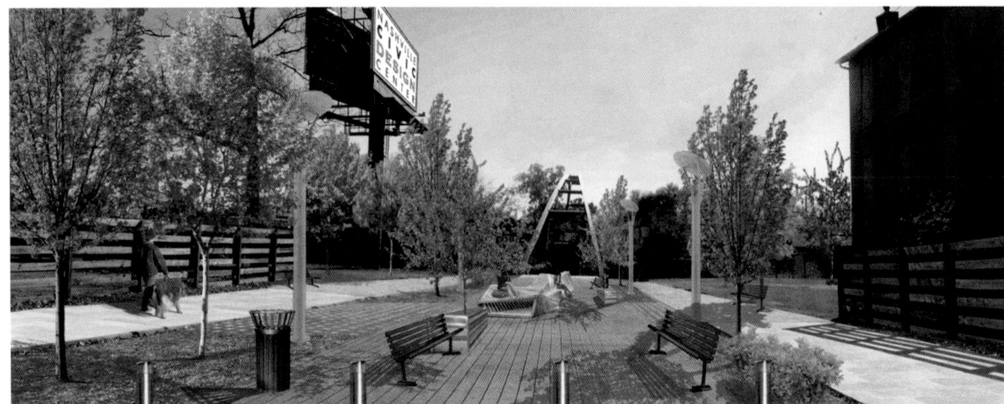

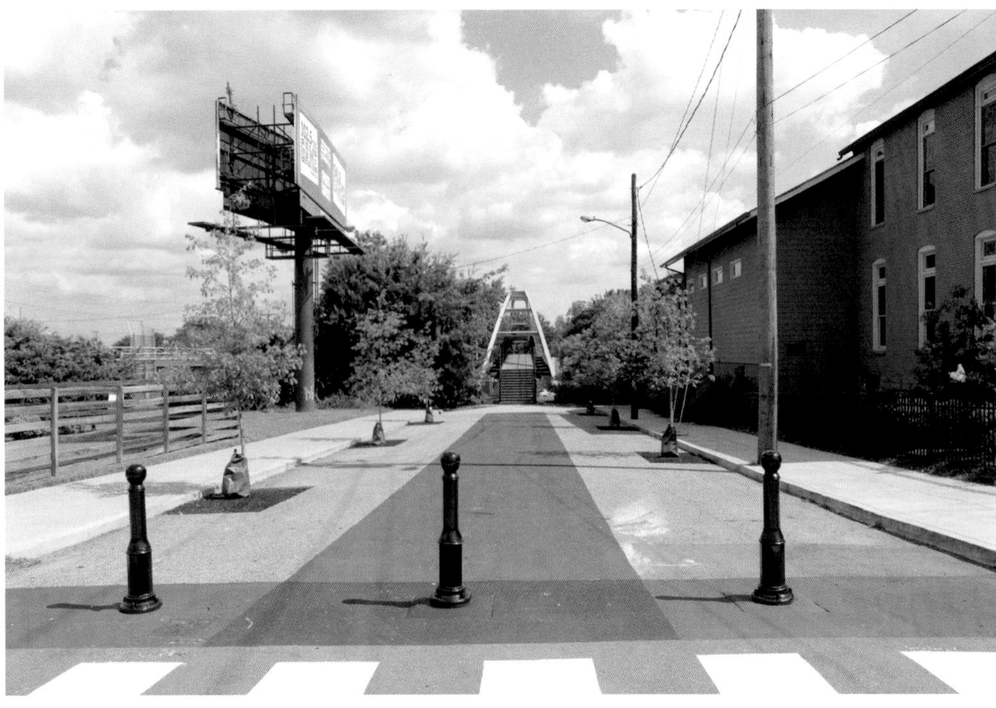

Academy Place, before, proposed, and after. The streetscape leading to the bridge over the interstate linking Rutledge Hill with Napier-Sudekum apartments had devolved into a weed-infested area lacking any pedestrian amenities. After NCDC visualized potential improvements, a private developer, Metro government, and the Tennessee Department of Transportation partnered to create a new parklet. *(2010; Visualization, 2010: Ron Yearwood, NCDC; 2015)*

Metropolitan Planning Organization's (MPO) *2040 Plan*,[2] the Metro Nashville Transit Authority's (MTA) *N-Motion 2015*,[3] the Nashville Area Chamber of Commerce plan called *Moving Forward*,[4] and the Tennessee Department of Transportation's (TDOT) ongoing statewide planning initiatives.

NCDC will coordinate and partner with these and other groups—such as the local chapter of the American Institute of Architects (AIA) and the Urban Land Institute (ULI), AARP, and Metro Nashville Public Schools (MNPS)—to integrate the strategies presented in *SHCN* into their respective planning and design efforts.

EDUCATION

Following the publication of *Shaping the Healthy Community*, NCDC staff will lead an intensive community education initiative through detailed presentations targeted to each transect zone—rural, suburban, urban, and downtown—with health-strategy content specific to the particular zone.

But attendance at a meeting or workshop is not necessary for individual and community group involvement. The checklists contained in this book provide the tools for self-assessments of specific neighborhood assets and needs. Neighborhood organizations and other community groups can then work with NCDC to develop detailed strategies and visualize improvements. These strategies and visualizations can be employed to lobby for change through Metro Council and state representatives, city and state government departments, and developers.

NCDC will also stage a citywide series of topic-based presentations focused on each of the six built environment factors that impact health: neighborhood design and development, transportation, walkability, food access, housing, and open space. This approach is intended to engage people across neighborhood boundaries and socioeconomic strata who perceive a particular need or have a special interest or expertise in, for example, public transit, pedestrian safety, etc.

A more expansive educational initiative targeted at Nashville's middle and high school students, as well as adult learners, is under development by NCDC in the form of a curriculum focused on architecture and civic design, with healthy design a key component. Students and community members will investigate how urban design concepts and practices affect the local environment and quality of life and develop ways to improve their neighborhoods. The goal is to grow, particularly in the rising generation, the civic skills necessary to participate substantively in the planning and design of communities.

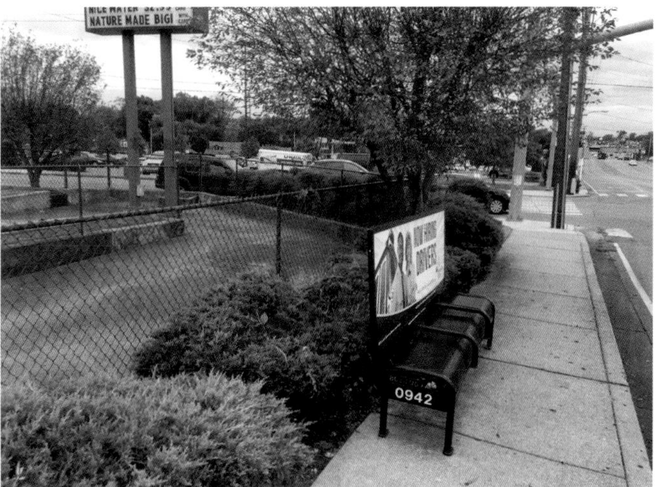

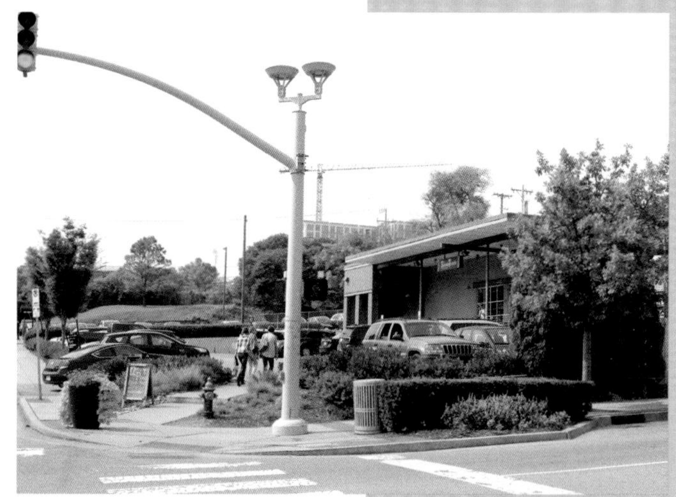

Two strikingly different ways to design access to corner commercial with high customer turnover.

This Walgreens on Gallatin Road in Inglewood virtually defines the car-centric approach. Fencing surrounds the corner, with the paving visible behind the fence solely for channeling polluted water runoff from the parking lot. Thus pedestrians approaching from the crosswalk, sidewalk, and bus stop must walk half a block then use vehicular curb cuts—or march through the landscaping—to access the store. *(2015)*

The Turnip Truck grocery in the Gulch features pedestrian-only paving from the corner, which is fed by sidewalk and crosswalk, reducing conflict with vehicles. *(2015)*

TRANSLATING PRECEPT INTO PRACTICE

Incorporating the recommendations and strategies presented in *SHCN* into public policies is a crucial aspect of implementation. Integrating a consideration of health impacts into planning and design will produce better decisions throughout the development process and lead to healthier outcomes. NCDC efforts in this regard will focus on specific initiatives.

Active Design Guidelines

Nashville needs guidelines that promote physical activity and a healthy environment at the level of individual building and site design. New York City's *Active Design* publication series, with its easy-to-comprehend explanations and checklists, can serve as a model for building and site assessments. Metro Nashville's government buildings and public schools are prime candidates for such guidelines. Due to their public profile and typically large square footage these buildings can serve as demonstration projects for the city. NCDC will also seek the support of the Middle Tennessee Chapter of the AIA.

Complete Streets 2.0

NCDC will convene a coalition of relevant organizations and departments to reinforce the application of complete streets policies to new and redeveloped streetscapes. The collaborative efforts of this coalition, which will include Metro's Public Works and Planning departments, MPO, MTA, MNPS, and TDOT, as well as nonprofit advocates such as Walk/Bike Nashville and Transit Now Nashville, can make the policies a reality on the ground.

Reclaiming Public Space

This NCDC program focuses on underutilized public spaces. Through the publication of case studies and best practices, as well as the analysis and visualization of improvements to specific sites, NCDC works to educate the Nashville community on the creation and rehabilitation of sustainable civic space.

Health Impact Assessments (HIA)

Checklists based on the policy recommendations and design strategies contained in *SHCN* (see pages 295–301) can be utilized by community members to assess the health factors of their neighborhoods' built environments. Larger scale developments merit a more detailed, individual assessment of health impacts through the agency of the Metro Nashville Public Health Department.

Recycling 2.0

Enabling Nashvillians to be better recyclers requires a comprehensive education program that Metro should undertake in coordination with Metro schools. Teaching people to sort before they toss and providing an ample supply of recycling receptacles in parks and other public spaces—the football stadium, the riverfront amphitheater, the arena—would reduce the waste going to landfills and the fees Metro pays to use them. A robust composting program for biowaste and more frequent pick-up of compostable materials such as yard waste would divert such items from landfills and convert them into rich, water-retaining soil. User fees levied on landfill-bound trash by bulk or weight, often called "pay as you throw," would provide financial support for recycling and composting programs and the education to use them.

The Health Impact Assessment: A Tool for Promoting Health in Public Policy

Health Impact Assessment (HIA) is a tool used to promote the consideration of health in decision-making. It is defined as "a combination of procedures, methods, and tools by which a policy, program, or project may be judged as to its potential effects on the health of a population, and the distribution of those effects within the population."[5] An HIA is typically conducted before a project or plan is implemented. Its purpose is to examine both the positive and negative potential impacts of an initiative on human health. An HIA provides recommendations for maximizing the health benefits of the initiative being assessed, while mitigating and managing any potential negative health impacts. It is a useful tool for including health in public policy decisions, particularly in non-health sectors that impact health but may not readily consider it as a factor in developing policies.

The first HIA in the United States was conducted in 1999. Since then it has grown in popularity, with hundreds completed and many more in progress. HIA aligns with a public health approach that recognizes the importance of social and environmental factors in a community's health. It is useful for evaluating potential changes to the built environment, including land-use planning, transportation, and urban design, but it is also relevant to education, criminal justice, food systems, and employment, among others. HIA is most often conducted by local health departments, planners, universities, community organizations, or policy makers. In most cases it is a collaborative effort, including stakeholders from different organizations and public agencies, as well as community members who may be affected by the proposed initiative. Collaboration in the HIA process is both a practical and an ethical consideration: it includes a range of relevant perspectives and information while seeking to promote social values including equity, democracy, and sustainability.[6]

The outcome of an HIA is a set of evidence-based recommendations for negating or minimizing any potential negative health impacts as well as promoting positive health impacts of the proposed initiative.[7] While the ultimate goal is to produce a healthier environment for the community, the HIA process itself also offers other benefits including increasing awareness and understanding of health conditions among community members and bringing together numerous stakeholders to foster collaboration and network development that can outlast the HIA process. However, collaboration can result in a time- and resource-intensive HIA process and should have the full commitment of all process partners in order to be successfully completed. Further, HIA is typically voluntary and should be carefully timed and planned to ensure the process and recommendations effectively inform decision-making.

HIA IN NASHVILLE

Several HIAs have been completed in the Nashville area. The Metro Nashville Public Health Department completed an HIA in 2012 examining the health benefits of the EasyRide program, which provides free or discounted Metro Transit Authority bus service for employees of major area employers.

The Nashville Area Metropolitan Planning Organization (MPO) has completed two HIAs to date. One examined the health impacts of locating a new school within a planned transit-oriented development (TOD) in Lebanon, Tennessee. It assessed the development on two potential health impacts: transportation options and food environments.[8] A second HIA examined the health impacts of locating a TOD in a northeast transit corridor in Madison, Tennessee.

In Nashville, opportunities for conducting HIAs may emerge from multiple places: academic researchers, community organizations or groups, state and local health departments, local or regional planning departments, the Metro Council, or others. Regardless of who initiates, funds, or manages the HIA, partnerships and collaboration are key. The sharing of resources, perspectives, political connections, and data can all contribute to an HIA's success. As Nashville continues to grow and develop in the coming years, HIA will be an important tool for evaluating proposed policy changes, programs, and developments. New local policies being discussed and proposed in housing, transportation, and other areas have the potential to improve or harm the health of residents, and HIA is a way to ensure those impacts are considered.

—JOHN VICK
Metro Public Health Department,
Division of Epidemiology and Research

SHAPING THE HEALTHY COMMUNITY

COMMUNITY ASSESSMENT CHECKLIST AND QUESTIONNAIRE BASED ON TRANSECT AND FILTERED BY FACTORS

HOW TO USE: This checklist provides a means for individuals and community groups to do a self-assessment of their communities. The questions are categorized by transect zone type and divided into categories based on the built environment factor groups explained in the text of the Transect chapter (pages 34–55). Two tools are provided. The first can be used by any individual to quickly assess his/her neighborhood health amenities. The second is lengthier and more detailed; some questions will require additional information from government or nonprofit organizations specializing in the topic area. Also included are questions government or nonprofit organization leaders may use to assess their respective policies and infrastructure support on a county-wide basis. A list of organizations that may be helpful in answering questions is provided at the end of the questionnaire.

TRANSECT ZONE - QUICK CHECKLIST AND QUESTIONNAIRE

What kind of community do you live in?

____ Rural
____ Suburban
____ Urban
____ Center
____ Downtown

Do you have a community or neighborhood organization?

What kind of walking infrastructure is used in your neighborhood? (Check all that apply)

____ Sidewalks
____ Crosswalks
____ Trails
____ Pedestrian signs
____ None of the above

The public transit in your neighborhood is: (Check all that apply)

____ Affordable
____ Reliable
____ Frequent
____ Convenient
____ None of the above

What kinds of public transit options are within a ½ mile of your home?

____ Bus
____ BRT (Bus Rapid Transit)
____ Light Rail
____ Commuter Rail
____ None of the above

For fresh food, I am able to walk or bike to a nearby:

____ Farmers' market
____ Grocery store
____ Convenience shop
____ Other; explain
____ None of the above

Do you have a park or public green space within walking distance?

Are natural areas and water sources well maintained and kept clean?

Does your neighborhood have pervious pavement, proper drainage, trees, rain gardens, or green roofs to help with flood control?

Does your neighborhood have recycling service? Do you use it?

Do new developments displace families, or is affordable housing integrated into new designs?

Does your community have a range of housing options to support and allow multiple generations to live in the neighborhood?

TRANSECT ZONE - DETAILED ASSESSMENT

NATURAL

Neighborhood Design and Development: Use greenways to link open spaces with each other and with commercial and residential development. (pg. 62)

Individual / Community Groups	Government / Organizations
Do greenways extend beyond the park and connect visitors to other activities?	*How many parks have residential neighborhoods surrounding the area?*

Transportation: Provide public transit access to natural areas. (pg. 65)

Individual / Community Groups	Government / Organizations
	How many bus lines connect to parks and greenways in the county?

Walkability: Create walking and hiking paths segregated from vehicular circulation. Make maps of trails in public open space easily accessible. (pg. 68)

Individual / Community Groups	Government / Organizations
Is the parking for the parks located on the perimeter? *Are park maps easy to read and located at intersections of trails?*	

RURAL

Neighborhood Design and Development: Strengthen the civic heart of rural communities. (pg. 78)

Individual / Community Groups	Government / Organizations
Does the center of your community have a variety of businesses within walking or biking distance to one another? *Do bike lanes and walking paths slow traffic near the community center and make it more walkable and bike friendly?* *Are there multiple housing options within the center of the community?*	

Transportation: Encourage transportation alternatives over single occupancy automobile trips. (pg. 79)

Individual / Community Groups	Government / Organizations
Do you have access to a vanpool system that provides transportation for daily commutes?	*Are railroad tracks used for commuting to work or for freight only?* *Are regional and local transit stops available in the heart of the town?*

Walkability: Create a safe network of pedestrian and bicycle paths connecting community resources. (pg. 80)

Individual / Community Groups	Government / Organizations
	How many walking paths lead to the center or to community resources such as stores and schools? *How many regional transit stations are within walking distance of the town center?* *How many miles of bike paths are located within the community?* *How many walking and biking fatalities occurred in the past year?*

Open Space: Create additional opportunities to connect regional parks and open spaces to surrounding communities. (pg. 84)

Individual / Community Groups	Government / Organizations
How many parks are connected by a trail or bikeway to the center of your community?	

Individual / Community Groups	Government / Organizations
SUBURBAN	
Neighborhood Design and Development: Strategically connect housing to schools, goods, services, and transportation. (pg. 105)	
Are retail stores and services located in a central location that can be reached by public transportation?	*How many students bike/walk to school daily?*
Transportation: Utilize road diets and complete streets policies to incorporate additional sidewalks, crosswalks, and bike lanes. (pg. 111)	
	How much funding was put into sidewalks, complete streets, and similar projects? Was it increased from previous years? *How many miles of bike lanes and/or sidewalks were added to the neighborhood in the past year?*
Food Access: Enable access to existing food resources with better connectivity to surrounding communities. (pg. 120)	
Are grocery stores and other fresh food resources scattered throughout the community or in a central location? *Are these resources accessible by sidewalk and/or bike lane?*	
Housing: Focus infill housing along commercial corridors to help preserve the character of existing neighborhoods and create a larger ridership pool for mass transit. (pg. 121)	
Do infill projects enhance transit, bike, and pedestrian options or promote driving?	*How many mass transit lines are within walking distance of residences? What is the frequency of service?*
URBAN	
Neighborhood Design and Development: Promote urban infill development in existing communities and use the urban design neighborhood form for new developments. (pg. 144)	
	Were any remediation or feasibility studies done for reuse of infill sites? *What is the amount of acreage zoned for mixed-use neighborhoods?* *Are there government programs, such as tax-increment financing, to encourage infill projects within the urban transect zone?*
Transportation: Utilize road diets and complete streets policies to incorporate additional sidewalks, crosswalks, and bike lanes. (pg. 150)	
	How much funding was put into complete streets, sidewalks, and similar projects? Was it increased from previous years? *How many miles of bike lanes were added to the neighborhood in the past year?*

Individual / Community Groups	Government / Organizations
Walkability: Increase pedestrian-accommodating infrastructure like sidewalks, crosswalks, human-scaled lighting, and signage. (pg. 156)	
Is signage that alerts drivers to pedestrians hidden by trees or difficult to see?	*How many sidewalks have been repaired in the past five years in the neighborhood?* *How many miles of new sidewalks have been added?* *How many new crosswalks have been added in the past five years?*
Food Access: Encourage access to fresh produce and nonprocessed foods in areas considered food deserts by promoting stores, pop-up markets, community gardens, and programs that provide healthy local foodstuffs. (pg. 157)	
How many fresh food options are within a 10-minute walk from your house? *During the summer months, can you walk to weekly farmers' markets or pop-up markets?* *Does your neighborhood have a community garden?*	
Open Space: Encourage community stewardship of existing and potential open spaces in urban neighborhoods. (pg. 169)	
How many urban and/or regional parks are in your neighborhood or within walking/biking distance? *Do these parks have an active Friends group?*	
CENTER	
Neighborhood Design and Development: Transform underdeveloped centers into complete centers that function as mixed-use areas with access to all the basic needs for living, working, and recreation. (pg. 192)	
	Are businesses located on separate sites with each business providing its own access from the road? *Are the buildings located along the sidewalk, or is the entranced preceded by a parking lot?* *Are there trees along the road?* *Is there a mixture of businesses that enable the area to be active throughout the day and week?*
Transportation: Establish public transit hubs in centers to anchor circulator routes in surrounding neighborhoods. (pg. 193)	
Is there a central location with the basic needs accessible by public transit?	*How wide are the streets? How much is devoted to automobiles compared to bike lanes / bike streets?*
Food Access: Ensure a wide variety of healthy food options in centers. (pg. 194)	
Are the healthy food options reasonably priced and of good quality?	*What is the ratio of healthy food sources to fast food outlets?* *When new projects are in the planning phase, are grocery stores considered and approached before construction begins?*

Individual / Community Groups	Government / Organizations
Housing: Increase the range of housing types and sizes within centers to ensure a wide variety of households and affordability. (pg. 195)	
How many types of housing options are in the center? (apartment, condo, duplex, single-family house, etc.) *Are affordable housing options available?* *Are there various developers and styles of housing to create a more appealing, less uniform center?*	*How much local, regional, and federal government funding contributed to affordable housing programs in the area?*
Open Space: Incorporate new public spaces and parks into centers, including areas for both active and passive recreation that are accessible to the entire community. (pg. 195)	
Do the parks provide space for various activities, or is their use restricted by rules or privatization? *Can you walk, bike, or take public transit to the parks in the center?*	
DOWNTOWN	
Neighborhood Design and Development: Focus on making downtown a complete neighborhood, with more residences and the necessities for daily life. Infill vacant lots, surface parking lots, and empty upper floors of existing buildings. Connect disjointed streets, sidewalks, and alleys. Extend Metro's recycling program to downtown. (pg. 225)	
Is the recycling service convenient and affordable?	*How many total acres of surface parking lots are within the core?* *Are there empty or abandoned buildings that can be restored for a different use?* *How many mixed-use buildings are in the downtown area?*
Transportation: Increase the frequency and hours of operation of the public transit service that operates from Music City Central. Enhance cycling safety for commuters and residents and create a network of protected bike routes through downtown. (pg. 228)	
Do buses have bike racks to store your bike during the ride?	*How many BRT or BRT-lite transit options are available? (15 minutes between buses)* *Is there a bike hub with shower and storage facilities?* *How many miles of bike lanes are located downtown?* *Is there a bike-share option? How many stations are located downtown?* *How many protected bike lanes or bike roads are located downtown?*
Walkability: Improve the pedestrian experience by upgrading the streetscape with more trees, benches, and public restrooms. Limit pedestrian/vehicular conflict by giving crosswalk priority to pedestrians over automobiles and limiting vehicular right turns on red lights. Enhance mobility for wheelchairs and strollers. (pg. 233)	
Do bus stops have benches and are they maintained? *Are stops protected from inclement weather?*	*How many complete streets are there in the core?*

Individual / Community Groups	Government / Organizations
Food Access: Develop a mid-size, full-service grocery store in the downtown core that features fresh produce and healthy take-out at prices reasonable for all shoppers. Increase healthy food options in the concessions of publicly owned venues such as Music City Central, Bridgestone Arena, and Nissan Stadium. (pg. 236)	
How many grocery stores are located downtown? *Do convenience stores provide fresh fruits and vegetables that are appealing and affordable?*	*How many healthy food stations are available at special event and sports venues?*
Housing: Increase housing diversity in terms of affordability and household types. (pg. 238)	
How many types of housing options are in the core? (apartment, condo, duplex, single-family house, etc.)	*Does legislation require affordable housing in new developments downtown?*
Open Space: Create new open spaces, parks, and recreational uses in the core, and activate existing underutilized spaces. (pg. 241)	
Do parks allow for multiple uses and have adequate land to enhance the experience downtown?	*How many parks are located downtown? What is the total acreage? Is public access to these parks restricted?* *Are vacant lots turned into parks that are open to the public?* *Do the parks attract locals and tourists alike?*
INDIVIDUAL BUILDING AND SITE DESIGN	
Design ground floors of buildings to be as "extroverted" as possible. Transparent glass at street level, for example, allows pedestrians to see interior activity. (pg. 277)	
Does the design allow for a mix of uses within the same building or block? *Is the front of the building maintained and kept clean?* *How many windows and glass doors are located on the ground level?* *Does the development provide protection from the weather with street trees or an awning on the front of the building?* *Is there access to fresh food nearby? If not, is there a way to incorporate a grocery store, food stand, or farmers' market in your building or to partner with others in the area?*	
Design buildings to encourage use of active transportation options. Rather than focusing on convenient car parking, prioritize accommodation for transit users and cyclists—including showers and lockers—whenever possible. (pg. 278)	
Are there bike stands or lockers on the building's site? *Is there is a bus stop within a five-minute walk? Does it have a shelter?*	

Individual / Community Groups	Government / Organizations
Design with nature. Orient buildings and sites relative to the sun; respect the body's need for natural light and vegetation. This saves energy while increasing comfort. (pg. 284)	
Do most rooms within the building have access to sunlight? *Do windows provide desirable views?* *Do windows open?* *Are there plants or natural materials within the building?*	
Make the staircase an obvious and attractive choice while backgrounding the elevator. (pg. 285)	
Does the building provide convenient access to highly visible stairs when entering? *Are the stairs appealing and used for more than a fire escape?*	
Build with materials that protect indoor air quality. (pg. 287)	
	Is the building LEED certified? *Are VOCs used within the building?* *Does the ventilation system provide fresh air throughout the building?* *Are GREENGAURD certified materials used within the building?*
Design buildings to enable growing food for both people and wildlife: green walls, rooftops, and gardens. (pg. 282)	
Is there green space in the site design? *Is there a community garden?* *Are there any green walls or vertical gardens that maximize green space and help insulate the building?*	*How many square feet of green roof is in the site design?*
Design ample opportunity for children's imaginative, physically active play. (pg. 284)	
Are there playgrounds for kids to play on or engaging exterior designs?	
Implement principles of Universal Design to allow anyone and everyone, regardless of age or ability, to use public and private interior environments safely and optimally. (pg. 290)	
Are the doorways and hallways wide and comfortable enough for wheelchairs to easily maneuver through the building? *Is the site attractive to a diverse age group?*	*Are facilities planned with handicap parking and accessible buildings?*

Government Departments and Organizations that may be able to provide resources to answering questions:

Departments of Metro Government—Metro Development and Housing Agency (MDHA), Parks and Recreation, Planning, Public Health, Public Works, Transit Authority.

Organizations—Community Food Advocates, Nashville Downtown Partnership, The Housing Fund, Transit Now Nashville, United States Green Building Council, Urban Green Lab, Walk / Bike Nashville.

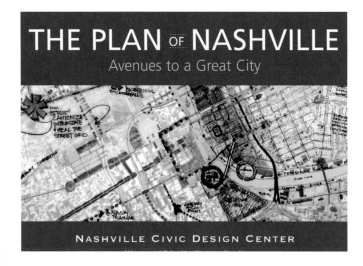

DOCUMENTING THE PROCESS

The Plan of Nashville: Avenues to a Great City established the Ten Principles to guide public policy, development practice, urban planning, and design. *Shaping the Healthy Community: The Nashville Plan* acts to implement these principles, viewed through the lens of public health.

The topic of health as an element of urban design is relatively new, coming to the forefront of community consciousness in the last decade. But the intentions of the Ten Principles are implicitly linked to the creation of a healthy city through their focus on walkability, open spaces, and transportation, even if the phrase "public health" was not directly addressed. And the vision for our city presented in *The Plan of Nashville* is the logical instrument for creating positive public health outcomes in our city.

WHO

Shaping the Healthy Community was orchestrated by the staff of the Nashville Civic Design Center (NCDC). Staff members organized and assigned tasks, staged programs, conducted research, and compiled images.

Christine Kreyling, writer and editor (2011–present)

Design Center staff

Patricia Conway, project manager (2011–2013)
Amy Eskind, research fellow (2011–2013)
Gary Gaston, design director (2008–2014); executive director (2015–present)
Matt Genova, research fellow (2014–present)
Eric Hoke, design fellow/urban designer (2013–present)
Julia Landstreet, executive director (2010–2014)
Joe Mayes, research fellow (2014–present)
Stephanie McCullough, communications and community outreach manager (2005–2014)
Janey Nachampasak, design fellow (2012–present)
Jill Robinson, research fellow (2011–present)
Kion Sawney, research fellow (2014–present)
Abby Wheeler, development manager (2014–present)
Billy White, digital fellow (2014–present)
Ron Yearwood, assistant design director (2010–2014); assistant director (2015–present)

Design Center interns

Vanessa Asaro, Vanderbilt University
Keaton Browder, Tennessee State University
Carrie Fry, Vanderbilt University
Meghan Fullham, Philadelphia University
Emma Grager, Vanderbilt University
David Heyburn, University of Cincinnati
Benjamin Jelsma, University of British Columbia, Vancouver
Kelsey Kaline, Vanderbilt University
Nora Kern, Williams College
Emily Kleinfelter, Hendrix College
Kristen McDaniel, Vanderbilt University
Caroline McDonald, University of Tennessee College of Architecture and Design
Tyler McSwain, Tennessee State University
Kiera Mitchell, Tennessee State University
Lauren Michele Murray, Vanderbilt University
Jonathan Nowlin, Syracuse University
Justin Ostrander, Syracuse University
Welsey Rhodes, Tennessee State University
Kathleen Russell, Vanderbilt University
Sonica Sundri, Vanderbilt University
Meghan Scholl, Westfield State University
Laura Schwinder, Vanderbilt University
Mary Ellen Smith, Lund University, Sweden

Alicia Meriwether Smith, University of Tennessee, Knoxville
Catherine Soudoplantoff, Watkins College of Art, Design and Film
Susan Steffenhagen, Georgia Tech
Chelsea Velaga, Vanderbilt University
Virginia (Ginny) Harr Webb, Virginia Tech
Whitney Youngblood, Watkins College of Art, Design and Film

Steering Committee

The Steering Committee was formed early in the process to provide advice and hands-on expertise.

Sandy Bivens, superintendent of nature centers, Metro Parks and Recreation
Jennifer Carlat, planning manager, Community Planning Division, Metro Planning Department
Hal Clark, associate principal, Civil Site Design Group
Ed Cole, executive director, Transit Alliance of Middle Tennessee
Laurel Creech, chief service officer and director of environment and sustainability, Office of the Mayor
Adriane Harris, economic development specialist, Metro Development and Housing Agency
Alisa Haushalter, director, Bureau of Population Health Programs, Metro Public Health Department
Chastity Hemmer-Mitchell, senior director, government relations, the American Heart Association; policy advocate, Tennessee Obesity Taskforce
Audra Ladd, project manager, Middle TN land use and open space, The Land Trust for Tennessee
Bert Mathews, developer, president of the Mathews Company; president of the Board of Directors of the Nashville Area Chamber of Commerce
Leslie Meehan, senior planner, Nashville Area Metropolitan Planning Organization; Tennessee Obesity Taskforce
Leslie Newman, attorney, commissioner, Tennessee Department of Commerce and Insurance
Toks Omishakin, deputy commissioner and environmental bureau chief, Tennessee Department of Transportation
Jeff Ockerman, director, Tennessee Division of Health Planning
Bill Paul, director, Metro Public Health Department
Douglas D. Perkins, professor of human and organizational development and director, PhD program in Community Research and Action, Peabody College, Vanderbilt University
Leslie Speller Henderson, professor of agriculture and human science, Tennessee State University

Metro Nashville departments and staff who served as consultants

Office of the Mayor: **Laurel Creech**
Metro Public Health Department: **Bill Paul, Alisa Haushalter, Tracy Buck, Jimmy Dills, Julie Fitzgerald, Joe Pinilla, John Vick**
Metro Planning Department: **Rick Bernhardt, Jennifer Carlat, Kathryn Withers, Anita McCaig, Michael Briggs, Stephanie McCullough, Cindy Wood**
Metro Parks Department: **Tim Netsche, Shain Dennison, Chris Koster**
Metro Transit Authority: **James McAteer**
Metro General Services: **Gary Layda, Dianna Stephens, Laura Burton**
Metro Public Works: **Mark Macy, Sharon Smith, Jenna Smith, Jennifer Smith**
Metro Water Services: **Rebecca Dohn**
Metro Arts Commission: **Caroline Vincent**
Nashville Farmers' Market: **Jolie Ayn Yockey, Laura Wilson**
Metro Historical Commission: **Tim Walker**
Metro Development and Housing Agency: **Joe Cain, Kaitlin Dastugue**
Metro Council: **Vice Mayor Diane Neighbors**
Nashville Archives: **Drew Mahan**
Metro Public Library: **Liz Coleman, Beth Odle**

Other government departments and staff who served as consultants

Nashville Area Metropolitan Planning Organization: **Michael Skipper, Leslie Meehan, Michelle Lacewell, Mary Beth Ikard**
Tennessee Department of Transportation: **Tanisha Hall, Larry McGoogin, Katy Braden**

Organizations whose staff served as consultants

Cumberland River Compact: **Paul Sloan, Mekayle Houghton**
Nashville Downtown Partnership: **Tamara Dickson, Andrea Champion**
Urban Land Institute: **Rose Fages-Easton**
US Green Building Council: **Heather Langford**
YMCA of Middle TN**: Ted Cornelius**

Professionals who served as consultants

Jay Everett, Transit Now Nashville
Veniece Jennings, US Forest Service
Kate Monaghan, Partnering Services
Mary Vavra, Lose and Associates

University Partnerships

Tennessee State University
Dr. David A. Padgett, associate professor of geography, geographic information systems

Vanderbilt University
Vanderbilt University faculty, students, and staff made major contributions to the research, editing, and production of this book.

Research:
Department of Human & Organizational Development
Community Research and Action Program
Center for Teaching

Several faculty members at Vanderbilt University incorporated aspects of research for *Shaping the Healthy Community* into their class curricula.

Paul Speer, professor of human and organizational development, Peabody College, Vanderbilt University
Students:
Saira Masood Ali
Mae Cooper
Carrie Fry
Jessica Gibbons-Benton
Laura Hardwicke
Judy Lewis
Christian Man
Rebecca Marchiafava
Annie Maselli
Tiffany McDole
Jera Niewoehner
Louise Riley
Robert Robinson
Kristyn Willis

Douglas D. Perkins, professor of human and organizational development and director, PhD

program in Community Research and Action, Peabody College, Vanderbilt University
Nikolay Mihaylov, graduate teaching assistant
Students:
Alexandria Baker
Rachel Bass
Cindy Basulto
Jeffrey Bond
Hanna Cutler
Honora Einhorn
Elissa Estopinal
Gabriella Flynn
Emily Francis
Catherine Garvey
Julia Geller
Erin Kelly
Christopher Kessenich
Ngoc-Thoa Khuu
Anna Liang
Nina Lim
Rebecca Matthews
James Reid
A'Yonnika Rogers
Erica Skurnik
Bethany Tuten
Grant Williams

Joe Bandy, assistant director of the Center for Teaching, and affiliated faculty in sociology, Vanderbilt University
Students:
Leia Andrew
Emma Applebome
Sara Boscacci
Patrick Burton
Tessa Chillemi
Evan Curran
Joseph Dow Jr.
Zachary Gellman
Matthew Genova
Audrey Jackson
Kelsey Kaline
Rachel Anne Kane
Monica Kumar
Julie Lapidot
Kevin Mink
Michael O'Connor
Kelly Anne Obranowicz
Cecily Parker
Katherine Pons
Courtney Rockwood
Alexandra Scavone
Sonica Sundri
Courtney van Stolk

Book production and distribution

Creative Services, Division of Public Affairs, Vanderbilt University: **Judy Orr,** assistant vice chancellor; **Deborah Hightower Brewington,** senior graphic designer
Vanderbilt University Press: **Michael Ames,** director; **Joell Smith-Borne**, managing editor; **Dariel Mayer,** design and production manager

WHAT

The goal of the process was to produce an action plan; that is, specific strategies for shaping the built environment that can be used by developers, design professionals, government officials, neighborhood and community organizations, educators, parents, and health conscious citizens.

This action plan relies on the vision presented in *The Plan of Nashville,* in particular the "Ten Principles" of *The Plan* intended to guide public policy, development practice, urban planning, and design.

WHERE

The focus was on Davidson County. Although the strategies have regional implications and applications, Metro Nashville within itself contains the basic forms of the built environment—rural, suburban, urban, core, etc.—to which these strategies are tailored.

Choosing the county as the boundary of study enabled a degree of specificity impossible when working at a regional scale. These specifics can be applied to communities throughout the region—and beyond.

Within each type of built environment—the transect zone—individual neighborhoods were selected as case studies to illustrate the necessity of considering the unique historical and physical characteristics of a community in devising and implementing strategies for a healthier environment.

WHEN: THE PROCESS

The project was structured in overlapping stages: research, programs to elicit community and professional input, plan organization and development, synthesis, writing, editing, and production.

2009

The city of Nashville received a grant as a part of the American Recovery and Reinvestment Act of 2009, administered through the Centers for Disease Control and Prevention. "Communities Putting Prevention to Work" (CPPW) was a $373 million community capacity-building program for instituting population-based policy, systems, and environmental change in communities and schools.

Nashville was one of only 44 cities nationwide to receive one of these highly competitive awards. The Metro Public Health Department (MPHD) received $7.5 million over a two-year timeframe to implement a multifaceted campaign to facilitate healthy eating and active living for everyone in Nashville.[1]

2010

In January, the Nashville Civic Design Center partnered with the University of Tennessee College of Architecture and Design to offer the "Health and the Built Environment: Whole-Community Wellness" lecture series. The six-part series focused on a range of topics including: an overview of how the built environment impacts public health; how urban design dictates activity levels;

the local manifestation of diabetes, cardiovascular problems, and lung disease on children and aging populations; and how evidenced-based design focused on outcomes in healthcare facilities further validates the importance of creating healing environments.

The first speaker in this series was Dr. Richard Jackson, a medical doctor formerly with the Centers for Disease Control and Prevention, who now crosses the country giving keynote speeches on the topic of the built environment and the role it plays in public health. Jackson's message served as the catalyst for NCDC to pursue the *Shaping the Healthy Community* project.

NCDC staff realized its natural partner for the project should be the Metro Nashville Public Health Department and approached the department with a proposal for a book in May 2010. Public Health embraced the proposal and began working with NCDC to help fund and inform the creation of the plan.

2011

Beginning in May 2011 NCDC focused the majority of its energy toward *Shaping the Healthy Community*. An intensive literature review on the topic of health and the built environment was conducted by NCDC staff, leading to the formation of a built environment factors list. The list consisted of six "factor groups" to serve as an ordering device for structuring the action plan by identifying health challenges presented by different neighborhoods, in both their form types and amenities.

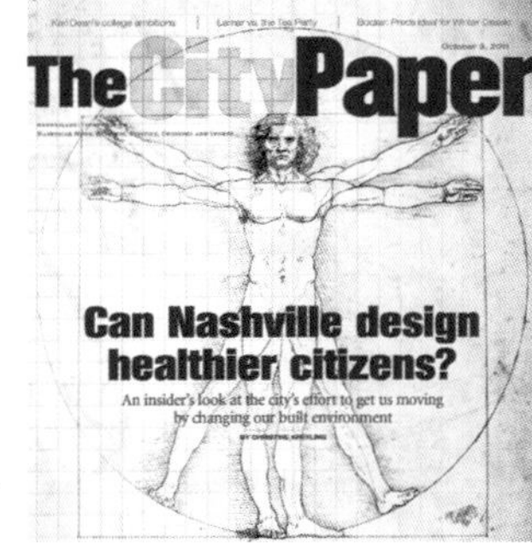
The City Paper
Can Nashville design healthier citizens?
An insider's look at the city's effort to get us moving by changing our built environment

Cover story in the *Nashville City Paper* (2011, Nashville City Paper)

NCDC staff then began the work of weaving together all the different elements that help create a healthy city in order to guide infrastructure investments and development projects to prioritize health impacts.

- Community Development Theory: Fall 2011
  Paul Speer, professor of human and organizational development, Peabody College, Vanderbilt University—Students reviewed a comprehensive list of all local plans related to the built environment done in Nashville between 2001 and 2011 to identify components that could be incorporated into strategies for *Shaping the Healthy Community*.
- Community Psychology: Fall 2011
  Douglas D. Perkins, professor of human and organizational development and director, PhD program in Community Research and Action, Peabody College, Vanderbilt University—Students visited specific neighborhoods in Nashville selected by NCDC staff to represent the various transect zones.

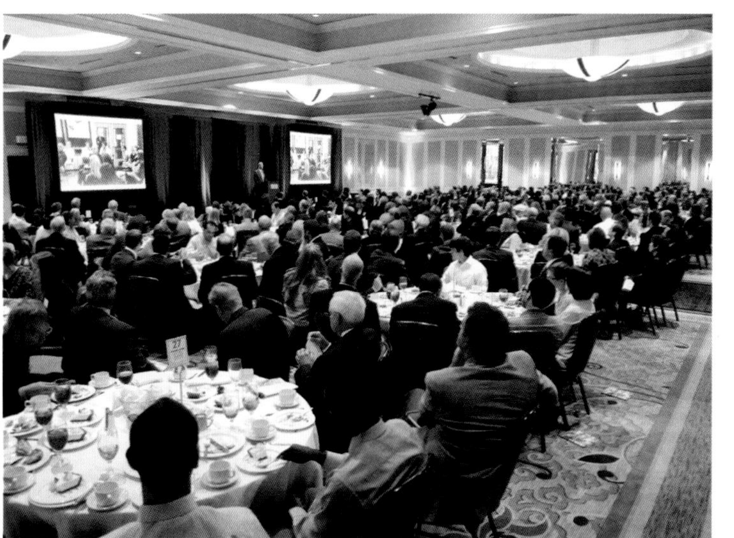

NCDC's annual luncheon, kicking off the *Shaping the Healthy Community* project. *(2011: Gary Layda)*

The students documented via photos, videos, and sketches the health-promoting and/or health-defeating factors in these built environments.

2012

- Environmental Inequality and Justice: Spring 2012
  Joe Bandy, assistant director of the Center for Teaching and affiliated faculty in sociology, Vanderbilt University—Students collaborated with NCDC staff to produce oral histories from eleven Nashville neighborhoods. Pairs of students researched the histories of their assigned communities, conducted interviews with neighborhood representatives, and produced short films or written reports on community health issues based on the factors of neighborhood design and development, transportation, walkability, housing, food resources, and open space. The class made presentations to their community representatives, which produced further insights for incorporation into this book. These oral histories supplied the materials for the Profile sections at the beginning of each chapter of the book.
- Designing Action
  NCDC received a grant from the National Endowment for the Arts to conduct the Designing Action International Design Competition to envision the many ways that infrastructure can promote active, healthy living. The site used for the competition is an industrial area along downtown Nashville's riverfront. NCDC received 133 entries from 29 countries. The finalist proposals were exhibited along the greenway overlooking the competition site.

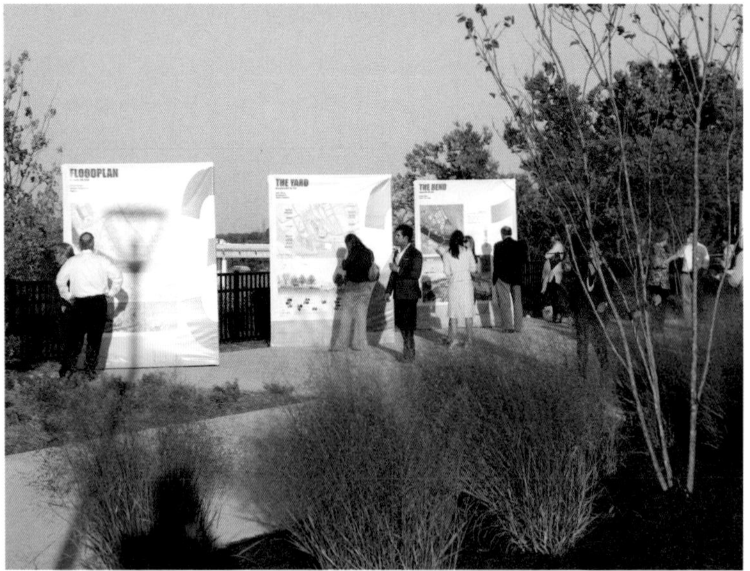

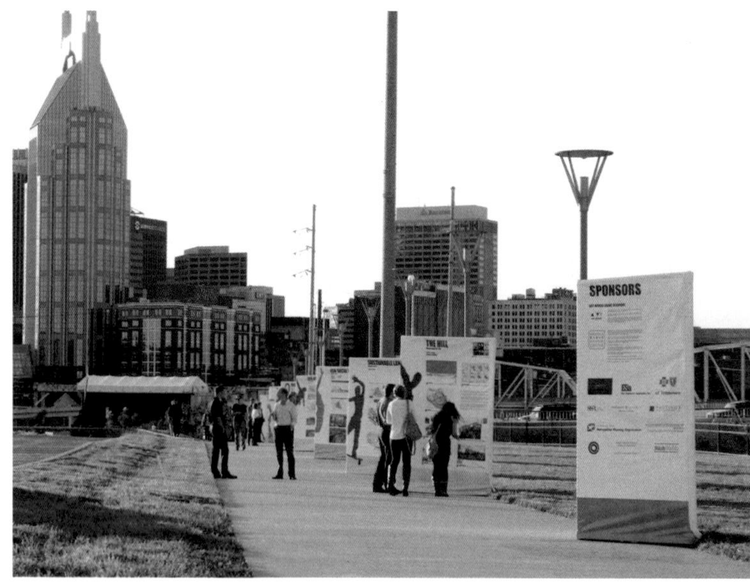

Designing Action Design Competition finalists on display along the Rolling Mill Hill greenway. *(2012)*

AIA 2012 December publication cover. *(2012: AIA)*

- American Institute of Architects
  Work of Nashville Civic Design Center was featured in AIA's December publication, *Local Leaders: Healthier Communities Through Design.*

2013

In January, the Metro Public Health Department, in partnership with NCDC, hosted the fourth annual Healthy Eating, Active Living Summit (HEALS) on the theme Health and the Built Environment. The theme was chosen in recognition that the built environment—including all of the human-made resources and infrastructure designed to support human activity, such as buildings, roads, neighborhoods, open space, food outlets, etc.—significantly impacts Nashville's health, especially in how individuals access opportunities for healthy eating and active living.

The keynote address was delivered by internationally renowned livable city strategist Gil (Guillermo) Penalosa. Penalosa is the Executive Director of 8–80 Cities, a Canadian nonprofit organization dedicated to transforming cities into places where people can walk, bike, access public transit, and visit vibrant parks, streets, and other public places. The 8–80 philosophy is that if you create a city that is good for an 8-year-old and good for an 80-year-old, you will create a successful city for everyone.

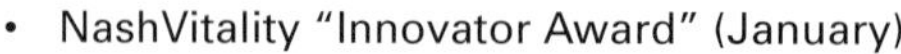

- NashVitality "Innovator Award" (January)
  NCDC received this award from the Metro Public Health Department for outstanding, innovative contributions to the promotion of healthy community design principles.
- January 17-May 19, Main Library Courtyard Gallery, Shaping • Building • Becoming: Setting the Tone for a Healthier Nashville—An exhibit organized by NCDC that illustrated the public health issues facing urban planners and citizens.

2014

- Value of Design: Design and Health Summit (May)
  Gary Gaston and Christine Kreyling were selected from a national call for proposals to present their work in Washington, DC, at the Value of Design: Design and Health Summit. This event was held at the national headquarters of the American Institute of Architects.

  The Value of Design: Design and Health Summit focused on five areas that are deemed essential in the dialogue between good design and health. These five areas include safety and social equity, physical activity, sensory experiences, environmental integrity, and access to nature. The goal of the summit was to engage the public in the discussion of design and how it influences health; to that end, it presented to a variety of architects, designers, and health practitioners.

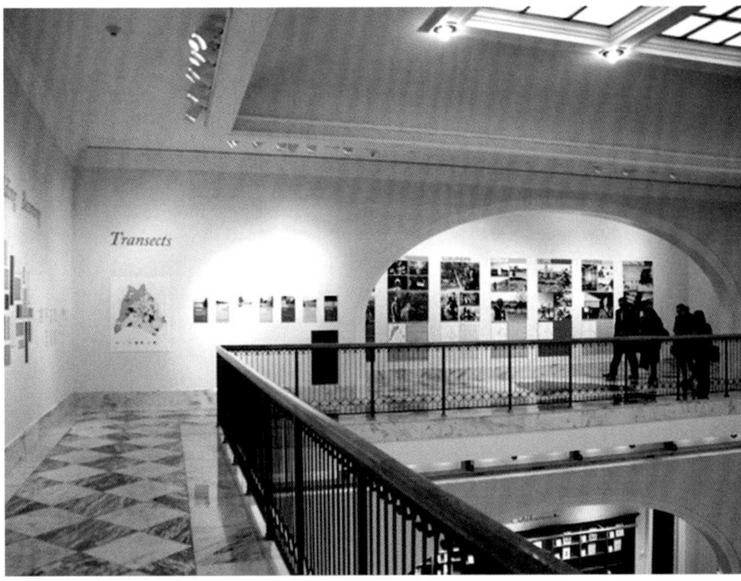

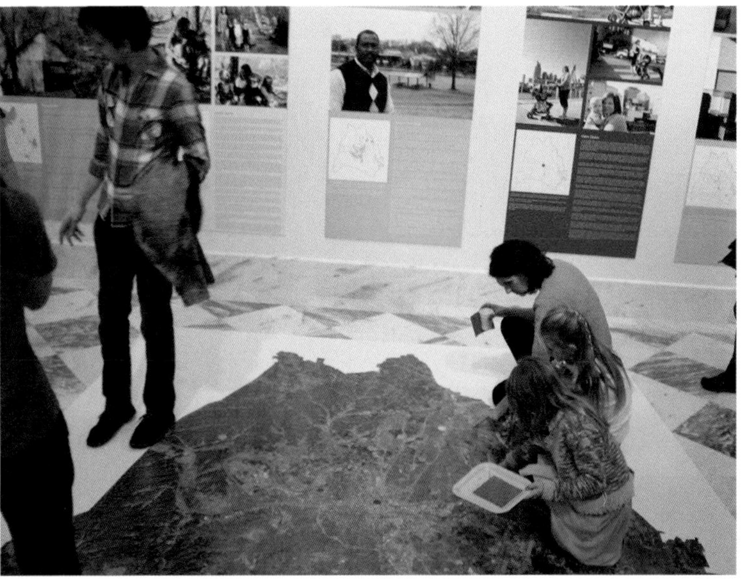

Downtown Nashville Public Library exhibition. *(2013)*

- Urban Land Institute—Urban Innovation Grant (June)

  The Urban Land Institute grant funded a half-day seminar and design workshop on how to build healthy places. The keynote speaker was Matthew Trowbridge, a physician, public health researcher, and assistant professor at the University of Virginia School of Medicine, whose work focuses on the impact of architecture, urban design, and transportation planning on public health issues.

  The design workshop focused on the Charlotte Pike corridor, an arterial roadway in Nashville that stretches from downtown to the rural and natural areas near the Davidson County line. More than 180 people attended the seminar and workshop.

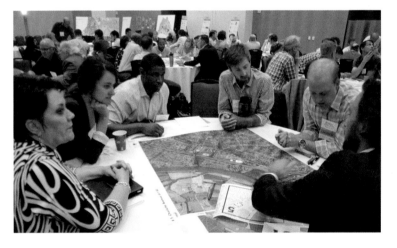

Design Workshop at the Music City Center Convention Center. *(2014)*

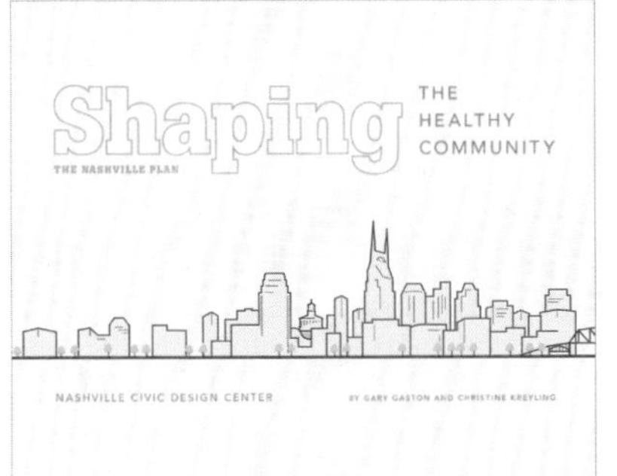

2015

- The Tennessee Public Health Association's 2015 Annual Meeting

  Themed Health by Design: Inspiring New Perspectives, the meeting highlighted built environments and their relationship to the health of the population. NCDC presented its work on the *Shaping the Healthy Community* project to more than 100 public health officials and medical practitioners.

2016

- Publication by Vanderbilt University Press of *Shaping the Healthy Community: The Nashville Plan*

GLOSSARY

GLOSSARY

affordable housing: Residential space that can be purchased, maintained or rented by a household with moderate, low, or very low income that costs less than 30 percent of the household's gross income. This percentage, defined by the US Department of Housing and Urban Development (HUD), includes utilities. HUD reports that "an estimated 12 million renter and homeowner households now pay more than 50 percent of their annual incomes for housing. A family with one full-time worker earning the minimum wage cannot afford the local fair-market rent for a two-bedroom apartment anywhere in the United States."

affordable housing tax credits: Federal tax credits that are awarded to developers of qualified rental projects as determined by HUD. Developers then sell these credits to investors to raise capital (or equity) for their projects, which reduces the debt that the developer would otherwise have to borrow. Because the debt is lower, a tax-credit property can be offered at lower rents. These tax credits provide the private market with an incentive to invest in affordable rental housing.

aging in place: The ability of people to live safely and relatively independently in the home or neighborhood of their choice, usually where they have lived for years, as they get older and their physical and/or financial circumstances change. This involves the provision of products, services, and assistance to enable them to remain living outside a health care environment or nursing home for as long as possible. Neighborhoods that feature a high level of walkability, pedestrian access to daily needs and community services, and good access to public transit and greenspace are most appropriate for aging in place.

agribusiness: Farming on an industrial scale. All elements and institutions of the food and fiber commodities chain are part of the agribusiness system, which involves the vertical integration of agrichemicals, animal breeding and maintenance, seed supply, crop production, farm machinery, food processing, distribution, marketing, and retail sales. Critics call this corporate farming, and have identified the practice with the overuse of chemicals in food production, unhealthy food content, pollution by animal waste, and animal cruelty. In recent years, conglomerates traditionally not involved in agricultural businesses have entered agribusiness by buying and operating large farms. Detractors say this is due to the tax breaks and price supports the US government provides to farming on this large scale.

agritourism: A growing form of niche tourism that brings visitors to a farm or ranch for a variety of activities: eating farm products, education in the cultivation and cooking of fresh foods, farm stays, observation of and/or participation in farm or ranch activities such as animal care or fruit and vegetable picking. The practice is especially useful for giving urban and suburban children—and adults—an understanding of the source of their food. The potential impacts are to promote the consumption of locally produced foodstuffs and improve the incomes and potential economic viability of small farms and rural communities.

alley: A narrow, public right-of-way not intended for general travel and primarily used as a means of vehicular and pedestrian access to the rear of abutting properties. Often used as a back lane by service vehicles like garbage trucks and for the placement of unsightly infrastructure, such as utility poles and lines.

arterial: A street that functions for longer trip length and higher volumes within the roadway network. Within the hierarchy of streets, the arterial takes traffic from collector streets and delivers it to limited-access highways: freeways and interstates.

avenue: A short-distance, medium speed corridor that traverses an urban area.

bike lane: Portion of a roadway designated for bicycles; the bike lane often lies between the sidewalk for pedestrians and car lanes. Bike lanes may be demarcated by different colored striping or signage, by street level, or by protective buffering such as bollards or landscaping.

bike rack: Stationary fixture to which bicycles can be securely attached; also known as bicycle stands. Bike racks should be placed where they will not impede pedestrian movement along the sidewalk.

bio-retention basin: Landscaped depression or shallow pond used to slow and filter pollutants from on-site storm water runoff. Storm water is directed to the basin and then percolates through the system for treatment by a number of physical, chemical, and biological processes. The cleaned water is then allowed to infiltrate adjacent soil or directed to nearby drains or receiving waters.

bioswale: A linear, landscaped channel with sloped sides that captures storm water runoff from adjacent surface areas. It contains vegetation and mulch designed to remove pollutants before the water infiltrates the soil. Bioswales are often integrated into parking lots and road medians and located parallel to roadways to filter and treat a portion of the stormwater volume.

blight: A physically and/or economically deteriorated condition in the built environment. The term derives from plant diseases and was, and still is, employed by the federal government to determine areas eligible for urban renewal programs.

block: A tract of land bounded on all sides by streets or by a combination of streets, public parks, and other rights-of-way.

blueway: Also known as a water trail, a blueway is a route along a river or across other bodies of water, such as a lake or salt water inlet, for people using small beachable boats like kayaks, canoes, day sailors, or rowboats. Water trails are most often identified by the land facilities that support water travel. These include launch and landing sites (trailheads), campsites, rest areas, and other points of interest.

body mass index (BMI): A measure of body fat that is the ratio of the weight of the body in kilograms to the square of its height in meters. An adult body mass index of 25 to 29.9 is considered an indication that the person is overweight; 30 or more indicates obesity.

bollard: A short vertical post. In street design bollards are used as a protective boundary between transportation modes, such as bikes and cars, and between vehicular and pedestrian traffic lanes.

boulevard: A wide, medium-speed vehicular corridor that traverses an urbanized area. It is frequently lined by parallel parking and wide sidewalks, divided by a median, and well landscaped.

buffer: In the built environment, a strip of land established to separate land uses or modes of transportation. It is typically landscaped.

build-to line: A distance designated by zoning statutes or restrictions in the deeds in various locales that determines how far a building must be set back from a street, flood plain, or other designated feature. These regulations help determine the size of a sidewalk, which can be a deciding factor in the walkability of a neighborhood.

built environment: That aspect of the environment that is made by humans. This includes buildings, roads, and other infrastructure.

bulk regulations: The combination of controls—lot size, floor area ratio, lot coverage, open space, yards, height, and setback—that determine the maximum size and placement of a building on a lot.

bus rapid transit (BRT): An enhanced mode within the bus system that operates in bus-only lanes in order to combine the flexibility of buses with travel speeds approaching that of rail.

central business district (CBD): The commercial and business center of a city.

chronic disease: A long-lasting condition that can be controlled, but not cured.

cohousing: A type of cooperative housing in which residents actively participate in the design and operation of their own neighborhood. Residents in these neighborhoods are consciously committed to living as a fully integrated community.

collector street: Within the roadway network, a street that collects or routes traffic from what are called local streets and delivers it to an arterial. Intended for trips of moderate length and moderate volume. Usually designed for speeds up to 35 mph, collectors have access from key community locations, such as churches and schools, as well as residential properties.

Communities Putting Prevention to Work (CPPW): A program of the federal Centers for Disease Control and Prevention that supports community efforts to reduce obesity and tobacco use, two top preventable causes of disability and death in the United States.

Community Health Improvement Plan (CHIP): A long-term, systematic effort to address public health problems in a community, based on the results of a community health assessment, usually performed by the local public health department.

community park: Land with full public access intended to provide recreation opportunities beyond those supplied by neighborhood parks. Community parks are larger in scale than neighborhood parks, but smaller than regional parks; examples in Nashville include Sevier Park and East Park.

community supported agriculture (CSA): A cooperative in which a consumer financially commits to purchasing a full season of produce from a farm or group of farms months in advance of the start of the growing season.

commuter rail: Trains running on rails also used by trains carrying heavy goods, that serve commuters and may operate only during peak commute hours. The Music City Star is an example of commuter rail in Middle Tennessee.

complete neighborhood: A neighborhood in which residents of all ages and abilities have safe and convenient access to the goods and services needed in daily life. These include a variety of housing options, grocery stores and other commercial services, quality public schools, public open spaces and recreational facilities, affordable active transportation options, and civic amenities.

complete street: Designed and built to serve pedestrians, bicyclists, transit users, drivers, people with disabilities, the elderly, and children equally well.

conservation easement: A voluntary contract between a landowner and a land trust, government agency, or another qualified organization in which the owner places permanent restrictions on the future uses of some or all of his property to protect scenic, wildlife, or agricultural resources. The landowner is often rewarded by a reduction in, or freezing of, property tax.

crosswalk: Portion of a roadway designated and marked for pedestrian crossing, typically at intersections, but also at some midblock locations.

cul-de-sac: A street closed at one end by a widened, semi-circular pavement of sufficient size for automotive vehicles to continue around and reverse direction.

curb bulb: Radial extensions of a sidewalk at an intersection used to shorten the crossing distance for pedestrians.

curb cut: An angled cut in the edge of a curb that permits vehicular access from a street to a driveway, garage, parking lot, or loading dock.

density: The number of dwelling units or residents within a designated land area, e.g., units per acre. More technically, density can also refer to the maximum number of dwelling units permitted on a zoning lot.

density bonus: The allocation of development rights that permits a parcel to accommodate additional square footage or residential units beyond the maximum for which the parcel is zoned, usually in exchange for the provision or preservation of an amenity at the same site or at another location. A form of incentive zoning that rewards developers for including features in the development deemed in the public interest, such as plazas and affordable housing.

design guidelines: A set of recommendations intended to guide development toward a desired form and level of quality relative to the context of development.

dog park: An enclosed area where dogs can be off-leash while supervised by their owners.

down-zoning: The rezoning of land to a more restrictive zone, for example, from multifamily residential to single-family residential or from commercial to agricultural. Down-zoning generally reduces the economic value of land, though it may serve a public benefit.

easement: The right to use property owned by another for specific purposes or to gain access to another property. Utility companies often have easements on private property to be able to install and maintain utility facilities. In Europe hiking trail easements allow the public to traverse private land.

empty nester: A parent whose children have grown up and no longer live in the family home.

epidemic: The rapid spread of a disease among a population within a short time. Although traditionally applied to infectious diseases, in 1997 the World Health Organization recognized obesity as a global epidemic.

farm-to-table: The movement promoting the production and consumption of food within the same locality; often associated with organic farming and community supported agriculture.

fast food: Food that is prepared and consumed quickly; often associated with unhealthy foodstuffs of low cost.

food desert: Geographic areas where residents' access to affordable, healthy food options, especially fresh fruits and vegetables, is limited or nonexistent due to the absence of full service grocery stores within a convenient traveling distance.

food truck: A portable restaurant in which food is prepared inside a vehicle or in a commissary kitchen, then served from the vehicle to customers immediately outside.

form-based code: A zoning code based on the physical form of development rather than the more traditional land-use basis for classification.

gentrification: The influx into a neighborhood of middle-class or affluent people who often displace poorer residents.

GREENGUARD: Certification program for low chemical and particle emission products for indoor use to improve air quality.

greenway: A corridor of undeveloped land for recreational use and/or environmental protection. Nashville's greenway system is concentrated within floodplains along the rivers, particularly the Cumberland; this focus delivers public benefits to land that is questionable for development.

health impact assessment (HIA): Combination of qualitative and quantitative methods used to assess the public health consequences of a policy, project, or program that does not have health as its primary objective. The design of an office building or the impacts of a road widening are two examples of projects for which an HIA can produce public benefits.

Healthy Nashville Leadership Council (HNLC): Group created by mayoral Executive Order No. 25 to mobilize community initiatives to achieve improvements in health, specifically to reduce the impact of three strategic issues: obesity, tobacco use, and disparities within the population in heart disease, diabetes, and cancer.

health defeating: Built environment factors that are detrimental to individual and environmental health.

health promoting: Built environment factors that enable better individual and environmental health.

heat island effect: Occurs as cities replace natural landscaping with streets, buildings, and other infrastructure. The average ambient temperatures within these areas can rise as much as 10 degrees F higher than surrounding, less developed areas. The effect increases the need for cooling energy, exacerbates pollution, and contributes to global warming. Expanding the urban forest can effectively reduce heat islands.

highway: A public roadway often associated with high speeds and long distance travel.

householder(s): The person or couple within a house or apartment who pays rent or claims ownership of the property.

impact fee: Also called a development fee and levied on the developer of a project by a city, county, or other public agency as compensation for otherwise unmitigated impacts the project will produce, such as traffic congestion or the need for school expansion.

infill: Development or redevelopment of land between existing structures to accommodate growth without expanding the boundaries of a neighborhood or city.

infrastructure: General term for public and quasi-public facilities and services, such as roads, sidewalks, transit systems, sewage-disposal systems, water-supply systems, and other utilities.

land use: The use of land for human purposes.

lane: A section of roadway accommodating a single line of vehicles.

Leader in Energy and Environmental Design (LEED): Rating and certification program developed by the US Green Building Council (USGBC) for new building development and the redevelopment of existing structures. The program evaluates the overall environmental performance during the lifecycle of a building and provides a tangible methodology for analyzing and applying environmental standards to building design and construction.

Leader in Energy and Environmental Design for Neighborhood Design (LEED-ND): Rating and certification program developed by the USGBC for new neighborhood development projects. The program evaluates the overall environmental performance during the lifecycle of a neighborhood project, similar to the LEED building standards. These large-scale design projects are rated on their innovation and design process, as well as the overall compactness, completeness, and connectivity of the project.

light rail transit (LRT): Public transit operating on a fixed rail system intended for light loads at high speeds.

limited-access highway: Within the network of streets, the roadway characterized by the highest volume and used for the longest trips. Access points, typically called interchanges, are spaced and limited to increase mobility. Designed for speeds of 50 to 80 mph. Originally planned to connect cities, traverse states and to lie in open land outside city limits, these highways spawned suburban development and were misguidedly brought into the heart of cities to be used by local commuters. In these circumstances, such highways have not performed well due to the amount of traffic concentrated onto a roadway that has limited ingress and egress. Also called expressways, freeways, and interstates.

local street: A street that is used primarily to gain access to the property bordering it, most often residences. Delivers traffic to collector streets; designed for low volume and speeds up to 30 mph.

market rate: The current price on the open market for goods and services. In market rate housing, characteristics such as size, location, and age are taken into consideration to determine the value of similar goods.

Metropolitan Planning Organization (MPO): A federally mandated and funded long-range transportation planning body composed of representatives from a region's local governments and transportation authorities.

micro-unit housing: Very small dwelling units—typically 200 to 300 square feet—developed to be affordable, especially for young people. These units often include features to save space, such as a fold-up bed or loft.

millennial: A person born in the 1980s or 1990s.

mixed-use development: A building or set of buildings with more than one type of land use. In the case of a single building, the mixture of land uses is integrated vertically; in a series of buildings, the integration is often horizontal.

mixed-use zoning: Permits various land uses, such as office, retail, institutional, light industrial, and residential to be combined in a single building or on a single site in an integrated development project. A street with shops at street level and dwelling units above is an example of vertical mixed use.

Mobilizing for Action through Planning & Partnerships (MAPP): A community-driven strategic planning process for improving community health, this tool was developed by the National Association of County and City Health Officials.

neighborhood park: Parks intended for use by local residents and/ workers; they frequently have a playground or athletic field. Typically smaller than community or regional parks, but size can vary depending on surroundings; examples in Nashville include Bass Park next to the Holly Street fire hall and Love Park at the top of Love Circle.

obesity: The excessive accumulation and storage of fat in the body; in an adult obesity is typically indicated by a body mass index of 30 or greater.

obesogenic environment: A society and physical environment that induces weight gain.

planting strip: A length of grass or other landscaping lying between a curb and a sidewalk or property line; often used for the planting of street trees.

pocket park: Small-scale urban green space, usually no more than a few house lots in size, that serves the immediately adjacent, local population; examples in Nashville include Church Street Park and Edmondson Park.

property tax abatement: The reduction or elimination of tax on a property for a designated period of time to provide assistance to low income households, elderly fixed-income households, or to encourage certain types of development, especially in areas that need revitalization.

pedestrian refuge: A raised area placed in the center of a roadway and separating opposing lanes of traffic to make it easier for pedestrians to cross wide streets; also called a pedestrian island.

regional park: Large public open space for recreation and passive enjoyment intended for patronage by citizens from across a region; examples in Nashville include Shelby Park and the Warner Parks.

road diet: The reduction in the number or width of lanes of a roadway. The technique is used to slow traffic and enhance safety; also used for the addition of features such as wider sidewalks, bike lanes, and/or planting strips.

sharrow: A shared-lane bicycle marking. This pavement marking includes a bicycle symbol and two white chevrons and is used to remind motorists that bicyclists are permitted to use the full lane. There are no designated bicycle lanes on streets marked with sharrows. However, with or without marked sharrows, bicyclists are encouraged to travel on streets and follow traffic laws just as any other vehicle on the road. This includes avoiding riding on sidewalks.

smart growth: Movement dedicated to achieving more compact, mixed-use, resource-efficient development.

snout house: A house with a garage that protrudes beyond the rest of the front façade. This design indicates the preference given to cars over pedestrian access to a dwelling. Because of the blank face the garage presents to the street, snout houses are criticized by proponents of traditional urban design and are currently banned in the city of Portland, OR.

sprawl: The process by which the spread of development across the landscape outpaces actual population growth. Sprawl creates landscapes with four characteristics: a population that is widely dispersed in low-density development; rigid separation of land uses, so that homes, commerce, and workplaces are segregated from one another; roads laid out to separate land into super blocks and offering poor access; a lack of well-defined commercial activity centers. Most of the other features usually associated with sprawl—a lack of transportation choices, relative uniformity of housing options, and difficulty walking from place to place—result from these conditions.

street furniture: Objects and pieces of equipment—such as benches, kiosks, planters, street signs—installed primarily on sidewalks. Their placement can enhance or impinge on the way pedestrians use the sidewalk.

street wall: The collective facades of buildings within a block that face the street.

streetcar: An historic transit mode that has experienced a recent revival and may be powered by gasoline, electricity, or a hybrid of the two. Typically single cars with a moderate level of capacity; also called a trolley.

streetscape: The entire system of streets, sidewalks, landscaping, street furniture, and open spaces by which people circulate through the built environment.

tax increment financing (TIF): A public financing tool used by redevelopment agencies—in Nashville it is the Metropolitan Development and Housing Agency—to support desired private development. The agency issues bonds for improvements, such as infrastructure, which are paid off over a designated period by the additional property tax revenues engendered by the development.

traditional neighborhood design (TND): A neighborhood with a variety of housing types, a mixture of land uses, an active center (e.g. small park or playground), a walkable design, and often a transit option within a compact neighborhood-scale area. TNDs can be developed either as infill in an existing developed area or as a new large-scale project. Also known as a village-style development.

traffic calming: The design of a roadway to slow vehicular traffic.

transit-oriented development (TOD): An area based around some form of public transit that is mixed-use, dense, and includes multiple housing options. These areas are typically found adjacent to railways, and they enhance the quality of life of their residents by encouraging walking, enhancing economic development, and creating community.

urban forest: The collection of trees in an urban area. Proponents advocate the expansion of the urban forest to shade sidewalks, cool the air, and to absorb stormwater runoff and carbon in the air.

urban renewal: Program of the federal government developed after World War II to revitalize urban areas designated as blighted. Typically combined with the construction of public housing and the interstate system, the program is today widely discredited for damaging the fabric of the built environment and for its disproportionately negative impact on low income, often minority, neighborhoods. Sarcastically called "Negro removal" by African Americans.

vacant: not filled, used, or lived in

vehicles: All motorized conveyances for street travel, and includes automobiles, vans, trucks, motorcycles, recreational vehicles, emergency vehicles, buses, and tractor-trailers.

viaduct: Elevated roadway that crosses land rather than water.

volatile organic compound (VOC): Material that emits a gas as the byproduct of a chemical process. Many building materials, such as particleboard, plywood, adhesives, paints, varnishes, carpet, drapes, and furniture are made with formaldehyde products that emit gas detrimental to air quality.

walkability: The measure of the overall walking conditions in an area (a place is walkable when it has characteristics that invite people to walk).

workforce housing: Housing that is affordable to working households that do not qualify for publicly subsidized housing, yet cannot afford appropriate market-rate housing in their communities. More specifically defined in terms of an area's median income (AMI). The Nashville Downtown Partnership's Workforce Housing Task Force defines workforce housing as dedicated to households earning between 80 and 150 percent of AMI.

years of potential life lost (YPLL): YPLL is defined as the number of years of potential life lost by each death occurring before a predetermined end point, set at age 65 years. CDC calculates YPLL over the age range from birth to 65 years using age-specific death rates for 15 selected causes and supplementary data on causes of infant mortality, provided yearly by the National Center for Health Statistics (NCHS).

NOTES

Introduction

1. Christine Kreyling, *The Plan of Nashville: Avenues to a Great City* (Nashville, TN: Vanderbilt University Press, 2005), 1.

2. US Environmental Protection Agency, *Our Nation's Air: Status and Trends Through 2010*, Washington, DC: United States Environmental Protection Agency, 2012, retrieved from *www.epa.gov/airtrends/2011/report/fullreport.pdf.*

3. Helen Lee, "The Making of the Obesity Epidemic," *Breakthrough Journal* 3 (Winter 2013), retrieved from *thebreakthrough.org/index.php/journal/issue-3/the-making-of-the-obesity-epidemic.*

4. Carrie Fry, "Public Health and Urban Planning: A History and Its Effects" (unpublished paper, Vanderbilt University, 2011).

5. American Public Health Association, "APHA History and Timeline" (web page), retrieved from *www.apha.org/news-and-media/newsroom/online-press-kit/apha-history-and-timeline.*

6. Robert Ivy, "10 Year Scope," in *Health + Urbanism*, eds. Alan M. Berger and Andrew Scott (Cambridge, MA: Massachusetts Institute of Technology, 2013), 3.

7. Richard Jackson and Chris Kochtitzky, *Creating a Healthy Environment: The Impact of the Built Environment on Public Health* (Washington, DC: Sprawl Watch Clearinghouse, 2001).

8. Reid Ewing and Barbara McCann, *Measuring the Health Effects of Sprawl: A National Analysis of Physical Activity, Obesity and Chronic Disease* (Washington, DC: Smart Growth America and the Surface Transportation Policy Project, 2003), 1.

9. Howard Frumkin, Lawrence Frank, and Richard Jackson, *Urban Sprawl and Public Health: Designing, Planning, and Building for Healthy Communities* (Washington, DC: Island Press, 2004).

10. Design, Community & Environment, et al., *Understanding the Relationship between Public Health and the Built Environment* (Washington, DC: LEED-ND Core Committee, 2006).

11. Andrew L. Dannenberg, Howard Frumkin, and Richard J. Jackson, eds., *Making Healthy Places: Designing and Building for Health, Well-Being and Sustainability* (Washington, DC: Island Press, 2011).

12. Richard Jackson, host, *Designing Healthy Communities* (PBS Video Series: 2011).

13. Alan M. Berger and Andrew Scott, eds., *Health + Urbanism* (Cambridge, MA: Massachusetts Institute of Technology, 2013).

14. Alan M. Berger, Casey Lance Brown, and Aparna Keshaviah, "Project Background," in Berger and Scott, *Health + Urbanism*, 7.

15. W. C. Perdue, L. O. Gostin, and L. A. Stone, "Public Health and the Built Environment: Historical, Empirical, and Theoretical Foundations for an Expanded Role," *Journal of Law, Medicine & Ethics* 31, no. 4 (2003): 557–66. Cited in Berger, Brown, and Keshaviah, "Project Background," 8.

16. John M. McDonald, et al., "The Effect of Light Rail Transit on Body Mass Index and Physical Activity," *American Journal of Preventive Medicine* 39, no. 2 (August 2010): 105–12.

17. Berger, Brown, and Keshaviah, "Project Background," 7.

18. Berger, Brown, and Keshaviah, "Project Background," 7.

19. The Potato Museum, "Couch Potato Gallery" (web page), retrieved from *potato-museum.com/index.php?option=com_content&view=article&id=26:artcounch&catid=19:catcontroversy&Itemid=48.*

20. F. Scott Fitzgerald, *The Great Gatsby* (New York: Charles Scribner's Sons, 1925, reprint, 2004), 180.

21. Jacob Riis, *How the Other Half Lives* (New York: Charles Scribner's Sons, 1890), 8, retrieved from *www.authentichistory.com/1898-1913/2-progressivism/2-riis.*

22. Frederick Law Olmsted Society of Riverside, "Maps of Riverside" (web page), retrieved from *www.olmstedsociety.org/resources/maps-of-riverside.*

23. Warren Winkelstein Jr., "History of Public Health," *Encyclopedia of Public Health*, 2002, retrieved from *www.enotes.com/public-health-encyclopedia/history-public-health.*

24. Martin Melosi, *The Sanitary City: Urban Infrastructure in America from Colonial Times to the Present* (Baltimore, MD: Johns Hopkins University Press, 1999), 187. Cited in Frumkin, Frank, and Jackson, *Urban Sprawl*, 52.

25. History from Jocelyn Pak Drummond, "Health + Urbanism Primer," in Berger and Scott, *Health + Urbanism*, unless otherwise noted.

26. J. A. Peterson, "The Impact of Sanitary Reform upon American Urban Planning, 1840–1890," *Journal of Social History* 13, no. 1 (1979): 83–103; David Vlahov and Sandro Galea, "Urbanization, Urbanicity, and Health," *Journal of Urban Health: Bulletin of the New York Academy of Medicine* 79, no. 4, suppl. 1 (2002): S1–S12. Cited in Drummond, "Health + Urbanism Primer," 14.

27. Joseph L. Arnold, "Riverside, IL," *Encyclopedia of Chicago*, retrieved from *www.encyclopedia.chicagohistory.org/pages/1080.html.*

28. Drummond, "Health + Urbanism Primer," 15.

29. John B. Thompson, "Disease in Nashville: A Short History," *Medical History in Nashville*, (symposium). A paper presented before the Nashville Academy of Medicine, September 14, 1982, 151–52.

30. Thompson, "Disease in Nashville," 151.

31. Thompson, "Disease in Nashville," 151.

32. Thompson, "Disease in Nashville," 152.

33. Thompson, "Disease in Nashville," 152.

34. Information on living conditions during this period from Don Doyle, *New Men, New Cities, New South: Atlanta, Nashville, Charleston, Mobile, 1860–1910* (Chapel Hill, NC: University of North Carolina Press, 1990), 39–108.

35. Don Doyle, *Nashville in the New South: 1880–1930* (Knoxville, TN: University of Tennessee Press, 1985), 83.

36. History of Nashville's water and sewer systems from Metropolitan Water Services, "History" (web page), retrieved from *www.nashville.gov/Water-Services/About-Us/History.*

37. Ivy, "Ten Year Scope," 5.

38. Metropolitan Water Services, "History."

39. Jocelyn Pak Drummond and Alan M. Berger, "Current Limitations," in Berger and Scott, *Health + Urbanism*, 29.

40. Lisa Wu, *Reducing Traffic-Related Air Pollution Exposure in the Built Environment: Recommendations for Urban Planners, Policymakers, and Traffic Engineers* (Los Angeles, CA: Los Angeles Sustainability Collaborative, 2014).

41. US Environmental Protection Agency, *Our Built and Natural Environments: A Technical Review of the Interactions among Land Use, Transportation, and Environmental Quality* (Washington, DC: United States Environmental Protection Agency, 2013), retrieved from *www.epa.gov/smartgrowth/built.htm*. Cited in Drummond and Berger, "Current Limitations," 26.

42. Quoted in Drummond and Berger, "Current Limitations,"26.

43. Steve Haruch, "Hot Problems: Climate Change Isn't Coming to Nashville—It's Already Here. And the Future Might Be Hotter than We Can Handle," *Nashville Scene*, August 26, 2010.

Scoping Nashville's Health

1. OECD, *Health at a Glance 2013: OECD Indicators* (Paris: OECD Publishing, 2013), 47, retrieved from *www.oecd.org/els/health-systems/health-at-a-glance.htm*.

2. Andrew P. Wilper, et al., "Health Insurance and Mortality in US Adults," *American Journal of Public Health* 99, no. 12 (December 2009): 2289–95, retrieved from *www.ncbi.nlm.nih.gov/pmc/articles/PMC2775760*.

3. J. Michael McGinnis, Pamela Williams-Russo, and James R. Knickman, "The Case for More Active Policy Attention to Health Promotion," *Health Affairs* 21, no. 2 (2002): 78–93.

4. See Paul Tough, *How Children Succeed: Grit, Curiosity, and the Hidden Power of Character* (Boston: Houghton Mifflin Harcourt, 2012), as described by David Brooks in "The Psych Approach," *New York Times* (September 28, 2012): A31.

5. Healthy Nashville Leadership Council, *Healthy Living Report* (Nashville, TN: Healthy Nashville, 2009), retrieved from *www.healthynashville.org/javascript/htmleditor/uploads/MPHDReportCard1_10.pdf*.

6. B. Rogers, B. McKelvey, and S. D. Thomas, *Davidson County Mortality Report for 2009* (Nashville, TN: Metropolitan Nashville Public Health Department, 2011).

7. Centers for Disease Control and Prevention, Division of Nutrition, Physical Activity, and Obesity, "Defining Adult Overweight and Obesity" (web page), retrieved from *www.cdc.gov/obesity/adult/defining.html*.

8. A. Ljungvall and F. J. Zimmerman, "Bigger Bodies: Long-Term Trends and Disparities in Obesity and Body-Mass Index among U.S. Adults, 1960–2008," *Social Science and Medicine* 75, no. 1 (2012), retrieved from *www.ncbi.nlm.nih.gov/pubmed/22551821*.109–19.

9. Ashleigh L. May, et al., "Vital Signs: Obesity Among Low-Income, Preschool-Aged Children—United States, 2008–2011," *Morbidity and Mortality Weekly Report* 62, no. 31 (August 9, 2013): 629–34.

10.Tennessee Department of Education, *A Summary of Weight Status Data: Tennessee Public Schools, 2012-2013 School Year* (Nashville, TN: Tennessee Department of Education), 18, retrieved from *www.tennessee.gov/education/schoolhealth/data_reports/doc/BMI_Sum_Data_State_Co_2013.pdf*.

11. D. G. Schlundt, M. K. Hargreaves, and L. McClellan, "Geographic Clustering of Obesity, Diabetes, and Hypertension in Nashville, Tennessee," *Journal of Ambulatory Care Management* 29, no. 2 (Apr–Jun 2006): 125–32.

12. Jarvis T. Chen, et al., "Mapping and Measuring Social Disparities in Premature Mortality: The Impact of Census Tract Poverty Within and Across Boston Neighborhoods, 1999–2001," *Journal of Urban Health* 83, no. 6 (November 2006): 1063–84.

13. Jens Ludwig, et al., "Neighborhoods, Obesity, and Diabetes—A Randomized Social Experiment," *New England Journal of Medicine* 365 (October 20, 2011): 1509–19.

14. T. Leventhal and J. Brooks-Gunn, "Moving to Opportunity: An Experimental Study of Neighborhood Effects on Mental Health," *American Journal of Public Health* 93, no. 9 (September 2003): 1576–82.

15. T. Laveist, et al., "Place, Not Race: Disparities Dissipate in Southwest Baltimore when Blacks and Whites Live under Similar Conditions," *Health Affairs* 30, no. 10 (2011): 1880–87.

16. "Highway Performance Monitoring System," retrieved from *www.tdot.state.tn.us/hpms*.

17. "America's Health Rankings," retrieved from *www.americashealthrankings.org*.

18. Trust for America's Health and Robert Wood Johnson Foundation, "Issue Brief: Bending the Obesity Cost Curve in Tennessee" (web page), retrieved from *healthyamericans.org/assets/files/obesity2012/TFAHSept2012_TN_ObesityBrief02.pdf*.

19. S. J. Olshansky, et al., "A Potential Decline in Life Expectancy in the United States in the 21st Century," *New England Journal of Medicine* 352, no. 11 (March 17, 2005): 1138–45.

20. United Health Foundation, *America's Health Rankings: 2014 Edition Tennessee* (Minnetonka, MN: United Health Foundation, 2015), retrieved from *cdnfiles.americashealthrankings.org/SiteFiles/StateProfiles/Tennessee-Health-Profile-2014.pdf*.

21. "Guide to Community Preventive Services," retrieved from *www.thecommunityguide.org/index.html*. Also see Committee on Accelerating Progress in Obesity Prevention, *Accelerating Progress in Obesity Prevention: Solving the Weight of the Nation* (Washington, DC: The National Academies Press, 2012).

22. Geoffrey Kabat, "Why Labeling Obesity as a Disease is a Big Mistake," *Forbes* (July 9, 2013), retrieved from *www.forbes.com/sites/geoffreykabat/2013/07/09/why-labeling-obesity-as-a-disease-is-a-big-mistake*.

23. Boyd A. Swinburn, et al., "The Global Obesity Pandemic: Shaped by Global Drivers and Local Environments," *Lancet* 378, no. 9793 (August 27, 2011): 804–14. *PubMed PMID: 21872749*.

24. Boyd A. Swinburn, Garry Egger, and Fezeela Raza, "Dissecting Obesogenic Environments: The Development and Application of a Framework for Identifying and Prioritizing Environmental Interventions for Obesity," *Preventive Medicine* 29, no. 6 (December 1999): 563–70.

25. Swinburn, et al., "The Global Obesity Pandemic," 804–14.

26. Gary Taubes, "What Really Makes Us Fat," *New York Times* (June 30, 2012). Reporting on Cara B. Ebbeling, et al., "Effects of Dietary Composition on Energy Expenditure During Weight Loss Maintenance," *Journal of the American Medical Association* 307, no. 24 (June 27, 2012): 2627–34.

27. Tara Parker-Pope, "The Fat Trap," *New York Times Magazine* (December 28, 2011).

28. Priya Sumithran, et al., "Long-Term Persistence of Hormonal Adaptations to Weight Loss," *New England Journal of Medicine* 365 (October 27, 2011): 1597–604.

29. Quoted in Parker-Pope, "The Fat Trap."

30. Susanna Y. Huh, et al., "Timing of Solid Food Introduction and Risk of Obesity in Preschool-Aged Children," *Pediatrics* 127, no. 3 (March 2011): e544–51.

31. Fabrizio Pasanisi, et al., "Benefits of Sustained Moderate Weight Loss in Obesity," *Nutrition, Metabolism and Cardiovascular Diseases* 11, no. 6 (December 2001): 401–6.

32. C. D. Lee, Andrew S. Jackson, and Steven N. Blair, "US Weight Guidelines: Is It Also Important to Consider Cardiorespiratory Fitness?" *International Journal of Obesity* 22, Suppl. 2 (1998): S2–S7.

The Transect

1. Chris Renwick, "The Practice of Spencerian Science: Patrick Geddes's Biosocial Program, 1876–1889," *Isis* 100, no. 1 (2009): 36–57.

2. For further information on the New Urbanist Transect, see: Center for Applied Tran-

sect Studies (*www.transect.org*) and "Building Community Across the Rural-to-Urban Transect" by Charles C. Bohl with Elizabeth Plater-Zyberk (*places.designobserver.com/media/pdf/Building_Commu_1336.pdf*).

3. The most up-to-date version of the code is available free to municipalities and planners from the Center for Applied Transect Studies (*www.transect.org/codes*).

4. "Doty Left His Mark," *Wisconsin State Journal* (June 26, 1976), retrieved from *www.newspapers.com/newspage/14893199*.

5. John Nolen, "Suggestive Plan for Madison, a Model City" (map, 1910), retrieved from *www.wisconsinhistory.org*.

6. The Trust for Public Land, "Annual City Parks Data Released by the Trust for Public Land" (web page), retrieved from *www.tpl.org/media-room/annual-city-parks-data-released-trust-public-land*.

7. Bicycling.com, "America's Top 50 Bike-Friendly Cities" (web page), retrieved from *www.bicycling.com/news/advocacy/america-s-top-50-bike-friendly-cities#snapback*.

8. Robert Woods Johnson Foundation, "How Healthy Is Your Community?" (web page), retrieved from *www.countyhealthrankings.org*.

9. "Race to Equity," retrieved from *racetoequity.net*.

10. Public Health Madison & Dane County, *The Health of Dane County 2013 Health Status Overview Report* (October 2013), retrieved from *www.publichealthmdc.com/documents/HealthDC-2013status.pdf*.

11. *racetoequity.net*.

12. Federal Highway Administration, *Summary Report: Evaluation of Lane Reduction 'Road Diet' Measures and Their Effects on Crashes and Injuries*, US Dept. of Transportation pub. # FHWA-HRT-04-082, March 2004, retrieved from *www.fhwa.dot.gov/publications/research/safety/humanfac/04082*.

See also Brian Teff, *Impact Speed and a Pedestrian's Risk of Severe Injury or Death* (Washington, DC: AAA Foundation for Traffic Safety, 2011), retrieved from *www.aaafoundation.org/sites/default/files/2011PedestrianRiskVsSpeed.pdf*.

13. Smart Growth America, National Complete Streets Initiative, "Benefits of Complete Streets: Economic Development" (web page), retrieved from *www.smartgrowthamerica.org/complete-streets/complete-streets-fundamentals/factsheets/economic-revitalization*.

14. City of Portland Bureau of Planning and Sustainability, *Portland Plan. Status Report: Twenty-Minute Neighborhoods* (Portland, OR: City of Portland Bureau of Planning and Sustainability, May 2009), retrieved from *www.cityofmadison.com/Sustainability/community/documents/20minNeigh.pdf*.

15. "Local Purchasing," retrieved from *cccfoodpolicy.org/working-group/local-purchasing*.

16. "Montana Wheat Farmers Improve Nutrient Use Efficiency through Research Collaboration," Sustainable Agriculture and Research, retrieved from *www.sare.org/Learning-Center/From-the-Field/Western-SARE-From-the-Field/Improving-Nutrient-Use-Efficiency-in-Montana-Wheat*.

17. Portland, OR; Seattle, WA; Vancouver, BC; San Diego, CA; San Francisco, CA; Boise, ID; and Cleveland, OH.

18. Abby White, "Everybody Knows Nashville Is Hurting for Affordable Housing. What Are We Gonna Do about It?" *Nashville Scene* (Nashville, TN: March 25, 2015), retrieved from *www.nashvillescene.com/nashville/everybody-knows-nashville-is-hurting-for-affordable-housing-what-are-we-gonna-do-about-it/Content?oid=4952842*.

19. Loretta Owens, *NashvilleNext Background Reports: Housing* (Nashville, TN: Metropolitan Planning Department, March 2013), retrieved from *www.nashville.gov/Portals/0/SiteContent/Planning/docs/NashvilleNext/next-report-Housing.pdf*.

20. Joint Center for Housing Studies of Harvard University, *Housing America's Older Adults* (Cambridge, MA: Joint Center for Housing Studies of Harvard University, 2014), retrieved from *www.jchs.harvard.edu/sites/jchs.harvard.edu/files/jchs-housing_americas_older_adults_2014.pdf*.

21. Joan Brasher, "Study: Frequent Moves Hinder Child's Early Education," *Research News at Vanderbilt University* (15 February 2013), retrieved from *news.vanderbilt.edu/2013/02/frequent-moves-study*.

22. Owens, *NashvilleNext*.

23. Chelsey Dulaney, "Nashville Rent Increases Have Residents Singing the Blues," *Wall Street Journal* (10 August 2014), retrieved from *www.wsj.com/articles/nashville-rent-increases-have-residents-singing-the-blues-1407708778*.

24. Stephen Goldsmith, William Eimicke, and Chris Pineda, *How City Hall Can Invigorate the Faith Community around a Citywide Housing Agenda* (Cambridge, MA: Harvard University Ash Institute for Democratic Governance and Innovation, Fall 2005), retrieved from *www.innovations.harvard.edu/sites/default/files/11119.pdf*.

25. Amie Thurber, Jyoti Gupta, James Fraser, and Doug Perkins, *Equitable Development: Promising Practices to Maximize Affordability and Minimize Displacement in Nashville's Urban Core*. A NashvilleNext report from the Housing resource team (Nashville, TN: Metropolitan Nashville Planning Department, September 2014), retrieved from *www.nashville.gov/Portals/0/SiteContent/Planning/docs/NashvilleNext/ResourceTeams/Housing_Gentrification_EquitableDevelopment.pdf*.

26. White, "Everybody Knows."

27. Brasher, "Study: Frequent Moves."

28. The Housing Fund, "Shared Equity: Our House" (web page), retrieved from *thehousingfund.org/loans/individual-assistance-programs/homeownership/shared-equity*.

29. Reconnecting America, *TOD 201. Mixed-Income Housing near Transit: Increasing Affordability with Location Efficiency* (Oakland, CA: Reconnecting America, 2009), retrieved from *ctod.org/pdfs/tod201.pdf*.

30. Enterprise Community Partners, Inc., "Denver Regional Transit-Oriented Development Fund" (web page), retrieved from *www.enterprisecommunity.com/financing-and-development/community-development-financing/denver-tod-fund*.

31. Bloomberg Philanthropies, "Bloomberg Philanthropies and Living Cities' CFE Fund Announce Five Cities Selected for $16.2 M in Financial Empowerment Center Grants," press release (Bloomberg online, January 8, 2013), retrieved from *www.bloomberg.org/press/releases/bloomberg-philanthropies-and-living-cities-cfe-fund-announce-five-cities-selected-for-16-2-m-in-financial-empowerment-center-grants*.

32. Metropolitan Government of Nashville and Davidson County, "Energy Efficiency Improvements Volunteer Opportunities" (program website, 2014), retrieved from *www.nashville.gov/Mayors-Office/Priorities/Volunteerism/Volunteer-Opportunities/Energy-Efficiency-Improvements.aspx*.

33. Metropolitan Government of Nashville and Davidson County, "Nashville Makes Progress Improving Energy Efficiency of Low-Income Homes" (program website, 2012), retrieved from *www.nashville.gov/News-Media/News-Article/ID/976/Nashville-Makes-Progress-Improving-Energy-Efficiency-of-LowIncome-Homes.aspx*.

34. American Planning Association, "Accessory Dwelling Units," *PAS Quicknotes* 19 (2009), retrieved from *www.planning.org/pas/quicknotes/pdf/QN19.pdf*.

35. William Williams, "Cottage-Style Infill Development Slated for East Side," *Nashville Post* (13 September 2013), retrieved from *www.nashvillepost.com/news/2013/9/13/cottage_style_infill_development_slated_for_east_side*.

36. Eliana Kampf Binelli, Henry L. Gholz, and Mary L. Duryea, *Chapter 4: Plant Succession and Disturbances in the Urban Forest Ecosystem*, Publication #FOR93 (Gainesville, FL: University of Florida, 2012), retrieved from *edis.ifas.ufl.edu/fr068*.

37. USDA Forest Service, *Weed of the Week: Exotic Bush Honeysuckles* (Newtown Square, PA: USDA Forest Service, Forest Health Staff, n.d), retrieved from *na.fs.fed.us/fhp/invasive_plants/weeds/bush_honeysuckle.pdf*.

38. For land stewardship performance benchmarks see Sustainable Sites Initiative (*www.sustainablesites.org*). For examples of specific stewardship programs see "Natural and Cultural Resource Management in Florida State Parks" (*www.dep.state.fl.us/parks/bncr/forms/LandManagement.pdf*); "A Plan for Sustainable Practices within NYC Parks" (*www.nycgovparks.org/sub_about/sustainable_parks/Sustainable_Parks_Plan*); and "Shelby Farms Park Master Plan" (*www.shelbyfarmspark.org/masterplan*).

Natural

1. Thomas Jefferson to Baron von Geismar, September 6, 1785.
2. Henry David Thoreau, "Spring," in *Walden* (1854), retrieved from *thoreau.eserver.org/walden17.html.*
3. Jim Rutenberg, "Speculators Rush In," *New York Times* (August 20, 2015), 10.
4. The Conservation Fund, *Nashville Open Space Plan: Creating, Enhancing and Preserving the Places that Matter. A Report of Nashville: Naturally.* (Nashville, TN: Metropolitan Government of Nashville and Davidson County, 2011), 6, retrieved from *www.conservationfund.org/images/projects/files/Nashville-Naturally-Green-Infrastructure-Plan-The-Conservation-Fund-2011.pdf.*
5. Metropolitan Planning Department, *Community Character Manual* (Nashville, TN: Metropolitan Government of Nashville and Davidson County, 2008), 111–12.
6. Email to Gary Gaston from Anita McCaig of Metropolitan Planning Department, Dec. 9, 2013.
7. Greenways Nashville, *The Greenways Master Plan* (Nashville, TN: Nashville Greenways website, 2013), retrieved from *www.nashville.gov/Parks-and-Recreation/Planning-and-Development/Park-Plans-and-Projects/County-Wide-Parks-Greenways-Master-Plan.aspx.*
8. Union of Concerned Scientists, "Car Emissions and Global Warming" (web page), retrieved from *www.ucsusa.org/our-work/clean-vehicles/car-emissions-and-global-warming.*
9. National Association of City Transportation Officials, "Pervious Pavement" (web page), retrieved from *nacto.org/publication/urban-street-guide/street-design-elements/stormwater-management/pervious-pavement.*
10. Urban Land Institute, *Intersections: Health and the Built Environment* (Washington, DC: Urban Land Institute, 2013), 70.
11. American Trails, "2013 RTP Achievement Awards: Beaman Park Accessible and Interpretive Trail (Tennessee)" (web page), retrieved from *www.americantrails.org/awards/CRT13awards/Beaman-Park-Accessible-Trail-CRT-award-2013.html.*
12. "Metro to Pay $8.2M for 600 Acres of Farmland along Stones River," *City Paper* (December 4, 2012), retrieved from *nashvillecitypaper.com/content/city-news/metro-pay-82m-600-acres-farmland-along-stones-river.*
13. Friends of Warner Parks, *A Master Plan for the Burch Reserve at Warner Parks* (Nashville, TN: Metropolitan Board of Parks and Recreation, 2011).

Rural

1. Metropolitan Planning Department, *Community Character Manual,* 123–25.
2. US Census Bureau, "TIGER / Line Shapefiles, 2010," retrieved from *www.census.gov/geo/maps-data/data/tiger.html.*
3. US Department of Agriculture, *2007 Census of Agriculture: County Profile: Davidson County, Tennessee* (Washington, DC: United States Department of Agriculture, 2007), retrieved from *www.agcensus.usda.gov/Publications/2007/Online_Highlights/County_Profiles/Tennessee/cp47037.pdf.*
4. Audra Ladd, e-mail message to Gary Gaston (NCDC), September 13, 2012.
5. The Conservation Fund, Nashville: *Naturally,* 6.
6. Thomas K. Davis, *The A.I.A. 150 Blueprint for America Visioning Workshop for Robertson County* (Springfield, TN: Cumberland Region Tomorrow, 2007), 11, retrieved from *www.cumberlandregiontomorrow.org/robertson/aia-150-robertson-county.*
7. Brookings Institution, *Average US Metro Areas* (Washington, DC: Brookings Institution, 2008).
8. Sarah A. Low and Stephen Vogel, *Direct and Intermediated Marketing of Local Foods in the United States*, Economic Research Report No. ERR-128 (Washington, DC: US Department of Agriculture, Economic Research Service, November 2011), retrieved from *www.ers.usda.gov/Publications/ERR128.*
9. Barham, James, et al., *Regional Food Hub Resource Guide* (Washington, DC: US Dept. of Agriculture, Agricultural Marketing Service, April 2012), retrieved from *ngfn.org/resources/ngfn-database/knowledge/FoodHubResourceGuide.pdf.*
10. Jean C. Buzby, et al., "The Value of Retail- and Consumer-Level Fruit and Vegetable Losses in the United States," *Journal of Consumer Affairs* 45, no. 3 (Fall 2011): 492–515.
11. Metropolitan Planning Department, "What Does My Zoning Allow?" (web page), retrieved from *www.nashville.gov/Planning-Department/Rezoning-Subdivision/What-your-zoning-allows.aspx.*
12. Nadejda Mishkovsky, et al., *Putting Smart Growth to Work in Rural Communities* (Washington, DC: International City/County Management Association, 2010), retrieved from *icma.org/en/icma/knowledge_network/documents/kn/Document/301483/Putting_Smart_Growth_to_Work_in_Rural_Communities.*
13. Justin Graham and Ian Hanou, *Metro Nashville Tree Canopy Assessment Project* (Nashville, TN: Metropolitan Government of Nashville and Davidson County, 2010).
14. US Census Bureau, "American Community Survey: 2010 Data Release" (web page), retrieved from *www.census.gov/acs/www/data_documentation/2010_release.*
15. Sources for information in this paragraph: Sandra Neely Peterson, "The Neely Family," *homepages.rootsweb.ancestry.com/~lpproots/Neeley/neelybnd.htm;* Mary Ellen Martin Walker, "From the book *The Neely's of Neelys Bend*, Davidson County, TN" (1996), (web page), retrieved from *homepages.rootsweb.ancestry.com/~lpproots/Neeley/samnb.htm.*
16. Richard Carlton Fulcher, *1770–1790 Census of the Cumberland Settlements* (Baltimore, MD: Genealogical Publishing Co. Inc., 1987).
17. United States Department of Agriculture Farm Service Agency, GIS Data, 2013.
18. Metropolitan Planning Department, *The Madison Community Plan: 2009 Update* (Nashville, TN: Metropolitan Planning Department, 2009), 26.
19. Metropolitan Planning Department, *Scottsboro/Bells Bend Detailed Neighborhood Design Plan* (Nashville, TN: Metropolitan Planning Department, 2008), 5.
20. Metropolitan Planning Department, *Scottsboro/Bells Bend*, 42.
21. The Conservation Fund, *Nashville Open Space Plan*, 3.
22. Nashville Area Chamber of Commerce, *Nashville-Davidson County Redevelopment Taskforce Summary of Year One Results* (Nashville, TN: Nashville Area Chamber of Commerce, 2012), 11–12.
23. David Price and Julie Coco, *Beaman Park to Bells Bend: A Community Conservation Project* (Nashville, TN: New South Associates & The Land Trust for Tennessee, 2007), 119.
24. US Census Bureau, "American Community Survey."
25. RPM Transportation Consultants, LLC., *Metro Nashville-Davidson County Strategic Plan for Sidewalks and Bikeways* (Nashville, TN: Metropolitan Government of Nashville and Davidson County, Tennessee, 2008), retrieved from *mpw.nashville.gov/IMS/Bikeways/StrategicPlan.aspx.*
26. Nashville Area Metropolitan Planning Organization, *2035 Nashville Area Regional Transportation Plan* (Nashville, TN: Metropolitan Nashville Government, 2010), 88–89; 96–99, retrieved from *www.nashvillempo.org/docs/lrtp/2035rtp/Docs/2035_Doc/2035Plan_Complete.pdf.*

Suburban

1. Urban Dictionary, *www.urbandictionary.com/define.php?term=suburb.*

2. Lewis Mumford, *The City in History* (New York: Harcourt Brace & Company, 1961. Reprint, 1989), 512.

3. Kreyling, *The Plan of Nashville*, 33.

4. Don Doyle, *Nashville Since the 1920s* (Knoxville, TN: University of Tennessee Press, 1985), 179.

5. Kreyling, *The Plan of Nashville*, 34.

6. Adie Tomer, "Where the Jobs Are: Employer Access to Labor by Transit," Metropolitan Policy Program (Washington, DC: Brookings Institution, July 2012), 1.

7. Jinwon Kim and David Brownstone, *The Impacts of Residential Density on Vehicle Usage and Fuel Consumption: Evidence from National Sample* (Irvine, CA: Department of Economics, University of California, Irvine, April 23, 2012), retrieved from *sites.uci.edu/jinwonkim/files/2012/05/paper_0423.pdf.*

8. Metropolitan Planning Department, *Community Character Manual*, 163–65.

9. US Census Bureau, "TIGER / Line Shapefiles, 2010."

10. Metropolitan Planning Department, *Subdivision Regulations* (Nashville, TN: Metropolitan Planning Department, 2011), retrieved from *www.nashville.gov/Portals/0/SiteContent/Planning/docs/subdivregs/2014%2001%2009%20ADOPTED%20Subdivision%20Regulation%20AmendmentsUPDATEDSEPT!.pdf.*

11. Rick Bernhardt, "Reforming the Arterials: Streets that Move Cars and Create Great Places," in Kreyling, *The Plan of Nashville*, 74.

12. Joseph Cortright, *Driven Apart: How Sprawl Is Lengthening Our Commutes and Why Misleading Mobility Measures are Making Things Worse* (Cleveland, OH: CEOs for Cities, 2010), retrieved from *www.infrastructureusa.org/wp-content/uploads/2010/09/technicalreport_drivenapart9-29-10.pdf.*

13. Data provided by Metro Nashville Public Works Department.

14. Lesa Rair, "Public Transit Riders Continue to Save as Gas Prices Remain High: Riding Public Transportation Saves Individuals on Average $10,126 a Year," (American Public Transportation Association, 2012), retrieved from *www.apta.com/mediacenter/pressreleases/2012/Pages/120418_AprilTransitSavings.aspx.*

15. A. Santos, et al., *Summary of Travel Trends: 2009 National Household Travel Survey* (Washington, DC: US Department of Transportation, Federal Highway Administration, 2011), retrieved from *nhts.ornl.gov/2009/pub/stt.pdf.*

16. Source for this data, unless otherwise noted in text: Benjamin Davis, Tony Dutzik, and Phineas Baxandall, *Transportation and the New Generation: Why Young People Are Driving Less and What It Means for Transportation Policy* (Boston: Frontier Group and US PIRG Education Fund, April 2012), 1–3, retrieved from *www.uspirg.org/reports/usp/transportation-and-new-generation.*

17. Office of Highway Policy Information, "National Household Travel Survey (NHTS)" (web page), retrieved from *www.fhwa.dot.gov/policyinformation/nhts.cfm.*

18. Henry Grabar, "The Urbanist Toolkit Bracket Challenge," *CityLab* (March 21, 2013), retrieved from *www.citylab.com/work/2013/03/urbanist-toolkit-bracket-challenge/5041.*

19. Dave Reid, "Car Culture: Freedom Brought to You by the American Auto Industry, Hello Officer, Put the Phone Down, and More," Video clip, *Urban Milwaukee* (April 26, 2012), retrieved from *www.urbanmilwaukee.com/2012/04/26/car-culture-freedom-brought-to-you-by-the-american-auto-industry-hello-officer-put-the-phone-down-and-more.*

20. Davis, Dutzik, and Baxandall, *Transportation and the New Generation*, 3–4.

21. RPM Transportation Consultants, *Metro Nashville-Davidson County.*

22. Sansone-Lauber Trial Lawyers, "Pedestrian Accidents and Injuries" (web page), retrieved from *www.missourilawyers.com/legal-services/car-accident-lawyer/pedestrian-accidents.*

23. Noreen C. McDonald, et al., "US School Travel, 2009: An Assessment of Trends," *American Journal of Preventive Medicine* 41, no. 2 (August 2011): 146–51, retrieved from *www.ajpmonline.org/article/S0749-3797(11)00263-7/abstract.*

24. Bill Purcell, interview by Christine Kreyling, March 18, 2013.

25. Joe Edgens, interview by Christine Kreyling, March 19, 2013.

26. "Our Infographic: Active Kids Do Better, Let's Move! Active Schools" (web page), retrieved from *www.letsmoveschools.org/infographic.*

27. Constance E. Beaumont and Elizabeth G. Pianca, *Why Johnny Can't Walk to School: Historic Neighborhood Schools in the Age of Sprawl*, 2nd edition (Washington, DC: National Trust for Historic Preservation, October 2002), 10–11.

28. Joe Cortright, *Walking the Walk: How Walkability Raises Home Values in US Cities* (Cleveland, OH: CEOs For Cities, 2009), retrieved from *www.reconnectingamerica.org/assets/Uploads/2009WalkingTheWalkCEOsforCities.pdf.*

29. US Census Bureau, "American Community Survey."

30. Historical information from Metropolitan Planning Department, *Bellevue Community Plan: 2011 Update* (Nashville, TN: Metropolitan Planning Department, 2011), 2–4.

31. "About Madison: Read about the History of Madison," Madison-Rivergate Area Chamber of Commerce, retrieved from *madisonrivergatechamber.com/about-madison.*

32. "Our Story," Amqui Station and Visitor Center, retrieved from *www.amquistation.org/#!about/c1se.*

33. "About Madison."

34. Source information for various plans: *Madison Community Plan*, Metro Planning Department, retrieved from *www.nashville.gov/Planning-Department/Community-Planning-Design/Community-Plans/Madison.aspx*; Nashville Civic Design Center, *The Livability Project: Building More Livable Communities. Public Charrette Workshop Report: Madison, Sylvan Park*, retrieved from *www.nashville.gov/Portals/0/SiteContent/Neighborhoods/Livability/LivabilityRptMay2011_MadisonSylvanPark.pdf*; "Developing with Transit," Nashville Civic Design Center, retrieved from *www.civicdesigncenter.org/projects/sm_files/Developing%20With%20Transit.pdf*; Urban Land Institute, *An Action Plan for Reinvestment and Revitalization in Madison, Tennessee*, retrieved from *nashville.uli.org/wp-content/uploads/sites/32/2013/01/ULI-Madison-TAP-Report-4-10-12.pdf.*

Urban

1. Source for information on early suburbs: Kreyling, *The Plan of Nashville*, 13–17.

2. Strategic Economics, *Fiscal Impact Analysis of Three Development Scenarios in Nashville-Davidson County, TN* (Washington, DC: Smart Growth America, April 2013), retrieved from *www.smartgrowthamerica.org/documents/fiscal-analysis-of-nashville-development.pdf.*

3. "Growth Trends and Forecasts," Nashville Area Metropolitan Planning Organization (December 15 2010), retrieved from *www.nashvillempo.org/growth.*

4. Belden Russonello and Stewart LLC, *Community Preference Survey: What Americans Are Looking for When Deciding Where to Live* (Washington, DC: National Association of Realtors, 2011), 3.

5. Bill Friskics-Warren, "One Street at a Time; Nashville's 12South," *New York Times* (June 15, 2003), retrieved from *www.nytimes.com/2003/06/15/magazine/one-street-at-a-time-nashville-s-12south.html.*

6. Conor Dougherty and Robbie Whelan, "Cities Outpace Suburbs in Growth," *Wall Street Journal* (June 28, 2012), retrieved from *online.wsj.com/article/SB10001424052702304830704577493032619987956.html.*

7. Conor Dougherty, "Which Cities Are Growing Faster than Their Suburbs," *The Wall Street Journal* (June 28, 2012), retrieved from *blogs.wsj.com/economics/2012/06/28/which-cities-are-growing-faster-than-their-suburbs.*

8. Metropolitan Planning Department, *Community Character Manual*, 237–39.

9. US Census Bureau, "TIGER / Line Shapefiles, 2010."

10. Kevin Ramsey, *Residential Construction Trends in America's Metropolitan Regions: 2012 Report* (Washington, DC: United States Environmental Protection Agency, 2013), 15, retrieved from *www.epa.gov/smartgrowth/pdf/residential_construction_trends.pdf.*

11. Kreyling, *The Plan of Nashville,* 73.

12. Metropolitan Historical Commission, "MHZC District Boundaries and Design Guidelines" (web page), retrieved from *www.nashville.gov/Historical-Commission/Services/Preservation-Permits/Districts-and-Design-Guidelines.aspx.*

13. Ann Roberts, "Phoenix Rising," in Kreyling, *The Plan of Nashville,* 174.

14. Julie Campoli and Alex S. MacLean, *Visualizing Density* (Cambridge, MA: Lincoln Institute of Land Policy, 2007), 16.

15. Capitol Region Council of Governments (CRCOG), "Chapter 5. Transit Oriented Development: Fact Sheet," in *Livable Communities Toolkit: A Best Practices Manual for Metropolitan Regions* (Hartford, CT: Capitol Region Council of Governments, 2002), 2, retrieved from *www.crcog.org/publications/CommDevDocs/TCSP/Ch05_FactSheet_TOD.pdf.*

16. Brian Hutchinson, "Forgotten 'Country Lane' Experiment Could Be Answer to Vancouver's Desire for More Green Space," *National Post* (July 13, 2002), retrieved from *news.nationalpost.com/2013/07/02/forgotten-country-lane-experiment-could-be-answer-to-vancouvers-desire-for-more-green-space.* Also see Jillian Glover, "Converting Alleways to Livable Laneways and Country Lanes," *This City Life* (blog), retrieved from *thiscitylife.tumblr.com/post/54683503256/converting-alleyways-to-livable-laneways-and-country.* Additional resources may be found at *www.facebook.com/LivableLaneways.*

17. Complete Streets is the policy established by Mayor Karl Dean's Executive Order #40 of 2010; the policy mandates that streets within Nashville be designed to accommodate multiple modes of transportation: cars, public transit, bicycles, and pedestrians.

18. Nashville MTA, "Consultants Present Phase 2 Summary: Preliminary Engineering and Design," news release (April 11, 2013), retrieved from *www.nashvillemta.org/pdf/fn22.pdf.*

19. Roger Geller, *Four Types of Cyclists* (Portland, OR: Portland Office of Transportation, n.d.), 2, retrieved from *www.portlandoregon.gov/transportation/article/264746.*

20. Chicago Department of Transportation, *Chicago Streets for Cycling Plan 2020* (Chicago, IL: Chicago Department of Transportation, 2012).

21. Angie Schmitt, "The Rise of the North American Protected Bike Lane," *Momentum Mag* (July 31, 2013), retrieved from *momentummag.com/features/the-rise-of-the-north-american-protected-bike-lane.*

22. Christine Kreyling, "Weaning Ourselves from the Highway: The Four-Step Program," in Kreyling, *The Plan of Nashville,* 77–84.

23. "Supermarket Facts," Food Market Institute (n.d.), retrieved from *www.fmi.org/research-resources/supermarket-facts.*

24. Campoli and MacLean, *Visualizing Density,* 16.

25. Jason Scully, "Rethinking Grocery Stores," *Urban Land* (May 16, 2011), retrieved from *urbanland.uli.org/Articles/2011/May/ScullyRethink.*

26. Mark Hinshaw and Brian Vanneman, "The Supermarket as a Neighborhood Building Block," *Planning Magazine* (March 2010), retrieved from *planning.org/planning/2010/mar.*

27. Michael Cass, "Most Residential Property Values See Drop," *Tennessean* (March 28, 2013).

28. Kreyling, *The Plan of Nashville,* 24–25.

29. "Virginia's Efforts to Promote Affordable Housing," *Breakthroughs* (May 2009), retrieved from *www.huduser.org/rbc/newsletter/vol8iss3_2.html.*

30. Bobby Lovett, *The African-American History of Nashville, Tennessee, 1780–1930* (Fayetteville, AR: University of Arkansas Press, 1999), 54–55.

31. "East Nashville History and Timeline," *Tennessean* (1 November 2006), retrieved from *archive.tennessean.com/article/99999999/MICRO0206/61027038/East-Nashville-history-timeline.*

32. Christopher Cotten, *Churches of Christ in East Nashville: Their Rise and Decline in the Twentieth Century,* August 2008, 13, retrieved from *ccotten.files.wordpress.com/2008/09/rough-draft.doc.*

33. US Census Bureau, "Community Facts, 2010" (web page), retrieved from *factfinder.census.gov/faces/nav/jsf/pages/community_facts.xhtml.*

34. Metropolitan Government of Nashville and Davidson County, "Interactive Map of Nashville's Tree Cover," retrieved from *maps.nashville.gov/UTC.*

35. Metropolitan Planning Department, *Community Character Manual,* 149.

36. US Census Bureau, "American Community Survey."

37. Centers for Disease Control and Prevention, "Healthy Places Terminology" (web page), retrieved from *www.cdc.gov/healthyplaces/terminology.htm.*

38. Lovett, *The African-American History,* 55.

39. Lovett, *The African-American History,* 54.

40. Metropolitan Development and Housing Agency (MDHA), "Family Housing" (web page), retrieved from *www.nashville-mdha.org/familyHousing.php#apt-17.*

41. MDHA, "Family Housing."

42. Nashville Civic Design Center, *Chestnut Hill Neighborhood, Formerly "Cameron Trimble," Findings and Recommendations* (Nashville, TN: Nashville Civic Design Center, 2005), 8–11.

43. Sources for this history: Gary Gaston, *The Historic Germantown Neighborhood, Nashville, TN,* policy brief (Nashville, TN: Nashville Civic Design Center, 2006); Nashville Civic Design Center, *Nashville's Neighborhoods,* policy brief (Nashville, TN: Nashville Civic Design Center, 2007); and Historical Commission of Metropolitan Nashville-Davidson County, *Nashville: Conserving A Heritage* (Nashville, TN: Historical Commission of Metropolitan Nashville-Davidson County, 1977), 35–36; 53–55.

44. John Lawrence Connelly, *North Nashville and Germantown Yesterday and Today* (Nashville, TN: The North High Association, Inc., Ambrose Printing Co., 1982).

45. National Park Service, *National Register of Historic Places Inventory: Nomination Form* (Washington, DC: National Park Service, 1979), retrieved from *www.nps.gov/nr/publications/forms.htm.*

46. Historic Germantown, "History of Germantown" (web page), retrieved from *historicgermantown.org/history.*

47. Randall Gross and Development Economics, *Market Analysis: Downtown/SoBro* (Nashville, TN: Metropolitan Development and Housing Authority, 2012), 68.

48. Cohousing Association of the United States, *What Is Cohousing?* (Mill Creek WA: Cohousing Association of the United States, 2013), retrieved from *www.cohousing.org/what_is_cohousing.*

49. Nashville Civic Design Center, *Cohousing: A Community Housing Type for Nashville* (Nashville, TN: Nashville Civic Design Center, 2010), retrieved from *www.sitemason.com/files/kqtHtm/NCDC_CoHousingWorkshopReport_web.pdf.*

50. Rebecca Dohn, Metro Water Services, email message to NCDC's Gary Gaston, May 24, 2013.

Center

1. Mumford, *The City in History,* 71.

2. Arlington County Government, "Projects and Planning: Planning and Development History" (web page), retrieved from *projects.arlingtonva.us/planning/history.*

3. Portland District Development Plan, *Pearl District Development Plan: A Future Vision for a Neighborhood in Transition* (Portland, OR: Portland Development Commission, 2011), retrieved from *www.pdc.us/Libraries/River_District/Pearl_District_Development_Plan_pdf.sflb.ashx.*

4. Metropolitan Planning Department, *Community Character Manual*, 321–22.

5. To encourage the adaptive reuse of commercial areas along arterials and collector streets for residential development, in 2005 the Planning Department created the "Adaptive Residential Development" policy to apply to properties within Nashville's Urban Zoning Overlay (see the text of Ordinance No. BL2004-492 at *www.nashville.gov/mc/ordinances/term_2003_2007/bl2004_492.htm*). In 2012 the change was expanded to include the entire Urban Services District (see the text of Ordinance No. BL2011-80 at *www.nashville.gov/mc/ordinances/term_2011_2015/bl2011_80.htm*).

6. Metropolitan Government of Nashville and Davidson County, *Specific Plan: Ordinance No. BL2005-762* (Nashville, TN: Metropolitan Government of Nashville and Davidson County, 2005).

7. US Census Bureau, "TIGER / Line Shapefiles, 2010."

8. Arthur C. Nelson, *Reshaping Metropolitan America: Development Trends and Opportunities to 2030* (Washington, DC: Island Press, 2013).

9. Nashville Area Metropolitan Planning Organization, *Regional Growth and Traffic Forecasts* (Nashville, TN: Nashville Area Metropolitan Planning Organization, March 2014), retrieved from *www.nashvillempo.org/docs/Presentations/MPO_XB_Forecasts_19MARCH14.pdf.*

10. Arthur C. Nelson, *Tear Up a Parking Lot and Rebuild Paradise: Development Trends and Opportunities for Nashville* (Nashville, TN: Nashville Civic Design Center, Remarks at Annual Luncheon, October 9, 2013).

11. Christine Cole Marshall and Joy Marshall, *Good Will and Affection for Antioch: Reminiscences of Antioch, Tennessee* (Franklin, TN: Providence House Publishers, 2002), 1–3.

12. Nashville Baptist Association, *Acorns to Oaks: The Story of the Nashville Baptist Association and Its Affiliated Churches* (Nashville, TN: Nashville Baptist Association, 1972), 69.

13. Marshall and Marshall, *Good Will and Affection*, 2.

14. Marshall and Marshall, *Good Will and Affection*, 4–6, 7.

15. Charles B. Castner Jr., *The Dixie Line: Nashville, Chattanooga & St. Louis Railway* (Newton, NJ: Carstens Publications, Inc., 1995), 7.

16. Marshall and Marshall, *Good Will and Affection*, 15.

17. Marshall and Marshall, *Good Will and Affection*, 12.

18. Clark Parsons, "An Antioch State of Mind: In Search of Nashville's Forgotten World," *The Nashville Scene* (7 October 1993), 14–18.

19. Marshall, *Good Will and Affection*, 47

20. Bobby Allyn, "Image, Growth Issues Challenge Antioch," *Tennessean* (May 11, 2012).

21. Bobby Allyn, "Hickory Hollow Tenants Given 30-Day Notice," *Tennessean* (June 2, 2012).

22. Nancy DeVille, "Classrooms Could Power Hickory Hollow Rebirth," *Tennessean* (July 24, 2011).

23. Joey Garrison, "Metro Council Finalizes Antioch Ice Rink Plans," *Tennessean* (August 7, 2013).

24. Getahn Ward, "Mall Opens With Global Flair," *Tennessean* (May 18, 2013).

25. Nashville Area Metropolitan Planning Organization, *Southeast Corridor High-Performance Transit Alternatives Study* (Nashville, TN: Nashville Area Metropolitan Planning Organization, 2007), 4–14.

26. The Conservation Fund, Nashville: *Naturally*, 6.

27. Dick Battle, "City of Harpeth Hills in the Making," *Nashville Banner* (October 24, 1956).

28. US Census Bureau, *Volume 1 of Sixteenth Census of the United States: 1940: Population, United States* (Washington, DC: Bureau of the Census, 1942), 1026–31.

29. "Little Journeys out of Nashville—the Hillsboro Pike," *Nashville Banner* (April 8, 1923).

30. George Zepp, "Cause of 1952 Fire that Gutted Hillsboro High School Still a Mystery," *Tennessean* (April 13, 2005), B.3.

31. "Work on Green Hills Village Expected to Start in 2 Weeks," *Nashville Banner* (July 29, 1953).

32. Taubman Centers, "The Mall at Green Hills" (web page), retrieved from *www.shopgreenhills.com/about_us.*

33. Renee Elder, "Green Hills Tries to Catch Its Breath," *Tennessean* (June 4, 1999).

34. "There Must Be Gold in That Thar Green Hills," *Tennessean* (July 23, 1965).

35. Elder, "Green Hills Tries."

36. Metropolitan Planning Department, *Green Hills UDO Design Guidelines, Bedford Avenue Urban Design Overlay* (Nashville, TN: Metropolitan Government of Nashville and Davidson County, 2003).

37. Nashville Civic Design Center, *The Livability Project: Green Hills* (Nashville, TN: Nashville Civic Design Center, 2012).

Downtown

1. US Census Bureau, "Historical Data: 2010s: Vintage 2012" (web page), retrieved from *www.census.gov/popest/data/historical/2010s/vintage_2012/index.html.*

2. Kreyling, *The Plan of Nashville*, 5–41.

3. Leland Johnson, *The Parks of Nashville* (Nashville, TN: Metro Nashville, 1986), 34–52.

4. Metropolitan Planning Department, *Community Character Manual*, 347–48.

5. Data provided by Metropolitan Planning Department.

6. Nashville Downtown Partnership, *Residential Report: July 2013* (Nashville, TN: Nashville Downtown Partnership, 2013), 4, retrieved from *www.nashvilledowntown.com/_files/docs/2013_residential_report.pdf.*

7. Randall Gross and Development Economics, *Market Analysis*, 94.

8. Randall Gross and Development Economics, *Market Analysis*, 122.

9. Nashville Downtown Partnership, *2012 Downtown Nashville Business Census: Report of Findings* (Nashville, TN: Nashville Downtown Partnership, 2012), retrieved from *www.nashvilledowntown.com/_files/docs/report-for-website.pdf.*

10. Data provided by Nashville Convention and Visitors Bureau.

11. Data provided by Nashville Downtown Partnership, from *Investment Listing, 2000–Present.*

12. Kim Hartley Hawkins, "Deadrick Green: Creating Tennessee's First Green Street," LandscapeOnline.com, retrieved from *www.landscapeonline.com/research/article.php/18146.*

13. Metropolitan Planning Department, *Nashville Downtown Code: Chapter 17.37 of the Metropolitan Nashville and Davidson County Zoning Code* (Nashville, TN: Metropolitan Planning Department, 2010), retrieved from *www.nashville.gov/Portals/0/SiteContent/Planning/docs/dtc/DTC_150819.pdf.*

14. Preservation Green Lab, *The Greenest Building: Quantifying the Environmental Value of Building Reuse* (Washington, DC: National Trust for Historic Preservation, 2011), vi, retrieved from *www.preservationnation.org/information-center/sustainable-communities/green-lab/lca/The_Greenest_Building_lowres.pdf.*

15. Data provided by Metropolitan Transit Authority.

16. US Census Bureau, "American Community Survey: 2010."

17. Brian C. Tefft, *Impact Speed and a Pedestrian's Risk of Severe Injury or Death* (Washington, DC: AAA Foundation for Traffic Safety, 2011), 12, retrieved from *www.aaafoundation.org/sites/default/files/2011PedestrianRiskVsSpeed.pdf.*

18. Rick Bernhardt, Nashville Planning Department, in email message to Gary Gaston, July 11, 2013.

19. Nashville Downtown Partnership, *Residential Report: July 2013.*

20. Elizabeth Mygatt, "Forest Cover: World's Forests Continue to Shrink," *Earth Policy Institute* (April 9, 2006), retrieved from *www.earth-policy.org/indicators/C56/forests_2006.*

21. National Geographic, "Deforestation" (web page), retrieved from *environment.nationalgeographic.com/environment/global-warming/deforestation-overview.*

22. Ryan Bell and Jennie Wheeler, *Talking Trees: An Urban Forestry Toolkit for Local Governments* (Oakland, CA: ICLEI—Local Governments for Sustainability, 2006), retrieved from *www.milliontreesnyc.org/downloads/pdf/talking_trees_urban_forestry_toolkit.pdf.*

23. Metropolitan Public Works, "Tree Canopy Assessment and Urban Tree Inventory" (web page), retrieved from *www.nashville.gov/Public-Works/Community-Beautification/Tree-Information/Inventory-and-Canopy-Assessment.aspx.*

24. Justin Graham and Ian Hanou, *Metropolitan Nashville and Davidson County: April 2010. Metro Nashville Tree Canopy Assessment Project* (Nashville, TN: Metro Tree Advisory Committee and Metropolitan Government of Nashville and Davidson County, 2010), retrieved from *www.nashville.gov/portals/0/SiteContent/pw/docs/beautification/tree_canopy/tc-assessment.pdf.*

25. "Chapter 17.24 - Landscaping, Buffering and Tree Replacement," *The Code of the Metropolitan Government of Nashville and Davidson County, Tennessee*, retrieved from *www.municode.com/library/tn/metro_government_of_nashville_and_davidson_county/codes/code_of_ordinances?nodeId=CD_TIT17ZO_CH17.24LABUTRRE.*

26. Kaitlin Dastugue, Metropolitan Development and Housing Agency, email message to NCDC's Gary Gaston, October 8, 2015.

27. "Annual Vehicle Crossings and Toll Revenues, FY 1938 to FY 2011," Golden Gate Bridge Highway and Transportation District, retrieved from *goldengatebridge.org/research/crossings_revenues.php.*

28. "Traffic History," Tennessee Department of Transportation (web page), retrieved from *www.tdot.tn.gov/APPLICATIONS/traffichistory.*

29. Nashville Civic Design Center, *Lafayette Neighborhood: Findings and Recommendations* (Nashville, TN: Nashville Civic Design Center, 2006).

30. Room in the Inn, *www.roomintheinn.org.*

31. Urban Design Associates, *South of Broadway Strategic Master Plan: Nashville, Tennessee* (Nashville, TN: Urban Design Associates, 2013).

32. Christine Kreyling, *The Plan for SoBro* (Nashville, TN: City Press Publishing, 1997), xv, 22–23.

33. National Health Care for the Homeless Council, *Homelessness & Health: What's the Connection?* Fact Sheet (Nashville, TN: National Health Care for the Homeless Council, June 2011), retrieved from *www.nhchc.org/wp-content/uploads/2011/09/Hln_health_factsheet_Jan10.pdf.*

34. US Interagency Council for Homelessness, "Fact Sheet: Chronic Homelessness," *Opening Doors: Federal Strategic Plan to Prevent and End Homelessness* (Washington, DC: US Interagency Council for Homelessness, 2010), retrieved from *usich.gov/resources/uploads/asset_library/FactSheetChronicHomelessness.pdf.*

35. Office of Community Planning and Development, *Defining Chronic Homelessness: A Technical Guide for HUD Programs* (Washington, DC: US Department of Housing and Urban Development, 2007), retrieved from *www.onecpd.info/resources/documents/DefiningChronicHomeless.pdf.*

36. National Health Care for the Homeless Council, *Homelessness & Health.*

37. James J. O'Connell, *Premature Mortality in Homeless Populations: A Review of the Literature* (Nashville, TN: National Health Care for the Homeless Council, 2005), retrieved from *santabarbarastreetmedicine.org/wordpress/wp-content/uploads/2011/04/PrematureMortalityFinal.pdf.*

38. National Health Care for the Homeless Council, *Homelessness & Health.*

39. Metropolitan Social Services – Planning & Coordination, *Community Needs Evaluation: 2012 Update – Davidson County, Tennessee* (Nashville, TN: Metropolitan Government of Nashville and Davidson County, 2012), retrieved from *www.nashville.gov/Portals/0/SiteContent/SocialServices/docs/cne/2012cne.pdf.*

40. Rent Jungle, "Rent trend data in Nashville, Tennessee" (web site), retrieved from *www.rentjungle.com/average-rent-in-nashville-rent-trends.*

41. "Subject: Transmittal of Fiscal Year (FY) 1998 Public Housing/Section 8 Income Limits," US Department of Housing and Urban Develpoment, huduser.gov (January 7, 1998), retrieved from *www.huduser.org/portal/datasets/il/fmr98/sect8.html.*

42. Micah Maidenberg, "Coming to a Block Near You: CHA Subsidized Housing?" *Crain's Chicago Business* (October 5, 1013), retrieved from *www.chicagobusiness.com/article/20131005/ISSUE01/310059985/coming-to-a-block-near-you-cha-subsidized-housing.*

District

1. Metropolitan Planning Department, *Community Character Manual*, 389–91.

2. US Census Bureau, "TIGER / Line Shapefiles, 2010."

3. Sasaki Associates, Inc., *Vanderbilt University Land Use and Development Plan* (Watertown, MA: Sasaki Associates, 2001), 3–4.

Active Building and Site Design

1. Many of the concepts in this chapter are derived from a seminal work on healthy building design: NY Department of Design and Construction, NY Department of Health and Mental Hygiene, NY Department of Transportation, NY Department of City Planning, and NY Office of the Mayor, *Active Design Guidelines: Promoting Physical Activity and Health in Design* (New York, NY: City of New York, 2010), retrieved from *centerforactivedesign.org/dl/guidelines.pdf.*

2. US Environmental Protection Agency, *Report to Congress on Indoor Air Quality. Volume 2. Assessment and Control of Indoor Air Pollution* (Washington, DC: US Environmental Protection Agency, 1989), 252.

3. Gautam Naik, "New Buildings Help People Fight Flab," *Wall Street Journal* (November 16, 2005), retrieved from *www.wsj.com/articles/SB113210855510098537.*

4. Beneficial Design, HDR, and Sprinkle Consulting, *Pedestrian Element Scottsdale Transportation Master Plan* (Scottsdale, AZ: City of Scottsdale, 2008), 10, retrieved from *www.scottsdaleaz.gov/Assets/Public+Website/traffic/Adopted+Transportation+Master+Plan/Pedestrian+Element.pdf.*

5. Gary Cudney, "Parking Structure Cost Outlook for 2014," *Industry Insights* (April 2014), retrieved from *www.carlwalker.com/wp-content/uploads/2014/04/April-Newsletter-2014.pdf.*

6. Donald Shoup, "The Trouble with Minimum Parking Requirements," *Transportation Research Part A: Policy and Practice* 33 (1999), 561.

7. NY Department of Planning, *Zoning for Bicycle Parking* (New York: New York City Department of Planning, 2008), retrieved from *www.nyc.gov/html/dcp/pdf/bicycle_parking/zoning_bike_parking.pdf.*

8. Nashville, TN, Ordinance No. BL2009-479 (2009), retrieved from *www.nashville.gov/mc/ordinances/term_2007_2011/bl2009_479.htm.*

9. Sustainable Sources, "Passive Solar Design" (web page), retrieved from *passivesolar.sustainablesources.com.*

10. Stephen R. Kellert and Edward O. Wilson, editors, *The Biophilia Hypothesis* (Washington, DC: Island Press, 1993).

11. Stephen R. Kellert, Judith H. Heerwagen, and Martin L. Mador, eds. *Biophilic Design: The Theory, Science, and Practice of Bringing Buildings to Life* (Hoboken, NJ: John Wiley & Sons, Inc., 2008).

12. Duro-Last Roofing, "White Roof Systems" (web page), retrieved from *www.duro-last.com/white_roofing*.

13. William McCoy, "Calories Burned Climbing One Flight of Stairs," *Livestrong* (January 16, 2014), retrieved from *www.livestrong.com/article/301539-calories-burned-climbing-one-flight-of-stairs*.

14. Wener Hoeger and Sharon Hoeger, *Fitness & Wellness*, 10th Edition (Belmont, CA: Cengage Learning, 2012).

15. Julia Gifford, "We Tested Standing Desks—Here's Proof They Make You More Productive," *ReadWrite* (September 26, 2013), retrieved from *www.readwrite.com/2013/09/26/standing-desks-productivity*.

16. Sally Augustin, *Place Advantage: Applied Psychology for Interior Architecture* (Hoboken, NJ: John Wiley & Sons, Inc., 2009).

17. L. Edwards and P. Torcellini, *A Literature Review of Effects of Natural Light on Building Occupants* (Oak Ridge, TN: US Department of Energy National Renewal Energy Laboratory, 2002).

18. GREENGUARD, "GREENGUARD Certification from UL Environment" (web page), retrieved from *www.greenguard.org*.

19. Janetta Mitchell McCoy and Gary W. Evans, "Physical Work Environment," in *Handbook of Work Stress*, Julian Barling, E. Kevin Kelloway and Michael R. Frone, eds. (Thousand Oaks, CA: Sage Publications, Inc., 2005).

20. Clarke Harris, "Building Planned as Hospital Has Been Office Center for Metro," *Tennessean* (4 May 2007), retrieved from *www.tennessean.com/article/20050608/COLUMNIST0102/105030008*.

21. P. A. Walsh "Fixed Equipment—A Time for Change," *Australian Journal of Early Childhood* 18, no. 2 (June 1993), 23–29.

22. A. C. Barbour, "The Impact of Playground Design on the Play Behaviors of Children with Differing Levels of Physical Competence," *Early Childhood Research Quarterly* 14, no. 1 (1999), 75–98.

23. National Association of Home Builders, "What is Universal Design?" (web page), retrieved from *www.nahb.org/generic.aspx?genericContentID=89934*.

Conclusion

1. NashvilleNext Health, Livability, and the Built Environment Resource Team, *NashvilleNext: Health, Livability, and the Built Environment Goals and Policies* (Nashville, TN: Metropolitan Planning Commission, 2015), retrieved from *www.nashville.gov/Portals/0/SiteContent/Planning/docs/NashvilleNext/ResourceTeams/next-rt-HLBE-GoalsPolicies_072114.pdf*.

2. Nashville Area Metropolitan Planning Organization, "2040 Regional Transportation Plan" (web page), retrieved from *www.nashvillempo.org/plans_programs/rtp/2040_rtp.aspx*.

3. Nashville nMotion, "Nashville MTA/RTA Strategic Plan" (web page), retrieved from *nmotion2015.com/project-schedule*.

4. Nashville Area Chamber of Commerce, "Moving Forward: Transit Solutions for Our Region" (web page), retrieved from *www.nashvillechamber.com/homepage/AboutUs/ChamberInitiatives/moving-forward*.

5. European Centre for Health Policy, *Health Impact Assessment: Main Concepts and Suggested Approach. Gothenburg Consensus Paper* (Brussels, Belgium: European Centre for Health Policy, 1999).

6. Rajiv Bhatia, *Health Impact Assessment: A Guide for Practice* (Oakland, CA: Human Impact Partners, 2011).

7. European Centre for Health Policy, *Health Impact Assessment*.

8. Sonia Sequeira and Leslie Meehan, *Hamilton Springs Transit-Oriented Development: School Siting Health Impact Assessment* (Nashville, TN: Nashville Area Metropolitan Planning Organization, 2013), retrieved from *www.nashvillempo.org/docs/Health/HIA_2013_FINAL.pdf*.

Documenting the Process

1. Metro Public Health Department, "Communities Putting Prevention to Work (CPPW)" (web page), retrieved from *www.nashville.gov/Health-Department/CPPW.aspx*.

BIBLIOGRAPHY

BIBLIOGRAPHY

Aboelata, Manal J. *The Built Environment and Health: 11 Profiles of Neighborhood Transformation.* Edited by Jessica DuLong. Oakland, CA: Prevention Institute, 2004.

Allyn, Bobby. "Hickory Hollow Tenants Given 30-Day Notice." *Tennessean*, June 2, 2012.

———. "Image, Growth Issues Challenge Antioch." *Tennessean*, May 11, 2012.

American Hospital Association. *A Call to Action: Creating a Culture of Health.* Chicago: American Hospital Association, 2011.

American Institute of Architects. *Local Leaders: Healthier Communities through Design.* Washington, DC: American Institute of Architects, 2012.

American Planning Association. *Integrating Planning and Public Health: Tools and Strategies to Create Healthy Places.* Chicago: American Planning Association, 2006.

———. "Accessory Dwelling Units." *PAS Quicknotes* 19 (2009). Retrieved from *www.planning.org/pas/quicknotes/pdf/QN19.pdf.*

American Psychological Association. "The Impact of Stress: 2012" (web page). Retrieved from *www.apa.org/news/press/releases/stress/2012/impact.aspx?item=2.*

American Public Health Association. "APHA History and Timeline" (web page). Retrieved from *www.apha.org/news-and-media/newsroom/online-press-kit/apha-history-and-timeline.*

American Trails. "2013 RTP Achievement Awards: Beaman Park Accessible and Interpretive Trail (Tennessee)" (web page). Retrieved from *www.americantrails.org/awards/CRT13awards/Beaman-Park-Accessible-Trail-CRT-award-2013.html.*

Arendt, Randall. *Envisioning Better Communities.* Chicago: The American Planning Association, 2010.

Arlington County Government. "Planning and Development History" (web page). Retrieved from *projects.arlingtonva.us/planning/history.*

Arnold, Joseph L. "Riverside, IL." *Encyclopedia of Chicago.* Retrieved from *www.encyclopedia.chicagohistory.org/pages/1080.html.*

Augustin, Sally. *Place Advantage: Applied Psychology for Interior Architecture.* Hoboken, NJ: John Wiley & Sons, Inc., 2009.

Barbour, Ann C. "The Impact of Playground Design on the Play Behaviors of Children with Differing Levels of Physical Competence." *Early Childhood Research Quarterly* 14, no. 1 (1999): 75–98.

Barham, James, Debra Tropp, Kathleen Enterline, Jeff Farbman, John Fisk, and Stacia Kiraly. *Regional Food Hub Resource Guide.* Washington, DC: US Dept. of Agriculture, Agricultural Marketing Service, 2012. Retrieved from *ngfn.org/resources/ngfn-database/knowledge/FoodHubResourceGuide.pdf.*

Battle, Dick. "City of Harpeth Hills in the Making." *Nashville Banner*, October 24, 1956.

Beaumont, Constance E., and Elizabeth G. Pianca. *Why Johnny Can't Walk to School: Historic Neighborhoods in the Age of Sprawl*, 2nd edition. Washington, DC: National Trust for Historic Preservation, 2002.

Bell, Ryan, and Jamie Wheeler. *Talking Trees: An Urban Forestry Toolkit for Local Governments.* Oakland, CA: ICLEI—Local Governments for Sustainability, 2006. Retrieved from *www.milliontreesnyc.org/downloads/pdf/talking_trees_urban_forestry_toolkit.pdf.*

Beneficial Design, HDR, and Sprinkle Consulting. *Pedestrian Element Scottsdale Transportation Master Plan.* Scottsdale, AZ: City of Scottsdale, 2008. Retrieved from *www.scottsdaleaz.gov/Assets/Public+Website/traffic/Adopted+Transportation+Master+Plan/Pedestrian+Element.pdf.*

Berger, Alan M., and Andrew Scott, editors, *Health + Urbanism.* Cambridge, MA: Massachusetts Institute of Technology, 2013.

Berger, Alan M., Casey Lance Brown, and Aparna Keshaviah. "Project Background." In *Health + Urbanism*, edited by Alan M. Berger and Andrew Scott, 7. Cambridge, MA: Massachusetts Institute of Technology, 2013. p. 7.

Berrigan, D., and R. A. McKinno. "Built Environment and Health." *Preventative Medicine* 47, no. 3 (September 2008): 239–40.

Berry, Sean. *Case Studies on Transit and Livable Communities in Rural and Small Town America.* Washington DC: Transportation for America, 2009.

Bhatia, Rajiv. *Health Impact Assessment: A Guide for Practice.* Oakland, CA: Human Impact Partners, 2011.

Bicycling.com. "America's Top 50 Bike-Friendly Cities" (web page). Retrieved from *www.bicycling.com/news/advocacy/america-s-top-50-bike-friendly-cities#snapback.*

Binelli, Eliana Kampf, Henry L. Gholz, and Mary L. Duryea. *Chapter 4: Plant Succession and Disturbances in the Urban Forest Ecosystem*, Publication #FOR93. Gainesville, FL: University of Florida, 2012. Retrieved from *edis.ifas.ufl.edu/fr068.*

Bloomberg Philanthropies. "Bloomberg Philanthropies and Living Cities' CFE Fund Announce Five Cities Selected for $16.2 M in Financial Empowerment Center Grants." Press Release. (Bloomberg online, January 8, 2013). Retrieved from *www.bloomberg.org/press/releases/bloomberg-philanthropies-and-living-cities-cfe-fund-announce-five-cities-selected-for-16-2-m-in-financial-empowerment-center-grants.*

Brasher, Joan. "Study: Frequent Moves Hinder Child's Early Education." *Research News at Vanderbilt University,* February 15, 2013. Retrieved from *news.vanderbilt.edu/2013/02/frequent-moves-study.*

Brookings Institution. *Average US Metro Areas.* Washington, DC: Brookings Institution, 2008.

Burden, Dan. *Street Design Guidelines for Healthy Neighborhoods.* Sacramento, CA: Local Government Commission, 2002.

Buzby, Jean C., Jeffrey Hyman, Hayden Stewart and Hodan F. Wells, "The Value of Retail- and Consumer-Level Fruit and Vegetable Losses in the United States." *Journal of Consumer Affairs* 45, no. 3 (Fall 2011), 492–515.

Campoli, Julie, and Alex S. MacLean. *Visualizing Density.* Cambridge, MA: Lincoln Institute of Land Policy, 2007.

Capitol Region Council of Governments (CRCOG). "Chapter 5. Transit Oriented Development: Fact Sheet," in *Livable Communities Toolkit: A Best Practices Manual for Metropolitan Regions.* Hartford, CT: Capitol Region Council of Governments, 2002. Retrieved from *www.crcog.org/publications/CommDevDocs/TCSP/Ch05_FactSheet_TOD.pdf.*

Cass, Michael. "Most Residential Property Values See Drop." *Tennessean,* March 28, 2013.

Castner, Charles B., Jr. *The Dixie Line: Nashville, Chattanooga & St. Louis Railway.* Newton, NJ: Carstens Publications, Inc., 1995.

Center for Environmental Policy and Management. *Schoolyards as Resources for Learning and Communities: A Design Handbook for Kentucky Schools.* Louisville, KY: University of Louisville, 2010.

Centers for Disease Control and Prevention. "Healthy Places Terminology" (web page). Retrieved from *www.cdc.gov/healthyplaces/terminology.htm.*

Centers for Disease Control and Prevention, Division of Nutrition, Physical Activity, and Obesity. "Defining Adult Overweight and Obesity" (web page). Retrieved from *www.cdc.gov/obesity/adult/defining.html.*

Cerin, E., B. E. Saelens, J. F. Sallis, and L. D. Frank. "Neighborhood Environment Walkability Scale: Validity and Development of a Short Form." *Medicine and Science in Sports and Exercise* (2006): 1682–91.

Cerin, Ester, Eva Leslie, Lorrine du Toit, Neville Owen, and Lawrence D. Frank. "Destinations that Matter: Associations with Walking for Transport." *Health and Place* 13 (2007): 713–24.

ChangeLab Solutions. *Creating Healthier Suburbs: Tools for Transforming Sprawl into Livable Communities.* Oakland, CA: ChangeLab Solutions, 2012.

Chatterjee, Anusuya, and Ross DeVol. *Best Cities for Successful Aging.* Washington, DC: Milken Institute, 2012.

Chen, Jarvis T., D. H. Rehkopf, P. D. Waterman, S. V. Subramanian, B. A. Coull, M. Ostrem, and N. Krieger. "Mapping and Measuring Social Disparities in Premature Mortality: The Impact of Census Tract Poverty Within and Across Boston Neighborhoods, 1999–2001." *Journal of Urban Health* 83, no. 6 (November 2006): 1063–84.

Chicago Department of Transportation. *The Chicago Green Alley Handbook.* Chicago: City of Chicago, 2010.

———. *Chicago Streets for Cycling Plan 2020.* Chicago, IL: Chicago Department of Transportation, 2012.

Chicago Metropolitan Agency for Planning. *Go to 2040: Comprehensive Regional Plan.* Chicago: Chicago Metropolitan Agency for Planning, 2010.

City CarShare. *Getting More with Less: Managing Residential Parking in Urban Developments with Carsharing and Unbundling Best Practices.* San Francisco: Nelson Nygaard, 2012.

City of Portland Bureau of Planning and Sustainability. *Portland Plan. Status Report: Twenty-Minute Neighborhoods.* Portland, OR: City of Portland Bureau of Planning and Sustainability, May 2009. Retrieved from *www.cityofmadison.com/Sustainability/community/documents/20minNeigh.pdf.*

Cobb, Rodney L., and Scott Dvorak. *Accessory Dwelling Units Model State Act and Local Ordinance.* Washington, DC: AARP Public Policy Institute, 2000.

Cohousing Association of the United States. "What Is Cohousing?" Mill Creek WA: Cohousing Association of the United States, 2013. Retrieved from *www.cohousing.org/what_is_cohousing.*

Colquhoun, Ian. *Design Out Crime: Creating Safe and Sustainable Communities.* Burlington, MA: Architectural Press, 2004.

Committee on Accelerating Progress in Obesity Prevention. *Accelerating Progress in Obesity Prevention: Solving the Weight of the Nation.* Washington, DC: The National Academies Press, 2012.

Congress for the New Urbanism. *Malls into Mainstreets: An In-Depth Guide to Transforming Dead Malls into Communities.* Chicago: Congress for the New Urbanism, 2005.

Connelly, John Lawrence. *North Nashville and Germantown Yesterday and Today.* Nashville, TN: The North High Association, Inc., Ambrose Printing Co., 1982.

The Conservation Fund. *Nashville Open Space Plan: Creating, Enhancing and Preserving the Places that Matter. A Report of Nashville: Naturally.* Nashville, TN: Metropolitan Government of Nashville and Davidson County, 2011. Retrieved from *www.conservationfund.org/images/projects/files/Nashville-Naturally-Green-Infrastructure-Plan-The-Conservation-Fund-2011.pdf.*

Cortright, Joseph. *Driven Apart: How Sprawl Is Lengthening Our Commutes and Why Misleading Mobility Measures are Making Things Worse.* Cleveland, OH: CEOs for Cities, 2010. Retrieved from *www.infrastructureusa.org/wp-content/uploads/2010/09/technicalreport_drivenapart9-29-10.pdf.*

———. *Walking the Walk: How Walkability Raises Home Values in US Cities.* Cleveland, OH: CEOs For Cities, 2009. Retrieved from *www.reconnectingamerica.org/assets/Uploads/2009WalkingTheWalkCEOsforCities.pdf.*

Cotten, Christopher. *Churches of Christ in East Nashville: Their Rise and Decline in the Twentieth Century.* August 2008. Retrieved from *ccotten.files.wordpress.com/2008/09/rough-draft.doc.*

Council of Educational Facility Planners International. *Schools for Successful Communities: An Element of Smart Growth.* Scottsdale, AZ: United States Environmental Protection Agency, 2004.

Cudney, Gary. "Parking Structure Cost Outlook for 2014," *Industry Insights* (April 2014). Retrieved from *www.carlwalker.com/wp-content/uploads/2014/04/April-Newsletter-2014.pdf.*

Cumberland Region Tomorrow. *Quality Growth Toolbox.* Nashville, TN: Cumberland Region Tomorrow, 2004.

Dannenberg, Andrew L. "The Impact of Community Design and Land-Use Choices on Public Health: A Scientific Research Agenda." *American Journal of Public Health* 93 (2003): 1500–08.

Dannenberg, Andrew L., Howard Frumkin, and Richard J. Jackson. *Making Healthy Places: Designing and Building for Health, Well-Being and Sustainability.* Washington, DC: Island Press, 2011.

Davis, Benjamin, Tony Dutzik, and Phineas Baxandall. *Transportation and the New Generation: Why Young People Are Driving Less and What It Means for Transportation Policy.* Boston: Frontier Group and US PIRG Education Fund (April 2012). Retrieved from *www.uspirg.org/reports/usp/transportation-and-new-generation.*

Davis, Thomas K. *The A.I.A. 150 Blueprint for America Community Assessment and Visioning Workshop for Kingston Springs.* Kingston Springs, TN: American Institute of Architects, 2008.

———. *The A.I.A. 150 Blueprint for America Visioning Workshop for Robertson County.* Springfield, TN: Cumberland Region Tomorrow, 2007. Retrieved from *www.cumberlandregiontomorrow.org/robertson/aia-150-robertson-county.*

———. *Micro Unit Housing: Downtown Nashville.* Knoxville, TN: The University of Tennessee, Knoxville, 2013.

Department of Health and Human Services. *Philadelphia 2035: Planning and Zoning for a Healthier City.* Philadelphia: City of Philadelphia, 2010.

Design for Health. *Planning Information Sheet: Influencing Mental Health with Comprehensive Planning and Ordinances.* Edited by Carissa Schively. Vers. 2.0. 2007. Retrieved from *www.designforhealth.net.*

Design Studio. *Living Alleys: Ideas for City Neighborhoods.* Nashville, TN: Metropolitan Nashville Planning Department, 2011.

Design, Community & Environment, Reid Ewing, Lawrence Frank and Company, Inc., and Richard Kreutzer. *Understanding the Relationship between Public Health and the Built Environment.* Washington, DC: LEED-ND Core Committee, 2006.

DeVille, Nancy. "Classrooms Could Power Hickory Hollow Rebirth." *Tennessean*, July 24, 2011.

Dills, James, Candace D. Rutt, and Karen G. Mumford. "Objectively Measuring Route-to-Park Walkability In Atlanta." *Environment and Behavior* 44 (November 2012): 841–60.

"Doty Left His Mark." *Wisconsin State Journal*, June 26, 1976. Retrieved from *www.newspapers.com/newspage/14893199.*

Dougherty, Conor. "Which Cities Are Growing Faster Than Their Suburbs." *Wall Street Journal*, June 28, 2012. Retrieved from *blogs.wsj.com/economics/2012/06/28/which-cities-are-growing-faster-than-their-suburbs.*

Dougherty, Conor, and Robbie Whelan. "Cities Outpace Suburbs in Growth." *Wall Street Journal*, June 28, 2012. Retrieved from *online.wsj.com/article/SB10001424052702304830704577493032619987956.html.*

Doyle, Don. *Nashville in the New South: 1880–1930.* Knoxville, TN: University of Tennessee Press, 1985.

———. *Nashville Since the 1920's.* Knoxville, TN: University of Tennessee Press, 1985.

———. *New Men, New Cities, New South: Atlanta, Nashville, Charleston, Mobile, 1860–1910.* Chapel Hill, NC: University of North Carolina Press, 1990.

Drummond, Jocelyn Pak. "Health + Urbanism Primer." In *Health + Urbanism,* edited by Alan M. Berger and Andrew Scott. Cambridge, MA: Massachusetts Institute of Technology, 2013.

Drummond, Jocelyn Pak, and Alan M. Berger. "Current Limitations." In *Health + Urbanism,* edited by Alan M. Berger and Andrew Scott. Cambridge, MA: Massachusetts Institute of Technology, 2013.

Duany, Andres, Elizabeth Plater-Zyberk, and Jeff Speck. *Suburban Nation.* New York: North Point Press, 2000.

Duany, Andres, Sandy Sorlien, and William Wright. *Smart Code Manual Version 9.* Ithaca, NY: New Urban New Publications, 2008.

Duany, Andrew, Jeff Speck, and Mike Lydon. *The Smart Growth Manual.* New York: McGraw Hill, 2010.

Dulaney, Chelsey. "Nashville Rent Increases Have Residents Singing the Blues." *Wall Street Journal,* August 10, 2014. Retrieved from *www.wsj.com/articles/nashville-rent-increases-have-residents-singing-the-blues-1407708778.*

Dunham-Jones, Ellen, and June Williamson. *Retrofitting Suburbia: Urban Design Solutions for Redesigning Suburbs.* Hoboken, NJ: John Wiley & Sons, 2009.

Duro-Last Roofing. "White Roof Systems" (web page). Retrieved from *www.duro-last.com/white_roofing.*

"East Nashville history and timeline." *Tennessean,* November 1, 2006. Retrieved from *archive.tennessean.com/article/99999999/MICRO0206/61027038/East-Nashville-history-timeline.*

Edwards, L., and P. Torcellini. *A Literature Review of Effects of Natural Light on Building Occupants.* Oak Ridge, TN: US Department of Energy National Renewable Energy Laboratory, 2002.

Edwards, Peggy, and Agis D. Tsuouros. *A Healthy City Is an Active City.* Copenhagen, Denmark: World Health Organization, 2008.

Egerton, John, and E. Thomas Wood, eds. *Nashville: An American Self-Portrait.* Nashville, TN: Beaten Biscuit Press, 2001.

Eitler, Thomas W., Edward T. McMahon, and Theodore C. Thoerig. *Ten Principles for Building Healthy Places.* Washington, DC: Urban Land Institute, 2013.

Elder, Renee. "Green Hills Tries to Catch Its Breath." *Tennessean,* June 4, 1999.

Enterprise Community Partners, Inc. "Denver Regional Transit-Oriented Development Fund" (web page). Retrieved from *www.enterprisecommunity.com/financing-and-development/community-development-financing/denver-tod-fund.*

———. *Preserving Affordable Housing Near Transit.* Edited by Leo Quigley. Oakland, CA: The National Housing Trust, 2010.

Ernst, Michelle, and Lilly Shoup. *Dangerous By Design: Solving the Epidemic of Preventable Pedestrian Deaths (And Making Great Neighborhoods).* Washington DC: Transportation For America, 2009.

European Centre for Health Policy. *Health Impact Assessment: Main Concepts and Suggested Approach. Gothenburg Consensus Paper.* Brussels, Belgium: European Centre for Health Policy, 1999.

Ewing, Reid, and Barbara McCann. *Measuring the Health Effects of Sprawl: A National Analysis of Physical Activity, Obesity and Chronic Disease.* Washington, DC: Smart Growth America and the Surface Transportation Policy Project, 2003.

Farber, Nicholas, and Douglas Shinkle. *Aging in Place: A State of Livability Policies and Practices.* Washington, DC: National Conference of State Legislatures, 2011.

Federal Highway Administration. *Summary Report: Evaluation of Lane Reduction 'Road Diet' Measures and Their Effects on Crashes and Injuries.* US Dept. of Transportation pub. # FHWA-HRT-04-082. March 2004. Retrieved from *www.fhwa.dot.gov/publications/research/safety/humanfac/04082.*

Fink, George. *Encyclopedia of Stress,* Vol. 1. San Diego, CA: Academic Press, 2000.

Fitzgerald, F. Scott. *The Great Gatsby.* 1925. Reprint, New York: Scribner, 2004.

Frank, Lawrence D., Martin A. Andresen, and Thomas L. Schmid. "Obesity Relationships with Community Design, Physical Activity, and Time Spent in Cars." *American Journal of Preventive Medicine* 27, no. 2 (August 2004): 87–96.

Frank, Lawrence D., Jacqueline Kerr, James F. Sallis, Rebecca Miles, and Jim Chapman. "A Hierarchy of Socio-demographic and Environmental Correlates of Walking and Obesity." *Preventative Medicine* 47, no. 2 (April 2008): 172–78.

Frank, Lawrence D., and Gary Pivo. *Impacts of Mixed Use and Density on Utilization of Three Modes of Travel: Single-Occupancy Vehicle, Transit, and Walking.* Seattle, WA: Transportation Research Record, 1994.

Frank, Douglas, Brian E. Saelens, Ken E. Powell, and James E. Chapman. "Stepping Towards Causation: Do Built Environments or Neighborhoods and Travel Preferences Explain Physical Activity, Driving, and Obesity?" *Social Science and Medicine* 65, no. 9 (November 2007): 1898–914.

Frank, Lawrence, D., James F. Sallis, Terry L. Conway, James E. Chapman, Brian E. Saelens, and Williams Bachman. "Many Pathways from Land Use to Health: Associations between Neighborhood Walkability and Active Transportation, Body Mass Index, and Air Quality." *Journal of the American Planning Association* 72, no. 1 (2006): 75–87.

Frank, Lawrence D., Thomas L. Schmid, James F. Chapman, James Sallis, and Brian E. Saelens. "Linking Objectively Measured Physical Activity with Objectively Measured Urban Form." *American Journal of Preventative Medicine* 28, no. 2 (2005): 117–25.

Frederick Law Olmsted Society of Riverside. "Maps of Riverside" (web page). Retrieved from *www.olmstedsociety.org/resources/maps-of-riverside.*

Friends of Warner Parks. *A Master Plan for the Burch Reserve at Warner Parks.* Nashville, TN: Metropolitan Board of Parks and Recreation, 2011.

Friskics-Warren, Bill. "One Street at a Time; Nashville's 12South." *New York Times,* June 15, 2003. Retrieved from *www.nytimes.com/2003/06/15/magazine/one-street-at-a-time-nashville-s-12south.html.*

Frumkin, Howard. "Guest Editorial: Health, Equity, and the Built Environment." *Environmental Health Perspectives* 115, no. 5 (2005): A290–91.

Frumkin, Howard, Lawrence Frank, and Richard Jackson. *Urban Sprawl and Public Health: Designing, Planning, and Building for Healthy Communities.* Washington, DC: Island Press, 2004.

Fry, Carrie. "Public Health and Urban Planning: A History and Its Effects." Unpublished paper, Vanderbilt University, 2012.

Fulcher, Richard Carlton. *1770–1790 Census of the Cumberland Settlements.* Baltimore, MD: Genealogical Publishing Co., Inc., 1987.

Garrison, Joey. "Metro Council Finalizes Antioch Ice Rink Plans." *Tennessean,* August 7, 2013.

Gaston, Gary. *The Historic Germantown Neighborhood, Nashville, TN.* Policy brief. Nashville, TN: Nashville Civic Design Center, 2006.

Gaston, Gary, and Ron Yearwood. *Moving Tennessee Forward: Models for Connecting Communities.* New Brighton, MN: Print Craft Inc., 2012.

Geller, Roger. *Four Types of Cyclists.* Portland, OR: Portland Office of Transportation, n.d. Retrieved from *www.portlandoregon.gov/transportation/article/158497.*

Gifford, Julia. "We Tested Standing Desks—Here's Proof They Make You More Productive." *ReadWrite,* September 26, 2013. Retrieved from *www.readwrite.com/2013/09/26/standing-desks-productivity.*

Glover, Jillian. "Converting Alleyways to Livable Laneways and Country Lanes." *This City Life* (blog). Retrieved from *thiscitylife.tumblr.com/post/54683503256/converting-alleyways-to-livable-laneways-and-country.*

Goldsmith, Stephen, William Eimicke, and Chris Pineda. *How City Hall Can Invigorate the Faith Community around a Citywide Housing Agenda.* Cambridge, MA: Harvard University Ash Institute for Democratic Governance and Innovation, Fall 2005. Retrieved from *www.innovations.harvard.edu/sites/default/files/11119.pdf.*

Goodstein, Anita Shafer. *Nashville 1780–1860: From Frontier to City.* Gainesville, FL: University of Florida Press, 1989.

Grabar, Henry. "The Urbanist Toolkit Bracket Challenge." *CityLab* (March 21, 2013). Retrieved from *www.citylab.com/work/2013/03/urbanist-toolkit-bracket-challenge/5041.*

Graham, Eleanor. *Nashville: A Short History and Selected Buildings.* Nashville, TN: Historical Commission of Metropolitan Nashville–Davidson County, 1974.

Graham, Justin, and Ian Hanou. *Metropolitan Nashville and Davidson County: April 2010. Metro Nashville Tree Canopy Assessment Project.* Nashville, TN: Metro Tree Advisory Committee and Metropolitan Government of Nashville and Davidson County, 2010. Retrieved from *www.nashville.gov/portals/0/SiteContent/pw/docs/beautification/tree_canopy/tc-assessment.pdf.*

GREENGUARD. "GREENGUARD Certification from UL Environment" (web page). Retrieved from *www.greenguard.org.*

Green Infrastructure Center. *Rural Preservation through Land Stewardship Tools.* Charlottesville, VA: Green Infrastructure Center, 2010.

Greenways for Nashville. *Greenways Master Plan.* Nashville, TN: Greenways Nashville, 2013. Retrieved from *www.greenwaysfornashville.org/maps-trails/sm_files/11x17%20map_master%20plan_2012_09_28.pdf.*

Gresham Smith and Partners. *Complete Streets Design Guidelines.* Knoxville, TN: Tennessee Department of Transportation, 2009.

Gross, Randall, and Development Economics. *Market Analysis: Downtown SoBro.* Nashville, TN: Metropolitan Development and Housing Authority, 2012.

Haggard, Merle, and Dean Holloway. "Big City." *Big City,* Epic Records, 1981. Copyright Sony/ATV Tree Publishing.

Hall, Kenneth B., and Gerald A. Porterfield. *Community by Design: New Urbanism for Suburbs and Small Communities.* New York: McGraw-Hill, 1995.

Hardwick, M. Jeffrey. *Mall Maker.* Philadelphia: University of Pennsylvania Press, 2004.

Hargreaves and Associates. *Nashville Riverfront.* Nashville, TN: Metropolitan Development and Housing Agency, 2011.

Harper, Garrett. *Nashville Region's Vital Signs 2013.* Nashville, TN: Nashville Area Chamber of Commerce, 2013.

Harrell, Rodney, Allison Brooks, and Todd Nedwick. *Preserving Affordability and Access in Livable Communities: Subsidized Housing Opportunities Near Transit and the 50+ Population.* Washington, DC: AARP, 2009.

Harris, Clarke. "Building Planned as Hospital Has Been Office Center for Metro." *Tennessean,* May 4, 2007. Retrieved from *www.tennessean.com/article/20050608/COLUMNIST0102/105030008.*

Haruch, Steve. "Hot Problems: Climate Change Isn't Coming to Nashville—It's Already Here. And the Future Might Be Hotter than We Can Handle." *Nashville Scene,* August 26, 2010.

Hawkins, Kim. "Deadrick Green: Creating Tennessee's First Green Street." Landscape-Online.com. Retrieved from *www.landscapeonline.com/research/article.php/18146.*

Healthy Nashville Leadership Council. *Healthy Living Report Card.* Nashville, TN: Healthy Nashville, 2009. Retrieved from *www.healthynashville.org/javascript/htmleditor/uploads/MPHDReportCard1_10.pdf.*

Hinshaw, Mark, and Brian Vanneman. "The Supermarket as a Neighborhood Building Block." *Planning Magazine,* March 2010. Retrieved from *planning.org/planning/2010/mar.*

Historical Commission of Metropolitan Nashville-Davidson County. *Nashville: Conserving A Heritage.* Nashville, TN: Historical Commission of Metropolitan Nashville-Davidson County, 1977.

Historic Germantown. "History of Germantown" (web page). Retrieved from *historicgermantown.org/history.*

Hoeger, Wener, and Sharon Hoeger. *Fitness & Wellness,* 10th Edition. Belmont, CA: Cengage Learning, 2012.

Holleman, Margaret. *The Evolution of Federal Housing Policy from 1892–1974 in Nashville, Tennessee.* Nashville, TN: Nashville Civic Design Center, 2002.

The Housing Fund. "Shared Equity: Our House" (web page). Retrieved from *thehousingfund.org/loans/individual-assistance-programs/homeownership/shared-equity.*

Huh, Susanna Y., Sheryl L. Rifas-Shiman, Elsie M. Taveras, Emily Oken, and Matthew W. Gillman. "Timing of Solid Food Introduction and Risk of Obesity in Preschool-Aged Children." *Pediatrics* 127, no. 3 (March 2011): e544–51.

Humphrey, Nancy P. "TRB Special Report. Does the Built Environment Influence Activity?: Examining the Evidence." *TR News* 237 (March-April 2005): 31–33.

Hutchinson, Brian. "Forgotten 'Country Lane' Experiment Could Be Answer to Vancouver's Desire for More Green Space." *National Post,* July 13, 2002. Retrieved from *news.nationalpost.com/2013/07/02/forgotten-country-lane-experiment-could-be-answer-to-vancouvers-desire-for-more-green-space.*

Institute of Medicine Committee on Sleep Medicine and Research. *Sleep Disorders and Sleep Deprivation: An Unmet Public Health Problem.* Edited by Harvey Colten and Bruce Altevogt. Washington, DC: The National Academies Press, 2006.

Ivy, Robert. "10 Year Scope." In *Health + Urbanism,* edited by Alan M. Berger and Andrew Scott, 3–5. Cambridge, MA: Massachusetts Institute of Technology, 2013.

Jackson, Richard, host. *Designing Healthy Communities.* PBS video series. 2011.

Jackson, Richard J. "The Impact of the Built Environment on Health: An Emerging Field." *American Journal of Public Health* 93, no. 9 (2003): 1382–84.

Jackson, Richard J., and Chris Kochtitzky. *Creating A Healthy Environment: The Impact of the Built Environment on Public Health.* Washington, DC: Sprawl Watch Clearinghouse, 2001.

Jackson, Richard, and Stacy Sinclaire. *Designing Healthy Communities.* San Francisco, CA: John Wiley and Sons, 2012.

Jacobs, Jane. *The Death and Life of Great American Cities.* New York: Random House, 1961; reprint, New York: Vintage Books, 1992.

Johnson, Leland. *The Parks of Nashville.* Nashville, TN: Metro Nashville, 1986.

Joint Center for Housing Studies of Harvard University. *Housing America's Older Adults.* Cambridge, MA: Joint Center for Housing Studies of Harvard University, 2014. Retrieved from *www.jchs.harvard.edu/sites/jchs.harvard.edu/files/jchs-housing_americas_older_adults_2014.pdf.*

Kabat, Geoffrey. "Why Labeling Obesity as a Disease is a Big Mistake." *Forbes* July 9, 2013. Retrieved from *www.forbes.com/sites/geoffreykabat/2013/07/09/why-labeling-obesity-as-a-disease-is-a-big-mistake.*

Kaplan, Alex, and Pearl Iams, editors. *Economic Development and Smart Growth.* Washington, DC: International Economic Development Council, 2006.

Kellert, Stephen, and Edward O. Wilson, editors. *The Biophilia Hypothesis.* Washington, DC: Island Press, 1993.

Kellert, Stephen, Judith H. Heerwagen, and Martin L. Mador, editors. *Biophilic Design: The Theory Science and Practice of Bringing Buildings to Life.* Hoboken, NJ: John Wiley and Sons, 2008.

Kerr, J., D. Rosenberg, J. F. Sallis, B. E. Saelens, L. D. Frank, and T. L. Conway. "Active

Commuting to School: Associations with Environment and Parental Concerns." *Medicine and Science in Sports and Medicine* 38, no. 4 (April 2006): 787–94.

Kim, Jinwon, and David Brownstone. *The Impacts of Residential Density on Vehicle Usage and Fuel Consumption: Evidence from National Sample.* Irvine, CA: Department of Economics, University of California, Irvine, April 2012. Retrieved from *sites.uci.edu/jinwonkim/files/2012/05/paper_0423.pdf.*

Kligerman, M., J. F. Sallis, S. Ryan, L. D. Frank, and P. R. Nader. "Association of Neighborhood Design and Recreation Environment Variables with Physical Activity and Body Mass Index in Adolescents." *American Journal of Health Promotion* 21, no. 4 (2005): 274–77.

Kostof, Spiro. *The City Shaped: Urban Patterns and Meanings Through History.* Boston: Bulfinch Press, Little, Brown and Co., 1991.

Kramer, Anita, Terry Lassar, Mark Federman, and Sarah Hammerschmidt. *Building for Wellness: The Business Case.* Washington, DC: Urban Land Institute, 2014.

Kreyling, Christine. *The Plan for SoBro.* Nashville, TN: City Press Publishing, 1997.

———. *The Plan of Nashville: Avenues to a Great City.* Nashville, TN: Vanderbilt University Press, 2005.

Kuhlman, Renee. *Helping Johnny Walk to School: Policy Recommendations for Removing Barriers to Community-Centered Schools.* Washington DC: National Trust for Historic Preservation, 2008.

Laveist, T., K. Pollack, R. Thorpe Jr., R. Fesahazion, and D. Gaskin. "Place, Not Race: Disparities Dissipate in Southwest Baltimore when Blacks and Whites Live under Similar Conditions." *Health Affairs* 30, no. 10 (2011): 1880–87.

Lee, C. D., Andrew S. Jackson, and Steven N. Blair, "US Weight Guidelines: Is It Also Important to Consider Cardiorespiratory Fitness?" *International Journal of Obesity* 22, Suppl. 2 (1998): S2–S7.

Lee, Helen. "The Making of the Obesity Epidemic: How Food Activism Led Public Health Astray." *Breakthrough Journal* 3 (Winter 2013). Retrieved from *thebreakthrough.org/index.php/journal/past-issues/issue-3/the-making-of-the-obesity-epidemic.*

Leventhal, T., and J. Brooks-Gunn. "Moving to Opportunity: An Experimental Study of Neighborhood Effects on Mental Health." *American Journal of Public Health* 93, no. 9 (September 2003): 1576–82.

Levy, Diane K., Zach McDade, and Kassie Dumlao. *Effects From Living In Mixed-Income Communities for Low-Income Families.* Washington, DC: Urban Institute, 2010.

Litman, Todd. *Parking Requirement Impacts on Housing Affordability.* Victoria, British Columbia: Victoria Transport Policy Institute, 2013.

"Little Journeys out of Nashville—The Hillsboro Pike." *Nashville Banner*, April 8, 1923.

Ljungvall, A., and F. J. Zimmerman. "Bigger Bodies: Long-Term Trends and Disparities in Obesity and Body-Mass Index among U.S. Adults, 1960–2008." *Social Science and Medicine* 75, no. 1 (2012). Retrieved from *www.ncbi.nlm.nih.gov/pubmed/22551821.*

Ludwig, Jens, Lisa Sanbonmatsu, Lisa Gennetian, Emma Adam, Greg J. Duncan, Lawrence F. Katz, Ronald C. Kessler, Jeffrey R. Kling, Stacy Tessler Lindau, Robert C. Whitaker, and Thomas W. McDade. "Neighborhoods, Obesity, and Diabetes—A Randomized Social Experiment." *New England Journal of Medicine* 365 (October 20, 2011):1509–19.

Lukez, Paul. *Suburban Transformations.* New York: Princeton Architectural Press, 2007.

Lovett, Bobby L. *The African-American History of Nashville, Tennessee, 1780–1930.* Fayetteville: University of Arkansas Press, 1999.

Low, Sarah A., and Stephen Vogel. *Direct and Intermediated Marketing of Local Foods in the United States.* Economic Research Report No. ERR-128. Washington, DC: US Department of Agriculture, Economic Research Service (November 2011). Retrieved from *www.ers.usda.gov/Publications/ERR128.*

Lydon, Mike, and Anthony Garcia. *Tactical Urbanism: Short-Term Action for Long-Term Change.* New York: Island Press, 2015.

Maidenberg, Micah. "Coming to a Block Near You: CHA Subsidized Housing?" *Crain's Chicago Business.* (October 5, 1013). Retrieved from *www.chicagobusiness.com/article/20131005/ISSUE01/310059985/coming-to-a-block-near-you-cha-subsidized-housing.*

Malone, Eileen, et al. *An Introduction to Evidence-Based Design: Exploring Healthcare and Design.* 2nd Edition. Concord, CA: The Center for Health Design, 2008.

Marshall, Christine Cole, and Jody Marshall. *Good Will and Affection for Antioch: Reminiscences of Antioch, Tennessee.* Franklin, TN: Providence House Publishers, 2002.

Massachusetts Department of Transportation. *Shared Use Paths and Greenways: Chapter 11.* Boston, MA: Massachusetts Department of Transportation, 2006.

May, Ashleigh L., Liping Pan, Bettylou Sherry, Heidi M. Blanck, Deborah Galuska, Karen Dalenius, Barbara Polhamus, Laura Kettel-Khan. "Vital Signs: Obesity Among Low-Income, Preschool-Aged Children—United States, 2008–2011." *Morbidity and Mortality Weekly Report* 62, no. 31 (August 9, 2013): 629–34.

McCann, Barbara A., and Reid Ewing. *Measuring the Health Effects of Sprawl: A National Analysis of Physical Activity, Obesity and Chronic Disease.* Washington, DC: Smart Growth America and the Surface Transportation Policy Project, 2003.

McCoy, Janetta Mitchell, and Gary W. Evans. "Physical Work Environment." In *Handbook of Work Stress*, edited by Julian Barling, E. Kevin Kelloway and Michael R. Frone. Thousand Oaks, CA: Sage Publications, Inc., 2005.

McCoy, William. "Calories Burned Climbing One Flight of Stairs." *Livestrong*, January 16, 2014. Retrieved from *www.livestrong.com/article/301539-calories-burned-climbing-one-flight-of-stairs.*

McDonald, John M., Robert J. Stokes, Deborah A. Cohen, Aaron Kofner, and Greg K. Ridgeway. "The Effect of Light Rail Transit on Body Mass Index and Physical Activity." *American Journal of Preventive Medicine* 39, no. 2 (August 2010): 105–12.

McDonald, Noreen C., Austin L. Brown, Lauren M. Marchetti, and Margo S. Pedrow. "US School Travel, 2009: An Assessment of Trends." *American Journal of Preventive Medicine* 41, no. 2 (August 2011): 146–51. Retrieved from *www.ajpmonline.org/article/S0749-3797(11)00263-7/abstract.*

McGinnis, J. Michael, Pamela Williams-Russo, and James R. Knickman. "The Case for More Active Policy Attention to Health Promotion." *Health Affairs* 21, no. 2 (2002): 78–93.

Melosi, Martin. *The Sanitary City: Urban Infrastructure in America from Colonial Times to the Present.* Baltimore, MD: Johns Hopkins University Press, 1999.

"Metro to Pay $8.2M for 600 Acres of Farmland along Stones River." *City Paper*, December 4, 2012. Retrieved from *nashvillecitypaper.com/content/city-news/metro-pay-82m-600-acres-farmland-along-stones-river.*

Metropolitan Board of Parks and Recreation. *Countywide Parks and Greenways Master Plan.* Nashville, TN: Metropolitan Council, 2002.

Metropolitan Development and Housing Agency (MDHA). "Family Housing" (web page). Retrieved from *www.nashville-mdha.org/familyHousing.php#apt-17.*

Metropolitan Government of Nashville and Davidson County. "Chapter 17.24 - Landscaping, Buffering and Tree Replacement." *The Code of the Metropolitan Government of Nashville and Davidson County, Tennessee.* Retrieved from *www.municode.com/library/tn/metro_government_of_nashville_and_davidson_county/codes/code_of_ordinances?nodeId=CD_TIT17ZO_CH17.24LABUTRRE.*

———. "Energy Efficiency Improvements Volunteer Opportunities" (program website, 2014). Retrieved from *www.nashville.gov/Mayors-Office/Priorities/Volunteerism/Volunteer-Opportunities/Energy-Efficiency-Improvements.aspx.*

———. "Executive Order #40." October 6, 2010. Retrieved from *www.nashville.gov/Metro-Clerk/Legal-Resources/Executive-Orders/Mayor-Karl-Dean/kd040.aspx.*

———. "Interactive Map of Nashville's Tree Cover" (web page). Retrieved from *maps.nashville.gov/UTC.*

———. "Nashville Makes Progress Improving Energy Efficiency of Low-Income Homes" (program website, 2012). Retrieved from *www.nashville.gov/News-Media/News-Article/ID/976/Nashville-Makes-Progress-Improving-Energy-Efficiency-of-LowIncome-Homes.aspx.*

———. *NashvilleNext.* Nashville, TN: Metropolitan Government of Nashville and Davidson County, 2015.

———. *Specific Plan: Ordinance No. BL2005-762.* Nashville, TN: Metropolitan Government of Nashville and Davidson County, 2005.

———. *The Strategic Plan to End Chronic Homelessness in Nashville.* Nashville, TN: Civil Service Commission, 2004.

Metropolitan Historical Commission. "MHZC District Boundaries and Design Guidelines" (web page). Retrieved from *www.nashville.gov/Historical-Commission/Services/Preservation-Permits/Districts-and-Design-Guidelines.aspx.*

———. *Nashville: Conserving A Heritage.* Nashville, TN: Historical Commission of Metropolitan Nashville-Davidson County, 1977.

Metropolitan Planning Commission of Nashville and Davidson County, Tennessee. *Scottsboro/Bells Bend Detailed Design Plan.* Nashville, TN: Metropolitan Planning Commission of Nashville and Davidson County, 2008.

———. *Concept 2010: A General Plan for Nashville and Davidson County.* Nashville, TN: Metropolitan Planning Commission of Nashville and Davidson County, Tennessee, 2010.

Metropolitan Planning Department. *Antioch / Priest Lake Community Plan.* Nashville: Metropolitan Planning Department, 2012.

———. *Bellevue Community Plan.* Nashville, TN: Metropolitan Planning Department, 2002.

———. *Bellevue Community Plan: 2011 Update.* Nashville, TN: Metropolitan Planning Department, 2011.

———. *Bordeaux/Whites Creek Community Plan Update.* Nashville, TN: Metropolitan Planning Department, 2003.

———. *Community Character Manual.* Nashville, TN: Metropolitan Government of Nashville and Davidson County, 2008.

———. *Donelson / Hermitage / Old Hickory Community Plan.* Nashville, TN: Metropolitan Planning Department, 2004.

———. *Downtown Community Plan.* Nashville, TN: Metropolitan Planning Department, 2007.

———. *East Nashville Community Plan.* Nashville, TN: Metropolitan Planning Department, 2006.

———. *Green Hills / Midtown Community Plan.* Nashville, TN: Metropolitan Planning Department, 2013.

———. *Green Hills UDO Design Guidelines, Bedford Avenue Urban Design Overlay.* Nashville, TN: Metropolitan Government of Nashville and Davidson County, 2003.

———. *Joelton Community Plan.* Nashville, TN: Metropolitan Planning Department, 2003.

———. *Madison Community Plan.* Nashville, TN: Metropolitan Planning Department, 2009.

———. *Nashville Downtown Code: Chapter 17.37 of the Metropolitan Nashville and Davidson County Zoning Code.* Nashville, TN: Metropolitan Planning Department, 2010. Retrieved from *www.nashville.gov/Portals/0/SiteContent/Planning/docs/dtc/DTC_150819.pdf.*

———. *Neighborhood Guidebook: A Resource Guide for the Neighborhood District Overlay.* Nashville, TN: Metropolitan Planning Department, 2003.

———. *North Nashville Community Plan.* Nashville, TN: Metropolitan Planning Department, 2002.

———. *Parkwood/Union Hill Community Plan.* Nashville, TN: Metropolitan Planning Department, 2006.

———. *Southeast Community Plan.* Nashville, TN: Metropolitan Planning Department, 2004.

———. *South Nashville Community Plan.* Nashville, TN: Metropolitan Planning Department, 2007.

———. *Subdivision Regulations.* Nashville, TN: Metropolitan Planning Department, 2011. Retrieved from *www.nashville.gov/Portals/0/SiteContent/Planning/docs/subdivregs/2014%2001%2009%20ADOPTED%20Subdivision%20Regulation%20AmendmentsUPDATEDSEPT!.pdf.*

———. *West Nashville Community Plan.* Nashville, TN: Metropolitan Planning Department, 2009.

———. "What Does My Zoning Allow?" (web page). Retrieved from *www.nashville.gov/Planning-Department/Rezoning-Subdivision/What-your-zoning-allows.aspx.*

Metropolitan Public Health Department. *Annual Report.* Nashville, TN: Metropolitan Health Department, 2010.

———. "Communities Putting Prevention to Work (CPPW)" (web page). Retrieved from *www.nashville.gov/Health-Department/CPPW.aspx.*

Metropolitan Public Works. "Tree Canopy Assessment and Urban Tree Inventory" (web page). Retrieved from *www.nashville.gov/Public-Works/Community-Beautification/Tree-Information/Inventory-and-Canopy-Assessment.aspx.*

Metropolitan Social Services. *Planning & Coordination. Community Needs Evaluation: 2012 Update – Davidson County, Tennessee.* Nashville, TN: Metropolitan Government of Nashville and Davidson County, 2012. Retrieved from *www.nashville.gov/Portals/0/SiteContent/SocialServices/docs/cne/2012cne.pdf.*

Metropolitan Water Services. *Green Infrastructure Master Plan.* Nashville, TN: The Metropolitan Government of Nashville and Davidson County, 2009.

———. "History" (web page). Retrieved from *www.nashville.gov/Water-Services/About-Us/History.*

Minicozzi, Joseph, and John Tyler Barnes. *Nashville Davidson: Local Solutions for a Regional Vision.* Asheville, NC: Urban3, 2014.

Mishkovsky, Nadejda, Matthew Dalbey, Stephanie Bertaina, Anna Read, and Tad McGalliard. *Putting Smart Growth to Work in Rural Communities.* Washington, DC: International City/County Management Association, 2010. Retrieved from *icma.org/en/icma/knowledge_network/documents/kn/Document/301483/Putting_Smart_Growth_to_Work_in_Rural_Communities.*

Mumford, Lewis. *The City in History.* New York: Harcourt, Brace and Co., 1961. Reprint, 1989.

Mygatt, Elizabeth. "Forest Cover: World's Forests Continue to Shrink." *Earth Policy Institute,* April 9, 2006. Retrieved from *www.earth-policy.org/indicators/C56/forests_2006.*

Naik, Gautam. "New Buildings Help People Fight Flab." *Wall Street Journal,* November 16, 2005. Retrieved from *www.wsj.com/articles/SB113210855510098537.*

Nashville Area Chamber of Commerce. "Moving Forward: Transit Solutions for Our Region" (web page). Retrieved from *www.nashvillechamber.com/homepage/AboutUs/ChamberInitiatives/moving-forward.*

———. *Nashville-Davidson County Redevelopment Taskforce Summary of Year One Results.* Nashville, TN: Nashville Area Chamber of Commerce, 2012.

Nashville Area Metropolitan Planning Organization. *2035 Nashville Area Regional Transportation Plan.* Nashville, TN: Nashville Area Metropolitan Planning Organization, 2010. Retrieved from *www.nashvillempo.org/docs/lrtp/2035rtp/Docs/2035_Doc/2035Plan_Complete.pdf.*

———. "2040 Regional Transportation Plan" (web page). Retrieved from *www.nashvillempo.org/plans_programs/rtp/2040_rtp.aspx.*

———. *Regional Growth and Traffic Forecasts.* Nashville, TN: Nashville Area Metropolitan Planning Organization, March 2014. Retrieved from *www.nashvillempo.org/docs/Presentations/MPO_XB_Forecasts_19MARCH14.pdf.*

———. *Southeast Corridor High-Performance Transit Alternatives Study.* Nashville, TN: Nashville Area Metropolitan Planning Organization, 2007.

Nashville Baptist Association. *Acorns to Oaks: The Story of the Nashville Baptist Association and Its Affiliated Churches.* Nashville, TN: Nashville Baptist Association, 1972.

Nashville Civic Design Center. *Buena Vista, East Germantown, Germantown, Hope Gardens and Salemtown.* Nashville, TN: Nashville Civic Design Center, 2002.

———. *Chestnut Hill Neighborhood.* Nashville, TN: Nashville Civic Design Center, 2005.

———. *Cohousing: A Community Housing Type for Nashville.* Nashville, TN: Nashville Civic Design Center, 2010. Retrieved from *www.sitemason.com/files/kqtHtm/NCDC_CoHousingWorkshopReport_web.pdf.*

———. *Lafayette Neighborhood: Findings and Recommendations.* Nashville, TN: Nashville Civic Design Center, 2006.

———. *The Livability Project: Building More Livable Communities. Public Charrette Workshop Report: Madison, Sylvan Park.* Nashville, TN: Nashville Civic Design Center, 2011. Retrieved from *www.nashville.gov/Portals/0/SiteContent/Neighborhoods/Livability/LivabilityRptMay2011_MadisonSylvanPark.pdf.*

———. *The Livability Project: Green Hills.* Nashville, TN: Nashville Civic Design Center, 2012.

———. *Nashville's Neighborhoods.* Nashville, TN: Nashville Civic Design Center, 2007.

———. *Rolling Mill Hill and The Rutledge Hill Neighborhood.* Nashville, TN: Nashville Civic Design Center, 2002.

Nashville Downtown Partnership. *2012 Downtown Nashville Business Census: Report of Findings.* Nashville, TN: Nashville Downtown Partnership, 2012. Retrieved from *www.nashvilledowntown.com/_files/docs/report-for-website.pdf.*

———. *Residential Report: July 2013.* Nashville, TN: Nashville Downtown Partnership, 2013. Retrieved from *www.nashvilledowntown.com/_files/docs/2013_residential_report.pdf.*

Nashville MTA. "Consultants Present Phase 2 Summary: Preliminary Engineering and Design." News Release, April 11, 2013. Retrieved from *www.nashvillemta.org/pdf/fn22.pdf.*

———. "The East-West Connector: Smart Transit for Nashville's Future." *Nashville MTA,* April 2011. Retrieved from *www.nashvillemta.org/pdf/fn23.pdf.*

Nashville nMotion. "Nashville MTA/RTA Strategic Plan" (web page). Retrieved from *nmotion2015.com/project-schedule.*

NashvilleNext Health, Livability, and the Built Environment Resource Team, *NashvilleNext: Health, Livability, and the Built Environment Goals and Policies* (Nashville, TN: Metropolitan Planning Commission, 2015). Retrieved from *www.nashville.gov/Portals/0/SiteContent/Planning/docs/NashvilleNext/ResourceTeams/next-rt-HLBE-GoalsPolicies_072114.pdf.*

Nashville, Tennessee, City Ordinance No. BL2004-492. 2004.

Nashville, Tennessee, City Ordinance No. BL2011-80. 2011.

National Association of City Transportation Officials. "Pervious Pavement" (web page). Retrieved from *nacto.org/publication/urban-street-guide/street-design-elements/stormwater-management/pervious-pavement.*

———. *Urban Street Design Guide.* New York: NACTO, 2013.

National Association of Home Builders. "What is Universal Design?" (web page). Retrieved from *www.nahb.org/generic.aspx?genericContentID=89934.*

National Association of Realtors. "Communities for All Generations." *On Common Ground* (Summer 2012). Washington, DC: National Association of Realtors, 2012.

National Center for Safe Routes to School. *Safe Routes to School Travel Data.* Chapel Hill, NC: SafeRoutes, 2010.

National Conference of State Legislatures, AARP Public Policy Institute. *Aging in Place: A State Survey of Livability Policies and Practices.* Washington, DC: AARP, 2011

National Geographic. "Deforestation" (web page). Retrieved from *environment.nationalgeographic.com/environment/global-warming/deforestation-overview.*

National Health Care for the Homeless Council. *Homelessness & Health: What's the Connection?* Fact Sheet. Nashville, TN: National Health Care for the Homeless Council, June 2011. Retrieved from *www.nhchc.org/wp-content/uploads/2011/09/Hln_health_factsheet_Jan10.pdf.*

National Park Service. "National Register of Historic Places Inventory: Nomination Form." (web page). Retrieved from *www.nps.gov/nr/publications/forms.htm.*

National Prevention, Health Promotion, and Public Health Council. *National Prevention Strategy: America's Plan for Better Health and Wellness.* Washington DC: National Prevention, Health Promotion, and Public Health Council, 2011.

Nelson, Arthur C. *Greater Nashville: Trends, Preferences and Opportunities: 2010 to 2025 and to 2040.* Nashville, TN: Metropolitan Planning Department, 2013.

———. *Reshaping Metropolitan America: Development Trends and Opportunities to 2030.* Washington, DC: Island Press, 2013.

———. *Tear Up a Parking Lot and Rebuild Paradise: Development Trends and Opportunities for Nashville.* Nashville, TN: Nashville Civic Design Center, Remarks at Annual Luncheon, October 9, 2013.

Nelson, Kevin. *Essential Smart Growth Fixes for Urban and Suburban Zoning Codes.* Washington DC: United States Environmental Protection Agency, 2009.

Nolen, John. "Suggestive Plan for Madison, a Model City." Map: 1910. Retrieved from *www.wisconsinhistory.org.*

Northridge, Mary E., Elliot D. Sclar, and Padmini Biswas. "Sorting Out the Connections Between the Built Environment and Health: A Conceptual Framework for Navigating Pathways and Planning Healthy Cities." *Journal of Urban Health* 80, no. 4 (December 2003): 556–68.

NY Department of Design and Construction, NY Department of Health and Mental Hygiene, NY Department of Transportation, NY Department of City Planning, and NY Office of the Mayor. *Active Design Guidelines: Promoting Physical Activity and Health in Design.* New York: City of New York, 2010. Retrieved from *centerforactivedesign.org/dl/guidelines.pdf.*

NY Department of Planning. *Zoning for Bicycle Parking.* New York: New York City Department of Planning, 2008. Retrieved from *www.nyc.gov/html/dcp/pdf/bicycle_parking/zoning_bike_parking.pdf.*

O'Connell, James J. *Premature Mortality in Homeless Populations: A Review of the Literature.* Nashville, TN: National Health Care for the Homeless Council, 2005. Retrieved from *santabarbarastreetmedicine.org/wordpress/wp-content/uploads/2011/04/PrematureMortalityFinal.pdf.*

OECD, *Health at a Glance 2013: OECD Indicators.* Paris: OECD Publishing, 2013. Retrieved from *www.oecd.org/els/health-systems/health-at-a-glance.htm.*

Office of Community Planning and Development. *Defining Chronic Homelessness: A Technical Guide for HUD Programs.* Washington, DC: US Department of Housing and Urban Development, 2007. Retrieved from *www.onecpd.info/resources/documents/DefiningChronicHomeless.pdf.*

Office of Highway Policy Information. "National Household Travel Survey (NHTS)" (web page). Retrieved from *www.fhwa.dot.gov/policyinformation/nhts.cfm.*

The Ohio State University. "Bike Sharrows" (web page). Retrieved from *ttm.osu.edu/bike-sharrows.*

Olshansky, S. J., D. J. Passaro, R. C. Hershow, J. Layden, B. A. Carnes, J. Brody, L. Hayflick, R. N. Butler, D. B. Allison, D. S. Ludwig. "A Potential Decline in Life Expectancy in the United States in the 21st Century." *New England Journal of Medicine* 352, no. 11 (March 17, 2005): 1138–45.

Owens, Loretta. *NashvilleNext Background Reports: Housing.* Nashville, TN: Metropolitan Planning Department, March 2013. Retrieved from *www.nashville.gov/Portals/0/SiteContent/Planning/docs/NashvilleNext/next-report-Housing.pdf.*

Parker-Pope, Tara. "The Fat Trap." *New York Times Magazine,* December 28, 2011.

Parsons, Clark. "An Antioch State of Mind: In Search of Nashville's Forgotten World." *Nashville Scene,* October 7, 1993.

Pasanisi, Fabrizio, Contaldo, G. de Simone, and M. Mancini. "Benefits of Sustained Moderate Weight Loss in Obesity." *Nutrition, Metabolism and Cardiovascular Diseases* 11, no. 6 (December 2001): 401–6.

Perdue, W. C., L. O. Gostin, and L. A. Stone. "Public Health and the Built Environment: Historical, Empirical, and Theoretical Foundations for an Expanded Role." *Journal of Law, Medicine & Ethics* 31, no. 4 (2003): 557–66.

Peterson, J. A. "The Impact of Sanitary Reform Upon American Urban Planning, 1840–1890." *Journal of Social History* 13, no. 1 (1979): 83–103.

Peterson, Sandra Neely. "The Neely Family" (web page). Retrieved from *homepages.rootsweb.ancestry.com/~lpproots/Neeley/neelybnd.htm.*

Philadelphia Department of Public Health. *Philadelphia 2035: Planning and Zoning a Healthier City.* Philadelphia: Philadelphia City Planning Commission, 2010.

The Potato Museum. "Couch Potato Gallery" (web page). Retrieved from *potatomuseum.com/index.php?option=com_content&view=article&id=26:artcounch&catid=19:catcontroversy&Itemid=48.*

Portland District Development Plan. *Pearl District Development Plan: A Future Vision for a Neighborhood in Transition.* Portland, OR: Portland Development Commission, 2011. Retrieved from *www.pdc.us/Libraries/River_District/Pearl_District_Development_Plan_pdf.sflb.ashx.*

Preservation Green Lab. *The Greenest Building: Quantifying the Environmental Value of Building Reuse.* Washington, DC: National Trust for Historic Preservation, 2011. Retrieved from *www.preservationnation.org/information-center/sustainable-communities/green-lab/lca/The_Greenest_Building_lowres.pdf.*

Price, David, and Julie Coco. *Beaman Park to Bells Bend: A Community Conservation Project.* Nashville, TN: New South Associates & The Land Trust for Tennessee, 2007.

Public Health Madison & Dane County. *The Health of Dane County 2013 Health Status Overview Report.* October 2013. Retrieved from *www.publichealthmdc.com/documents/HealthDC-2013status.pdf.*

Rair, Lesa. "Public Transit Riders Continue to Save as Gas Prices Remain High: Riding Public Transportation Saves Individuals on Average $10,126 a Year." American Public Transportation Association, 2012. Retrieved from *www.apta.com/mediacenter/pressreleases/2012/Pages/120418_AprilTransitSavings.aspx.*

Ramsey, Kevin. *Residential Construction Trends in America's Metropolitan Regions: 2012 Edition.* Washington, DC: United States Environmental Protection Agency, 2012.

Reconnecting America. *TOD 101: Transit-Oriented Development and Why Now?* Oakland, CA: Reconnecting America, 2007.

———. *TOD 201. Mixed-Income Housing near Transit: Increasing Affordability with Location Efficiency.* Oakland, CA: Reconnecting America, 2009. Retrieved from *ctod.org/pdfs/tod201.pdf.*

———. *TOD 204. Planning for TOD at the Regional Scale: The Big Picture.* Oakland, CA: Reconnecting America, 2011.

Reconnecting America's Center for Transit-Oriented Development. *Realizing the Potential: Expanding Housing Opportunities Near Transit.* Washington DC: U.S. Department of Transportation, 2007.

Reid, Dave. "Car Culture: Freedom Brought to You by the American Auto Industry, Hello Officer, Put the Phone Down, and More." Video Clip. *Urban Milwaukee,* April 26, 2012. Retrieved from *www.urbanmilwaukee.com/2012/04/26/car-culture-freedom-brought-to-you-by-the-american-auto-industry-hello-officer-put-the-phone-down-and-more.*

The Reinvestment Fund. *Pennsylvania Fresh Food Financing Initiative.* Philadelphia: The Reinvestment Fund, 2010.

Rent Jungle. "Rent Trend Data in Nashville, Tennessee" (web page). Retrieved from *www.rentjungle.com/average-rent-in-nashville-rent-trends.*

Renwick, C. "The Practice of Spencerian Science: Patrick Geddes's Biosocial Program, 1876–1889." *Isis,* 100, no. 1 (2009): 36–57.

Research Division, Metropolitan Planning Commission. *History and Physical Setting: Nashville and Davidson County, Tennessee.* Vol. 1. Nashville, TN: Planning Commission of the Metropolitan Government of Nashville and Davidson County, 1965.

Riis, Jacob. *How the Other Half Lives.* New York: Charles Scribner's Sons, 1890. Retrieved from *www.authentichistory.com/1898-1913/2-progressivism/2-riis.*

Robert Woods Johnson Foundation. "How Healthy Is Your Community?" (web page). Retrieved from *www.countyhealthrankings.org.*

Rogers, B., B. McKelvey, and S. D. Thomas. *Davidson County Mortality Report for 2009.* Nashville, TN: Metropolitan Nashville Public Health Department, 2011.

Roof, Karen, and Robert Glandon. "Tool Created to Assess Health Impacts of Development Decisions in Ingham County, Michigan." *Journal of Environmental Health* 71, no. 1 (July/August 2008): 35–38.

RPM Transportation Consultants, LLC. *Metro Nashville-Davidson County Strategic Plan for Sidewalks and Bikeways.* Nashville, TN: Metropolitan Government of Nashville and Davidson County, Tennessee, 2008. Retrieved from *mpw.nashville.gov/IMS/Bikeways/StrategicPlan.aspx.*

Russonello, Belden, and Stewart LLC. *Community Preference Survey: What Americans Are Looking for When Deciding Where to Live.* Washington, DC: National Association of Realtors, 2011.

Rutenberg, Jim. "Speculators Rush In." *New York Times,* August 20, 2015, 10.

Rutt, Candace, Andrew Dannenburg, and Christopher Kochtitzky. "Using Policy and Built Environment Interventions to Improve Public Health." *Journal of Public Health Management and Practice* 14, no. 3 (May/June 2008): 221–23.

Sallis, James F., et al. "Neighborhood Built Environment and Income: Examining Multiple Health Outcomes." *Social Science and Medicine* 68, no. 7 (April 2009): 1285–93.

Sallis, James F., Lawrence D. Frank, Brian E. Saelens, and M. Katherine Kraft. "Active Transportation and Physical Activity: Opportunities for Collaboration on Transportation and Public Health Research." *Transportation Research Part A: Policy and Practice* 38, no. 4 (May 2004): 249–68.

Sansone-Lauber Trial Lawyers. "Pedestrian Accidents and Injuries" (web page). Retrieved from *www.missourilawyers.com/legal-services/car-accident-lawyer/pedestrian-accidents.*

Santos, A., N. McGuckin, H. Y. Nakamoto, D. Gray, and S. Liss. *Summary of Travel Trends: 2009 National Household Travel Survey.* Washington, DC: US Department of Transportation, Federal Highway Administration, 2011. Retrieved from *nhts.ornl.gov/2009/pub/stt.pdf.*

Sasaki Associates, Inc. *Vanderbilt University Land Use and Development Plan.* Watertown, MA: Sasaki Associates Inc., 2001.

Schlundt, D. G., M. K. Hargreaves, and L. McClellan. "Geographic Clustering of Obesity, Diabetes, and Hypertension in Nashville, Tennessee." *Journal of Ambulatory Care Management* 29, no. 2 (Apr–Jun 2006): 125–32.

Schmitt, Angie. "The Rise of the North American Protected Bike Lane." *Momentum Mag,* July 31, 2013. Retrieved from *momentummag.com/features/the-rise-of-the-north-american-protected-bike-lane.*

Scully, Jason. "Rethinking Grocery Stores." *Urban Land,* May 16, 2011. Retrieved from urbanland.uli.org/Articles/2011/May/ScullyRethink.

Seattle Parks and Recreation; Seattle School District No. 1. *An Agreement for the Joint Use of Facilities Between The Seattle School District No. 1 and Seattle Parks and Recreation.* Seattle, WA: Seattle Parks and Recreation, 2005.

Sequeira, Sonia, and Leslie Meehan. *Hamilton Springs Transit-Oriented Development: School Siting Health Impact Assessment.* Nashville, TN: Nashville Area Metropolitan Planning Organization, 2013. Retrieved from *www.nashvillempo.org/docs/Health/HIA_2013_FINAL.pdf.*

Shoup, Donald. *The High Cost of Free Parking.* Washington, DC: American Planning Association, 2011.

———. "The Trouble with Minimum Parking Requirements." *Transportation Research Part A: Policy and Practice* 33 (1999): 549–74.

Skolnik, Lisa. *Sleeping Spaces: Designs for Rest and Renewal.* Gloucester, MA: Rockport Publishers, Inc., 2000.

Smart Growth America, National Complete Streets Initiative. "Benefits of Complete Streets: Economic Development" (web page). Retrieved from *www.smartgrowthamerica.org/complete-streets/complete-streets-fundamentals/factsheets/economic-revitalization.*

Smart Growth Network. *Putting Smart Growth to Work in Rural Communities.* Washington DC: ICMA, 2010.

Squatriti, Paolo. *Nature's Past: The Environment and Human History.* Ann Arbor, MI: University of Michigan Press, 2007.

Strategic Economics. *Fiscal Impact Analysis of Three Development Scenarios in Nashville-Davidson County, TN.* Washington, DC: Smart Growth America, April 2013. Retrieved from *www.smartgrowthamerica.org/documents/fiscal-analysis-of-nashville-development.pdf.*

Sumithran, Priya, Luke A. Prendergast, Elizabeth Delbridge, Katrina Purcell, Arthur Shulkes, Adamandia Kriketos, and Joseph Proietto. "Long-Term Persistence of Hormonal Adaptations to Weight Loss." *New England Journal of Medicine* 365 (October 27, 2011): 1597–604.

Sustainable Cities Institute. "Traditional Neighborhood Development" (web page). Retrieved from *www.sustainablecitiesinstitute.org/topics/land-use-and-planning/traditional-neighborhood-development-(tnd).*

Sustainable Sources. "Passive Solar Design" (web page). Retrieved from *passivesolar.sustainablesources.com.*

Swinburn, Boyd A., Gary Sacks, Kevin D. Hall, Klim McPherson, Diane T. Finegood, Marjory L. Moodie, and Steven L. Gortmaker. "The Global Obesity Pandemic: Shaped by Global Drivers and Local Environments." *Lancet* 378 no. 9793 (August 27, 2011): 804–14.

Swinburn, Boyd A., Garry Egger, and Fezeela Raza. "Dissecting Obesogenic Environments: The Development and Application of a Framework for Identifying and Prioritizing Environmental Interventions for Obesity." *Preventive Medicine* 29 no. 6 (December 1999): 563–70.

Tachieva, Galina. *Sprawl Repair Manual.* Washington, DC: Island Press, 2010.

Taubman Centers. "The Mall at Green Hills" (web page). Retrieved from *www.shopgreenhills.com/about_us.*

Taubes, Gary. "What Really Makes Us Fat." *New York Times,* June 30, 2012.

Technical Assistance Panel, ULI Nashville. *An Action Plan for Reinvestment and Revitalization in Madison, Tennessee.* Nashville, TN: Urban Land Institute, 2012.

Tefft, Brian C. *Impact Speed and a Pedestrian's Risk of Severe Injury or Death.* Washington, DC: AAA Foundation for Traffic Safety, 2011. Retrieved from *www.aaafoundation.org/sites/default/files/2011PedestrianRiskVsSpeed.pdf.*

Tennessee Department of Education. "A Summary of Weight Status Data: Tennessee Public Schools, 2000–2012 School Year." Retrieved from *www.tennessee.gov/education/schoolhealth/data_reports/doc/BMI_Sum_Data_State_Co_2013.pdf.*

Tennessee Department of Finance and Administration. *Bicentennial Mall Urban Plan: The Making of a District.* Nashville, TN: The Associates, 1998.

"There Must Be Gold in That Thar Green Hills." *Tennessean,* July 23, 1965.

Thompson, John B. "Disease in Nashville: A Short History." *Medical History in Nashville,* (symposium). A paper presented before the Nashville Academy of Medicine, September 14, 1982.

Tomer, Adie. *Where the Jobs Are: Employer Access to Labor by Transit.* Washington, DC: Brookings Institution, Metropolitan Policy Program, July 2012.

Thoreau, Henry David. "Spring." *Walden,* 1854. Retrieved from *thoreau.eserver.org/walden17.html.*

Thurber, Amie, Jyoti Gupta, James Fraser, and Doug Perkins. *Equitable Development: Promising Practices to Maximize Affordability and Minimize Displacement in Nashville's Urban Core.* A NashvilleNext report from the Housing resource team. Nashville, TN: Metropolitan Nashville Planning Department, September 2014. Retrieved from *www.nashville.gov/Portals/0/SiteContent/Planning/docs/NashvilleNext/ResourceTeams/Housing_Gentrification_EquitableDevelopment.pdf.*

Torres, Gretchen, and Mary Pittman. *Active Living Through Community Design.* Princeton, NJ: Robert Wood Johnson Foundation, 2001.

Tough, Paul. *How Children Succeed: Grit, Curiosity, and the Hidden Power of Character.* Boston: Houghton Mufflin Harcourt, 2012.

Transportation for America. *Aging in Place, Stuck without Option: Fixing the Mobility Crisis Threatening the Baby Boom Generation.* Washington, DC: AARP Public Policy Institute, 2010.

Trust for America's Health and Robert Wood Johnson Foundation. "Issue Brief: Bending the Obesity Cost Curve in Tennessee" (web page). Retrieved from *healthyamericans.org/assets/files/obesity2012/TFAHSept2012_TN_ObesityBrief02.pdf.*

The Trust for Public Land. "Annual City Parks Data Released by the Trust for Public Land" (web page). Retrieved from *www.tpl.org/media-room/annual-city-parks-data-released-trust-public-land.*

Underground 2020. *The Power to Change the Face of America . . . Converting Overhead Utilities to Underground.* Okahumpka, FL: Underground 2020, 2009.

Union of Concerned Scientists. "Car Emissions and Global Warming" (web page). Retrieved from *www.ucsusa.org/our-work/clean-vehicles/car-emissions-and-global-warming.*

United Health Foundation. *America's Health Rankings: 2014 Edition Tennessee.* Minnetonka, MN: United Health Foundation, 2015. Retrieved from *cdnfiles.americashealthrankings.org/SiteFiles/StateProfiles/Tennessee-Health-Profile-2014.pdf.*

University of Oregon. *Planning for Schools and Livable Communities: The Oregon School Siting Handbook.* Eugene, OR: Oregon Transportation and Growth Management, 2005.

Urban Design Associates. *South of Broadway Strategic Master Plan.* Nashville, TN: Urban Design Associates, 2013.

Urban Land Institute, Technical Assistance Panel. *An Action Plan for Reinvestment and Revitalization in Madison, Tennessee.* Nashville, TN: Urban Land Institute. Retrieved from *nashville.uli.org/wp-content/uploads/sites/32/2013/01/ULI-Madison-TAP-Report-4-10-12.pdf.*

Urban Land Institute. *Intersections: Health and the Built Environment.* Washington, DC: Urban Land Institute, 2013.

———. "Urban Land Institute Nashville" (web page). Retrieved from *www.nashville.uli.org/events/urban-magnet.*

US Census Bureau. "American Community Survey: 2010 Data Release" (web page). Retrieved from *www.census.gov/acs/www/data_documentation/2010_release.*

———. "Community Facts, 2010" (web page). Retrieved from *factfinder.census.gov/*

faces/nav/jsf/pages/community_facts.xhtml.

———. "Historical Data: 2010s: Vintage 2012" (web page). Retrieved from *www.census.gov/popest/data/historical/2010s/vintage_2012/index.html.*

———. "TIGER / Line Shapefiles, 2010." Retrieved from *www.census.gov/geo/maps-data/data/tiger.html.*

———. *Volume 1 of Sixteenth Census of the United States: 1940: Population, United States.* Washington, DC: Bureau of the Census, 1942.

USDA Forest Service. *Weed of the Week: Exotic Bush Honeysuckles.* Newtown Square, PA: USDA Forest Service, Forest Health Staff, n.d.. Retrieved from *na.fs.fed.us/fhp/invasive_plants/weeds/bush_honeysuckle.pdf.*

US Department of Agriculture. *2007 Census of Agriculture: County Profile: Davidson County, Tennessee.* Washington, DC: United States Department of Agriculture, 2007. Retrieved from *www.agcensus.usda.gov/Publications/2007/Online_Highlights/County_Profiles/Tennessee/cp47037.pdf.*

US Department of Transportation. *Non-Motorized User Safety: A Manual for Local Rural Road Owners.* Washington DC: Office of Safety, 2012.

US Environmental Protection Agency. *Our Built and Natural Environments: A Technical Review of the Interactions among Land Use, Transportation, and Environmental Quality.* Washington, DC: United States Environmental Protection Agency, 2013. Retrieved from *www.epa.gov/smartgrowth/built.htm.*

———. *Our Nation's Air: Status and Trends Through 2010.* Washington, DC: United States Environmental Protection Agency, 2012. Retrieved from *www.epa.gov/airtrends/2011/report/fullreport.pdf.*

———. *Report to Congress on Indoor Air Quality. Volume 2. Assessment and Control of Indoor Air Pollution.* Washington, DC: US Environmental Protection Agency, 1989.

———. *Travel and Environmental Implications of School Siting.* Research Triangle Park, NC: Office of Air Quality Planning and Standards, 2003.

US Interagency Council for Homelessness. "Fact Sheet: Chronic Homelessness." *Opening Doors: Federal Strategic Plan to Prevent and End Homelessness.* Washington, DC: US Interagency Council for Homelessness, 2010. Retrieved from *usich.gov/resources/uploads/asset_library/FactSheetChronicHomelessness.pdf.*

"Virginia's Efforts to Promote Affordable Housing." *Breakthroughs,* May 2009. Retrieved from *www.huduser.org/rbc/newsletter/vol8iss3_2.html.*

Vlahov, David, and Sandro Galea. "Urbanization, Urbanicity, and Health." *Journal of Urban Health: Bulletin of the New York Academy of Medicine* 79, no. 4, suppl. 1 (2002): S1–S12.

Walker, Mary Ellen Martin. "From the book *The Neely's of Neelys Bend,* Davidson County, TN" (1996), (web page). Retrieved from *homepages.rootsweb.ancestry.com/~lpproots/Neeley/samnb.htm.*

Waller, William. *Nashville in the 1890's.* Nashville, TN: Vanderbilt University Press, 1970.

———. *Nashville, 1900–1910.* Nashville, TN: Vanderbilt University Press, 1972.

Walsh, P. A.. "Fixed Equipment—A Time for Change." *Australian Journal of Early Childhood* 18, no. 2 (June 1993): 23–29.

Ward, Getahn. "Mall Opens with Global Flair." *Tennessean,* May 18 , 2013.

Wernham, Aaron. "Health Impact Assessments Are Needed in Decision-Making about Environmental and Land-Use Policy." *Health Affairs* 30, no. 5 (2011): 947–56.

White, Abby. "Everybody Knows Nashville Is Hurting for Affordable Housing. What Are We Gonna Do about It?" *Nashville Scene,* March 25, 2015. Retrieved from *www.nashvillescene.com/nashville/everybody-knows-nashville-is-hurting-for-affordable-housing-what-are-we-gonna-do-about-it/Content?oid=4952842.*

Williams, William. "Cottage-Style Infill Development Slated for East Side." *Nashville Post,* September 13, 2013. Retrieved from *www.nashvillepost.com/news/2013/9/13/cottage_style_infill_development_slated_for_east_side.*

Wilper, Andrew P., Steffie Woolhandler, Karen E. Lasser, Danny McCormick, David H. Bor, and David U. Himmelstein. "Health Insurance and Mortality in US Adults." *American Journal of Public Health* 99, no. 12 (December 2009): 2289–95. Retrieved from *www.ncbi.nlm.nih.gov/pmc/articles/PMC2775760.*

Winkelstein, Warren, Jr. "History of Public Health." *Encyclopedia of Public Health.* 2002. Retrieved from *www.encyclopedia.com/doc/1G2-3404000428.html.*

"Work on Green Hills Village Expected to Start in 2 Weeks." *Nashville Banner,* July 29, 1953.

World Health Organization. *Global Age-Friendly Cities: A Guide.* Geneva, Switzerland: WHO Press, 2007.

Wu, Lisa. *Reducing Traffic-Related Air Pollution Exposure in the Built Environment: Recommendations for Urban Planners, Policymakers, and Traffic Engineers.* Los Angeles: Los Angeles Sustainability Collaborative, 2014.

Zepp, George. "Cause of 1952 Fire that Gutted Hillsboro High School Still a Mystery." *Tennessean,* April 13, 2005.

Zimmerman, Erich. *The Most for Our Money: Taxpayer Friendly Solutions for the Nation's Transportation Challenges.* Transportation for America, Washington DC: Taxpayers for Common Sense, 2011.

INDEX

INDEX

The Nashville Civic Design Center was founded in 2000 as a nonprofit organization dedicated to elevating the quality of Nashville's built environment and to promoting public participation in the creation of a more beautiful and functional city for all.

Shaping the Healthy Community: The Nashville Plan is the second publication by the Nashville Civic Design Center in partnership with Vanderbilt University Press. *The Plan of Nashville: Avenues to a Great City* was published in 2005.

Gary Gaston, co-author, is the NCDC executive director, lecturer with the University of Tennessee College of Architecture and Design, and co-author of *Moving Tennessee Forward: Models for Connecting Communities.*

Christine Kreyling, co-author and editor, is the author of *The Plan of Nashville: Avenues to a Great City.* As the architecture and urban planning critic for the *Nashville Scene,* she received three awards from the American Planning Association for best writing in the nation.

Ron Yearwood, NCDC assistant director and co-author of *Moving Tennessee Forward,* served as images editor.

Deborah Hightower Brewington, Creative Services, Vanderbilt University, was the art director.

Eric Hoke, NCDC design fellow, supplied graphic illustrations.

Joe Mayes, NCDC research fellow, served as research assistant.

Joell Smith-Borne, Vanderbilt University Press, served as managing editor.

Cover illustration: Eric Hoke
Cover design: Deborah Hightower Brewington

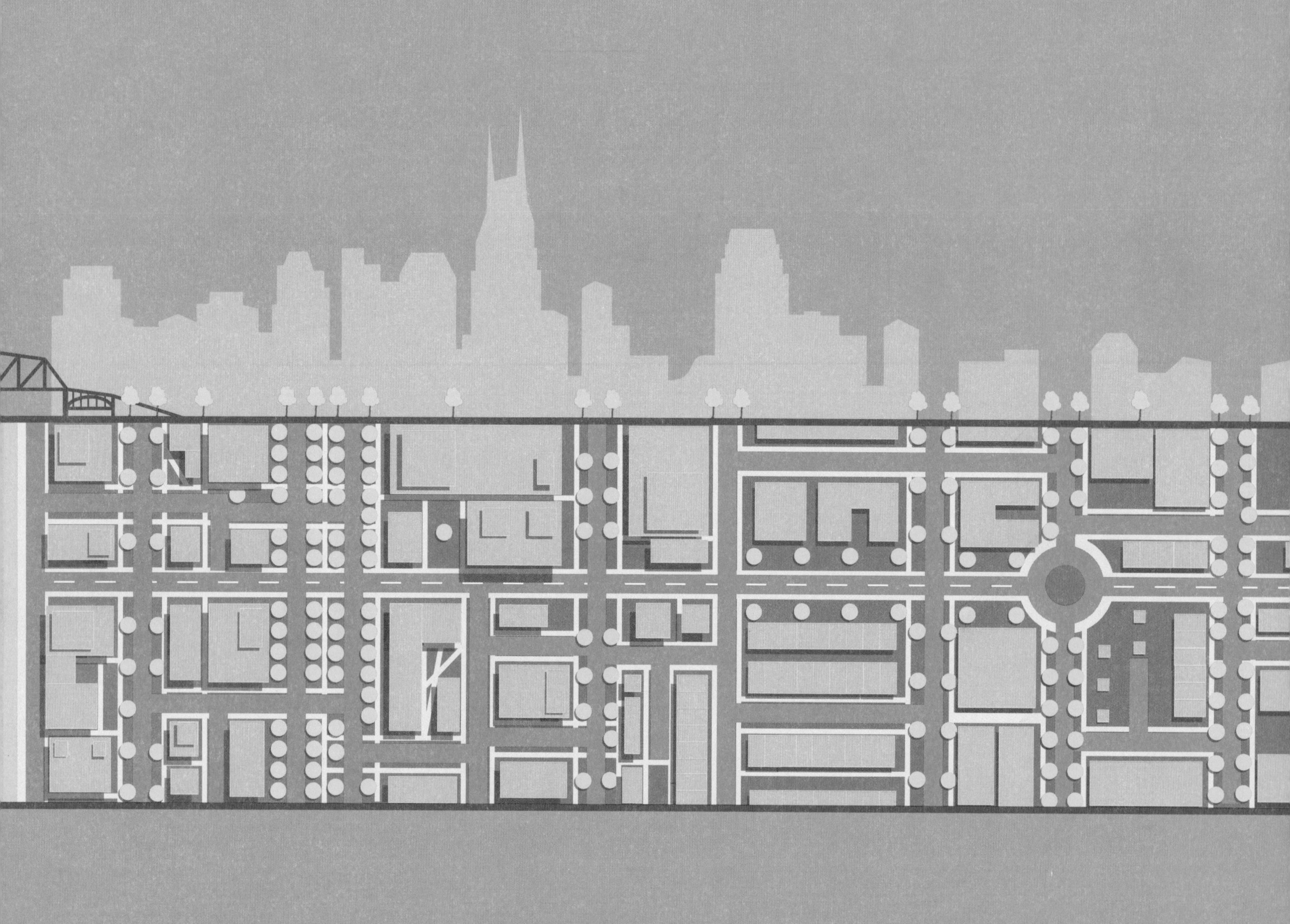